SLEEP MEDICINE

SERIES EDITOR
EVA FELDMAN, MD, PHD, FAAN, FANA
Russell N. DeJong, Professor of Neurology
University of Michigan

Contemporary Neurology Series

76 PERIPHERAL NEUROPATHIES IN CLINICAL PRACTICE
Steven Herskovitz, MD, Stephen N. Scelsa, MD, and Herbert H. Schaumburg, MD

77 CLINICAL NEUROPHYSIOLIOGY OF THE VESTIBULAR SYSTEM
Fourth Edition
Robert W. Baloh, MD, FAAN, and Kevin A. Kerber, MD

78 THE NEURONAL CEROID LIPOFUSCINOSES (BATTEN DISEASE)
Second Edition
Sara E. Mole, PhD, Ruth D. Williams, MD, and Hans H. Goebel, MD, Editors

79 PARANEOPLASTIC SYNDROMES
Robert B. Darnell, MD, PhD, and Jerome B. Posner, MD

80 JASPER'S BASIC MECHANISMS OF THE EPILEPSIES
Jeffrey L. Noebels, MD, PhD, Massimo Avoli, MD, PhD, Michael A. Rogawski, MD, PhD, Richard W. Olsen, PhD, and Antonio V. Delgado- Escueta, MD

81 MYASTHENIA GRAVIS AND MYASTHENIC DISORDERS
Second Edition
Andrew G. Engel, MD

82 MOLECULAR PHYSIOLOGY AND METABOLISM OF THE NERVOUS SYSTEM
Gary A. Rosenberg, MD

83 SEIZURES AND EPILEPSY
Second Edition
Jerome Engel, Jr., MD, PhD

84 MULTIPLE SCLEROSIS
Moses Rodriguez, MD, Orhun H. Kantarci, MD, and Istvan Pirko, MD

85 FRONTOTEMPORAL DEMENTIA
Bruce L. Miller, MD

86 AUTONOMIC NEUROLOGY
Eduardo E. Benarroch, MD

87 EVALUATION AND TREATMENT OF MYOPATHIES
Second Edition
Emma Ciafaloni, MD, Patrick F. Chinnery, FRCP, FMedSci, and Robert C. Griggs, MD, Editors

88 MOTOR NEURON DISEASE IN ADULTS
Mark Bromberg, MD

89 HYPERKINETIC MOVEMENT DISORDERS
Roger M. Kurlan, MD, Paul E. Green, MD, and Kevin M. Biglan, MD, MPH

90 THE NEUROLOGY OF EYE MOVEMENTS
Fifth Edition
R. John Leigh, MD, FRCP, and David S. Zee, MD

91 MIGRAINE
Third Edition
David W. Dodick, MD, and Stephen D. Silberstein, MD, FACP, FAHS, FAAN

92 CLINICAL NEUROPHYSIOLOGY
Fourth Edition
Devon Rubin, MD, and Jasper Daube, MD, Editors

93 NEUROIMMUNOLOGY
Bibiana Bielekova, MD, Gary Birnbaum, MD, and Robert P. Lisak, MD, FRCP

94 PLUM AND POSNER'S DIAGNOSIS AND TREATMENT OF STUPOR AND COMA
Fifth Edition
Jerome B. Posner, MD, Clifford B. Saper, MD, PhD, Nicholas D. Schiff, MD, and Jan Claassen, MD, PhD

95 CLINICAL NEUROPHYSIOLOGY
Fifth Edition
Devon I. Rubin

96 PARKINSON DISEASE
Roger L. Albin, MD

97 NEUROLOGIC COMPLICATIONS OF CRITICAL ILLNESS
Fourth Edition
Eelco F. M. Wijdicks, MD, PhD, FACP

98 JASPER'S BASIC MECHANISMS OF THE EPILEPSIES
Fifth Edition
Jeffrey L. Noebels, MD, PhD, Massimo Avoli, MD, PhD, Michael A. Rogawski, MD, PhD, Annamaria Vezzani, PhD, and Antonio V. Delgado-Escueta, MD, Editors

99 THE DYSTONIAS
H. A. Jinnah, MD, PhD, Bettina Balint, MD, PhD, and Victor S. C. Fung, PhD, FRACP

SLEEP MEDICINE

Second edition

Edited by

Douglas Kirsch

OXFORD
UNIVERSITY PRESS

OXFORD
UNIVERSITY PRESS

Oxford University Press is a department of the University of Oxford.
It furthers the University's objective of excellence in research, scholarship,
and education by publishing worldwide. Oxford is a registered trade mark of
Oxford University Press in the UK and in certain other countries.

Published in the United States of America by Oxford University Press
198 Madison Avenue, New York, NY 10016, United States of America.

Library of Congress Cataloging-in-Publication Data
Names: Kirsch, Douglas B. author
Title: Sleep medicine / Douglas Kirsch.
Description: New York, NY : Oxford University Press, [2025] |
Series: Contemporary neurology series |
Includes bibliographical references and index. |
Identifiers: LCCN 2025016120 (print) | LCCN 2025016121 (ebook) |
ISBN 9780197550823 hb | ISBN 9780197550830 |
ISBN 9780197550847 epub | ISBN 9780197550854
Subjects: LCSH: Sleep disorders | Sleep—Physiological aspects
Classification: LCC RC547.K57 2025 (print) | LCC RC547 (ebook) |
DDC 616.8/498—dc23/eng/20250730
LC record available at https://lccn.loc.gov/2025016120
LC ebook record available at https://lccn.loc.gov/2025016121

DOI: 10.1093/med/9780197550823.001.0001

Printed by Integrated Books International, United States of America

The manufacturer's authorized representative in the EU for product safety is
Oxford University Press España S.A., Parque Empresarial San Fernando de Henares,
Avenida de Castilla, 2 – 28830 Madrid (www.oup.es/en or product.safety@oup.com).
OUP España S.A. also acts as importer into Spain of products made by the manufacturer.

MIX
Paper
FSC FSC® C183721

Contents

SECTION V. THE ADULT SLEEP PATIENT IN THE CLINIC AND LABORATORY

SECTION VI. SLEEP AND OTHER ASPECTS OF MEDICINE

SECTION VII. THE FIELD OF SLEEP MEDICINE

Foreword

As I write this Foreword, chapters are being submitted and galley proofs generated, and I am honored to share my excitement for the upcoming publication of *Sleep Medicine*, edited by Douglas B. Kirsch, MD. This book represents a complete rewrite of the celebrated first edition of *Sleep Medicine*, written 25 years ago by Michael S. Aldrich, MD. for the Contemporary Neurology Series. A consummate sleep medicine educator, physician, and educator, Dr. Aldrich single-authored the original monograph, bringing years of skill as a writer, editor, and mentor to the task of summarizing a young field that he had helped to build. As sleep medicine has grown substantially since then, *Sleep Medicine* is now authored by a number of widely recognized experts, rather than one, but many remain grateful for past training or mentorship in the program Dr. Aldrich founded at the University of Michigan, and have built on his legacy in education.

The first section of *Sleep Medicine* offers an overview of key topics in normal sleep and biological rhythms. Fascinating in their own right, these four chapters—each written by thought leaders in these topics—provide the common language that will be useful to understand the remainder of the book, and gain fluency in terminology that permeates the field of sleep medicine. The second section delves into the "bread and butter" of any sleep medicine practice: sleep-disordered breathing. Although several dozen sleep disorders are defined in the *International Classification of Sleep Disorders*, 3rd edition, text revision (2023), sleep-disordered breathing and obstructive sleep apnea in particular are encountered so commonly that this area is an excellent place to start any discussion of pathological sleep. The four separate chapters on treatment for obstructive sleep apnea reflect traditional approaches as well as modern strategies still undergoing rapid development, showing a broad variety of therapeutic options for a condition in which the saying "one size fits all" could not be farther from reality. The authors are leaders in clinical sleep medicine, dentistry, or surgery who have helped to shape the field and have had central roles in education as well.

The third section of the book explores disorders for which abnormal sleep patterns or excessive daytime sleepiness are key defining features. Sleep deprivation, insomnia, and circadian rhythm disorders are part of the human experience in many if not most lifetimes, and some knowledge about how to diagnose and treat these conditions is important for any clinician. Hypersomnias such as narcolepsy are less widespread, and many affected patients wait years for diagnosis, in part because formal training of most clinicians still does not include much time on sleep medicine. The fourth section of the book focuses on sleep-related movement disorders, including restless legs syndrome, another highly common and often under-addressed sleep disorder, as well as parasomnias that can affect the young, old, and all ages in between. Both the third and fourth sections are written by superb, experienced clinicians and leaders in the field of sleep medicine.

The book turns in Section V to the clinical knowledge and skills necessary for successful practice in a sleep clinic or sleep laboratory setting, or in a practice that refers to these facilities. The chapters include an overview of the approach to patients; questionnaires that can bring validated screening or assessment to larger numbers of patients; laboratory-based and home-testing methods; and some of the latest devices and wearables that promise to give insight into sleep patterns over days, weeks, or months in the natural environment. Each chapter is authored by a national leader in sleep medicine education, testing for sleep disorders, or novel technology that is changing the field.

In the sixth section, another highly accomplished set of academic clinicians illustrate why sleep medicine increasingly has central relevance to the practice of so many other fields of medicine, including neurology, psychiatry, cardiology, pulmonary medicine, pediatrics, and occupational health. Increasingly, research findings on the sleep of women and underserved populations will help clinicians provide more patient-centered care. The final section of the book includes a look back to see where sleep medicine has been, and then a look forward to see where it is likely to go as a field. The authors are two individuals who have themselves done much to innovate and improve training and practice in sleep medicine.

In short, *Sleep Medicine* provides an overview of the field that should prove worthwhile to sleep specialists and non-specialists alike. Its thoughtfully organized content covers fundamental principles, tools and tests, nosology, diagnosis, treatment, relationships to common medical conditions, and the field itself, with a modern approach and timely topics within a rapidly evolving specialty. The book has been edited by one of the most accomplished physicians and educators in sleep medicine. Dr. Kirsch is the Medical Director for Sleep Medicine at Atrium Health, in Charlotte, NC, where he also serves as a Clinical Professor of Neurology at the Wake Forest University School of Medicine. Before that, he held faculty appointments at Brigham and Women's Hospital/Harvard Medical School, and at the University of Michigan. Dr. Kirsch is a widely sought-after speaker and author. He has chaired multiple committees and task forces for the American Academy of Sleep Medicine (AASM), leading to his service on the Board of Directors and then as president from 2018 to 2019.

I take no small amount of pride in noting that Dr. Kirsch shares something else in common with many of the other chapter authors for *Sleep Medicine*. They each spent formative years in the training programs or on the faculty of the University of Michigan (UM) sleep program. Founded in the mid-1980s by Dr. Aldrich, the UM Sleep Disorders Centers have had a tradition ever since of emphasis on education as a vital, central mission no less important than its patient care or research ambitions. With one of the largest training programs nationally—graduating 7 new sleep physicians annually—this program has trained some of the most productive and influential clinicians and clinical educators in the field today. These individuals populate the committees of sleep professional societies, rosters of faculty around the country, websites of leading sleep disorders centers, line-ups of speakers at national meetings, and authorship lists for books that record the knowledge of our field. *Sleep Medicine* is no exception. While not all its accomplished authors have University of Michigan ties—and that would include several who also are renowned past presidents of the AASM or Sleep Research Society—those who do have roots in Ann Arbor, past or present, showcase my point. As should this book itself, which like its editors and all its authors, follows in a long tradition of excellence in sleep medicine education.

January 2024

Ronald D. Chervin, MD, MS
Professor of Neurology and Chief, Division of Sleep Medicine
Michael S. Aldrich Collegiate Professor of Sleep Medicine
Director, Sleep Disorders Centers
University of Michigan Health

Acknowledgments

Writing a book like this is a team endeavor and many people deserve plaudits:

To the entire University of Michigan Sleep Medicine program, to whom I am indebted in many ways. I am grateful not just for my introductory training in Sleep Medicine and mentoring as a young faculty member, but also for all the UM clinicians contributing chapters for this text which honors the work of Dr. Michael Aldrich, the founder of the University of Michigan Sleep Medicine program and author of the original version of this text. You are the Leaders and the Best!

To the non-Michigan clinicians around the country who were willing to spend their incredibly valuable non-clinical time lending their expertise to this text, this book wouldn't have been nearly as good without your assistance.

To Dr. Raman Malhotra, who was crucial to bringing an early version of this text to fruition, I am grateful for his help and guidance in this work and for his long-standing support.

To the Oxford team, particularly Craig Panner, who helped shepherd this long-delayed text to the finish line.

To Dr. Eva Feldman, editor of the Contemporary Neurology Series, whose guidance and assistance were essential to this book arriving at the finish line.

And lastly to my family, Erin, Ryan, and Kira; thank you for sparing our precious family time for this project. Team Kirsch always guides me to true north; whether a dance party, soccer game, or trip for bubble tea, there is no one I would rather take our yearly journey around the sun with.

Douglas Kirsch, MD, FAAN, FAASM
Medical Director, Sleep Medicine,
Atrium Health Clinical Professor,
Department of Neurology,
Wake Forest School of Medicine

Contributors

Sabra M. Abbott, MD, PhD
Department of Neurology
Northwestern University, Feinberg School of Medicine
Center for Circadian and Sleep Medicine
Northwestern University, Feinberg School of Medicine

J. Todd Arnedt, PhD
Professor, Departments of Psychiatry and Neurology
Co-Director, Sleep and Circadian Research Laboratory
Michigan Medicine, University of Michigan

Abdullah Arjomand, MD
Pulmonary and Critical Care Medicine
University of South Florida

Elda Arrigoni, PhD
Associate Professor of Neurology
Beth Israel Deaconess Medical Center
Harvard Medical School

Alon Y. Avidan, MD, MPH, FAAN, FAASM
Director, UCLA Sleep Disorders Center
Professor, UCLA Department of Neurology
David Geffen School of Medicine at UCLA

Salma Batool-Anwar, MD
Division of Sleep and Circadian Disorders
Brigham and Women's Hospital
Harvard Medical School

Sara Benjamin, MD
Johns Hopkins University

Tiffany J. Braley, MD, MS
Holtom-Garrett Family Professor of Neurology
Section Head, Multiple Sclerosis
Associate Professor of Neurology
University of Michigan Medical School

Gwendolyn C. Carlson, PhD
Department of Mental Health, VA (Veteran Affairs)
VA Health Services Research and Development Service (HSR&D)
Center for the Study of Healthcare Innovation, Implementation and Policy
VA Greater Los Angeles Healthcare System
Department of Psychiatry and Biobehavioral Sciences
University of California, Los Angeles (UCLA)
David Geffen School of Medicine

Libby Cardoni, MS
Sleep and Circadian Research Laboratory
Department of Psychiatry
Michigan Medicine, University of Michigan

Lauren Castner, DO
Pulmonologist, Children's Wisconsin
Assistant Professor, Medical College of Wisconsin

Chandra M. Cherukuri, MD, MS
Clinical Assistant Professor
Department of Family Medicine
Hennepin Healthcare

Nancy Collop, MD
Department of Pulmonary, Critical Care and Sleep Medicine
Emory University

Charles Davies, MD, PhD
Clinical Associate Professor
Carle Illinois College of Medicine

Gail Demko, DMD
Sleep Apnea Dentists of New England (ret.)

Matthew Dennis, MD
Assistant Professor
UNMC Division of Pulmonology and Sleep Medicine

Abbey Dunn, MD
Sleep Medicine
ProMedica Physicians

Mohan Dutt, MD
Sleep Medicine
ProMedica Physicians

Lawrence J. Epstein, MD
Division of Sleep and Circadian Disorders
Brigham and Women's Hospital
Harvard Medical School

Barry G. Fields, MD, MSEd
Program Director, Emory Sleep Medicine Fellowship Program
Associate Professor of Medicine, Emory University School of Medicine

Patrick M. Fuller, PhD, MS
Professor
Director, Laboratory of Systems Neuroscience
Neurological Surgery
University of California, Davis School of Medicine

Charlene Gamaldo, MD
Vice Chair, Faculty Development, Department of Neurology
Professor of Neurology
Johns Hopkins University

Susan L. Garetz, MD, MS
Professor Emeritus
Department of Otolaryngology-Head and Neck Surgery and Neurology Sleep Disorders Center Michigan Medicine
University of Michigan

Rupendra Ghatak, MD
Sleep Medicine Physician
Riverside Pulmonary and Sleep Specialists
Riverside Health

Cathy Goldstein, MD
Clinical Professor of Neurology
University of Michigan

Raphael Golebiowski
Psychiatry and Sleep Medicine
District Medical Group

Sasikanth Gorantla, MD
Clinical Assistant Professor
Department of Neurology
University of Illinois College of Medicine Peoria

John Harrington, MD
Associate Professor, UNMC Division of Pulmonary, Critical Care & Sleep Medicine
Program Director, UNMC Sleep Medicine Fellowship
University of Nebraska

Fauziya Hassan, MD, MS
Clinical Associate Professor, Sleep Disorders Center
Department of Neurology, Division of Pediatric Pulmonology
Department of Pediatrics, University of Michigan

Shelley Hershner, MD
Associate Professor of Neurology
Division of Sleep Medicine
University of Michigan

Paul T. Hoff, MD, MS
Adjunct Associate Clinical Professor
Department of Otolaryngology-Head and Neck Surgery
Michigan Medicine
University of Michigan

Michael Howell, MD
Division Director, Sleep Medicine
Professor, Department of Neurology
University of Minnesota

Stephanie D. Ivins, MD
Department of Neurology
Northwestern University, Feinberg School of Medicine
Center for Circadian and Sleep Medicine
Northwestern University
Feinberg School of Medicine

Gnanaraj Joseph, MD
Assistant Professor of Medicine
Pulmonary, Allergy, and Critical Care Medicine
Duke University School of Medicine

Neeraj Kaplish, MD
Clinical Associate Professor
Sleep Disorders Center
Department of Neurology
University of Michigan

Shakira King, BS
University of Pennsylvania School of Medicine

Douglas Kirsch, MD, FAAN, FAASM
Medical Director, Atrium Health Sleep Medicine
Clinical Professor, Wake Forest School of Medicine

Bhanu Prakash Kolla, MBBS, MD
Vice Chair for Education, Department of Psychiatry & Psychology
Professor of Psychiatry
Mayo Clinic

David Kuhlmann, MD, FAASM
Medical Director, Sleep Medicine
Bothwell Regional Health Center

Sandhya Kumar, MD
Program Director, Sleep Medicine Fellowship
Associate Professor, Neurology
Wake Forest School of Medicine

Christopher J. Lettieri, MD, FCCP, FAASM
Professor of Medicine
Uniformed Services
University of the Health Sciences

Mitchell Levine, DMD, CAGS, MS
Clinical Associate Professor, Adams School of Dentistry
University of North Carolina

Raman Malhotra
Section Chief - Section of Sleep Medicine
Professor of Neurology
Washington University

Meghna P. Mansukhani
Professor of Family Medicine
Mayo Clinic

Jennifer L. Martin, PhD
Geriatric Research, Education and Clinical Center
VA Greater Los Angeles Healthcare System
Department of Medicine
University of California, Los Angeles (UCLA)
David Geffen School of Medicine

Sheila Maurer, MD, MS, BSN
Clinical Adjunct Faculty, Pediatrics – Pulmonary
Wake Forest School of Medicine

Syed Kamal Nasser, MD
Department of Neurology
University of Michigan

Shalini Paruthi, MD, FAASM
Sleep Medicine Attending Physician, John Cochran VA Hospital
Adjunct Professor, Saint Louis University School of Medicine

Alberto R. Ramos, MD, MS, FAASM, FAAN
Professor of Neurology
University of Miami
Miller School of Medicine

Subhendu Rath, MD
Assistant Professor of Neurology
University of Kentucky

Kyle Rexer, PhD
Psychologist
VA Ann Arbor Healthcare System

Ilene M. Rosen, MD, MSCE
Associate Dean for Graduate Medical Education, Perelman School of Medicine
Designated Institutional Official, University of Pennsylvania Health System
Vice President for Graduate Medical Education, University of Pennsylvania Health System
Associate Professor of Medicine (Sleep Medicine) at the Hospital of the University of Pennsylvania

Helena Schotland, MD
Professor of Medicine
Icahn School of Medicine at Mount Sinai

Ejaz A. Shamim, MD, MS, MBA, FAAN
Chief, Department of Neurology
Mid-Atlantic Permanente Medical Group
Chair, Mid-Atlantic Kaiser Permanente Neuroscience Institute
Associate Investigator, Mid-Atlantic Permanente Research Institute
Special Volunteer, NINDS, National Institutes of Health
Assistant Professor, Department of Neurology
The George Washington University
Associate Professor, Penn State College of Medicine

Qurratul (Afifa) Shamim-Uzzaman, MD, MS, FAASM
Chief, Sleep Medicine
Director, AAVA Sleep Disorders Center
VA Ann Arbor Healthcare System
Associate Professor, Departments of Internal Medicine & Neurology
University of Michigan Medical School

Surina Sharma, MD
Department of Pulmonary, Critical Care and Sleep Medicine
Emory University

Anita V. Shelgikar, MD, MHPE
Program Director, Sleep Medicine Fellowship
Clinical Professor, Neurology
University of Michigan

Andrew R. Spector, MD, FAASM, FAAN
Associate Professor of Neurology
Duke University School of Medicine

Lee A. Surkin, MD, FACC, FCCP, FASNC
President, Empire Sleep Medicine
President, CardioSleep Diagnostics
Founder, American Academy of Cardiovascular Sleep Medicine

Sheila C. Tsai, MD
Professor, Department of Medicine
National Jewish Health

Matthew Wilson, MD
Pulmonary/Critical Care, Prisma Health
Assistant Professor of Clinical Medicine
University of South Carolina School of Medicine

Sarah Zallek, MD
Clinical Professor
Department of Neurology
University of Illinois College of Medicine Peoria

Phyllis C. Zee, MD, PhD
Department of Neurology
Center for Circadian and Sleep Medicine
Northwestern University
Feinberg School of Medicine

Introduction

Douglas Kirsch and Raman Malhotra

The last several decades have witnessed remarkable growth in our understanding of sleep as a fundamental determinant of health and disease. What was once considered a passive, poorly understood physiologic state is now recognized as an active, highly regulated process essential to neurologic function, metabolic regulation, immune system defense, and psychological well-being. Sleep medicine has evolved from a niche clinical interest into a robust multidisciplinary field that touches nearly every domain of modern healthcare.

The clinical practice of Sleep Medicine has emerged as a critical subspecialty at the intersection of neurology, pulmonology, psychiatry, pediatrics, anesthesia, otolaryngology, and internal medicine. This text is designed to serve as a comprehensive clinical and scientific reference for all medical practitioners, both Sleep Medicine-specialized and those with interest in care of sleep disorders, as well as researchers doing work within sleep and circadian science. *Sleep Medicine* integrates foundational concepts in sleep physiology with evidence-based approaches to clinical care while also addressing the evolving technological and societal dimensions of the field.

As noted in the Foreword to this text, this book is the second edition of the Sleep Medicine text for the Contemporary Neurology Series. The first edition was written solely by Dr. Michael Aldrich, the founder of the Sleep Medicine program at the University of Michigan. As the breadth of information in Sleep Medicine has significantly expanded over time, experts from across the field of Sleep Medicine were involved in the creation of this text, many of whom have a connection with the University of Michigan Sleep Medicine program.

This book is divided into seven sections to help organize the extensive information.

Section I begins by establishing the biological underpinnings of normal sleep. It reviews fundamental questions such as "What is sleep?," outlines developmental variations in sleep across the lifespan, and introduces essential concepts from chronobiology and neurobiology. These chapters form the basis for understanding the pathophysiology underlying sleep disorders.

Section II addresses abnormal sleep-related breathing. Several chapters are focused on obstructive sleep apnea, one of the most commonly diagnosed disorders in Sleep Medicine. These include a focus on epidemiology, clinical presentation, and systemic impact, followed by a comprehensive review of therapeutic modalities including positive airway pressure therapies, oral appliances, surgical interventions, and pharmacologic strategies. Central sleep apnea and hypoventilation syndromes are also reviewed in detail.

Section III covers abnormal sleep patterns, including the topics of sleep deprivation, insomnia, circadian rhythm disturbances, and hypersomnia disorders. This section includes both pharmacological and non-pharmacological treatment modalities for insomnia, with attention to diagnostic differentiation and individualized treatment planning.

Section IV examines abnormal sleep behaviors, including movement disorders such as restless legs syndrome and periodic limb movements, as well as parasomnias arising from both non-rapid eye movement (NREM) and rapid eye movement (REM) sleep. Emphasis is placed on differential diagnosis, clinical features, and therapeutic considerations.

Section V focuses on the evaluation of the sleep patient in both clinical and laboratory settings. Practical chapters address the approach to a patient in a sleep medicine clinic, validated survey tools in Sleep Medicine, diagnostic modalities including polysomnography and home sleep apnea testing, the clinical utility of actigraphy, and emerging consumer technologies.

Section VI explores the bidirectional relationship between sleep and various medical conditions. The chapters detail the interaction of sleep with neurological diseases, cognitive and emotional health, psychiatric disorders, cardiopulmonary conditions, and special populations including pediatric, occupation-specific, women, and underserved groups.

Section VII concludes the text with an overview of the field itself—its historical development and the anticipated future of sleep medicine, including technological advances, evolving diagnostic paradigms, and new therapeutic frontiers.

SECTION I

Normal Sleep

Chapter 1

What Is Sleep?

Shalini Paruthi

Sleep is essential for life! The brain is highly active during sleep, as the physical body is allowed to rest, repair, and rejuvenate. Sleep is required for optimal cognition, emotional regulation, physical performance, immune function, cardiovascular function, and hormonal function. Sleep is associated with quality of life, as well as mental and physical health.

Sleep has been succinctly distinguished from wake by these criteria: "1. reduced motor activity, 2. decreased response to stimulation, 3. stereotypic postures (e.g. in humans, lying down with eyes closed, 4. relatively easy reversibility (distinguishing it from coma, hibernation, and estivation), 5. homeostatic regulation (i.e. sleep deprivation is followed by sleep rebound), . . . 6. loss of consciousness of the environment."[1p52]

The quest to learn more about human sleep became possible in the early 1900s when electroencephalograms (EEG) were first recorded in awake humans. Prior to this, most interest and research in human sleep focused on dream interpretations. The EEG led to the recognition of different brain wave morphologies, and in the 1930s, waves such as spindles were named during sleep. Later in the 1950s, researchers were able to fully record all night, overnight, noting there were clear changes in the EEG occurring in cycles through the night. It is interesting to recall that sleep was a new frontier; there were no standardized measurements of sleep, much was trial and error during recordings, there were no sleep labs, and items required to record overnight sleep, such as enormous amounts of paper, were expensive. On the other hand, clinically, sleep disorder syndromes were being described and identified as early as 1880, with the description of signs and symptoms of narcolepsy. Sleep disorders are still being clarified today as to etiologies, best tests for diagnosis, and treatments best suited for each individual. In-depth details about the history of the sleep medicine field can be found in Chapter 32.

The exact moment of falling asleep can be ascertained with EEG. Sleep begins when alpha waves transition to theta waves, signifying the brain transitioning from a state of alertness to now a light stage of sleep. During this transition, the person loses awareness of self and the environment. The waves continue to slow as they transition to delta waves and deeper sleep is achieved.

As an adult or child (>1 year of age) falls asleep, they often transition from wake into N1 sleep. Infants under 1 year of age may enter sleep through N1 or REM (rapid eye movement) sleep. Sleep is classified into 4 stages: N1, N2, N3, also known as non-REM (NREM) sleep, and REM sleep. The technical specifications of how to score these stages of sleep on a polysomnogram (sleep study) can be found in the American Academy of Sleep Medicine *Manual for the Scoring of Sleep and Associated Events*.[2] Sleep cycles typically last 60–90 minutes in duration as the person transitions through N1, N2, N3, then a brief period of REM sleep.

Within the circadian system, sleep is driven by a homeostatic factor called process S, and this factor causes a person to feel sleepier the longer they have been awake. Process S accumulates during the waking hours and dissipates during sleep. On the other hand, Process C causes alertness, and is regulated by the suprachiasmatic nucleus. The basic science of chronobiology is further explored in Chapter 3.

Biochemicals and neurotransmitters such as adenosine, prostaglandin D2, muramyl dipeptides, tumor necrosis factor-alpha, gamma-aminobutyric acid (GABA), and galanin are sleep-inducing.

Wake-promoting neurotransmitters include acetylcholine, serotonin, dopamine, norepinephrine, histamine, orexin A, and orexin B. Sleep is achieved by GABA and galanin inhibition of regions of the brain that promote wakefulness. Wake-promoting neurotransmitters decrease during NREM and REM sleep; although acetylcholine levels rise again during REM sleep. During wake, acetylcholine and the other wake-promoting neurotransmitters reduce the activity of the inhibitory neuron cells in the cortex, thereby causing arousal and alertness. Chapter 4 reviews the neurobiology of sleep in greater detail.

Furthermore, sleep patterns have been studied to determine what is within normal ranges for different stages of life. Infants may sleep 12–16 hours per 24-hour period. Toddlers need 10–13 hours of sleep per 24 hours, including their overnight sleep and nap sleep. Grade-school children need 9–12 hours of sleep nightly; teens need 8–10 hours of sleep nightly. A consensus panel of pediatric sleep clinicians and sleep scientists reviewed published sleep medical literature and found:

> sleeping the number of recommended hours on a regular basis is associated with better health outcomes including: improved attention, behavior, learning, memory, emotional regulation, quality of life, and mental and physical health. Regularly sleeping fewer than the number of recommended hours is associated with attention, behavior, and learning problems. Insufficient sleep also increases the risk of accidents, injuries, hypertension, obesity, diabetes, and depression. Insufficient sleep in teenagers is associated with increased risk of self-harm, suicidal thoughts, and suicide attempts. Regularly sleeping more than the recommended hours may be associated with adverse health outcomes such as hypertension, diabetes, obesity, and mental health problems.[3p785]

Similarly, a consensus panel of sleep clinicians and sleep scientists reviewed published sleep medicine literature and found:

> Adults should sleep 7 or more hours per night on a regular basis to promote optimal health. Sleeping less than 7 hours per night on a regular basis is associated with adverse health outcomes, including weight gain and obesity, diabetes, hypertension, heart disease and stroke, depression, and increased risk of death. Sleeping less than 7 hours per night is also associated with impaired immune function, increased pain, impaired performance, increased errors, and greater risk of accidents.[4p591]

Once normal sleep patterns across the life span were established, disorders of sleep became better recognizable. Over the last 40+ years, sleep clinicians have organized the sleep disorders into six main categories within the International Classification of Sleep Disorders (3rd ed.-TR).[5] There are over 70 distinct sleep disorders identified thus far. Sleep disorders are categorized into insomnia disorders, sleep-related breathing disorders, central disorders of hypersomnolence, circadian rhythm sleep-wake disorders, parasomnias, and sleep-related movement disorders. These disorders, including diagnosis and management in children and adults, are covered in great detail in later chapters throughout this textbook.

An objective sleep test is used to diagnose the majority of sleep disorders. These tools include the gold-standard, in-lab, overnight polysomnogram, which is used to accurately measure sleep through electrooculography, EEG, electrocardiography, nasal and oral respiratory sensors, thoracic and abdominal excursion, plethysmography and pulse oximetry, capnography, chin and limb electromyography, and snore microphone sensor. Home sleep apnea tests can be used outside of the sleep center in appropriately selected patients with a high pre-test probability of sleep apnea. Hypersomnia can be objectively measured with the Multiple Sleep Latency Test or the Maintenance of Wakefulness Test. Actigraphy (accelerometers) can clarify sleep and wake periods to assist with detection of circadian rhythm disorders or insomnia. Several questionnaires have been developed and validated to improve screening for sleep disorders and to monitor for improvements or worsening of the sleep disorder when the questionnaires are answered serially over time. These sleep tests, pertinent genetic tests, lab tests, and questionnaires are reviewed within sections describing each sleep disorder and within Section V.

Evidence-based sleep medicine, coupled with shared decision-making with the patient, fully captures the art of sleep medicine. To assist healthcare professionals, there are several clinical practice guidelines published by the American Academy of Sleep Medicine and other leading physician organizations. Additionally, there are patient education and advocacy groups for many sleep disorders, which provide excellent resources for patients and healthcare professionals. Sleep partners in the pharmaceutical industry and sleep equipment industry lead the way for improved sleep-disorder diagnosis and effective treatments. Additionally, consumer technologies such as wearables and nearables perhaps will provide sleep researchers with huge data sets of sleep and wake behaviors which may help to unlock future strategies for improved sleep health or treatment of sleep disorders.

REFERENCES

1. Siegel JM. Introduction/defining sleep. In: *Principles and Practice of Sleep Medicine*. 7th ed. Philadelphia, PA: Elsevier; 2022:569–578.
2. Troester MM, Quan SF, Berry RB, et al.; for the American Academy of Sleep Medicine. *The AASM Manual for the Scoring of Sleep and Associated Events: Rules, Terminology and Technical Specifications*. Version 3. American Academy of Sleep Medicine; 2023.
3. Paruthi S, Brooks LJ, D'Ambrosio C, et al. Recommended amount of sleep for pediatric populations: A consensus statement of the American Academy of Sleep Medicine. *J Clin Sleep Med*. 2016;12(6): 785–786.
4. Watson NF, Badr MS, Belenky G, et al. Recommended amount of sleep for a healthy adult: A joint consensus statement of the American Academy of Sleep Medicine and Sleep Research Society. *J Clin Sleep Med*. 2015;11(6): 591–592.
5. American Academy of Sleep Medicine. *International Classification of Sleep Disorders*. 3rd ed., text revision. American Academy of Sleep Medicine; 2023.

Chapter 2

Sleep Patterns over the Life Span

John Harrington and Matthew Dennis

INTRODUCTION

The dynamic nature of sleep "maturation" requires a thorough discussion of sleep patterns, duration, and architecture across the ages. This is needed to allow the sleep clinician to discern appropriate from inappropriate sleep habits in patients of all ages. Even the clinician whose focus is on the care of mature adults will be faced with the normal changes in sleep habits that occur during advanced years.

THE STUDY OF EARLY SLEEP DEVELOPMENT

The following definitions from the American Academy of Sleep Medicine (AASM) *Manual for the Scoring of Sleep and Associated Events* regarding premature infant nomenclature are imperative to the discussion of premature infants:

> Conceptional age (CA) is gestational age (GA) at birth plus the number of weeks postpartum. GA is the time elapsed between the first day of the mother's last menstrual period and the day of delivery expressed in completed weeks. If the pregnancy was achieved using assisted reproductive technology, GA is calculated by adding 2 weeks to the CA. Chronological age (or postnatal or legal age) is the time elapsed since birth (can be expressed in days, months, or years).[1p39]

The ex utero infant, whether term or preterm, can undergo full polysomnographic assessment, whereas the in utero infant cannot. Multiple studies have utilized prenatal ultrasound to identify behavioral sleep states, and the accuracy of this methodology has been promising when compared to postnatal behavioral and polysomnographic assessments in term and preterm infants.[2] However, this form of assessment has limitations when compared with full polysomnography, as often the nature of sleep development in utero in term infants is extrapolated from ex utero preterm infants. This approach makes presumptions that sleep measures, and in particular the EEG recording, will develop in similar fashion whether the development takes place in utero or ex utero. This hypothesis is supported by a recent review which revealed that when premature infants were assessed at subsequent conceptional ages their electroencephalogram (EEG) patterns were similar to those of infants born at a similar level of maturity (i.e., infants with CA "x" had similar EEGs to infants with GA "x").[3] In one study by Sher et al., 13 healthy premature infants and a total of 25 EEG recordings were included. Although the study patients were premature and spent time in a neonatal intensive care unit (NICU), they were considered healthy as they did not have "major medical illness," did not require ventilatory assistance or have "clinical neonatal depression or signs of encephalopathy." This study demonstrated no significant differences between EEG and obstetric/ultrasound estimation of gestational age.[4p215] It is hard to ignore the obvious environmental differences between in utero versus ex utero development (especially in a premature infant with likely intensive care needs). That being said, a study involving 25 premature infants who were all ventilator dependent, and who ultimately died, showed an agreement between EEG and anatomic estimation of GA in 23 of 25 patients (92%).[5] The Collaborative Home Infant Monitoring Evaluation (CHIME) study offered valuable information regarding not only the differences in development between preterm and term infants, but also the effects of ventilatory support (an estimate of morbidity) on sleep development. In brief, "asymptomatic" preterm infants did not show statistically significant differences in sleep patterns when compared to term infants with the same CA, with three exceptions. The exceptions were the number of quiet sleep episodes ≥ 10 minutes, the mean duration of indeterminate epochs, and the longest indeterminate epoch. The infants who required ventilatory support demonstrated no difference in percentage of quiet sleep, but had more active sleep: 42% (±13.0%) in the ventilator group versus 34.4% (±12.5%) in the control group (P <.001).[6]

The hypothesis that the maturation of sleep is primarily dependent on CA, and not on GA, is commonly used in clinical practice. However, given the profound environmental differences between in utero versus ex utero development, and the possible effects of complex intensive care, this remains an interesting subject for further study.

FETAL AND NEONATAL SLEEP

The sleep states of infants with conceptual ages of 37–48 weeks are defined as follows: wake; non-rapid eye movement (NREM) sleep (aka quiet sleep); rapid eye movement (REM) (aka active sleep); and transitional (aka indeterminate). These infant-specific definitions are applied during the first 2 months of post-term life because waveforms used to stage typical N2 and N3 in children and adults (e.g., sleep spindles, K-complexes, slow wave activity) are not appreciable until approximately 2–3 months of post-term life.[1] Similar definitions are commonly applied to the staging of infants with conceptual ages of <37 weeks. However, as will be described, not all of these states are appreciable in early prematurity, particularly <30 weeks CA.[7,8]

Early in development, from 24 to 29 weeks CA, the EEG may be entirely flat or demonstrate trace discontinu (TD). Low voltage irregular (LVI), high voltage slow (HVS), and mixed (M) waveform patterns are not present at this time, but clear sleep-wake cycles do not occur. From 29 to 32 weeks CA, tardive discontinu becomes established with an interburst interval (IBI) of 6–35 seconds. LVM and M continuous activity is rarely present, but if present is it associated with active sleep and wakefulness. The REMs of active sleep can be observed at this point. Respirations begin to exhibit a regular pattern during quiet sleep and an irregular pattern during wake and active sleep. That being said, the majority of the EEG remains indeterminate (i.e., transitional). From 32 to 35 weeks CA, the IBI of TD becomes shorter (<10 seconds) and less frequent. The continuous activity of active sleep and wakefulness (i.e., LVI and M) may be seen, but large portions of the EEG remain indeterminate (i.e., transitional). From 35 to 37 weeks CA, the TD of quiet sleep begins to transition to the Trace alternant (TA). Specifically, the amplitude of the high voltage bursts decreases from 50–300 uV to 50–150 uV, the amplitude of the interburst activity increases from <25 uV to 25–50 uV, and the IBI decreases to 4–6 seconds. The continuous activity of active sleep and wakefulness (i.e., LVI and M) is typically present. From 37 to 44 weeks CA, the continuous activity of active sleep and wakefulness (i.e., LVI and M) becomes the majority of the recording. The

TA of quiet sleep transitions to the HVS pattern of quiet sleep during this time.[1,7,8]

Quiet sleep usually cannot be identified until around 35 weeks CA, but once recognizable, the percentage of quiet sleep increases while the percentage of active (REM) sleep decreases.[9ch3] Around term CA, active (REM) sleep makes up roughly 50% of total sleep time, but by 52 weeks CA, active (REM) sleep has decreased below 40% of total sleep time.[8] Hoppenbrouwers and colleagues recorded this gradual increase in percentage quiet sleep and gradual decrease in percentage active sleep during late preterm development. *Paraphrasing their data as percentages of total sleep time*: At 34–37 weeks CA, the mean amount of quiet sleep was 27%, and the mean amount of active sleep was 61%. By 50–53 weeks CA, the mean amount of quiet sleep was 64% and the mean amount of active sleep was 28%.[6] Coons et al. demonstrated similar reductions in active (REM) sleep and increases in quiet sleep during postnatal development in term infants (i.e., this pattern was not specific to preterm infants only). Differences in sleep staging methodology between these studies limit the propriety of direct quantitative data comparisons; however, comparisons of the trends can be made. At 3 weeks postnatal age, the mean amount of quiet sleep was 31.0% of total sleep time and the mean amount of REM sleep was 31.6% of total sleep time. At 12 weeks postnatal age, the mean amount of NREM sleep was 68.1% of total sleep time and the mean amount of REM sleep was 28.0% of total sleep time.[10]

The development of sleep onset parallels this overall change from predominantly REM sleep to predominantly NREM sleep. Around term CA, approximately 80% of sleep onset includes active (REM) sleep, but by 52 weeks CA, sleep onset typically involves NREM sleep.[8]

MATURATION OF SLEEP PERIODS

The post-term neonate lacks a clear nocturnal-diurnal pattern, with sleep relatively evenly distributed across the day and night. This is in part related to their short periods of sleep (2–5 hours) and wakefulness (1–2 hours).[9,11,12] Anders studied infant sleep-wake patterns by use of in-home, overnight time-lapse video somnography and parental questionnaires. They found that 2-week-old full-term infants' longest sustained sleep period was on average 3.89 hours, and only 46% of the longest sustained sleep periods were between 12:00 AM and 5:00 AM.[13] Gradually, over the course of several weeks, the longest periods of sleep and wakefulness lengthen, with the former consolidating to nighttime hours and the latter consolidating to daytime hours. This leads to the development of a nocturnal-diurnal pattern consistency of longer periods of sleep at night, and longer periods of wake admixed with shorter naps during the day, around 3–4 months of age. At this point the longest period of sustained sleep is around 8–9 hours, and the longest sustained period of wakefulness is around 3–4 hours.[9] Anders observed complementary findings by use of their in-home, overnight time-lapse video somnography and parental questionnaires. They found that at 2 months of age the mean longest sustained sleep period was 6.18 hours, and 76% of longest sustained sleep periods were between 12:00 AM and 5:00 AM. At 6 months of age, the mean longest sustained sleep period had increased to 7.03 hours and 81% of longest sustained sleep periods were occurring between 12:00 AM and 5:00 AM. By 9 months of age, the mean longest sustained sleep period had risen to 7.43 hours and 89% of longest sustained sleep periods were occurring during the 12:00 AM to 5:00 AM interval.[13]

A major milestone, certainly in the context of family dynamics, is when infants begin "sleeping through the night." This milestone, which is defined as when parents perceive the infant to be sleeping at least 8 hours without parental intervention, typically occurs around 6–9 months of age.

At this point (around 6–9 months of age), daytime napping patterns remain quite variable. Some infants have consolidated their naps to 2 naps, whereas others continue to take several short naps spread throughout the day. It is important for the clinician to highlight the variability in napping patterns to parents, as to prevent pressure for infants to conform to a "normal" napping routine. Naps are typically consolidated down to 1 nap per day around 12–18 months of age. Eventually, daytime napping becomes extinct between 3 and 5 years of age.[11,12] Iglowstein found that 87% of 2-year-olds, 50% of 3-year-olds, 35% of 4-year-olds, and 8% of 5-year-olds took daytime naps.[14]

SLEEP DURATION

A common question posed by parents is "how much should my infant sleep?" Answering this can be challenging since although the average total sleep time throughout infancy remains relatively constant at 14 hours a day, wide variability exists.[11,12] This variability in total sleep time is most significant during infancy. In one instance the standard deviation for total sleep time at 6 months was ± 1.9 hours versus ± 0.8 hours for the average of ages 1–10 years (Oskar 2009). Iglowstein found that at 6 months of age the 2nd percentile for total sleep time was as low as 10.4 hours, and the 98th percentile for total sleep time was as high as 18.1 hours.[14] The 2016 AASM consensus guideline recommends that infants ages 4–12 months get 12–16 hours of sleep per 24-hour period.[15]

Throughout toddlerhood and childhood there is a gradual reduction in total sleep time. During toddler years the nighttime sleep duration declines only slightly, while the decline in daytime sleep duration is the predominant contributor to the gradual reduction of total sleep time.[11,12] Iglowstein found the following at 1 year of age: mean total sleep time of 13.9 hours, mean nighttime sleep time of 11.7 hours, and mean daytime sleep time of 2.4 hours. At 2 years of age these values had decreased to the following: mean total sleep time of 13.2 hours, mean nighttime sleep time of 11.5 hours, and mean daytime sleep time of 1.8 hours. By 4 years of age these values had decreased to the following: mean total sleep time of 11.8 hours, mean nighttime sleep time of 11.2 hours, and mean daytime sleep time of 1.5 hours. By 6 years of age only 5% of the studied children were napping, so the mean total sleep time and the mean nighttime sleep time were essentially the same. The mean total sleep time at ages 6, 8, 10, and 12 were 11.0, 10.4, 9.9, and 9.3 hours, respectively.[14] A meta-analysis by Kocevska identified similar findings, with a mean total sleep time of 11.6 hours for 3- to 5-year-olds, and a mean total sleep time of 10.6 for 6- to 13-year-olds.[16] The 2016 AASM consensus guideline recommends total sleep time per 24 hours similar to Iglowstein's findings: 11–14 hours for ages 1–2 years, 10–13 hours for ages 3–5 years, and 9–12 hours for ages 6–12 years.[15]

Iglowstein observed a continued decreased in total sleep time during adolescence, with a mean total sleep time of 9.3 hours at 12 years and a mean total sleep time of 8.1 hours at 16 years.[14] However, as was described in the seminal study by Carskadon, unconstrained total sleep time (clinically equated to total sleep requirement) actually remains relatively stable at 9.25 hours throughout adolescence. The decrease in adolescent total sleep times that is often observed can be attributed to extrinsic constraints on sleep time compounded by the natural circadian phase delay of adolescence.[12,17] The 2016 AASM consensus guideline recommends 8–10 hours of sleep per 24-hour-period for adolescents ages 13–18 years.[15]

SLEEP ARCHITECTURE

As described previously, during late preterm gestation (around 35 weeks CA) the percentage of quiet sleep increases, while the percentage of active (REM) sleep decreases.[9] Coons demonstrated that by 3 months postnatal age, the mean amount of NREM sleep had increased to 68.1% of total sleep time and the mean amount of REM sleep had decreased to 28.0% of total sleep time. At 6 months the mean amount of NREM sleep had risen further to 74.9% of total sleep time and the mean amount of REM sleep had decreased further to 23.6% of total sleep time.[10]

Scholle obtained normative polysomnography data by looking at single polysomnogram data on 209 healthy German children. The subjects were grouped into the following age (in years) categories: 1.4 ± 0.3, 2.9 ± 0.5, 5.1 ± 0.5, 8.1 ± 1.4 (Tanner stage 1), 11.5 ± 1.2 (Tanner stage 2), 12.8 ± 1.6 (Tanner stage 3), 15.2 ± 1.4 (Tanner stage 4), and 16.9 ± 0.9 (Tanner stage 5). In terms of sleep stage architecture, the percentage of N1 was relatively the same, at approximately 7% of total sleep time, throughout the studied age groups. When moving from the younger to older age groups, the percentage of N2 sleep gradually increased: 31.1% at 1 year of age, and 49.4% at Tanner stage 5. The percentage of N3 sleep increased when moving from the 1-year-old group (34.9%) to the 3-year-old group (38.4%). Stage N3 sleep subsequently decreased when moving from the young childhood groups to the older adolescent groups, and was 22.9% in the Tanner stage

5 group. This higher quantity and intensity of slow wave sleep in younger children serve as an explanation for why some pre-pubertal children "skip" REM sleep during their first sleep cycle. The percentage of REM sleep gradually decreased when moving from younger to older age groups: 25.6% at 1 year of age, and 19.0% at Tanner stage 5.[18]

Sleep latency and sleep efficiency were essentially unchanged when moving from childhood to adolescence. Sleep cycle duration, on the other hand, did change when moving from childhood to adolescence. Specifically, it increased from an average of 64.7 minutes at 1 year of age to 91.4 minutes at Tanner stage 5. This was accompanied by an increase in REM sleep latency: average of 83.9 minutes at 1 year of age, average of 132.7 minutes at Tanner stage 5. This change was somewhat intuitive, as if the sleep cycle gets longer, it will take more time to get to the REM sleep phase of the sleep cycle (certainly if the general pattern of sleep cycles is maintained). Another intuitive finding was that with elongation of sleep cycle duration (in the setting of decreased total sleep), the number of sleep cycles per sleep period decreased: average of 7.5 cycles/sleep period at 1 year of age, 4.9 cycles/sleep period at Tanner stage 5.[12,18]

YOUNG ADULT SLEEP

While many young adults report sleep durations of about 8 hours per night, the actual duration of nocturnal sleep is quite variable and is influenced by a variety of genetic and behavioral factors and underlying sleep and health disorders. Some examples of these barriers to adequate sleep are listed in Table 2.1.

Table 2.1 **Barriers to Adequate Sleep**

- Social norms
- Electronic use
- Work obligations
- Family obligations
- Substance use
- Physical environment
- Comorbid health disorders

SLEEP DURATION

Overall nighttime sleep duration decreases from adolescence into adulthood. The 2012 Bedroom Poll found that younger adults (age 25–55 years) tend to sleep about 6.75 hours and 7.5 hours on weeknights and weekends, respectively.[19] Similarly, in a study of healthy adults by Dijk et al.,[20] older subjects, aged 66–83 years, slept about 20 minutes less than middle-aged subjects aged 40–55 years, who in turn slept 23 minutes less than youngest group at 20–30 years of age. These decrements in sleep duration were primarily related to increased awakenings and duration of wake after sleep onset and not increased sleep latency. Approximate sleep efficiencies of young (92%), middle-aged (87%), and older adults (82%) were significantly different across age groups.

Sleep duration variations are influenced by gender. The SIESTA database included polysomnographic findings from 160 data sets of healthy subjects aged 20–90 years. The analysis of this data demonstrated age-dependent sleep architectural differences between age groups and genders, with decrease of total sleep time of approximately 8 minutes per decade in males and 10 minutes in females. These changes were primarily related to increased wake after sleep onset and not other variables.[21] In a large meta-analysis, Kocevska and colleagues included data from 34 population-based studies from the Netherlands (n = 200,358), United States (n = 409,617), and United Kingdom (n = 471,759). Just over 50% of those aged 14–17 years reported sleep durations of less than 8–10 hours per night. While sleep efficiency declined into adulthood, one-quarter of those over age 65 years reported 95% sleep efficiency. Adult women reported longer total sleep time and somewhat lower sleep efficiencies compared to men. In women 41–65 years of age the average reported nighttime sleep duration was 7.1 ± 1.1 hours each night, compared to 6.9 ± 1 hours to men of similar age. Despite reported increased sleep durations, women reported sleep efficiencies of 89 ± 10% compared to 92 ± 9% in men.[16] A recent literature review of studies published between 1960 and 2013 evaluated reported objectively measured sleep duration among over 6000 healthy adults aged 18–88 years. Despite reported limitations of the included studies, these authors concluded relatively consistent sleep durations across age groups and sexes.[22] A recent consensus statement from the American Academy of Sleep Medicine (AASM) recommends that adults should sleep 7 or more hours per night on a consistent basis to promote optimal health. The panel of sleep experts found that consistently sleeping less than 7 hours per night was associated with a variety of adverse health and performance outcomes, while regularly sleeping longer than 9 hours may have uncertain effects on health.

SLEEP ARCHITECTURE

A large meta-analysis by Ohayon et al. attempted to better describe age-related changes in sleep. The finding of modestly increased sleep latency with age was noted but was only significantly different in comparison between very young adults and older adults with a resultant increase of less than 10 minutes. Comparisons of sleep latencies between other age groups of adults were more or less comparable.[23] Stage N1 sleep was noted to increase across adulthood with significant changes noted between young, middle-aged, and older adults. Stage N2 likewise increased during adulthood until age 60 years. Stage R sleep was found to decrease with advancing age from young adulthood to middle-aged adults but stabilized in adults older than 60 years of age. There were consistent reductions in total sleep time and sleep efficiency with age. Wake after sleep onset was also increased with age during adulthood. Sleep efficiency was the only sleep metric that continued to significantly decrease into advanced age while other parameters remained stable. These findings were moderated by psychiatric and medical conditions and sleep disorders, such as sleep apnea. These authors found that most age-related changes in sleep architecture occurred before the age of 60 years, with only minor changes in stages N1, N3, and R sleep. However, there were consistent reductions in sleep efficiency well into late life. Other measures of sleep architecture revealed linear declines in total sleep time, stage R sleep, slow wave sleep, and wake after sleep onset.[23] However, a later analysis by Floyd and colleagues found that there was a 2.9% decline in stage R percentage from age 19 to 75 years but an approximate 1.6% recovery of stage R sleep from age 76 to 85.[24]

The prospective Sleep Heart Health Study (SHHS) included 2685 participants, aged 37 to 92 years. Redline et al. found that percentages of stage N1 and N2 sleep were significantly higher in individuals older than 61 years compared to those 54 and younger.[25] Slow wave sleep was significantly lower in those older than 54 years of age compared to younger adults. Stage R sleep was also significantly decreased among those older than 61 years compared to younger participants. Age-related reductions in sleep efficiency were noted within advancing age. Differences in sleep architectural variables between genders was also noted, with men having significantly higher stage N1 sleep percentage with age; this change was not noted in women. Similar increases in stage N2 sleep percentages in men were noted, again without age-related increases in women. Slow wave sleep was significantly lower in men with age, but this was not noted in women. Arousal index was significantly increased in those older than 55 compared to younger subjects. Sleep efficiency was significantly lower in older versus younger participants. A study by Bonnet and Anand of 76 subjects (age 18–70 years) found that subjects younger than 31 years had significantly less arousals compared to older groups and those age 31–50 years had significantly less arousal indices compared to older groups.[26] Other gender differences included increased stage N1 in men of about 2% per decade that primarily corresponded to decreased N3 sleep, while stage N2 sleep remained unchanged. In women, there was also an increase in stage N1 sleep, albeit smaller at 1.1%, and increased N2 sleep of 0.9%, which was explained by decreased stage R sleep (−1.4%) without change in stage N3 sleep.[21]

In adults there is a marked decrease in stage N3 sleep compared to children. Slow wave sleep by age of 60 years is much reduced, particularly in men. The amount of stage R sleep as a total of nocturnal sleep remains generally consistent into later life, though it can be greatly diminished in those with neurodegenerative disorders.[27] Sleep consolidation can diminish with age as arousals increase substantially. Wakefulness increases with age and may be idiopathic or related to an underlying sleep disorder. Slow wave sleep percentage was significantly higher in the young compared to both the middle-aged (P = 0.0004) and older age group (P = 0.0015), but the difference between the middle-aged and older age groups was not statistically significant.[20]

OLDER ADULT SLEEP

Sleep Duration

Sleep duration among older adults is more consistent compared to younger adults. Older adults (age 55–84 years) in one survey reported more consistent sleep durations of 7–7.1 hours durations over the entire week. This same poll noted somewhat more consistent bedtimes of 10 PM to 12 AM in 74% of older respondents throughout the week, compared to younger adults who tended to go to bed later on weekends.[28]

Sleep Architecture

Sleep architecture among the elderly may differ compared to younger adults. Slow wave sleep percentage was significantly higher in the young adults compared to both the middle-aged (P = 0.0004) and older age groups (P = 0.0015), but the difference between these two older groups was not significant.[20] Sleep in older adults is marked by increased nighttime arousals, awakenings, and sleep stage shifts.[29–31] In addition, the duration of awakenings at night is increased. These features contribute to age-related reductions in total sleep time, sleep efficiency, and slow wave sleep.[23] Other studies have demonstrated longer sleep latency in older subjects.[29] While older adults in a study by Klerman woke up from sleep about 2.7 times the rate as younger subjects, they fell back to sleep at a rate similar to young subjects,[32] and despite significantly reduced nighttime slow wave sleep and increased nocturnal awakenings with advancing age, objectively measured sleepiness was significantly decreased among healthy older adults compared to younger adults.[20]

Age-related changes in stage R sleep are often seen in older adults when compared to younger persons. These changes include reduced percentage of stage R sleep, decreased stage R sleep latency, longer duration of the 1st stage R episode. In a study by van Cauter et al., stage R sleep was decreased by as much as one-half in late life compared to younger adults,[31] and there is some evidence that stage R sleep density is decreased in older adults.[33] In a prospective study by Mitterling and colleagues, polysomnographic sleep variables among 100 healthy adults (age 19–77 years) were evaluated. Age-related decrements in total sleep time, sleep efficiency, and N3 sleep and stage R sleep percentages were noted in subjects older than 60 years compared to those less than or equal to 30 years, but wake after sleep onset percentage increased in older subjects. There was no significant difference in total arousals or arousals from NREM, N2, and N3 sleep between younger and older age groups, but stage R sleep arousal index did increase with age, and this finding remained significant after adjustment for gender.[34] The lack of increase in arousal index among older subjects was not consistent compared to findings of earlier studies.[26,35,36]

Sleep Architecture

Age-related changes in sleep architecture are predominantly characterized by reductions in sleep efficiency, N3 sleep, and stage R sleep.[37] There is also age-related dampening of the circadian sleep-wake rhythms, and these are associated with concurrent reduction in melatonin secretion amplitude and core body temperature.[38] The deterioration of the suprachiasmatic nucleus (SCN) contributes to diminished and altered rhythms.[39,40] These alterations may contribute to increased daytime sleepiness and decreased nighttime sleep efficiency. Sleep onset tends to occur earlier in older adults relative to their melatonin secretory phase, and then older adults wake up from sleep with increased melatonin levels compared to younger adults. This suggests alterations in the relationships between internal phase and output of the SCN.[41,42] Older adults also tend to have less bright light exposure, which can contribute to circadian rhythm abnormalities.[40]

Phase advancement of circadian rhythms is common in older subjects and contributes to early morning awakenings and hypersomnolence earlier in the evening.[31] Other studies have found that reductions in circadian rhythm amplitude[38,43] may increase susceptibility of arousing circadian signals and decreased homeostatic sleep pressure.[44] While there is evidence to support earlier circadian phases in older subjects, the data supporting reductions in circadian rhythm amplitude and period length, which are postulated to contribute to increased nocturnal awakenings and daytime hypersomnolence among healthy older adults, are not consistent.[45]

COMORBIDITIES

Sleep quality and architecture change not only with aging but also with medical and psychiatric conditions commonly associated with advancing age. Depression may increase sleep onset latency, sleep fragmentation and total sleep time, and early morning awakenings. Sleep stage findings in depressed adults may include increased stage N1 and N2 sleep and decreased N3 sleep. Stage R sleep changes include decreased stage R latency but with increased first R period, REM density, and percentage.[46–48] In addition, older women with depressive symptoms may have increased actigraphically measured wake after sleep onset (WASO), nighttime wake periods longer than 5 minutes in duration, and nap episodes.[49] Adults with anxiety may demonstrate increase wakefulness after sleep onset.[50] Objective sleep measures in older adults with GAD revealed decreased sleep durations and efficiency due to increased awakenings and sleep onset latencies.[51] Post-traumatic stress disorder (PTSD) may be associated with increased N1 sleep and REM density with decreased N3 sleep.[52]

Various medical disorders can contribute to sleep architectural changes among adults. Chronic pain in older adults may result in increased sleep onset latencies, WASO, and decreased sleep efficiencies.[53,54] Gastroesophageal reflux disease (GERD) in older adults is often associated with insomnia and associated sleep,[55,56] and nocturnal reflux events were noted to occur during periods of wakefulness and arousals were much more likely to precede rather than follow reflux events.[57]

Thirty-seven percent of older patients hospitalized with acute coronary syndrome reported moderate-to-severe insomnia, and WASO durations of 76 minutes were noted in approximeatly 20%.[58] Congestive heart failure (CHF) patients may have reduced sleep durations, efficiencies, and stages R and N3 sleep with higher WASO.[59] Mild-to-moderate chronic obstructive pulmonary disease (COPD) is associated with decreased sleep efficiency, total sleep time, and increased insomnia symptoms.[60] In moderate-to-severe COPD, longer sleep latencies, decreased sleep efficiencies, increased stage N1 sleep, and decreased stage R sleep with reasonably preserved N3 sleep have been reported.[61]

Patients on dialysis generally have increased nighttime arousals with decreased total sleep time and sleep efficiencies. While there was variability in the distribution of sleep stages, increased N1 and N2 sleep and decreased N3 and stage R sleep were often reported.[62] Sleep disturbances of increased stage N1 and stage R sleep in nondialyzed patients with chronic kidney disease may not be directly related to their decrements in glomerular filtration rate but rather their underlying sleep-disordered breathing severity.[63] However, reduced total sleep and stage R durations remained significant after adjusting for sleep apnea and other factors in a cross-sectional study.[64]

Primary sleep disorders may be associated with sleep architectural alterations. Sleep apnea may suppress stages N3 or R sleep[28] and increased N1 sleep.[65] Restless legs syndrome and insomnia are often associated with delays in sleep onset latencies.

NAPPING

Actigraphic measured napping has been reported in 45% adults over 65 years of age.[66] A more recent analysis of those aged 65 and older found that 23.3% intentionally took naps, while 28.4% napped unintentionally but with only 20.1% of those naps longer than 1 hour duration.[67] Napping is common among older men and women. In a large sample of community-dwelling older women 79–96 years of age, 23% reported napping for at least 1 hour each time and 43% were objectively classified as nappers.[68] Among older men, napping was also prevalent, with overall mean nap durations of 40.2 minutes.[69]

Some studies have found that napping may worsen subsequent nighttime sleep efficiency and nocturnal total sleep time[70] or could be associated with increased depression and mortality[71] and cognitive impairment in those who nap longest.[69] Other investigators have reported the potential benefits of short daytime napping, such as improved subsequent nighttime sleep and daytime functioning[70,72,73] and improved cognitive and psychomotor performance.[74]

SUMMARY

It is evident that sleep patterns change across one's lifetime. However, it is less clear why and how these changes occur, or what the consequences of these specific variations in sleep architecture are. Are these findings simply a limitation of using imprecise technology available today to measure EEG activity? Do they reflect differences in the function of sleep among the very young and the very old, and in every age in between? Are they the product of brain maturation and eventual senescence? And do these variations confer any survival benefit or performance advantage, or the converse?

It is essential to understand the effect of different sleep habits on altering the sleep architecture among the various cultures, life stations (student, worker, retiree), careers (shift worker, submarine crew), lifestyle choices (alcohol, caffeine or substance use, voluntary sleep restriction, sedentary or active living), social determinants of health (nutrition, home environment), medical conditions (insomnia, chronic renal failure, stress), and medications (antidepressants, opioids). As understanding of these changes in sleep architecture increases, we may better understand the impact on an individual's life quality and longevity.

REFERENCES

1. Berry RB, Brooks R, Gamaldo CE, et al.; for the American Academy of Sleep Medicine. *The AASM Manual for the Scoring of Sleep and Associated Events: Rules, Terminology and Technical Specifications*. Version 2.6. www.aasmnet.org. American Academy of Sleep Medicine; 2020.
2. Mirmiran M, Maas YG, Ariagno RL. Development of fetal and neonatal sleep and circadian rhythms. *Sleep Med Rev*. 2003 Aug;7(4):321–334.
3. Scher MS. Ontogeny of EEG-sleep from neonatal through infancy periods. *Sleep Med*. 2008 Aug;9(6):615–636.
4. Scher MS, Martin JG, Steppe DA, Banks DL. Comparative estimates of neonatal gestational maturity by electrographic and fetal ultrasonographic criteria. *Pediatr Neurol*. 1994 Oct;11(3):214–218.
5. Scher MS, Barmada MA. Estimation of gestational age by electrographic, clinical, and anatomic criteria. *Pediatr Neurol*. 1987;3(5):256–262.
6. Hoppenbrouwers T, Hodgman JE, Rybine D, et al.; CHIME Study Group. Sleep architecture in term and preterm infants beyond the neonatal period: The influence of gestational age, steroids, and ventilatory support. *Sleep*. 2005 Nov;28(11):1428–1436.
7. Berry RB. Sleep staging in infants and children. In: Berry RB, *Fundamentals of Sleep Medicine*. Elsevier Saunders; 2012:65–77.
8. Marcuse LV, Fields MC, Yoo J. The normal EEG from neonates to adolescents. In: Marcuse LV, Fields MC, Yoo J, eds. *Rowan's Primer of EEG*. 2nd ed. Elsevier Saunders; 2016:67–86.
9. Sheldon, SH. Development of sleep in infants and children. In: Sheldon SH, Ferber, R, Kryger MH, Gozal D, eds. *Principles and Practice of Pediatric Sleep Medicine*. 2nd ed. Elsevier Saunders; 2014:17–23.
10. Coons S, Guilleminault C. Development of sleep-wake patterns and non-rapid eye movement sleep stages during the first six months of life in normal infants. *Pediatrics*. 1982 Jun;69(6):793–798.
11. Owens JA. Sleep medicine. In: Kliegman RM, St Geme JW, Blum NJ, Shah SS, Tasker RC, Wilson KM, eds. *Nelson Textbook of Pediatrics*. 21st ed. Elsevier; 2020:174.
12. Oskar JG, Carskadon MA. Life cycles: Infants and children. In: Amlaner CJ, Fuller PM, eds. *Basics of Sleep Guide: Sleep Research Society*. 2nd ed. Sleep Research Society; 2009:33–42.
13. Anders TF, Keener M. Developmental course of nighttime sleep-wake patterns in full-term and premature infants during the first year of life. I. *Sleep*. 1985;8(3):173–192. doi:10.1093/sleep/8.3.173. PMID: 4048734.
14. Iglowstein I, Jenni OG, Molinari L, Largo RH. Sleep duration from infancy to adolescence: Reference values and generational trends. *Pediatrics*. 2003 Feb;111(2):302–307.
15. Paruthi S, Brooks LJ, D'Ambrosio C, et al. Recommended amount of sleep for pediatric populations: A consensus statement of the American Academy of Sleep Medicine. *J Clin Sleep Med*. 2016 Jun 15;12(6):785–786.
16. Kocevska D, Lysen TS, Dotinga A, et al. Sleep characteristics across the lifespan in 1.1 million people from the Netherlands, United Kingdom and United States: A systematic review and meta-analysis. *Nat Hum Behav*. 2021 Jan;5(1):113–122.
17. Carskadon MA, Harvey K, Duke P, Anders TF, Litt IF, Dement WC. Pubertal changes in daytime sleepiness. *Sleep*. 1980;2(4):453–460.
18. Scholle S, Beyer U, Bernhard M, et al. Normative values of polysomnographic parameters in childhood and adolescence: Quantitative sleep parameters. *Sleep Med*. 2011 Jun;12(6):542–549.
19. Watson NF, Badr MS, Belenky G, et al. Recommended amount of sleep for a healthy adult: A

joint consensus statement of the American Academy of Sleep Medicine and Sleep Research Society. *J Clin Sleep Med*. 2015;11(6):591–592.
20. Dijk DJ, Groeger JA, Stanley N, Deacon S. Age-related reduction in daytime sleep propensity and nocturnal slow wave sleep. *Sleep*. 2010 Feb;33(2):211–223.
21. Dorffner 2015 Dorffner G, Vitr M, Anderer P. The effects of aging on sleep architecture in healthy subjects. *Adv Exp Med Biol*. 2015;821:93–100.
22. Youngstedt SD, Goff EE, Reynolds AM, et al. Has adult sleep duration declined over the last 50+ years? *Sleep Med Rev*. 2016;28:69–85.
23. Ohayon MM, Carskadon MA, Guilleminault C, Vitiello MV. Meta-analysis of quantitative sleep parameters from childhood to old age in healthy individuals: Developing normative sleep values across the human lifespan. *Sleep*. 2004 Nov 1;27(7):1255–1273.
24. Floyd JA, Janisse JJ, Jenuwine ES, Ager JW. Changes in REM-sleep percentage over the adult lifespan. *Sleep*. 2007 Jul;30(7):829–836.
25. Redline S, Kirchner HL, Quan SF, Gottlieb DJ, Kapur V, Newman A. The effects of age, sex, ethnicity, and sleep-disordered breathing on sleep architecture. *Arch Intern Med*. 2004;164(4):406–418.
26. Bonnet MH, Arand DL. EEG arousal norms by age. *J Clin Sleep Med*. 2007 Apr 15;3(3):271–274.
27. Prinz PN, Peskind ER, Vitaliano PP, et al. Changes in the sleep and waking EEGs of nondemented and demented elderly subjects. *J Am Geriatr Soc*. 1982 Feb;30(2):86–93.
28. Foley D, Ancoli-Israel S, Britz P, Walsh J. Sleep disturbances and chronic disease in older adults: Results of the 2003 National Sleep Foundation Sleep in America Survey. *J Psychosom Res*. 2004 May;56(5):497–502.
29. Floyd JA, Medler SM, Ager JW, et al. Age-related changes in initiation and maintenance of sleep: A meta-analysis. *Res Nurs Health*. 2000;23(2):106–117.
30. Phillips B, Ancoli-Israel S. Sleep disorders in the elderly. *Sleep Med*. 2001;2:99–114.
31. Van Cauter E, Leproult R, Plat L. Age-related changes in slow wave sleep and REM sleep and relationship with growth hormone and cortisol levels in healthy men. *JAMA*. 2000;284(7):861–868.
32. Klerman EB, Davis JB, Duffy JF, Dijk DJ, Kronauer RE. Older people awaken more frequently but fall back asleep at the same rate as younger people. *Sleep*. 2004 Jun 15;27(4):793–798.
33. Darchia N, Campbell IG, Feinberg I. Rapid eye movement density is reduced in the normal elderly. *Sleep*. 2003;26(8):973–977.
34. Mitterling T, Högl B, Schönwald SV, et al. Sleep and respiration in 100 healthy Caucasian sleepers: A polysomnographic study according to American Academy of Sleep Medicine standards. *Sleep*. 2015;38:867–875.
35. Mathur R, Douglas NJ. Frequency of EEG arousals from nocturnal sleep in normal subjects. *Sleep*. 1995 Jun;18(5):330–333.
36. Boselli M, Parrino L, Smerieri A, et al. Effect of age on EEG arousals in normal sleep. *Sleep*. 1998;21:351–357.
37. Anoli-Israel S. Life cycles: Sleep in the older adult. In: Amlaner CJ, Fuller PM, eds. *Basics of Sleep Guide*. 2nd ed. Sleep Research Society; 2009.
38. Huang YL, Liu RY, Wang QS, et al. Age-associated difference in circadian sleep-wake and rest activity rhythms. *Physiol Behav*. 2002;76:597–603.
39. Swaab DF, Fliers E, Partiman TS. The suprachiasmatic nucleus of the human brain in relation to sex, age and senile dementia. *Brain Res*. 1985;342:37–44.
40. Turek FW, Penev P, Zhang Y, van Reeth O, Zee P. Effects of age on the circadian system. *Neurosci Biobehav Rev*. 1995 Spring;19(1):53–58.
41. Duffy J, Zeitzer JM, Rimmer OW, Klarman EB, Oljk O, Czeisler CA. Peak of circadian melatonin rhythm occurs later within the sleep of older subjects. *Am J Physiol Endocrinol Metab*. 2002;282:E297–E303.
42. Benarroch EE. Suprachiasmatic nucleus and melatonin: Reciprocal interactions and clinical correlations. *Neurology*. 2008;19;71:594–598.
43. Buysse DJ, Browman KE, Monk TH, et al. Napping and 24-hour sleep/wake patterns in healthy elderly and young adults. *J Am Geriatr Soc*. 1992; 40(8):779–786.
44. Dijk DJ, Duffy JF, Czeisler CA. Contribution of circadian physiology and sleep homeostasis to age-related changes in human sleep. *Chronobiol Int*. 2000;17(3):285–311.
45. Monk TH. Aging human circadian rhythms: Conventional wisdom may not always be right. *J Biol Rhythms*. 2005;20:366–374.
46. Benca RM, Obermeyer WH, Thisted RA, et al. Sleep and psychiatric disorders: A meta-analysis. *Arch Gen Psychiatry*. 1992;49:651–668.
47. Reynolds CF 3rd, Kupfer DJ, Houck PR, et al. Reliable discrimination of elderly depressed and demented patients by electroencephalographic sleep data. *Arch Gen Psychiatry*. 1988;45:258–264.
48. Thase ME. Depression, sleep, and antidepressants. *J Clin Psychiatry*. 1998;59(Suppl 4):55–65.
49. Maglione JE, Ancoli-Israel S, Peters KW, et al. Depressive symptoms and subjective and objective sleep in community-dwelling older women. *J Am Geriatr Soc*. 2012;60:635–643.
50. Spira AP, Friedman L, Aulakh JS, et al. Subclinical anxiety symptoms, sleep, and daytime dysfunction in older adults with primary insomnia. *J Geriatr Psychiatry Neurol*. 2008;21:149–153.
51. Barczi SR, Teodorescu MC. Psychiatric and medical comorbidities and effects of medications in older adults In: Kryger MH, Roth T, Dement WC, eds. *Principles and Practice of Sleep Medicine*. 6th ed. Elsevier; 2017.
52. Kobayashi I, Boarts JM, Delahanty DL. Polysomnographically measured sleep abnormalities in PTSD: A meta-analytic review. *Psychophysiology*. 2007;44:660–669.
53. Blagestad T, Pallesen S, Lunde LH, et al. Sleep in older chronic pain patients: A comparative polysomnographic study. *Clin J Pain*. 2012;28:277–283.
54. Lunde LH, Pallesen S, Krangnes L, et al. Characteristics of sleep in older persons with chronic pain: A study based on actigraphy and self-reporting. *Clin J Pain*. 2010;26:132–137.
55. Jansson C, Nordenstedt H, Wallander MA, et al. A population-based study showing an association between gastroesophageal reflux disease and sleep problems. *Clin Gastroenterol Hepatol*. 2009;7:960–965.

56. Orr WC. Sleep and gastroesophageal reflux disease: A wake-up call. *Rev Gastroenterol Disord.* 2004;4(Suppl. 4):S25–S32.
57. Shepherd K, Ockelford J, Ganasan V, et al. Temporal relationship between night-time gastroesophageal reflux events and arousals from sleep. *Am J Gastroenterol.* 2020;115:697–705.
58. Coryell VT, Ziegelstein RC, Hirt K, et al. Clinical correlates of insomnia in patients with acute coronary syndrome. *Int Heart J.* 2013;54:258–265.
59. Redeker NS, Adams L, Berkowitz R, et al. Nocturia, sleep and daytime function in stable heart failure. *J Card Fail.* 2012;18:569–575.
60. Valipour A, Lavie P, Lothaller H, et al. Sleep profile and symptoms of sleep disorders in patients with stable mild to moderate chronic obstructive pulmonary disease. *Sleep Med.* 2011;12:367–372.
61. McSharry DG, Ryan S, Calverley P, Edwards JC, McNicholas WT. Sleep quality in chronic obstructive pulmonary disease. *Respirology.* 2012 Oct;17(7):1119–1124.
62. Parker KP. Sleep disturbances in dialysis patients. *Sleep Med Rev.* 2003;7:131–143.
63. Marrone O, Cibella F, Roisman G, et al.; ESADA study group. Effects of sleep apnea and kidney dysfunction on objective sleep quality in nondialyzed patients with chronic kidney disease: An ESADA study. *J Clin Sleep Med.* 2020 Sep 15;16(9):1475–1481.
64. Elias RM, Chan CT, Bradley TD. Altered sleep structure in patients with end-stage renal disease. *Sleep Med.* 2016 Apr;20:67–71.
65. Shahveisi K, Jalali A, Moloudi MR, Moradi S, Maroufi A, Khazaie H. Sleep architecture in patients with primary snoring and obstructive sleep apnea. *Basic Clin Neurosci.* 2018;9(2):147–156.
66. Ancoli-Israel S, Kripke DF, Mason W, Kaplan OJ. Sleep apnea and periodic movements in an aging sample. *J Gerontol.* 1985;40:419–425.
67. Owusu JT, Wennberg AMV, Holingue CB, et al. Napping characteristics and cognitive performance in older adults. *Int J Geriatr Psychiatry.* 2019 Jan;34(1):87–96.
68. Leng Y, Stone K, Ancoli-Israel S, et al. Who takes naps? Self-reported and objectively measured napping in very old women. *J Gerontol A Biol Sci Med Sci.* 2018 Mar;73(3):374–379.
69. Leng Y, Redline S, Stone KL, et al. Objective napping, cognitive decline, and risk of cognitive impairment in older men. *Alzheimers Dement.* 2019 Aug;15(8):1039–1047.
70. Monk TH, Buysse DJ, Carrier J, et al. Effects of afternoon "siesta" naps on sleep, alertness, performance, and circadian rhythms in the elderly. *Sleep.* 2001;24:680–686.
71. Hays JC, Blazer DG, Foley DJ. Risk of napping: Excessive daytime sleepiness and mortality in an older community population. *J Am Geriatr Soc.* 1996;44:693–698.
72. Tamaki M, Shirota A, Tanaka H, et al. Effects of a daytime nap in the aged. *Psychiatry Clin Neurosci.* 1999;53:273–275.
73. Tamaki M, Shirota A, Hayashi M, Hori T. Restorative effects of a short afternoon nap (<30 min) in the elderly on subjective mood, performance and EEG activity. *Sleep Res Online.* 2000;3:131–139.
74. Campbell SS, Murphy PJ, Stauble TN. Effects of a nap on nighttime sleep and waking function in older subjects. *J Am Geriatr Soc.* 2005;53:48–53.

Chapter 3

The Chronobiology of Sleep

Alberto R. Ramos and Douglas Kirsch

INTRODUCTION

Sleep can be defined as a reversible behavioral state characterized by detachment and unresponsiveness to the environment. The function of sleep is not fully understood.[1] However, sleep is known to impact memory consolidation, brain plasticity,[2,3] and oxidative stress,[4] as well as a possible proto-consciousness (the primordial state of brain organization that forms the building blocks of consciousness).[5] The circadian rhythm is a central driver for sleep to occur at a certain time in the solar day-night cycle. This chapter will review the history of the understanding of the circadian rhythm and the neurobiology and physiology that keep humans on time.

Circadian rhythms, driven by the suprachiasmatic nucleus (SCN), integrate environmental light cues to regulate metabolism, cognition, and physical activity. Feeding cues also entrain circadian rhythms, highlighting the interaction between diet, circadian timing, and metabolic health. Circadian rhythms and sleep significantly affect immune system regulation, with sleep disorders linked to inflammatory response dysregulation. Factors like shift work and nighttime light exposure disrupt these rhythms, underscoring the importance of circadian and sleep health in the broader context of public health.

THE 2-PROCESS MODEL FOR SLEEP

Sleep supports a myriad of vital functions from organismal development to metabolism. Sleep is pivotal for synaptic plasticity, which is integral to memory consolidation. Sleep-wake cycles are regulated by a 2-process model: the homeostatic drive, known as sleep propensity, or Process S; and the circadian signal, or Process C. Process S increases as the duration of wakefulness is prolonged, driven at least in part by climbing levels of adenosine. Thus, sleep occurs when Process S is highest, and wake occurs when Process S is lowest. Process C is driven primarily by the 24-hour solar day-night cycle and the light signals through the retina to the SCN.[6] It is the mismatch between Process S and Process C which creates sleeping difficulty in situations such as shift work and jet lag.

SLEEP NEUROBIOLOGY BASICS

Sleep is a complex physiological state, marked by unique cerebral activities that oscillate between non-rapid eye movement (NREM) and rapid eye movement (REM) phases. Sleep, far from a passive state, requires intricate coordination of biological and chemical systems. The interplay between neurotransmitters and brain regions shapes the sleep-wake cycle.[7]

Sleep is classified into REM and NREM phases, which, along with quiet wakefulness, represent different "brain states" with signature neurophysiologic, metabolic, endocrine, and autonomic system correlates.[8] During sleep, humans cycle through periods of NREM and REM sleep approximately every 90 minutes. The electroencephalogram (EEG) of REM sleep is characterized by desynchronized EEG activity with faster oscillations and lower amplitude. The electrooculogram captures the REM, while the electromyogram shows muscle atonia (skeletal muscle paralysis). In contrast, human NREM sleep is subdivided into three stages (N1–N3). The N1 stage consists of synchronous waveforms in the theta frequency, with occasional vertex sharp waves and electrooculogram-defined roving eye movements. The N2 stage has sleep spindles (12–14 Hz), which are bursts of sinusoidal high-frequency activity, and K-complexes that are negative, sharp waves followed by a positive wave lasting more than 0.5 seconds. The N3 stage, also known as deep or delta sleep, is defined by synchronized high amplitude (>75 microvolts), low frequency delta waves (0.5–2 Hz).[9]

AN EARLY HISTORY OF CIRCADIAN SCIENCE

The study of plants was likely the first scientific exploration of biological rhythms. In the early 1700s, Jean Jacques d'Ortous de Mairan observed the mimosa plant, which would open and close its leaves in a set pattern in the absence of the light-dark cycle.[10] This finding suggested an internal clock in the plant that did not require an external time marker to maintain a rhythm. The circadian period of this plant was later measured by Augustin Pyramus De Candolle in 1832, suggesting the internal clock was approximately 22 hours coming "from within the plant."[11] A potential genetic basis for circadian rhythms was demonstrated in experiments on bean plants by Erwin Bunning in the 1930 where crossing plants with different length leaf-movement rhythms resulted in a plant with an intermediate length rhythm.[12]

Evaluation of the circadian clock in humans in controlled environments was first done by one of the fathers of modern sleep medicine, Nathaniel Kleitman, in the late 1930s:

> So he has to take his beds, with their instruments, recording every move of a sleeper, down under the earth to one of the chambers of Mammoth Cave. There the darkness is an unvarying 100 percent throughout the 24 hours, the temperature remains at exactly 54 degrees Fahrenheit whether it is noon or night, no football, no honk or motor horn, no radio, and not even thunder can penetrate. . . . One hour of the 24 is precisely like any of the others, therefore he could ignore even the sun, turning night to day.[13]

Kleitman's project using body temperature and sleep movement assessed the impact of a 28-hour circadian day on himself and his colleague, Bruce Richardson. Findings of this study were mixed; one participant maintained a near 24-hour biological rhythm, while the other deviated toward the 28-hour day. Michel Siffre in the early 1960s descended into a cavern in the Alps for 63 days, eliminating any clear zeitgebers. He tracked his sleep-wake patterns and demonstrated a free-running pattern, experiencing 42 physiological days compared to 58 day-night cycles above ground.[14] The understanding of the impact of the intensity and wavelength of light on the circadian rhythm was elucidated in dinoflagellates by Hastings and Sweeney in the late 1950s.[15] This approach was later applied to humans in seminal work by Dr. Charles Czeisler and colleagues in the mid-1980s.[16]

NEUROBIOLOGY OF THE CIRCADIAN RHYTHM

The SCN, the central circadian pacemaker, is in the anterior hypothalamus, lateral to the third ventricle and dorsal to the optic chiasm. Some consider the geography of the SCN to be defined in 2 portions, the core (ventrolateral) and shell (dorsomedial). These regions are defined based on the presence of the neuron type: the core is composed of mostly vasoactive intestinal polypeptide (VIP)-containing neurons, while the shell consists of arginine vasopressin (AVP)-containing neurons.[17]

The SCN synchronizes the body's 24-hour rhythm with environmental light cycles, mediated by melanopsin-containing retinal ganglion cells which project to the SCN core. These cells influence not only circadian rhythms but also mood through various retina-brain pathways. Gamma-aminobutyric acid (GABA) and various neuropeptides expressed by the SCN neurons modulate circadian outputs. Melatonin, interacting with MT-1 and MT-2 receptors, provides timing cues to this nucleus, influencing alertness. The SCN also connects with the dorsomedial hypothalamic nucleus, linking with the lateral hypothalamic orexin system.[18] The initial connections of the circadian rhythm are demonstrated in Figure 3.1.[19]

Central and peripheral circadian oscillators are fundamental in organizing mammalian physiology, tracking the day-night cycle, and governing behavioral and physiological rhythms. Gene transcription within the SCN is controlled by a positive-negative feedback mechanism. The SCN is entrained by the light-dark cycle, with retinal ganglion cells conveying light information to the SCN, impacting various physiological processes including sleep.[19] Circadian rhythmicity is conveyed from the SCN to other brain structures, regulating functions such as sleep, body temperature, and hormone levels. Melatonin from the pineal gland

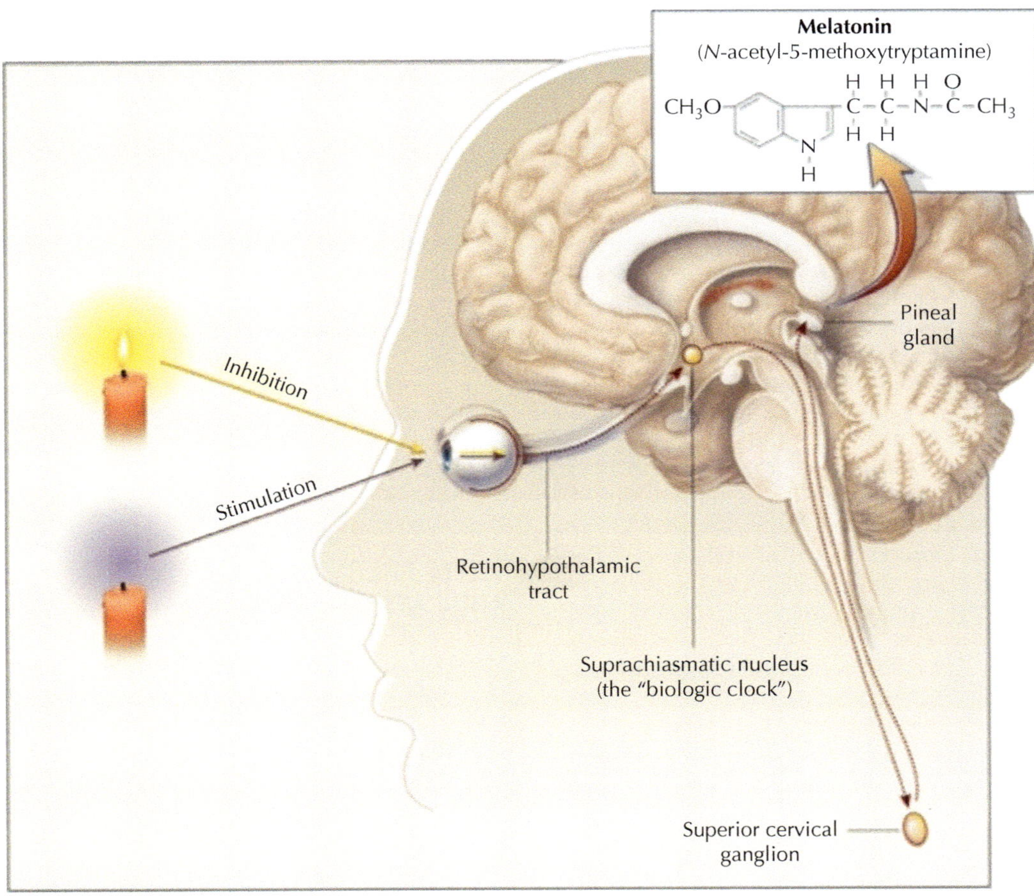

Figure 3.1. Physiology of Melatonin Secretion. Melatonin (inset) is produced in the pineal gland. The production and) secretion of melatonin are mediated largely by postganglionic retinal nerve fibers that pass through the retinohypothalamic tract to the suprachiasmatic nucleus, then to the superior cervical ganglion, and finally to the pineal gland. This neuronal system is activated by darkness and suppressed by light. The activation of a1- and ß1-adrenergic receptors in the pineal gland raises cyclic AMP and calcium O concentrations and activates arylalkylamine N-acetyltranferanse, initiating the synthesis and release of O melatonin. The daily rhythm of melatonin secretion is also controlled by an endogenous, free-running pacemaker located in the suprachiasmatic nucieus.

Reproduced from Brzezinski A. Melatonin in humans. N Eng J Med 1997; 336:186–195 (with kind permission from The Publishing Division of the Massachusetts Medical Society, Waltham, Massachusetts).

and other neuromodulators like acetylcholine provide feedback to the SCN, influencing its responsiveness to light. The ventrolateral preoptic area (VLPO) of the hypothalamus, receiving circadian output, promotes NREM sleep by inhibiting various arousal systems. Sleep onset is triggered by circadian and homeostatic signals, with adenosine playing a role in indicating sleep need based on wake duration. An ultradian oscillator in the mesopontine junction controls the alternation between REM and NREM sleep, involving complex interactions between various neurotransmitters. The 2017 Nobel Prize in Physiology or Medicine was awarded for discoveries of molecular mechanisms controlling the circadian rhythm.[6]

Biological clocks in living organisms, including humans, are adapted to the Earth's rotation, helping to anticipate and adapt to the day's regular rhythm. Fruit fly research was used to identify 3 mutant alleles of a single gene (period); mutations of this gene lead to either increasing or decreasing the circadian period or eliminated circadian rhythmicity.[20] The protein encoded by the "period" gene, *PER*, accumulates at night and degrades during the day, thus influencing the circadian rhythm. A feedback loop involving PER protein was hypothesized to generate and sustain circadian oscillations, regulating its own synthesis in a cyclic rhythm.

The understanding of the complexity of the circadian system has increased over time and includes both gene transcription and gene translation aspects. CLOCK and BMAL (proteins synthesized from the genes *Clock* and *Bmal*) combine as heterodimers and activate the synthesis of PER and cryptochrome (CRY). The feedback loop occurs in the presence of PER and CRY proteins, which prevent their own production from *Per* genes (*Per1*, *Per2*, *Per3*) and *Cry* genes (*Cry1*, *Cry2*). The production of PER and CRY protein then begins to occur when the intranuclear level of PER and CRY is low due to degradation of these proteins.[21]

Given the importance of the SCN in regulating aspects of behavior, physiology, and metabolism, the size and number of outputs are limited. There are several output pathways from the SCN, which include: (1) a rostral pathway to the medial preoptic area to the thalamus and eventually on to the medial prefrontal cortex, (2) a caudal pathway that runs to the retrochiasmatic area and into the ventromedial nucleus, and (3) a large dorsal and caudal pathway innervating the ventral subparaventricular zone and dorsal subparaventricular zone. The subparaventricular zone appears to amplify the signals coming from the SCN and may be the control point of whether the animal is diurnal or nocturnal.[22]

While the SCN is the most important of the circadian regulators, several other brain regions and most organs have autonomous circadian oscillations, using the same core *Clock* genes. However, these non-SCN-based oscillators depend on the SCN signal and its connection to the retina to maintain stable circadian rhythms. Glucocorticoid secretion, controlled by the SCN, also synchronizes peripheral circadian oscillators; glucocorticoids act through transcriptional regulation via glucocorticoid receptors in the *Per* genes sequences.[22]

Advancements in molecular biology and neurophysiology have elucidated the complex circadian pathways contributing to sleep neurobiology. The SCN, acting as a master circadian clock, orchestrates sleep-wake cycles and physiological rhythms in response to the light-dark cycle. The integration of circadian signals with homeostatic sleep drivers initiates and maintains sleep states. This internal clock regulates critical functions such as behavior, hormone levels, body temperature, and metabolism. Disruptions in these pathways—whether due to environmental factors, aging, or disease—can lead to sleep and metabolic disorders. Understanding these intricate mechanisms is crucial for the development of treatments for circadian rhythm sleep disorders and for enhancing overall sleep quality, and potentially impacts treatments of other medical conditions.

ZEITGEBERS AND THE CIRCADIAN CLOCK

Zeitgebers are the environmental agents which serve as the external timekeepers for the circadian clock. The endogenous period of a circadian rhythm for an individual creature is expressed in the absence of any external zeitgebers. To determine the endogenous rhythm in humans, studies were initially done in caves or bunkers, as discussed above, where conditions could be kept constant, with estimated endogenous rhythms of 25 hours.[23] However, more recent studies with advanced forced desynchrony protocols of 40 hours, with constant routine, derived endogenous body temperature rhythms of 24.18 hours.[24] Differences between sexes may have a small role in circadian control, as data suggest that women have a rhythm of 24.1 hours, with men having a slightly longer rhythm of 24.2 hours.[25]

The most common and powerful zeitgeber is light, which throughout most of human history was the sun. The presence of light at solar dawn is the most important photic cue to reset the circadian clock. However, the introduction of artificial light during periods of typical darkness has introduced complexity to the previous astronomically driven pattern. The phase-response curve to light (Figure 3.2)[19] details how the timing of light impacts the forward or backward movement of the internal body clock. Light exposure slightly before the typical time of awakening tends to pull the circadian clock earlier, whereas light exposure around dusk (or early evening) in the cycle will push the circadian clock later, prolonging wake time and delaying sleep. Thus, the introduction of non-natural light sources (room lights, television, computers, personal electronic devices) during solar night and the presence of artificially dark rooms (e.g., with use of light-blocking curtains) can disconnect the human clock from the biological rhythm of the sun, and in some cases, can cause clinically significant sleep disruption.

While light is the strongest zeitgeber, there are several non-photic zeitgebers that also influence the circadian pattern. Availability of food, social schedules, and even the Earth's magnetic field all can influence an organism's body clock. These influence the circadian system, not using the SCN system, but via peripheral circadian systems.[26]

PHYSIOLOGY OF THE CIRCADIAN RHYTHM

Many human body functions have a relationship to the circadian rhythm, including body temperature, cardiac rhythms, endocrine function, and metabolism. Human core body temperature (CBT) fluctuates during the 24-hour solar day, dropping during our typical sleeping period and rising as we get ready to wake for the day. CBT correlates with neurobehavioral functioning, with less strong cognitive performance first thing in the morning, which improves during circadian daytime. The CBT minimum is often used as a marker of circadian phase, typically occurring about 2 hours before an individual spontaneously wakes for the day.[27]

Many essential endocrine functions are impacted by sleep and circadian rhythms. There is a complex relationship between circadian phase and actual sleep, in which some aspects of endocrine physiology are impacted by the presence and type of sleep during the appropriate circadian phase, and some are solely circadian rhythm-specific (isolated from the presence or absence of sleep). Melatonin is synchronized with light, with onset near sunset and offset around sunrise; however,

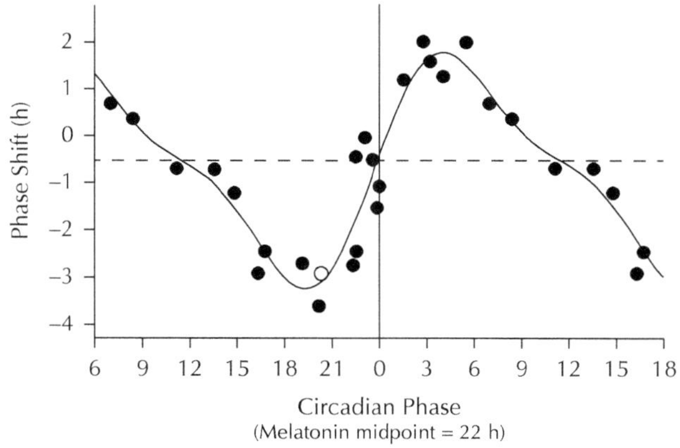

Figure 3.2. The PRC to the bright light stimulus using melatonin midpoints as the circadian phase marker. Phase advances (positive values) and delays (negative values) are plotted against the timing of the centre of the light exposure relative to the melatonin midpoint on the pre-stimulus constant routine (defined to be 22 h), with the core body temperature minimum assumed to occur 2 h later at 0 h. Data points from circadian phases 6-18 are double plotted. The filled circles represent data from plasma melatonin, and the open circle represents data from salivary melatonin in subject 18Ki? from whom blood samples were not acquired. The solid curve is a dual harmonic function fitted through all of the data points. The horizontal dashed line represents the anticipated 0.54 h average delay drift of the pacemaker between the pre-and post-stimulus phase assessments.

Reproduced from: Khalsa SBS, Jewett ME, Cajochen C, Czeisler CA. A phase response curve to single bright light pulses in human subjects. J Physiol 2003; 549: 945–952 (with kind permission of Wiley-Blackwell, Oxford, UK)

even if a person stays awake all through the night, the melatonin pattern remains the same. Similarly, cortisol is typically lowest at sleep onset, which is independent of the presence of sleep, though cortisol would be elevated the following day if sleep does not occur. Dim light melatonin onset (DLMO) is another method of marking an individual's circadian rhythm, typically occurring about 2–3 hours before sleep onset (and about 6 hours before CBT minimum).[28] Measurement of the DLMO can occur by plasma, saliva, or urine; however, measurement is most effective in light- and behavior-controlled circumstances.[29] An example of melatonin measurement in a control patient and one with delayed sleep phase syndrome under a research protocol is listed in Figure 3.3.[30]

Other hormones are more sensitive to the presence of sleep. Thyroid stimulating hormone (TSH) production is lower during sleep and higher during wakefulness (notably high right before sleep onset), but if sleep does not occur, TSH levels are elevated. This blockade of TSH is correlated specifically with the presence of slow-wave sleep.[31] Conversely, growth hormone, prolactin, and parathyroid hormone are all increased during circadian-based sleep time. Ghrelin and leptin have some circadian rhythmicity, though they are somewhat more variable given the impact of energy intake and expenditure.

Circadian disorders, driven in part by the impact on this physiology, are commonly experienced in modern society. Air travelers often acutely experience the conflict of internal circadian time and external zeitgebers when crossing multiple time zones. Fatigue or sleepiness, impaired physical and mental performance, and gastrointestinal discomfort are common symptoms of jet leg, though typically these symptoms resolve with multiple days at the same location.[32] Shift workers, however, are particularly prone to sleeping off-cycle from their circadian phase, with a host of negative effects on health and functioning.[33] Impairment of or complete absence of sight (thus reduction of light into the SCN and the circadian system) can have dramatic impact on human sleep, in some cases creating a free-running sleep pattern.[34]

SUMMARY

The study of circadian rhythms has been ongoing for centuries, with increasing illumination of neurobiology and physiology in plants, nonhuman animals, and humans. The 2017 Nobel Prize recognized groundbreaking work elucidating the inner workings of the circadian clock, revealing the molecular mechanisms by which organisms, including humans, synchronize their biological rhythm

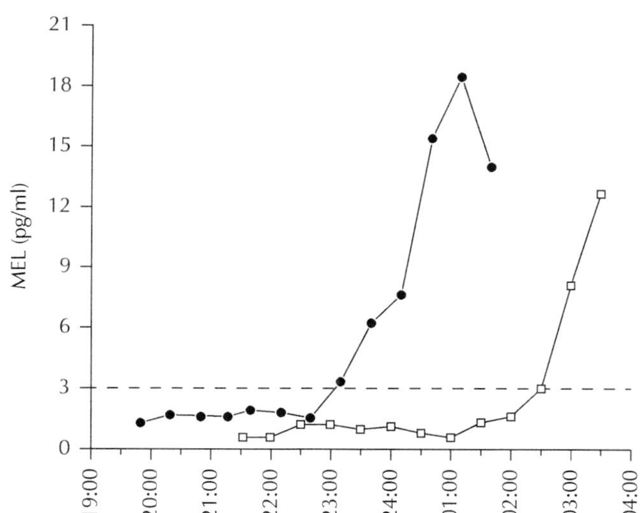

Figure 3.3. Examples of salivary melatonin (MEL) levels, obtained under the dim-light melatonin onset (DLMO) protocol, for a prototypi- cal patient with delayed sleep phase syndrome (DSPS) (open squares) and a control subject (filled circles). DLMO was estimated from saliva samples to be the clock time at which melatonin reached a 3-pg/mL threshold, based on linear interpolation of adjoining points.

with the Earth's cycles. This research has profound implications for our understanding of how the internal clock regulates vital physiological processes and the consequences of its misalignment, offering insights into the treatment of circadian disorders and their impact on overall health.

REFERENCES

1. Siegel J. Sleep viewed as a state of adaptive inactivity. Nature Reviews Neuroscience. 2009;10:747–753.
2. Tononi G, Cirelli C. Sleep and the price of plasticity: From synaptic and cellular homeostasis to memory consolidation and integration. *Neuron*. 2014;81:12–34.
3. Komaroff AL. Does sleep flush wastes from the brain? *JAMA*. 2021;325:2153–2155.
4. Vaccaro A, Kaplan Dor Y, Nambara K, et al. Sleep loss can cause death through accumulation of reactive oxygen species in the gut. *Cell*. 2020;181:1307–1328, e1315.
5. Hobson JA. REM sleep and dreaming: Towards a theory of protoconsciousness. *Nat Rev Neurosci*. 2009;10:803–813.
6. Falup-Pecurariu C, Diaconu Ş, Ţînţ D, Falup-Pecurariu O. Neurobiology of sleep (Review). *Exp Ther Med*. 2021 Mar;21(3):272. doi:10.3892/etm.2021.9703. Epub 2021 Jan 25. PMID: 33603879; PMCID: PMC7851648.
7. Wolpert EA. A manual of standardized terminology, techniques and scoring system for sleep stages of human subjects. *Arch Gen Psychiatry*. 1969;20:246–247.
8. Hobson JA. Sleep is of the brain, by the brain and for the brain. *Nature*. 2005;437:1254–1256.
9. Carskadon MA, Dement WC. Monitoring and staging human sleep. In MH Kryger, T Roth, WC Dement (Eds.), *Principles and practice of sleep medicine*, 5th edition. St. Louis: Elsevier Saunders; 2011:16–26.
10. De Mairan M. *Historie de l'Academie Royale des Sciences*. Paris; 1729. Observation botanique; p. 1.
11. De Candolle A. *Physiologie vegetale, ou Exposition des forces et des fonctions vitals des vegetaux, Bechet jeune*. Paris; 1832.
12. Sehgal A. Physiology flies with time. *Cell*. 2017;171(6):1232–1235.
13. American Weekly. Need we sleep away 1/3 of our lives? April 2, 1939. Nathaniel Kleitman; Papers (Box 53) Hanna Holborn Gray Special Collections Research Center, University of Chicago.
14. Hussey KD. Timeless spaces: Field experiments in the physiological study of circadian rhythms, 1938–1963. *Hist Philos Life Sci*. 2023 Apr 19;45(2):17. doi:10.1007/s40656-023-00571-w. PMID: 37076757; PMCID: PMC10115684.
15. Hastings JW, Sweeney BM. A persistent diurnal rhythm of luminescence in Gonyaulax polyedra. *Biol Bull*. 1958;115:440.
16. Czeisler CA, Allan JS, Strogatz SH, et al. Bright light resets the human circadian pacemaker independent of the timing of the sleep-wake cycle. *Science*. 1986;233(4764):667–671.
17. Moore RY, Speh JC, Leak RK. Suprachiasmatic nucleus organization. *Cell Tissue Res*. 2002;309:89–98.
18. España RA, Scammell TE. Sleep neurobiology from a clinical perspective. *Sleep*. 2011;34:845–858.
19. Shirani A, St. Louis EK. Illuminating rationale and uses for light therapy. *J Clin Sleep Med*. 2009;5(2):155–163. https://jcsm.aasm.org/doi/10.5664/jcsm.27445.
20. Konopka RJ, Benzer S. Clock mutants of Drosophila melanogaster. *Proc Natl Acad Sci USA*. 1971;68:2112–2116.
21. Reppert SM, Weaver DR. Coordination of circadian timing in mammals. *Nature*. 2002 Aug 29;418(6901):935–941.
22. Sollars P, Pickard G. *Psychiatr Clin North Am*. 2015 Dec;38(4):645–665. doi:10.1016/j.psc.2015.07.003.
23. Aschoff J. Circadian rhythms in man. *Science*. 1965 Jun 11;148:1427–1432.
24. Scheer FA, Wright KP Jr, Kronauer RE, et al. Plasticity of the intrinsic period of the human circadian timing system. *PLoS ONE*. 2007 Aug 8;2(1):e721.
25. Czeisler CA, Duffy JF, Shanahan TL, et al. Stability, precision, and near-24-hour period of the human circadian pacemaker. *Science*. 1999 Jun 25;284(5423):2177–2181. doi:10.1126/science.284.5423.2177.
26. Schulz P, Steimer T. Neurobiology of circadian systems. *CNS Drugs*. 2009;23(Suppl 2):3–13. doi:10.2165/11318620-000000000-00000. PMID: 19708721.
27. Duffy, JF, Dijk, DJ, Klerman, EB. Czeisler CA. Later endogenous circadian temperature nadir relative to an earlier wake time in older people. *Am J Physiol*. 1998;275:R1478–R1487.
28. Schwartz W, Klerman E. Circadian neurobiology and the physiologic regulation of sleep and wakefulness. *Neurologic Clin*. 2019 Aug 1;37(3):475–486.
29. Rzepka-Migut B, Paprocka J. Melatonin-measurement methods and the factors modifying the results: A systematic review of the literature. *Int J Environ Res Public Health*. 2020 Mar 15;17(6):1916. doi:10.3390/ijerph17061916. PMID: 32183489; PMCID: PMC7142625.
30. Wyatt JK, Stepanski EJ, Kirkby J, et al. Circadian phase in delayed sleep phase syndrome predictors and temporal stability across multiple assessments. *Sleep*. 2006;29(8):1075–1080.
31. Goichot B, Brandenberger G, Saini J, et al. Nocturnal plasma thyrotropin variations are related to slow-wave sleep. *J Sleep Res*. 1992;1:186–190.
32. Janse van Rensburg DC, Jansen van Rensburg A, Fowler PM, et al. Managing travel fatigue and jet lag in athletes: A review and consensus statement. *Sports Med*. 2021 Oct;51(10):2029–2050. doi:10.1007/s40279-021-01502-0. Epub 2021 Jul 14. PMID: 34263388; PMCID: PMC8279034.
33. Boivin DB, Boudreau P, Kosmadopoulos A. Disturbance of the circadian system in shift work and its health impact. *J Biol Rhythms*. 2022 Feb;37(1):3–28. doi:10.1177/07487304211064218. Epub 2021 Dec 30. PMID: 34969316; PMCID: PMC8832572.
34. Hartley S, Dauvilliers Y, Quera-Salva MA. Circadian rhythm disturbances in the blind. *Curr Neurol Neurosci Rep*. 2018 Aug 6;18(10):65. doi:10.1007/s11910-018-0876-9. PMID: 30083814.

Chapter 4

The Neurobiology of Sleep

Elda Arrigoni and Patrick M. Fuller

INTRODUCTION

Substantial advancements have been achieved in identifying and characterizing the intricate brain circuits responsible for regulating sleep, wakefulness, and their cyclic patterns. This progress owes much to the recent development of genetically engineered tools, which has allowed researchers to manipulate neuronal activity with unparalleled spatial and temporal precision. These tools have, in addition, facilitated the mapping of circuit nodes with unprecedented specificity.

A fundamental model of sleep-wake regulation posits that reciprocal inhibitory interactions between sleep-promoting neurons in the preoptic area and wake-promoting neurons in the brainstem and hypothalamus govern the dynamics of sleep-wake states and the rapid transitions between them.[1,2] While this model has served as a valuable interpretive framework in sleep-wake research, achieving a more comprehensive understanding of the brain circuitry underlying sleep-wake regulation necessitates a deeper exploration of its constituent elements.

This chapter aims to provide a comprehensive overview of the current understanding of the functional organization of brain circuits involved in regulating sleep and arousal.

REGULATION OF AROUSAL

A heightened level of arousal, synonymous with wakefulness or conscious awareness, serves as an essential prerequisite for nearly all nonvegetative neurobiological functions. This state of arousal is orchestrated and sustained during waking periods by the concerted activity of various neurochemically distinct subcortical cell populations distributed across the medullary and pontine brainstem, midbrain, hypothalamus, basal forebrain, and thalamus.

Canonical models of arousal regulation emphasize neurons utilizing histamine, serotonin, noradrenaline, dopamine, acetylcholine, and hypocretin/orexin as pivotal neurotransmitters in this process. These arousal systems are believed to exert their influence on neocortical activity, thereby impacting electroencephalography (EEG) and neurobehavioral arousal, both indirectly through projections to the thalamus, lateral hypothalamus, or basal forebrain, and directly via projections to the cortex.

However, recent investigations have proposed that monoaminergic and cholinergic systems primarily assume a modulatory role in sleep-wake regulation, with the fundamental framework of the wake-sleep regulatory system relying on fast neurotransmitters like glutamate and gamma-aminobutyric acid (GABA).[2] Both glutamate and GABA may interact with the classical monoaminergic modulatory systems through various mechanisms, including presynaptic modulation of transmitter release, as well as by modulating the activity of target neurons, such as those in the cerebral cortex.

REGULATION OF SLEEP

Sleep is a dynamic process that necessitates the coordinated activity of various sleep-active neuronal groups. These groups must effectively suppress multiple arousal-promoting neuronal systems within seconds to minutes to facilitate the transition from wakefulness to sleep. As outlined in the introduction to this chapter, the reciprocal inhibitory interaction between sleep-promoting neurons, such as those in the preoptic area, and wake-promoting neurons in the brainstem and hypothalamus serves as the foundation for explaining the swift transitions between the behavioral states of wakefulness and sleep, as well as their maintenance. Moreover, as discussed later in the section on rapid eye movement (REM) sleep, a comparable reciprocal inhibitory interaction between REM sleep-generating neurons and GABAergic REM sleep-suppressing neurons in the brainstem has been proposed to govern the onset and cessation of REM sleep.

Alongside the network of sleep-promoting neurons, many of which are GABAergic and exert potent inhibitory control over key arousal systems, the initiation and sustenance of sleep are regulated by the interplay between two processes: (1) the gradual accumulation and dissipation of sleep need, which occurs through the buildup and breakdown of somnogens during prolonged wakefulness and subsequent sleep; somnogens promote sleep by inhibiting wake-promoting circuits and contribute to what is known as the homeostatic sleep drive; and (2) the output of the circadian clock in the suprachiasmatic nucleus, which orchestrates wakefulness and sleep patterns at different times of the day.

This chapter will delve into the primary sleep-promoting circuits and will examine somnogens such as adenosine, prostaglandins, and cytokines. For a comprehensive understanding of the circadian regulation of sleep, readers are encouraged to consult reviews on the topic.[3–6]

Sleep-Promoting Circuits

Over the past three decades, researchers have identified several key neuronal groups involved in regulating sleep, primarily through direct neuronal recordings during sleep and wakefulness, as well as via sleep-related expression of c-Fos. The functional significance of these sleep-active neurons has been largely validated through various studies, including lesion studies to assess loss-of-function effects, as well as gain- and loss-of-function studies utilizing chemogenetic and optogenetic techniques.

PREOPTIC HYPOTHALAMIC NEURONS

The preoptic area encompasses two clusters of sleep-active neurons that hold significant functional importance: one located in the ventrolateral preoptic area (VLPO) as identified by Sherin and colleagues,[7,8] and the other in the median preoptic nucleus (MnPO) as highlighted by subsequent research.[9] Both the VLPO and MnPO neurons demonstrate heightened discharge rates during both non-rapid eye movement (NREM) and REM sleep compared to wakefulness, and they are responsive to sleep pressure.[10]

Within the VLPO, the sleep-active neurons are primarily GABAergic and express the inhibitory neuropeptide galanin.[7] Lesions in the VLPO region of animals result in chronic insomnia, while in humans, the loss of galanin-expressing neurons in the VLPO contributes to sleep fragmentation and loss in the elderly.[11,12] Recent investigations have revealed that optogenetic activation of VLPO galanin neurons prolongs the duration of NREM sleep,[13] while optogenetic stimulation of inputs from the later hypothalamus originating from orexin and GABAergic neurons, or from the locus coeruleus to the VLPO, induces rapid awakening from sleep, indicating that the inhibition of VLPO sleep-promoting neurons is sufficient to promote arousal.[14–16]

In the MnPO, both GABAergic and glutamatergic neurons play roles in sleep regulation. GABAergic neurons in the MnPO promote sleep in response to homeostatic sleep pressure, whereas glutamatergic neurons in this region are implicated in the modulation of sleep following exposure to stressors.[17]

NUCLEUS ACCUMBENS

The nucleus accumbens (NAc) is a brain region well known for its involvement in motivation, pleasure, and positive reinforcement functions. However, recent studies have shed light on an additional role for the NAc in regulating the sleep-wake cycle.[18] Within the NAc, researchers have identified two distinct groups of sleep-wake regulatory neurons. The first group, when stimulated, rapidly awakens mice from sleep, and these neurons express adenosine A_1 and dopamine D_1 receptors. Conversely, the second group promotes sleep; these neurons are GABAergic and express adenosine A_{2A} and dopamine D_2 receptors.[18,19] Despite these findings, the precise mechanism by which the NAc induces sleep remains incompletely understood.

PARAFACIAL ZONE NEURONS IN THE ROSTRAL MEDULLA

A novel group of sleep-active neurons has recently been uncovered in the rostral medulla, marking a significant departure from historical focus on forebrain circuitry in studies of NREM sleep. These newly discovered medullary NREM-active neurons are GABAergic and reside in the parafacial zone (PZ), situated lateral and dorsal to the facial nerve.[20] Initially identified through c-Fos immunoreactivity, subsequent single-unit recordings have confirmed that roughly 40% of recorded PZ neurons exhibit an increase in firing rate during NREM sleep. Analogous to the sleep-active neurons found in the VLPO and MnPO, PZ neurons commence their firing rate escalation prior to the onset of NREM sleep, underscoring their probable involvement in NREM sleep initiation.[21]

Chemogenetic activation of PZ GABA neurons promptly induces sustained periods of NREM sleep, affirming not only their sleep-active status but also their role as promoters of sleep. Despite significantly prolonging NREM sleep duration upon activation, REM sleep is diminished, suggesting their preferential influence on NREM sleep.[20] PZ neurons project to and inhibit wake-promoting neurons in the parabrachial nucleus. Furthermore, they likely facilitate sleep by inhibiting other wake-promoting systems, including the lateral hypothalamus, basal forebrain, and thalamus, although the precise functional implications of these additional projections remain to be elucidated.[22]

Sleep Pressure and Endogenous Somnogenic Substances

Throughout the waking day, our need for sleep intensifies, a phenomenon referred to as “sleep pressure” or heightened homeostatic sleep need/drive. Following prolonged wakefulness, both humans and other mammals, whether diurnal or nocturnal, compensate for sleep loss by extending subsequent sleep periods (sleep rebound). After sleep deprivation, individuals not only sleep longer but also fall asleep more rapidly during subsequent sleep. This is accompanied by deeper NREM sleep, characterized by a higher arousal threshold and increased EEG δ power (0.5 to 4 Hz range).

Homeostatic sleep pressure gradually builds up and diminishes over time, accumulating during prolonged wakefulness and dissipating during subsequent sleep, much like a capacitor. The intricate dynamics of sleep homeostasis are believed to be governed by endogenous somnogenic substances, among which adenosine, prostaglandins, and cytokines play crucial roles. These somnogens, whose levels rise during wakefulness, function as paracrine mediators that facilitate sleep induction by suppressing wake-promoting circuits and presumably activating or disinhibiting sleep-promoting neurons.

ADENOSINE

Adenosine stands out as one of the most well-known endogenous somnogens, steadily accumulating in the extracellular space during wakefulness and periods of sleep deprivation, followed by a decline during subsequent recovery sleep.[23] The central administration of adenosine and its analogs has been shown to increase the time spent asleep and to enhance EEG slow-wave activity. Perhaps the most compelling evidence supporting the sleep-promoting effects of adenosine comes from the action of caffeine, as caffeine acts as a competitive antagonist for adenosine receptors.

The specific cellular source of adenosine, whether it originates from neurons or glia, is still a subject of investigation and debate. However, recent research suggests that astrocytes likely play a key role in adenosine release, which is functionally significant in regulating homeostatic sleep.[24] This conclusion is supported by studies demonstrating that blocking the release of gliotransmitters, including ATP and adenosine, from astrocytes diminishes homeostatic responses to sleep deprivation. Moreover, mice deficient in glial adenosine kinase, the primary enzyme responsible for adenosine catabolism, exhibit enhanced homeostatic responses to sleep deprivation, whereas knockout of neuronal adenosine kinase has no effect on homeostatic sleep need.[25]

In the brain, adenosine exerts its effects through two types of receptors: adenosine A_1 receptors, which are inhibitory and distributed throughout the brain, and A_{2A} receptors, which are excitatory and predominantly found in the striatum and NAc.[26] Both receptor types are believed to play a role in mediating the effects of adenosine on sleep.[26] At the cellular and circuit levels, adenosine is thought to promote sleep by inhibiting several, if not all, known wake-promoting groups and disinhibiting the VLPO sleep-promoting neurons primarily via A_1 receptors.[27,28] Additionally, adenosine activates NAc sleep-promoting neurons via A_{2A} receptors.[18]

Despite its widespread consumption by humans, the precise mechanism underlying caffeine's stimulant effects was long debated. However, research using adenosine receptor knockout mice has clarified this issue. It was found that the arousal effect of caffeine remains unaffected in A_1 receptor knockout mice but is lost in A_{2A} receptor knockout mice, indicating that A_{2A} receptors, rather than A_1 receptors, mediate caffeine's arousal effect.[29] Furthermore, the selective deletion of A_{2A} receptors limited to the NAc is sufficient to block the effects of caffeine.[26]

PROSTAGLANDINS

Prostaglandins (PGs) are lipid compounds released as part of inflammatory responses. Among them, PGD_2 holds particular significance in mammalian brains as it is the most abundant prostaglandin and is recognized for its sleep-promoting properties, likely achieved through the facilitation of adenosine release. A key distinction between prostaglandins and adenosine lies in their respective sites of action. While injections of adenosine in various brain regions consistently induce sleep, prostaglandins are effective only when infused into the lateral ventricles or the subarachnoid space at the base of the forebrain, rather than when injected into the brain parenchyma.[30] This disparity can be attributed to the fact that adenosine receptors are predominantly expressed in neurons, whereas receptors for PGD_2 (DP_1) are primarily found in the leptomeninges of the ventral surface of the rostral basal forebrain, precisely where injections of PGD_2 exert their sleep-promoting effects.[30]

PGD_2 is synthesized in the leptomeninges and progressively accumulates in the extracellular space during wakefulness and sleep deprivation.[31] Elevated levels of PGD_2 during inflammation are also believed to mediate the sleepiness associated with infections and inflammation.[32] Intriguingly, mice lacking DP_1 receptors exhibit regular sleep and wake patterns but display an attenuated rebound of NREM sleep following sleep deprivation, suggesting that endogenous PGD_2 may not be implicated in the regular alternation of sleep and wake, but rather in the homeostatic regulation of NREM sleep.[33]

One prevailing model concerning the cellular mechanisms underlying PGD_2's sleep-promoting effects proposes that PGD_2 acts via DP_1 receptors on the leptomeninges to induce the production of adenosine, which subsequently activates VLPO sleep-promoting neurons.[26]

CYTOKINES

Cytokines, such as interleukin-1β (IL-1β) and tumor necrosis factor-α (TNF-α), are released in response to inflammation. Elevated levels of these cytokines are also detected during prolonged wakefulness, prompting the hypothesis that they could serve as homeostatic sleep factors. Findings from both whole-animal and in vitro recordings indicate that the mechanisms underlying cytokine-induced sleep may entail a combination of inhibiting arousal systems and activating preoptic sleep-regulatory neurons.[34–36]

REM SLEEP

REM sleep represents a distinct behavioral state characterized by cortical activation, marked by low amplitude and fast EEG activity, reminiscent of wakefulness. Due to these EEG similarities with wakefulness, some researchers prefer terms like *paradoxical sleep* or *active sleep* to describe REM sleep. In nonpathological conditions, REM sleep is invariably preceded by one or several NREM sleep periods, and individuals typically undergo several NREM-REM cycles per night, often awakening from REM sleep.

During REM sleep, there is a notable increase in hippocampal theta activity within the 4–7 Hz range, alongside the suppression of muscle activity in postural muscles, termed *muscle atonia*. Individuals often experience phasic muscle twitches in distal limb and orofacial muscles, as well as phasic bursting of oculomotor muscles, leading to rapid eye movements (REMs). While respiratory-related muscles are tonically suppressed during REM sleep, the degree of suppression varies; for instance, the diaphragm is minimally affected, whereas the genioglossus muscle of the tongue is completely suppressed. Autonomic activation, a lowered arousal threshold, and bursts of large waves known as PGO-waves, originating in the pons and propagating to the lateral geniculate nucleus and occipital cortex, are also characteristic of REM sleep. Similar to NREM sleep, REM sleep is subject to homeostatic control, as REM sleep deprivation results in an increased duration and shortened onset delay during REM rebound.

As detailed in the subsequent sections, the brain circuitry governing REM sleep is primarily located in the pontine brainstem and encompasses ascending and descending projections regulating the EEG and motor components of REM sleep.

Circuits of REM Sleep

PONTINE GLUTAMATERGIC REM SLEEP-GENERATING NEURONS

Transection studies conducted in the 1960s provided pivotal insights indicating that the rostral pons plays a critical role in the generation of REM sleep. Subsequent investigations, including unit recordings, c-Fos studies, and more recent calcium imaging studies, have contributed to the identification of two distinct groups of REM sleep-generating neurons in the rostral dorsal pons.[37,38] One group resides ventral to the locus coeruleus (LC) in the sublaterodorsal tegmental nucleus (SLD), while the second group is situated in the medial parabrachial and precoeruleus region (PB/PC). Both of these neuronal populations are adjacent to each other and consist of glutamatergic neurons. While active during REM sleep (REM-on neurons), they are believed to drive different aspects of REM sleep.[38,39]

Specifically, SLD neurons are responsible for inducing muscle atonia, whereas those in the PB/PC region are thought to contribute to cortical activation. The presence of these two distinct cell groups mediating the EEG and muscle atonia components of REM sleep forms the basis for the pathological dissociation observed in conditions such as cataplexy, sleep paralysis, and REM sleep behavior disorder (RBD).[40] It is widely acknowledged that SLD glutamatergic neurons promote muscle atonia during REM sleep through their descending projections, which activate glycinergic premotor neurons in the ventromedial medulla and/or spinal cord. These premotor neurons, in turn, inhibit motor neurons, resulting in loss of muscle tone.[41,42]

In contrast, the identity of REM-generating neurons responsible for EEG desynchronization is less well understood. The prevailing view suggests that these neurons are located in the PB/PC region and drive cortical desynchronization during REM sleep through projections to the basal forebrain and intralaminar thalamic nuclei.[38,40,43]

BRAINSTEM GABAERGIC REM-SUPPRESSING NEURONS

The mechanisms underlying the activation and termination of REM sleep by pontine REM-generating neurons remain the subject of ongoing investigation. The current hypothesis posits that during wakefulness, and to a lesser extent during NREM sleep, REM-generator neurons in the SLD and PB/PC are subject to strong inhibitory input from GABAergic neurons. The activation of these REM-generator neurons occurs in response to the withdrawal of this inhibitory input, a process known as disinhibition.

This model was initially proposed based on findings demonstrating that local application of $GABA_A$ antagonists in the pontine region rapidly induces a long-lasting REM sleep-like state.[37] Additionally, it is believed that the GABAergic input originates from the ventrolateral periaqueductal gray (vlPAG) and lateropontine tegmentum (LPT), regions housing GABA neurons that are active during wakefulness but silent during REM sleep (REM-off neurons).[39,44] Accordingly, lesions or inhibition of the vlPAG/LPT increase the duration of REM sleep and elicit episodes of muscle atonia during wakefulness. Conversely, optogenetic activation of vlPAG GABA neurons has been shown to terminate REM sleep.[45]

One proposed model for the switch between NREM and REM sleep involves reciprocal inhibitory interactions between the GABAergic vlPAG/LPT neurons (REM-off) and the GABA neurons in the SLD and PB/PC, which, like the REM-on glutamate neurons, are active during REM sleep. During wakefulness, REM sleep is prevented by the inhibition of REM-generating neurons. In REM sleep, the firing of SLD and PB/PC GABA neurons stabilizes REM sleep by inhibiting the GABAergic vlPAG/LPT REM-off neurons. This intricate interplay between inhibitory circuits helps regulate the initiation and termination of REM sleep.[1]

CATAPLEXY: A DYSFUNCTION OF PONTINE CIRCUIT FOR REM SLEEP MUSCLE ATONIA

In addition to excessive daytime sleepiness, individuals with narcolepsy, caused by the loss of orexin neurons, may also experience cataplexy, characterized by sudden muscle paralysis triggered by intense positive emotions. In severe cases, narcoleptic patients may collapse, rendered temporarily unable to speak or move while remaining conscious.[46] Cataplexy is believed to stem from dysfunction within the pontine circuit responsible for controlling muscle atonia during REM sleep. This dysfunction leads to inappropriate disinhibition, resulting in the activation of SLD REM sleep atonia neurons during wakefulness.[47]

Supporting this hypothesis, chemogenetic activation of SLD exacerbates cataplexy in narcoleptic mice and notably can induce cataplexy in mice with intact orexin signaling.[48] This provides further evidence for the involvement of the pontine circuitry controlling REM sleep muscle atonia in the manifestation of cataplexy in narcolepsy.

Cholinergic and Monoaminergic Modulation of REM Sleep

CHOLINERGIC REGULATION

Anticholinergic drugs are known for their potent suppression of REM sleep, and muscarinic cholinergic receptors M_1 and M_3 have been identified as essential for REM sleep regulation.[49,50] However, the precise sites where acetylcholine (ACh) promotes REM sleep have not been fully elucidated. Initially, it was thought that pontine cholinergic neurons in the laterodorsal tegmental and pedunculopontine tegmental nuclei (LDT/PPT) played a direct role in the initiation of REM sleep, with their activity in REM sleep being necessary for the activation of "cholinoceptive" REM-generating neurons in the pons. This model was supported by findings demonstrating that microinjections of carbachol (a cholinergic agonist) into the pontine tegmentum induced a prolonged REM-like state, and that LDT/PPT ACh neurons were active during REM sleep.[51,52]

However, this model has been re-examined over time, with subsequent research yielding inconsistent results regarding the effects of carbachol injections in the pons and showing that chemogenetic activation of ACh LDT/PPT neurons does not significantly impact REM sleep duration.[53] Furthermore, while blocking the GABAergic input in the dorsal pontine tegmentum, where REM-generating neurons are located, strongly promotes REM sleep,[37] blocking cholinergic signaling does not have the expected effect on REM sleep.[54]

Although cholinergic agonists can directly excite the SLD REM-generator neurons, this excitation alone may not be sufficient to promote REM sleep. The current understanding suggests that REM sleep production requires the disinhibition of pontine REM-generator neurons from a strong GABAergic input, while cholinergic activation may serve an ancillary role in reinforcing transitions from NREM to REM sleep.

NORADRENALINE AND SEROTONIN REGULATION

Two groups of monoaminergic neurons, the noradrenergic neurons of the locus coeruleus (LC) and the serotonin neurons of the dorsal raphe nucleus (DRN), have long been recognized for their robust behavioral state-dependent activity. These neurons exhibit high activity levels during wakefulness but become nearly silent during REM sleep, suggesting their involvement in preventing the onset of REM sleep during wakefulness. Consequently, drugs that elevate serotonin and noradrenaline levels, such as selective serotonin reuptake inhibitors and tricyclic antidepressants, are known to have potent REM sleep-suppressing effects in humans.[50]

The precise mechanism by which the activity of LC and DRN neurons suppresses REM sleep is not fully understood. One potential mechanism involves their projections to the SLD and PB/PC, where local application of noradrenaline has been shown to inhibit REM sleep-active neurons and suppress REM sleep.[55] However, lesions or photoinhibition of LC neurons do not increase REM sleep, nor do they induce muscle tone loss as observed in cataplexy.[56] This suggests that while low levels of monoaminergic activity may be necessary for REM sleep to occur, they are not sufficient to initiate REM sleep.

DOPAMINERGIC REGULATION

While noradrenaline and serotonin have been implicated in suppressing REM sleep, recent research suggests that dopamine may play a role in promoting REM sleep. Specifically, emerging evidence indicates that ventral tegmental area (VTA) dopaminergic neurons may positively regulate REM sleep.[57]

First, VTA dopaminergic neurons display activity during both wakefulness and REM sleep, with their firing rate being notably higher during REM sleep compared to wakefulness.[58] Moreover, optogenetic stimulation of VTA dopaminergic neurons has been shown to rapidly awaken mice.[58] Additionally, optogenetic stimulation of VTA dopaminergic terminals in the basolateral amygdala can induce a swift transition from NREM to REM sleep.[57]

However, several questions regarding this circuitry remain unanswered. For instance, it is still unclear how this circuit integrates with pontine REM circuits, and notably, why drugs that increase extracellular dopamine, such as modafinil, which is prescribed to enhance wakefulness in idiopathic hypersomnia and narcolepsy, have no effect on REM sleep. Given that this area of research is relatively recent, future studies are required to address these unresolved questions and further elucidate the role of dopamine in REM sleep regulation.

Forebrain Regulation of REM Sleep

The core of the brainstem REM-generating circuits is intricately regulated by descending inputs from sleep- and arousal-regulatory hypothalamic neuronal systems, with orexin/hypocretin signaling playing a pivotal role.

OREXIN/HYPOCRETIN

It is well established that orexin signaling acts to suppress REM sleep. Central administration of orexin prevents REM sleep for several hours, and chemogenetic activation of orexin neurons effectively blocks REM sleep. Conversely, orexin receptor antagonists enhance REM sleep and reduce its latency.[59] Narcoleptic patients, who have poor regulation of REM sleep, often experience REM sleep occurring at any time of day, accompanied by cataplexy and dream-like hallucinations intruding into wakefulness.[46,47]

Orexin neurons are notably active during waking states, where they exert a suppressive effect on REM sleep and its components, such as muscle atonia. Consequently, with intact orexin signaling, cataplexy does not typically occur. However, during NREM sleep when neuronal activity of orexin is low, the REM-generating circuits become disinhibited, facilitating the transition from NREM to REM sleep.[46,47] Thus, orexin signaling serves as a crucial regulator of REM sleep dynamics, modulating its occurrence and maintaining its integrity across different states of arousal.

MELANIN-CONCENTRATING HORMONE (MCH) NEURONS

The melanin-concentrating hormone (MCH) neurons, situated in the posterior lateral hypothalamus alongside orexin neurons, exhibit elevated firing discharge during REM sleep, suggesting a potential positive regulatory role in REM sleep dynamics.[60] These neurons, contrary to initial assumptions, release glutamate but not GABA[61,62] and project to brainstem nuclei involved in REM sleep control.

Supporting their role in promoting REM sleep, central administration of MCH has been shown to double the amount of REM sleep, and both chemogenetic and optogenetic activation of MCH neurons increase REM sleep.[65–67] However, while activation of MCH neurons can effectively drive REM sleep, it remains uncertain whether these neurons are necessary for spontaneous REM sleep, as neither their ablation nor inhibition affects REM sleep amount or episode duration. Thus, while MCH neurons demonstrate the capacity to modulate REM sleep, their precise role in the initiation and maintenance of REM sleep warrants further investigation.[68,69]

PREOPTIC NEURONS

Lesion studies have provided evidence suggesting the presence of two distinct populations of galanin-expressing neurons within the VLPO. Those clustered in the core of the VLPO are believed to primarily regulate NREM sleep, while those situated in the dorsal extended VLPO have been implicated in REM sleep and its homeostatic regulation.[70]

Supporting this model, neurons active during REM sleep have been identified in the dorsal extended VLPO.[10,71] However, it remains unclear whether these REM-on neurons express galanin. Nonetheless, the galanin neurons in the extended VLPO are predominantly GABAergic and project to various regions known to suppress REM sleep, including the ventrolateral periaqueductal gray (vlPAG), dorsal raphe nucleus (DRN), and locus coeruleus (LC). Therefore, these neurons may play a positive regulatory role in REM sleep by disinhibiting the pontine REM sleep-generating neurons.[28] Further research is necessary to elucidate the precise mechanisms by which galanin-expressing neurons in the extended VLPO contribute to REM sleep modulation.

REFERENCES

1. Saper CB, Fuller PM, Pedersen NP, Lu J, Scammell TE. Sleep state switching. *Neuron*. 2010;68:1023–1042.
2. Saper CB, Fuller PM. Wake-sleep circuitry: An overview. *Curr Opin Neurobiol*. 2017;44:186–192.
3. Fuller PM, Gooley JJ, Saper CB. Neurobiology of the sleep-wake cycle: Sleep architecture, circadian regulation, and regulatory feedback. *J Biol Rhythms*. 2006;21:482–493.
4. Kim, MJ, Lee JH, Duffy JF. Circadian rhythm sleep disorders. *J Clin Outcomes Manag*. 2013;20:513–528.
5. Saper CB. The central circadian timing system. *Curr Opin Neurobiol*. 2013;23:747–751.
6. Videnovic A, Lazar AS, Barker RA, Overeem S. "The clocks that time us": Circadian rhythms in neurodegenerative disorders. *Nat Rev Neurol*. 2014;10:683–693.
7. Sherin JE, Shiromani PJ, McCarley RW, Saper CB. Activation of ventrolateral preoptic neurons during sleep. *Science*. 1996;271:216–219.
8. Sherin JE, Elmquist JK, Torrealba F, Saper CB. Innervation of histaminergic tuberomammillary neurons by GABAergic and galaninergic neurons in the ventrolateral preoptic nucleus of the rat. *J Neurosci*. 1998;18:4705–4721.
9. Gong H, McGinty D, Guzman-Marin R, et al. Activation of c-Fos in GABAergic neurones in the preoptic area during sleep and in response to sleep deprivation. *J Physiol*. 2004;556:935–946.
10. Alam MA, Kumar S, McGinty D, Alam MN, Szymusiak R. Neuronal activity in the preoptic hypothalamus during sleep deprivation and recovery sleep. *J Neurophysiol*. 2014;111:287–299.
11. Lim AS, Ellison BA, Wang JL, et al. Sleep is related to neuron numbers in the ventrolateral preoptic/intermediate nucleus in older adults with and without Alzheimer's disease. *Brain*. 2014;137:2847–2861.
12. Lu J, Greco MA, Shiromani P, Saper CB. Effect of lesions of the ventrolateral preoptic nucleus on NREM and REM sleep. *J Neurosci*. 2000;20:3830–3842.
13. Kroeger D, Absi G, Gagliardi C, et al. Galanin neurons in the ventrolateral preoptic area promote sleep and heat loss in mice. *Nat Commun*. 2018;9:4129.
14. Venner A, De Luca R, Sohn LT, et al. An inhibitory lateral hypothalamic-preoptic circuit mediates rapid

arousals from sleep. *Curr Biol.* 2019;29(24):4155–4168.e5. doi:10.1016/j.cub.2019.10.026.
15. Liang Y, Shi W, Xiang A, et al. The NAergic locus coeruleus-ventrolateral preoptic area neural circuit mediates rapid arousal from sleep. *Curr Biol.* 2021;31(17):3729–3742.e5. doi:10.1016/j.cub.2021.06.031.
16. De Luca R, Nardone S, Grace KP, et al. Orexin neurons inhibit sleep to promote arousal. *Nat Commun.* 2022;13:4163.
17. Machado NLS, Todd WD, Kaur S, Saper CB. Median preoptic GABA and glutamate neurons exert differential control over sleep behavior. *Curr Biol.* 2022;32:2011–2021.e3.
18. Oishi Y, Suzuki Y, Takahashi K, et al. Activation of ventral tegmental area dopamine neurons produces wakefulness through dopamine D2-like receptors in mice. *Brain Struct Funct.* 2017;222:2907–2915.
19. Luo Y-J, Li YD, Wang L, et al. Nucleus accumbens controls wakefulness by a subpopulation of neurons expressing dopamine D1 receptors. *Nat Commun.* 2018;9:1576.
20. Anaclet C, Ferrari L, Arrigoni E, et al. The GABAergic parafacial zone is a medullary slow wave sleep-promoting center. *Nat Neurosci.* 2014;17:1217–1224.
21. Alam MA, Kostin A, Siegel J, et al. Characteristics of sleep-active neurons in the medullary parafacial zone in rats. *Sleep.* 2018;41(10):zsy130. doi:10.1093/sleep/zsy130.
22. Su Y-T, Gu M-Y, Chu X, Feng X, Yu Y-Q. Whole-brain mapping of direct inputs to and axonal projections from GABAergic neurons in the parafacial zone. *Neurosci Bull.* 2018;34:485–496.
23. Porkka-Heiskanen T, Strecker RE, Thakkar M, et al. Adenosine: A mediator of the sleep-inducing effects of prolonged wakefulness. *Science.* 1997;276:1265–1268.
24. Halassa MM, Florian C, Fellin T, Munoz JR, Lee SY, Abel T, Haydon PG, Frank MG. Astrocytic modulation of sleep homeostasis and cognitive consequences of sleep loss. *Neuron.* 2009;61:213–219.
25. Bjorness TE, Dale N, Mettlach G, et al. An adenosine-mediated glial-neuronal circuit for homeostatic sleep. *J Neurosci.* 2016;36:3709–3721.
26. Lazarus M, Chen J-F, Huang Z-L, Urade Y, Fredholm BB. Adenosine and sleep. *Handb Exp Pharmacol.* 2019;253:359–381.
27. Fredholm BB, Battig K, Holmen J, Nehlig A, Zvartau EE. Actions of caffeine in the brain with special reference to factors that contribute to its widespread use. *Pharmacol Rev.* 1999;51:83–133.
28. Arrigoni E, Fuller PM. The sleep-promoting ventrolateral preoptic nucleus: What have we learned over the past 25 years? *Int J Mol Sci.* 2022;23:2905.
29. Hong ZY, Huang ZL, Qu WM, et al. An adenosine A receptor agonist induces sleep by increasing GABA release in the tuberomammillary nucleus to inhibit histaminergic systems in rats. *J Neurochem.* 2005;92:1542–1549.
30. Matsumura H, Nakajima T, Osaka T, et al. Prostaglandin D2-sensitive, sleep-promoting zone defined in the ventral surface of the rostral basal forebrain. *Proc Natl Acad Sci U S A.* 1994;91:11998–12002.
31. Ram A, Pandey HP, Matsumura H, et al. CSF levels of prostaglandins, especially the level of prostaglandin D2, are correlated with increasing propensity towards sleep in rats. *Brain Res.* 1997;751:81–89.
32. Urade Y, Hayaishi O. Prostaglandin D2 and sleep/wake regulation. *Sleep Med Rev.* 2011;15:411–418.
33. Mizoguchi A, Eguchi N, Kimura K, et al. Dominant localization of prostaglandin D receptors on arachnoid trabecular cells in mouse basal forebrain and their involvement in the regulation of non-rapid eye movement sleep. *Proc Natl Acad Sci U S A.* 2001;98:11674–11679.
34. Alam MN, McGinty D, Bashir T, et al. Interleukin-1beta modulates state-dependent discharge activity of preoptic area and basal forebrain neurons: Role in sleep regulation. *Eur J Neurosci.* 2004;20:207–216.
35. Baker FC, Shah S, Stewart D, et al. Interleukin 1beta enhances non-rapid eye movement sleep and increases c-Fos protein expression in the median preoptic nucleus of the hypothalamus. *Am J Physiol Regul Integr Comp Physiol.* 2005;288:R998–R1005.
36. Brambilla D, Barajon I, Bianchi S, Opp MR, Imeri L. Interleukin-1 inhibits putative cholinergic neurons in vitro and REM sleep when microinjected into the rat laterodorsal tegmental nucleus. *Sleep.* 2010;3:919–929.
37. Boissard R, Gervasoni D, Schmidt MH, et al. The rat ponto-medullary network responsible for paradoxical sleep onset and maintenance: A combined microinjection and functional neuroanatomical study. *Eur J Neurosci.* 2002;16:1959–1973.
38. Lu J, Sherman D, Devor M, Saper CB. A putative flip-flop switch for control of REM sleep. *Nature.* 2006;441:589–594.
39. Sapin E, Lapray D, Bérod A, et al. Localization of the brainstem GABAergic neurons controlling paradoxical (REM) sleep. *PLoS One.* 2009;4:e4272.
40. Fuller PM, Saper CB, Lu J. The pontine REM switch: Past and present. *J Physiol.* 2007;584:735–741.
41. Arrigoni E, Chen MC, Fuller PM. The anatomical, cellular and synaptic basis of motor atonia during rapid eye movement sleep. *J Physiol.* 2016;594:5391–5414.
42. Luppi P-H, Fort P. Sleep-wake physiology. *Handb Clin Neurol.* 2019;160:359–370.
43. Valencia Garcia S, Libourel PA, Lazarus M, et al. Genetic inactivation of glutamate neurons in the rat sublaterodorsal tegmental nucleus recapitulates REM sleep behaviour disorder. *Brain.* 2017;140:414–428.
44. Weber F, Hoang Do JP, Chung S, et al. Regulation of REM and non-REM sleep by periaqueductal GABAergic neurons. *Nat Commun.* 2018;9:354.
45. Peever J, Luppi PH, Montplaisir J. Breakdown in REM sleep circuitry underlies REM sleep behavior disorder. *Trends Neurosci.* 2014;37:279–288.
46. Mahoney CE, Cogswell A, Koralnik IJ, Scammell TE. The neurobiological basis of narcolepsy. *Nat Rev Neurosci.* 2019;20:83–93.
47. Burgess CR, Scammell TE. Narcolepsy: Neural mechanisms of sleepiness and cataplexy. *J Neurosci.* 2012;32:12305–12311.
48. Torontali ZA, Fraigne JJ, Sanghera P, Horner R, Peever J. The sublaterodorsal tegmental nucleus functions to couple brain state and motor activity during REM sleep and wakefulness. *Curr Biol.* 2019;29:3803–3813.e5.
49. Niwa Y, Kanda GN, Yamada RG, et al. Muscarinic acetylcholine receptors Chrm1 and Chrm3 are essential for REM sleep. *Cell Rep.* 2018;24:2231–2247 e7.

50. Espana RA, Scammell TE. Sleep neurobiology from a clinical perspective. *Sleep*. 2011;34:845–858.
51. Baghdoyan HA, Rodrigo-Angulo ML, McCarley RW, Hobson JA. A neuroanatomical gradient in the pontine tegmentum for the cholinoceptive induction of desynchronized sleep signs. *Brain Res.* 1987;414:245–261.
52. Boucetta S, Cisse Y, Mainville L, Morales M, Jones BE. Discharge profiles across the sleep-waking cycle of identified cholinergic, GABAergic, and glutamatergic neurons in the pontomesencephalic tegmentum of the rat. *J Neurosci.* 2014;34:4708–4727.
53. Kroeger D, Ferrari LL, Petit G, et al. Cholinergic, glutamatergic, and GABAergic neurons of the pedunculopontine tegmental nucleus have distinct effects on sleep/wake behavior in mice. *J Neurosci.* 2017;37:1352–1366.
54. Grace KP, Vanstone LE, Horner RL. Endogenous cholinergic input to the pontine REM sleep generator is not required for REM sleep to occur. *J Neurosci.* 2014;34:14198–14209.
55. Crochet S, Sakai K. Effects of microdialysis application of monoamines on the EEG and behavioural states in the cat mesopontine tegmentum. *Eur J Neurosci.* 1999;11:3738–3752.
56. Carter ME, Yizhar O, Chikahisa S, et al. Tuning arousal with optogenetic modulation of locus coeruleus neurons. *Nat Neurosci.* 2010;13:1526–1533.
57. Hasegawa E, Miyasaka A, Sakurai K, et al. Rapid eye movement sleep is initiated by basolateral amygdala dopamine signaling in mice. *Science*. 2022;375:994–1000.
58. Eban-Rothschild A, Rothschild G, Giardino WJ, Jones JR, de Lecea L. VTA dopaminergic neurons regulate ethologically relevant sleep-wake behaviors. *Nat Neurosci.* 2016;19:1356–1366.
59. Scammell TE, Arrigoni E, Lipton JO. Neural circuitry of wakefulness and sleep. *Neuron*. 2017; 93:747–765.
60. Hassani OK, Lee MG, Jones BE. Melanin-concentrating hormone neurons discharge in a reciprocal manner to orexin neurons across the sleep-wake cycle. *Proc Natl Acad Sci U S A.* 2009;106:2418–2422.
61. Chee MJ, Arrigoni E, Maratos-Flier E. Melanin-concentrating hormone neurons release glutamate for feedforward inhibition of the lateral septum. *J Neurosci*. 2015;35:3644–3651.
62. Mickelsen LE, Kolling FW 4th, Chimileski BR, et al. Neurochemical heterogeneity among lateral hypothalamic hypocretin/orexin and melanin-concentrating hormone neurons identified through single-cell gene expression analysis. *eNeuro.* 2017;4(5):ENEURO.0013-17.2017.
63. Bittencourt JC. Anatomical organization of the melanin-concentrating hormone peptide family in the mammalian brain. *Gen Comp Endocrinol.* 2011;172:185–197.
64. Luppi PH, Clement O, Fort P. Paradoxical (REM) sleep genesis by the brainstem is under hypothalamic control. *Curr Opin Neurobiol.* 2013;23:786–792.
65. Vetrivelan R, Kong D, Ferrari LL, et al. Melanin-concentrating hormone neurons specifically promote rapid eye movement sleep in mice. *Neuroscience*. 2016;336:102–113.
66. Varin C, Luppi PH, Fort P. Melanin-concentrating hormone-expressing neurons adjust slow-wave sleep dynamics to catalyze paradoxical (REM) sleep. *Sleep*. 2018;41:1–12.
67. Verret L, Goutagny R, Fort P, et al. A role of melanin-concentrating hormone producing neurons in the central regulation of paradoxical sleep. *BMC Neurosci.* 2003;4:1–10.
68. Jego S, Glasgow SD, Herrera CG, et al. Optogenetic identification of a rapid eye movement sleep modulatory circuit in the hypothalamus. *Nat Neurosci.* 2013;16:1637–1643.
69. Tsunematsu T, Ueno T, Tabuchi S, et al. Optogenetic manipulation of activity and temporally controlled cell-specific ablation reveal a role for MCH neurons in sleep/wake regulation. *J Neurosci.* 2014;34:6896–6909.
70. Lu J, Bjorkum AA, Xu M, et al. Selective activation of the extended ventrolateral preoptic nucleus during rapid eye movement sleep. *J Neurosci.* 2002;2:4568–4576.
71. Szymusiak R, Alam N, Steininger TL, McGinty D. Sleep-waking discharge patterns of ventrolateral preoptic/anterior hypothalamic neurons in rats. *Brain Res.* 1998;803:178–188.

SECTION II

Abnormal Sleep-Related Breathing

Chapter 5

The Obstructive Sleep Apnea Patient

Epidemiology, Symptoms and Signs, and Impact of the Disorder

Lauren Castner and Anita V. Shelgikar

INTRODUCTION

Obstructive sleep apnea (OSA) is characterized by repetitive interruptions in airflow during sleep due to pharyngeal narrowing and collapse.[1,2] OSA a common disorder that, without treatment, is associated with neurocognitive and cardiovascular sequelae,[3] along with economic and societal burdens.[3] Untreated OSA can contribute to poor health outcomes; treatment generally reduces associated adverse clinical outcomes and improves sleep-related quality of life.[3] OSA often remains undiagnosed and untreated, even in developed countries with efforts to effectively diagnose and treat OSA.[3] This chapter aims to identify the common signs and symptoms of OSA, discuss OSA screening tools, and review the impact of disease on the general population, the concerns within the public health sector, and the burden of disease among patients with additional comorbidities. While it is recognized that OSA also has a significant burden of disease upon the pediatric population, this chapter will focus on OSA in the adult population. Effective assessment and treatment of OSA may help reduce healthcare costs and the burden of chronic diseases, and improve related negative health consequences.[3]

EPIDEMIOLOGY

Rates of Obstructive Sleep Apnea

As of 2007, the World Health Organization (WHO) estimated that more than 100 million individuals were affected by OSA worldwide with a prevalence between 1% and over 6% of the adult population,[2] although recent estimates are suggestive that OSA affects nearly 1 billion individuals.[3] The estimated number of individuals with OSA is highest in China, followed by the United States, Brazil, and India, which reflects the overall population of these countries.[3] The number of individuals with moderate to severe OSA (apnea-hypopnea index >15/hr) is estimated to be 425 million worldwide.[3] The global prevalence of OSA is likely to increase further due to the worldwide obesity pandemic and aging populations.[3]

The Wisconsin Sleep Cohort Study, which studied men and women in the United States age 30–60 years, found that 9% of women and 24% of men had an apnea index greater than 5 per hour on full polysomnography.[4] However, when assessing symptomatic patients, the prevalence was 2% of women and 4% of men who had an apnea index of greater than 5 events/hr and excessive daytime sleepiness.[2] Peppard et al. realized that with the continuing obesity epidemic, the initial findings of the Wisconsin Sleep Cohort Study were likely underrepresenting the prevalence of OSA. Utilizing the data from the Wisconsin Sleep Cohort Study and National Health and Nutrition Examination Survery (NHANES) data sets' body mass index (BMI) classifications, models of OSA for the entire U.S. population were created.[5] It was estimated that the overall prevalence of mild to severe OSA was 26% among individuals 30–70 years of age, with an overall prevalence of moderate to severe OSA of 10%.[5]

China has been estimated to have the highest number of individuals with OSA. When assessing the Hong Kong Special Administrative Region, China, the prevalence of symptomatic OSA was over 4% in men and over 2% of women age 30–60 years.[6,7]

Gender Disparities Among Patients with Obstructive Sleep Apnea

In order to create systematic change regarding health disparities and healthcare inequalities, one must first be aware of and understand current inequalities. Current literature aims to assess the disparities within sleep medicine among different populations based on age, gender, race, and ethnicities. While there are differences between populations of different genders and races, the results are also intertwined, creating a complex field to navigate. This section aims to highlight these disparities separately, but we acknowledge that there is a great deal of intersectionality between sleep health disparities, race/ethnicity, and gender.

A health disparity is defined as:

> a health difference that adversely affects populations designated as disadvantaged, based on one or more of the following health outcomes: higher incidence or prevalence of disease, including earlier onset or more aggressive progression; premature or excessive mortality from specific conditions; greater global burden of disease, such as disability, adjusted life years, as measured by population health metrics; poor health behaviors and clinical outcomes related to the aforementioned information; and worse outcomes on validated self-reported measures that reflect daily functioning or symptoms from specific health difference conditions.[8p435]

A limited number of studies assess the intersectionality, or overlapping and interdependent systems, of sex/gender differences or disparities. However, assessments of sleep disparities by racial/ethnic and additional social identities stratified by sex/gender identify that men are more likely to be diagnosed with OSA. These sex/gender differences could exist, at least in part, due to differences in sex-related hormones and/or fat distribution that contribute to differences in pathophysiological manifestations.[8] Androgens may promote upper airway collapsibility, while progesterone leads to an augmented ventilatory response.[9]

Population-based studies have found a 2:1, male-female ratio of prevalence of OSA,[10] with a male-female ratio of 9:1 when assessing utilization data for referral to sleep centers; these data indicate reduced consideration of OSA in the female population.[10] Peppard et al. estimated that approximately 13% of men and 6% of women age 30–70 years have OSA.[5] Post-menopausal women have an increased OSA occurrence, especially when adjusted for age, BMI, and other health parameters[11] and the estimated prevalence also increases with age based on the Wisconsin Sleep Cohort Study.[5] Progesterone, a reproductive hormone, has a stimulatory effect on ventilation drive and expansion of the upper airway tract and may thus yield a protective effect prior to menopause.[11] Post-menopausal changes in fat distribution may increase neck circumference, and increased fat mass in the trunk and abdomen could increase the likelihood of developing OSA.[11]

Racial/Ethnic Disparities Among Patients with Obstructive Sleep Apnea

Members from racial/ethnic minorities are less likely to report poor sleep despite having poorer sleep characteristics, such as reduced total sleep time, lower sleep efficiency, reduced time in slow wave sleep, greater variability in sleep timing, higher likelihood of circadian misalignment, and greater daytime sleepiness.[12–16] This mismatch makes it difficult to fully interpret self-reported data as an objective measure of sleep.[8] Blacks/African Americans, Hispanics/Latinos, and Asians appear to be particularly susceptible and are more likely to have OSA, as demonstrated by the following results.[8,17,18] Black children have an OSA prevalence that is 3.5–6 times greater than that of white children.[8,19] Black women generally have a higher prevalence and severity of OSA than white women, along with an earlier age of incidence, which can result in greater health sequelae with time.[8,17] The Hispanic/Latino population also has a high OSA prevalence, with almost one-third of men and 18% of women being affected by OSA, after accounting for age and obesity.[8] Within Hispanic/Latino heritage groups, women of Puerto Rican background and men of Cuban background have the highest prevalence of OSA.[8,18]

Racial and ethnic minorities, especially Black women, experience a disproportionate risk of both suboptimal sleep and obesity.[8] The *Hispanic Community Health Study/Study of Latinos* demonstrated that OSA was associated with a 90% increase in diabetes mellitus prevalence and a 50% increase in hypertension prevalence, independent of obesity, which suggests that Hispanic/Latino patients may have a large burden of cardiometabolic disease possibly caused by untreated OSA.[8,18] The same study found an association between neurocognitive dysfunction in all tested neurocognitive domains and sleep apnea; this association was worse in women, especially those 45–55 years of age.[8]

There are still limitations in the current literature. There is variability in the quality of data when assessing various sleep dimensions and racial/ethnic groups. Many studies are observational, some with small population sizes, especially for racial/ethnic minorities, which can impact inferences made regarding disparities. There is also underrepresentation of certain racial/ethnic minorities, such as native Hawaiian/Pacific islanders, and rarely do studies assess groups within a certain population (e.g., Black women).

Risk Factors for Obstructive Sleep Apnea

Many patients do not report sleep-related symptoms to their primary care provider.[10] The prevalence of OSA is increased in certain populations, and there are patient characteristics that can increase the risk of OSA as well. These patients, as listed in Box 5.1, would be well served with regular assessments of their sleep and further evaluation based on responses. The American Academy of Sleep Medicine (AASM) recommends the screening of patients with a positive family history for OSA and those with retrognathia.[10,20] The elderly population is also more commonly affected by OSA.[21,22] Although many patients may be asymptomatic, there is evidence of adverse prognosis when an elderly patient has OSA.[22]

Obesity is a major risk factor for OSA, and excess weight is responsible for 41% of all cases and 58% of moderate to severe cases.[10] Patients of East Asian heritage are at risk for OSA at lower levels of obesity due to differences in facial bone structure.[10] Weight gain over time is associated with OSA incidence, and a 10% increase in weight predicts a 6-fold increase in the likelihood of developing clinically significant OSA.[10,23]

SIGNS AND SYMPTOMS OF OBSTRUCTIVE SLEEP APNEA

The AASM recommends asking all adults whether they are dissatisfied with their sleep, or have daytime sleepiness, as a part of routine

Box 5.1 Risk Factors for Obstructive Sleep Apnea

Obesity, especially with body mass index >35 kg/m^2
Family history of obstructive sleep apnea
Retrognathia
Treatment-resistant hypertension
Congestive heart failure
Atrial fibrillation
Stroke
Type 2 diabetes
Polycystic ovary syndrome
Acromegaly
Trisomy 21
Nocturnal dysrhythmias
Pulmonary hypertension

health maintenance exams.[10] Further screening by using clinical history or screening tools can be utilized if there is a positive response to these questions. Due to the risks of public health effects, commercial truck drivers and public transit operators should be screened regularly, along with any patient with a history of a recent motor vehicle accident or near miss due to sleepiness.[10] Screening for OSA should be considered for patients with common comorbidities of OSA, such as hypertension, atrial fibrillation, heart failure, stroke, and type 2 diabetes.[10] Additional symptom assessments and specific examinations for OSA will aid in guiding further decisions about testing for OSA.

Common Symptoms of Obstructive Sleep Apnea

Obtaining a history from a bedpartner or cohabitant can be particularly helpful, as many OSA symptoms may not be apparent to the patient. Common symptoms are detailed in Box 5.2. Snoring has the highest sensitivity for OSA but is a nonspecific symptom. Details about snoring volume and if it is bothersome to others can help differentiate OSA from primary snoring.[10] Excessive daytime sleepiness, while also a nonspecific finding, is critical to determine at initiation of OSA therapy and to follow the response to therapy. Explicit questioning about drowsiness or falling asleep while driving and use of caffeine or other stimulants is imperative to understand the extent of the patient's sleepiness.[10] Patients may also express "brain fog" or difficulties with concentrating rather than explicit sleepiness.[10]

Choking or gasping during sleep and the presence of a morning headache are highly specific for moderate to severe OSA, but these findings have low sensitivity.[10] Additional symptoms of untreated OSA may include depressive symptoms, decreased libido, and frequent nocturnal awakenings.[10] OSA can present atypically as well, with insomnia and fatigue as the predominant symptoms, especially in women. Sleep-maintenance insomnia is more likely to be related to OSA than sleep-onset insomnia.[10]

Common Physical Exam Findings Associated with Obstructive Sleep Apnea

The physical examination should include the respiratory, cardiovascular, and neurologic systems. The presence and degree of obesity

Box 5.2 Common Symptoms of Obstructive Sleep Apnea

Loud, frequent, bothersome snoring
Witnessed episodes of apnea
Choking/gasping during sleep
Excessive daytime sleepiness
Drowsy driving—recent motor vehicle accident or near miss associated with sleepiness
Unrefreshing sleep
Frequent nocturnal awakenings
Sleep-maintenance awakening—prolonged wake after sleep onset
Nocturia
Morning headache
Decreased concentration—"brain fog"
Depressed mood
Irritability
Decreased libido

should also be noted. Indications of upper airway narrowing may include: an enlarged neck circumference (>16 inches in women and >17 inches in men); a modified Mallampati score of 3 or 4 (Figure 5.1); macroglossia; tonsillar hypertrophy; an enlarged or elongated uvula; a high or arched palate; signs of nasal obstruction (polyps, septal deviation, turbinate hypertrophy, significant congestion); and retrognathia.[10,20]

Screening Instruments and Applications

Although there are several screening questionnaires available, they typically identify high-risk patients and are not as accurate as formal sleep testing.[10] The STOP-Bang and Berlin Questionnaire are widely used and well-validated tools for OSA screening.

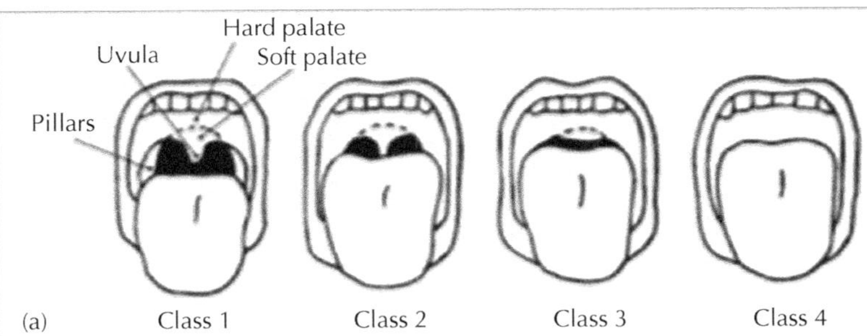

The Mallampati score:
Class 1. Complete visualization of the soft palate
Class 2. Complete visualization of the uvula
Class 3. Visualization of only the base of the uvula
Class 4. Soft palate is not visible at all

Figure 5.1. Modified Mallampati classification. Image from Sankal A, Halemani, KR, Bhadrinath N, et al. Assessment of the Effect of Supine Posture and Phonation on Modified Mallampati Grading and its Applicability in Prediction of Difficult Airway. J Mahatma Gandhi Inst Med Sci. 2018;23(1):19–24.

Table 5.1 **STOP-Bang Questionnaire**

A set of 8 questions to assess for OSA. A score of 3 or more "yes" answers demonstrates a high risk for OSA. A score of 5 or more "yes" answers is predictive of moderate to severe OSA.24

1. **S**noring: Do you snore loudly (loud enough to be heard through closed doors)?	Yes	No
2. **T**ired: Do you often feel tired, fatigued, or sleepy during daytime?	Yes	No
3. **O**bserved: Has anyone observed you stop breathing during your sleep?	Yes	No
4. Blood **P**ressure: Do you have or are you being treated for high blood pressure?	Yes	No
5. **B**MI: BMI more than 35 kg/m^2?	Yes	No
6. **A**ge: Age over 50 years old?	Yes	No
7. **N**eck circumference: Neck circumference >40 cm?	Yes	No
8. **G**ender: Male?	Yes	No

The STOP-Bang screening test (Table 5.1) was developed by an anesthesiologist to assess patients for OSA during the preoperative period. It is an 8-item tool, with the acronym STOP-Bang, that assigns 1 point for each positive answer.[24] A score of 3 or higher among preoperative patients had a sensitivity of 84% for predicting any OSA, and a score of 5 or higher was more predictive of clinically relevant OSA, typically moderate to severe.[24]

The Berlin Questionnaire (Table 5.2) asks about risk factors for sleep apnea, particularly snoring characteristics, waketime sleepiness or fatigue, and the presence of obesity or hypertension.[25] Patients with persistent and frequent symptoms in any 2 of the 3 domains

Table 5.2 **Berlin Questionnaire**

Questionnaire to elicit factors or behaviors that consistently predict the presence of OSA[25,26]

Category 1					
1. Do you snore?	Yes	No	Don't know		
2. Your snoring is:	Slightly louder than breathing	As loud as talking	Louder than talking		
3. How often do you snore?	Almost every day	3–4 times per week	1–2 times per week	1–2 times per month	Rarely or never
4. Has your snoring ever bothered other people?	Yes	No	Don't know		
5. Has anyone noticed that you stop breathing during your sleep?	Almost every day	3–4 times per week	1–2 times per week	1–2 times per month	Rarely or never
Category 2					
6. How often do you feel tired or fatigued after your sleep?	Almost every day	3–4 times per week	1–2 times per week	1–2 times per month	Rarely or never
7. During your waking time, do you feel tired, fatigued, or not up to par?	Almost every day	3–4 times per week	1–2 times per week	1–2 times per month	Rarely or never
8. Have you ever nodded off or fallen asleep while driving a vehicle?	Yes	No			
9. If you answered "yes": How often does this occur?	Almost every day	3–4 times per week	1–2 times per week	1–2 times per month	Rarely or never
Category 3					
10. Do you have high blood pressure?	Yes	No	Don't know		
Height:	Weight:	Age:	Male or Female		

Table 5.3 **Epworth Sleepiness Scale**

Subjective assessment of likelihood to doze off or fall asleep during common daily activities.[27] A score of 11 or greater indicates increased sleepiness.

0 = would *never* doze	1 = *slight* chance of dozing	2 = *moderate* chance of dozing	3 = *high* chance of dozing
Sitting and reading			
Watching television			
Sitting, inactive in a public place (e.g., a theater or a meeting)			
As a passenger in a car for an hour without a break			
Lying down to rest in the afternoon when circumstances permit			
Sitting and talking to someone			
Sitting quietly after a lunch without alcohol			
In a car, while stopped for a few minutes in traffic			

were at high risk for OSA.[26] In the primary care setting, there was a sensitivity of 86% for OSA with a positive screening, and more than a third of respondents were at high risk for OSA.[25]

The Epworth Sleepiness Scale (ESS) is an 8-item scale (Table 5.3) that quantifies the propensity for dozing off during everyday activities.[10] It is a self-administered questionnaire using a 0–3 rating system based upon how likely they are to doze off or fall asleep based upon their usual way of life.[27] High ESS scores are not diagnostic of any particular sleep disorder;[27] correlation with objective measures of sleepiness is inconsistent, and correlation with OSA severity is poor.[10] The ESS can help to standardize the evaluation of the patient's subjective perceptions.[10]

When to Refer for Evaluation

A consultation with a sleep specialist may not be necessary prior to evaluation for uncomplicated OSA. In order to reduce sleep study no-show and cancellation rates, the referring clinician should be able to adequately counsel patients on the rationale for diagnostic testing, OSA-related health risks, and what to expect with a sleep study, and also should be able to address concerns regarding subsequent management.[10] Evaluation by a sleep specialist is particularly recommended when there is concern for complex forms of sleep-disordered breathing (e.g., suspected nocturnal hypoventilation due to chronic lung disease or neuromuscular disorders, or central apnea), or when non-respiratory sleep disorders (e.g., parasomnia, narcolepsy) are a part of the differential, so that the most appropriate testing can be arranged.

There are multiple testing methods to diagnose OSA, a diagnosis which requires formal testing to document obstructive respiratory events during sleep. When a clinician has a high index of suspicion for OSA due to the presence of risk factors for OSA, positive screening tests, and/or concerning physical exam findings, further testing or evaluation at a sleep center should be performed. Historically, all testing was performed in a sleep laboratory with a technologist present; the use of home sleep apnea testing (HSAT), followed by initiation of home-based treatment, can lead to equivalent outcomes for patients with uncomplicated OSA.[10] A home-based strategy may be less expensive, may lead to more rapid initiation of treatment, and broadens access for patients who would have turned down laboratory-based test or who live in remote or underserved areas.[10] There is currently no evidence to support the use of overnight oximetry to screen patients for obstructive sleep apnea.[10]

Although an HSAT is useful in evaluating a patient for OSA much of the time, it is not indicated in all circumstances. In less straightforward cases, an in-laboratory sleep study should be pursued. Patients with unstable housing or cognitive or physical disabilities that would prevent the self-application of the monitoring device are not considered appropriate candidates for home-based testing.[10] An HSAT has a relative contraindication in patients with other causes of oxyhemoglobin desaturations such as chronic lung disease, congestive heart failure, or high likelihood of central sleep apnea since the accuracy of a HSAT in these settings has not been well evaluated.[10] An in-laboratory sleep study should be considered when the differential diagnosis includes other sleep-related breathing disorders such as central sleep apnea or obesity hypoventilation syndrome.[10] An in-laboratory sleep study includes limited electroencephalography (EEG) monitoring, which can be expanded to a full EEG montage when indicated (e.g., differentiating parasomnias from sleep-related seizures). In cases of severe OSA, an in-laboratory sleep study enables a sleep lab technologist to initiate intervention if indicated.

There is no high-level evidence to support testing for OSA in asymptomatic patients.[10] It may be reasonable to test patients with morbid obesity who are asymptomatic but are scheduled for bariatric surgery given the high prevalence of OSA in the population and the risks of adverse perioperative outcomes with untreated OSA.[10] Due to the high prevalence of OSA in patients with treatment-refractory hypertension on 5 or more medications, the evaluation and treatment of OSA, even when otherwise asymptomatic, may be beneficial in clinically significant reduction of blood pressure.[10]

IMPACT OF OBSTRUCTIVE SLEEP APNEA

OSA is associated with many adverse sequelae, both behavioral and physical. Behavioral consequences include daytime sleepiness, impaired concentration, and neuropsychological dysfunction.[28] Physical consequences include cardiovascular disorders, especially hypertension.[29–32] It is known that excessive daytime sleepiness and other associated behavioral consequences are reversible with appropriate treatment of OSA, and there is growing evidence that cardiovascular disorders also benefit from therapy.[33–35]

Health Risks of Obstructive Sleep Apnea

There is a statistically significant independent association of increased risk or prevalence of hypertension and habitual sleep duration, OSA, insomnia, restless legs syndrome, and periodic limb movement disorder when assessing epidemiological studies.[16] More than 30% of patients with hypertension have OSA, approximately 50% of patients with OSA are hypertensive, and OSA is present in up to 90% of patients with treatment-resistant hypertension.[16,36] Blood pressure will typically decrease by approimately 10% while sleeping, but there is an increased risk of cardiovascular disease when the blood pressure does not decrease during sleep.[37] OSA may cause endothelial dysfunction, which is primarily driven by intermittent hypoxia.[38] In addition, OSA can trigger a cascade of acute hemodynamic, autonomic, chemical, inflammatory, and metabolic effects leading to chronic after-effects that initiate or exacerbate cardiovascular disease.[23] In addition, the cycles of hypoxia and carbon dioxide retention lead to fluctuations in cardiac parasympathethic and sympathetic nervous activity, affecting heart rate along with the sympathetically mediated peripheral vasoconstriction that raises systemic blood pressure.[23] In addition to initiating or exacerbating hypertension, the presence of OSA can lead to treatment resistance due to biochemical features of primary aldosteronism, leading to oxidative stress, inflammation, and ventricular fibrosis and hypertrophy.[23]

There is a 2.38 times increase in the likelihood of having heart failure that is associated with OSA independent of of confounders.[23] In patients with heart failure, there is a prevalence of OSA with an apnea hypopnea index (AHI) greater than 10–15 events/hr of 11%–53%, but it is important to note that there is a greater prevalence of central apnea associated with heart failure as well.[23] The provider must differentiate between the sleep-disordered breathing types due to the important differences in pathophysiology and potential treatments needed. One hypothesized reason for increased OSA in patients with heart failure is that there is fluid redistribution from edematous legs to peripharyngeal tissues during the position change required for sleep, which then can impinge upon the pharyngeal lumen and lead to collapse during sleep.[23]

Atrial fibrillation (AF) is the most common sustained cardiac arrhythmia, and lifetime prevalence is 1 in 4 for men and women over the age of 40 years.[39] Those with AF are at an increased risk for cardiovascular disease such as stroke and myocardial infarctions, along with death.[39–41] OSA has been associated with an increased risk for AF, especially within the first 5 years of diagnosis.[42] Through multiple pathophysiological mechanisms, OSA may trigger or maintain AF due to repetitive and prolonged hypoxemia, exaggerated intrathoracic pressure oscillations with increased cardiac wall stress, systemic inflammation, sympathetic and parasympathetic imbalances, and diastolic dysfunction.[42] Worsening severity of nocturnal oxygen desaturation associated with OSA independently correlates with increasing risk of incident AF.[42] In addition to AF, OSA may predispose patients to additional arrhythmias, including nonsustained ventricular tachycardia and complex ventricular ectopy, especially during periods of sleep.[43] These nocturnal arrhythmias in the setting of OSA, especially severe untreated OSA, could lead to an increased incidence of fatal and nonfatal cardiovascular events.[43]

OSA is highly prevalent before stroke, but also in post-stroke patients.[44] OSA is an independent risk factor for cerebrovascular disease, and is associated with post-stroke mortality.[44] In addition to being a risk factor for incident strokes, OSA after a stroke predicts an increased risk for another ischemic stroke, especially with increased severity of OSA.[44] The treatment of OSA may represent a modifiable risk factor for poor stroke outcomes.[44]

Alzheimer disease (AD) is a neurodegenerative disease and the most common cause of dementia, which shares risk factors and neuropathological features with cerebrovascular disease, which may ultimately promote and lead to the progression of disease.[45] Parkinson disease (PD) is another neurodegenerative condition that affects approximately 630,000 people in the United States and may be associated with cerebrovascular disease.[45] Cerebrovascular risk factors for neurocognitive diseases include prior strokes, atrial fibrillation, coronary heart disease, hyperlipidemia, hypertension, diabetes mellitus, heart failure, peripheral vascular disease, chronic kidney disease, chronic obstructive pulmonary disease (COPD), valvular heart disease, OSA, tobacco use, and alcohol abuse.[45] In a single study assessing the associations of cerebrovascular risk factors and the subsequent development of PD, OSA was one of the risk factors with the strongest association.[45] Potential mechanisms for the relationship between AD, PD, and cerebrovascular dysfunction could include insufficient delivery of cerebral blood flow during neural activity, cerebral endothelial dysfunction, and altered cerebrovascular autoregulation.[45] These cerebral blood flow abnormalities may lead to impaired clearance of β-amyloid and possibly tau in AD, while PD pathology could promote cerebral ischemia and stroke.[45]

Morbidity and Mortality

The primary cause of morbidity and mortality in OSA is related to the cardiovascular system.[2] There is a significant overlap between cardiovascular risk factors in patients with OSA, which makes the assessment of the independent contribution of OSA in cardiovascular disease difficult.[2] The Sleep Heart Health study evaluated over 6000 subjects with in-home polysomnography, and there was a modest independent association with hypertension, which increased with more severe OSA.[29] There was a stronger correlation identified between OSA and hypertension identified in the Wisconsin Cohort Study.[30] The Sleep Heart Health Study cohort revealed that OSA is an independent risk factor for congestive cardiac failure, cerebrovascular disease, and coronary artery disease.[46] Long-term cardiovascular outcome studies have found that effective continuous positive airway pressure decreases cardiovascular morbidity and mortality.[31,33,34]

Effects of Excessive Daytime Sleepiness

Excessive daytime sleepiness reportedly affects 40.5%–58% of individuals with OSA.[47] In addition to excessive daytime sleepiness, patients with OSA report lack of concentration, memory impairment, and at times psychological disturbances.[47,48] These symptoms and the additional functional impairments lead to many patients with OSA reporting a poor quality of life in social, emotional, and physical domains.[48] When assessing quality of life with the use of the SF-36 questionnaire for self-reported perceptions of functional status, well-being, and overall health, it was found that all questionnaire respondents with a diagnosis of OSA had decreased health status in all domains of the SF-36 compared to age-matched control subjects, and there was not a correlation between the severity of a patient's OSA.[48]

Excessive daytime sleepiness is believed to be due to episodic, intermittent hypoxia and sleep fragmentation which are associated with neuronal injury and degeneration in wake-promoting brain regions.[47] Sleep-disordered breathing also affects sleep architecture, which is variable depending upon the respiratory disturbance index (RDI).[49] There is an increase in the percentage of stages 1 and 2 sleep along with decreased sleep efficiency and stage 3 sleep.[49]

Economic Impact

Evidence exists that patients with OSA have higher healthcare costs than matched control subjects prior to diagnosis.[50–53] One study reported an annual healthcare cost of 2720 US dollars for OSA patients prior to diagnosis when compared to matched controls (1384 US dollars).[53] In a 10-year period prior to diagnosis, patients with OSA used more than twice as many healthcare services compared to controls, which amounted to an excess of approximately 4265 Canadian dollars per patient.[50] There was a significant reduction in healthcare costs in the same population with the initiation of continuous positive airway pressure.[52]

Although there are greater healthcare costs prior to diagnosis and treatment of OSA, there is also a significant economic cost of obtaining diagnosis and treatment.[2] A traditional approach to diagnosis requires an overnight sleep study in a dedicated sleep laboratory, which is resource intensive.[54] There is increasing emphasis and use of limited diagnostic techniques, such as HSAT, that often focus solely on cardio-respiratory variables.[55] Despite the economic burden of diagnosis and treatment, the management of OSA is likely not just cost effective, but cost saving due to the reduction of major complications and additional health expenses.[3,56]

From a public health perspective, there are significant economic costs associated with untreated OSA. There is an increased risk of road traffic accidents in untreated patients, with an increased accident rate between 3 and 7 times that of the general population.[57–59] Suboptimal sleep contributes to poor performance in everyday activities such as work-related productivity.[16] Due to the recognition that sleep deficiency and poor sleep have a significant impact on the population, Healthy People 2020 has created sleep health objectives: increase in the proportion of adolescents obtaining adequate sleep (baseline 31%); increase in the proportion of adults obtaining adequate sleep (baseline 63%); decrease in the number of motor vehicle incidents attributed to drowsy driving (baseline 2.7/100 million miles); and increase in the proportion of adults with apnea symptoms seeking medical attention (baseline 10%).[16,60]

OBSTRUCTIVE SLEEP APNEA AND SPECIFIC COMORBIDITIES

In addition to OSA being associated with worsened outcomes in certain diseases, such as cardiovascular conditions, there are additional disease processes that are intermingled with OSA. These disorders may be causative of OSA, such as neuromuscular disease, or may be associated with poorer outcomes for both OSA and the primary condition when present together, such as diabetes. Table 5.4 summarizes multiple disease processes and their relationship with OSA and outcomes of treatment.

CONCLUSION

Obstructive sleep apnea can affect a patient's sleep quality, impair quality of life, and yield effects on major health and economic outcomes. The multifactorial pathophysiology of OSA can cause significant and varied effects on overall health. Health disparities can also influence access to care and OSA treatment outcomes. Ongoing research on the diagnosis and treatment of OSA is needed to enhance awareness and early identification of OSA to mitigate disease burden and development of comorbidities while also addressing inequities in care.

Table 5.4 Comorbid Conditions Associated with Obstructive Sleep Apnea

Disease State	Epidemiology	Relationship to OSA	Outcomes
Obesity hypoventilation syndrome (OHS)	In 20% of patients with obesity of BMI >30 kg/m^2 and 30% of those with BMI >40 kg/m^2 OSA is associated with awake hypercapnia in the absence of other causes of hypoventilation and is known as obesity-hypoventilation syndrome.[61] Prevalence in the general population is unknown due to lack of testing, but is likely increasing as the prevalence of obesity is increasing.	Must be associated with sleep-disordered breathing, either OSA or sleep-related hypoventilation.[62] Typically have severe obesity, severe OSA with AHI >30 events/hour, and have excessive daytime sleepiness.[62] More likely to report dyspnea, manifest corpulmonale, and have worse quality of life than patients with eucapnic OSA.[62]	Treatment includes weight loss and PAP therapy. Weight loss is aimed at 25%–30% of actual body weight in order to reverse OHS.[62] Treat with CPAP or consider noninvasive ventilation in order to treat the sleep-disordered breathing. PAP improves daytime sleepiness, quality of life, and dyspnea along with gas exchange.[62]
Chronic obstructive pulmonary disease (COPD)	Affects 210 million individuals worldwide.[63] COPD is associated with additional comorbidities such as pulmonary hypertension, malnutrition, anxiety, sleep-related disorders, osteoporosis, obesity, diabetes, metabolic syndrome, and others.[64]	Moderate-to-severe COPD is associated with an increased mortality risk in patients with OSA,[65] likely due to OSA exacerbating pathophysiologic mechanisms leading to progression of COPD due to chronic intermittent hypoxia and sleep disruption.[65]	The use of PAP therapy can interrupt and treat the pathophysiological overlaps of hypoxemia and hypercapnia that worsen overall outcomes and can improve quality of life.[64]
Asthma	Affects 300 million people worldwide: 7.5% of adults in the United States and approximately 8.7% of Black, 7.6% of whites, and 5.8% of Hispanics/Latinos.[66] Asthma is also the most common chronic disease in children.[63]	OSA is frequently associated with asthma, particularly neutrophilic asthma.[66]	Treatment of OSA improves asthma symptoms, reduces the use of bronchodilators, and overall improves quality of life from an asthma perspective.[66]
Chronic rhinitis	Affects 400 million people worldwide.[63]	Associated with both asthma and OSA. Both can lead to airflow limitation within the upper airways, along with create chronic inflammation of the airways.[63]	Treating rhinitis can reduce upper airway resistance and improve both asthma and OSA symptoms.[66]
Diabetes	34.2 million people of all ages, 10.5% of the U.S. population, have diabetes as of 2018 CDC data. Diabetes affects 13% of all U.S. adults. The percentage of adults with diabetes increases with age.[67]	Quantity and quality of sleep can significantly predict the risk of type 2 diabetes. Snoring and OSA are also associated with abnormal glucose control and risk of diabetes.[16]	Some evidence that treatment of OSA improves the risk of diabetes.[16]

Continued

Table 5.4 *Continued*

Disease State	Epidemiology	Relationship to OSA	Outcomes
Metabolic syndrome	Metabolic syndrome comprises co-occurring conditions that increase the risk of diabetes and cardiovascular disease, including abdominal obesity, high blood pressure, hyperglycemia, and dyslipidemia.[68] It is estimated that one-fifth of the adult population in the Western countries have metabolic syndrome.[69]	Both can independently increase risks of diabetes and cardiovascular diseases. There is a close relationship between metabolic syndrome and OSA with increased risk for OSA as more components of metabolic syndrome are met.[68] Alternatively, OSA can lead to metabolic syndrome due to repeated obstructive events, hypoxia, and arousals.[68]	Further research on outcomes is needed, but benefits are likely if patients with OSA are treated with PAP therapy and weight loss, along with management of additional comorbidities due to the overlap of multiple conditions and syndromes.
Duchenne muscular dystrophy (DMD)	DMD is an X-linked recessive disorder with a prevalence of 15.9 to 19.5 per 100,000 live male births. It is caused by the absence or deficiency of functional dystrophin protein that ultimately leads to progressive neuromuscular weakness. With the use of noninvasive positive pressure ventilation and therapy advances, life expectancy for boys born today can be beyond age 40.[70]	Due to decreased muscle tone and ventilatory drive during sleep, most often sleep-disordered breathing presents before other respiratory complications, including OSA.[70] Initially OSA is due to adenotonsillar hypertrophy in the early years, but due to chronic systemic steroid use, obesity and fat deposits in the tongue and neck are a proposed mechanism for OSA.[70] Sleep-disordered breathing can progress as the disease progresses to include central sleep apnea and nocturnal hypoventilation.	Treatment of OSA depends upon the age of the patient, with an adenotonsillectomy being performed in early childhood. along with treatments for mucociliary airway clearance.[70] It is generally recommended to initiate noninvasive ventilation with bilevel pressure as opposed to CPAP due to potential to worsen hypoventilation with disease progression. Patients will likely progress to needing positive pressure ventilation, either noninvasive or via tracheostomy.[70] Disease progression is not halted, but there can be improvements in quality of life and respiratory complications.
Amyotrophic lateral sclerosis (ALS)	ALS is a progressive and fatal neurodegenerative disease that presents with bulbar or limb weakness. There is increasing evidence that it affects cognition, behavior, sleep, pain, and fatigue.[71] The associated respiratory muscle weakness is one of the major causes of morbidity and premature death due to chronic hypercapnic respiratory failure or respiratory tract infection.[72] There is a prevalence between 4.1 and 8.4 per 100,000 persons.[73]	ALS is associated with sleep-disordered breathing, including OSA, central sleep apnea, and nocturnal hypoventilation. OSA may be further promoted in the ALS patient by posterior tongue displacement and reduced pharyngeal tone.[72] Sleep apnea is more common in patients with bulbar dysfunction.[72]	Noninvasive ventilation has significant impact on both quality of life and life expectancy; therefore early diagnosis and treatment of sleep-disordered breathing is of great importance.[72] Due to comorbid nocturnal hypoventilation, noninvasive ventilation is recommended with care titration.[72]

REFERENCES

1. Khor YH, Ryerson CJ, Landry SA, et al. Interstitial lung disease and obstructive sleep apnea. *Sleep Med Rev*. 2021;58:101442.
2. Global surveillance, prevention and control of chronic respiratory diseases: A comprehensive approach. Brochure. World Health Organization. Accessed 11 March 2021. https://iris.who.int/bitstream/handle/10665/43776/9789241563468_eng.pdf?sequence=1
3. Benjafield AV, Ayas NT, Eastwood PR, et al. Estimation of the global prevalence and burden of obstructive sleep apnoea: A literature-based analysis. *Lancet Respir Med*. 2019;7:687–698.
4. Young T, Palta M, Dempsey J, et al. The occurrence of sleep-disordered breathing among middle-aged adults. *N Engl J Med*. 1993;328:1230–1235.
5. Peppard PE, Young T, Barnet JH, et al. Increased prevalence of sleep-disordered breathing in adults. *Am J Epidemiol*. 2013;177:1006–1014.
6. Ip MS, Lam B, Lauder IJ, et al. A community study of sleep-disordered breathing in middle-aged Chinese men in Hong Kong. *Chest*. 2001;119:62–69.
7. Ip MS, Lam B, Tang LWH, et al. A community study of sleep-disordered breathing in middle-aged Chinese women in Hong Kong: Prevalence and gender differences. *Chest*. 2004;125:127–134.
8. Jackson CL, Powell-Wiley TM, Gaston SA, et al. Racial/ethnic disparities in sleep health and potential interventions among women in the United States. *J Womens Health (Larchmt)*. 2020;29:435–442.
9. Cistulli PA, Sullivan CE. Sleep apnea in Marfan's syndrome. Increased upper airway collapsibility during sleep. *Chest*. 1995;108:631–635.
10. Patel SR. Obstructive sleep apnea. *Ann Intern Med*. 2019;171:ITC81–ITC96.
11. Zolfaghari S, Yao C, Thompson C, et al. Effects of menopause on sleep quality and sleep disorders: Canadian Longitudinal Study on Aging. *Menopause*. 2020;27:295–304.
12. Johnson DA, Jackson CL, Williams NJ, Alcántara C. Are sleep patterns influenced by race/ethnicity—a marker of relative advantage or disadvantage? Evidence to date. *Nat Sci Sleep*. 2019;11:79–95.
13. Stepnowsky CJ, Moore PJ, Dimsdale JE. Effect of ethnicity on sleep: Complexities for epidemiologic research. *Sleep*. 2003;26:329–332.
14. Profant J, Ancoli-Israel S, Dimsdale JE. Are there ethnic differences in sleep architecture? *Am J Hum Biol*. 2002;14:321–326.
15. Eastman CI, Tomaka VA, Crowley SJ. Circadian rhythms of European and African-Americans after a large delay of sleep as in jet lag and night work. *Sci Rep*. 2016;6:36716.
16. Jackson CL, Redline S, Emmons KM. Sleep as a potential fundamental contributor to disparities in cardiovascular health. *Annu Rev Public Health*. 2015;36:417–440.
17. Meetze K, Gillespie MB, Lee FS. Obstructive sleep apnea: A comparison of black and white subjects. *Laryngoscope*. 2002;112:1271–1274.
18. Redline S, Stores-Alvarez D, Loredo J, et al. Sleep-disordered breathing in Hispanic/Latino individuals of diverse backgrounds: The Hispanic Community Health Study/Study of Latinos. *Am J Respir Crit Care Med*. 2014;189:335–344.
19. Redline S, Tishler PV, Schluchter M, et al. Risk factors for sleep-disordered breathing in children: Associations with obesity, race, and respiratory problems. *Am J Respir Crit Care Med*. 1999;159:1527–1532.
20. Epstein LJ, Kristo D, Strollo Jr PJ, et al. Clinical guideline for the evaluation, management and long-term care of obstructive sleep apnea in adults. *J Clin Sleep Med*. 2009;5:263–276.
21. Ancoli-Israel S, Kripke DF, Klauber MR, et al. Sleep-disordered breathing in community-dwelling elderly. *Sleep*. 1991;14:486–495.
22. Cohen-Zion M, Stepnowky C, Marler, et al. Changes in cognitive function associated with sleep disordered breathing in older people. *J Am Geriatr Soc*. 2001;49:1622–1627.
23. Bradley TD, Floras JS. Obstructive sleep apnoea and its cardiovascular consequences. *Lancet*. 2009;373:82–93.
24. Chung F, Subramanyam R, Liao P, et al. High STOP-Bang score indicates a high probability of obstructive sleep apnoea. *Br J Anaesth*. 2012;108:768–775.
25. Netzer NC, Stoohs RA, Netzer CM, Clark K, Strohl KP. Using the Berlin Questionnaire to identify patients at risk for the sleep apnea syndrome. *Ann Intern Med*. 1999;131:485–491.
26. Thurtell MJ, Bruce BB, Rye DB, Newman NJ, Biousse V. The Berlin Questionnaire screens for obstructive sleep apnea in idiopathic intracranial hypertension. *J Neuroophthalmol*. 2011;31:316–319.
27. Johns MW. A new method for measuring daytime sleepiness: The Epworth sleepiness scale. *Sleep*. 1991;14:540–545.
28. Engleman HM, Douglas NJ. Sleep 4: Sleepiness, cognitive function, and quality of life in obstructive sleep apnoea/hypopnoea syndrome. *Thorax*. 2004;59:618–622.
29. Nieto FJ, Young TB, Lind BK, et al. Association of sleep-disordered breathing, sleep apnea, and hypertension in a large community-based study: Sleep Heart Health Study. *JAMA*. 2000;283:1829–1836.
30. Peppard PE, Young T, Palta M, Skatrud J. Prospective study of the association between sleep-disordered breathing and hypertension. *N Engl J Med*. 2000;342:1378–1384.
31. Peker Y, Hedner J, Norum J, Kraiczi H, Carlson J. Increased incidence of cardiovascular disease in middle-aged men with obstructive sleep apnea: A 7-year follow-up. *Am J Respir Crit Care Med*. 2002;166:159–165.
32. Arzt M, Young T, Finn L, Skatrud JB, Bradley TD. Association of sleep-disordered breathing and the occurrence of stroke. *Am J Respir Crit Care Med*. 2005;172:1447–1451.
33. Doherty LS, Kiely JL, Swan V, McNicholas WT. Long-term effects of nasal continuous positive airway pressure therapy on cardiovascular outcomes in sleep apnea syndrome. *Chest*. 2005;127:2076–2084.
34. Marin JM, Carrizo SJ, Vicente E, Agusti AG. Long-term cardiovascular outcomes in men with obstructive sleep apnoea-hypopnoea with or without treatment with continuous positive airway pressure: An observational study. *Lancet*. 2005;365:1046–1053.
35. Becker HF, Jerrentrup A, Ploch T, et al. Effect of nasal continuous positive airway pressure treatment on blood pressure in patients with obstructive sleep apnea. *Circulation*. 2003;107:68–73.
36. Worsnop CJ, Naughton MT, Barter CE, et al. The prevalence of obstructive sleep apnea in hypertensives. *Am J Respir Crit Care Med*. 1998;157:111–115.
37. Dolan E, Stanton A, Thijs L, et al. Superiority of ambulatory over clinic blood pressure measurement in predicting mortality: The Dublin outcome study. *Hypertension*. 2005;46:156–161.

38. Walia HK, Li H, Rueschman M, et al. Association of severe obstructive sleep apnea and elevated blood pressure despite antihypertensive medication use. *J Clin Sleep Med*. 2014;10:835–843.
39. Lloyd-Jones DM, Wang TJ, Leip EP, et al. Lifetime risk for development of atrial fibrillation: The Framingham Heart Study. *Circulation*. 2004;110:1042–1046.
40. Wolf PA, Abbott RD, Kannel WB. Atrial fibrillation as an independent risk factor for stroke: The Framingham Study. *Stroke*. 1991;22:983–988.
41. Soliman EZ, Safford MM, Muntner P, et al. Atrial fibrillation and the risk of myocardial infarction. *JAMA Intern Med*. 2014;174:107–114.
42. Gami AS, Hodge DO, Herges RM, et al. Obstructive sleep apnea, obesity, and the risk of incident atrial fibrillation. *J Am Coll Cardiol*. 2007;49:565–571.
43. Mehra R, Benjamin EJ, Shahar E, et al. Association of nocturnal arrhythmias with sleep-disordered breathing: The Sleep Heart Health Study. *Am J Respir Crit Care Med*. 2006;173:910–916.
44. Brown DL, Shafie-Khorassani F, Kim S, et al. Sleep-disordered breathing is associated with recurrent ischemic stroke. *Stroke*. 2019;50:571–576.
45. Kummer BR, Diaz I, Wu X, et al. Associations between cerebrovascular risk factors and Parkinson disease. *Ann Neurol*. 2019;86:572–581.
46. Shahar E, Whitney CW, Redline S, et al. Sleep-disordered breathing and cardiovascular disease: Cross-sectional results of the Sleep Heart Health Study. *Am J Respir Crit Care Med*. 2001;163:19–25.
47. Lal C, Weaver TE, Bae CJ, Strohl KP. Excessive daytime sleepiness in obstructive sleep apnea: Mechanisms and clinical management. *Ann Am Thorac Soc*. 2021;18:757–768.
48. D'Ambrosio C, Bowman T, Mohsenin V. Quality of life in patients with obstructive sleep apnea: effect of nasal continuous positive airway pressure: A prospective study. *Chest*. 1999;115:123–129.
49. Redline S, Kirchner HL, Quan SF, et al. The effects of age, sex, ethnicity, and sleep-disordered breathing on sleep architecture. *Arch Intern Med*. 2004;164:406–418.
50. Ronald J, Delaive K, Roos L, et al. Health care utilization in the 10 years prior to diagnosis in obstructive sleep apnea syndrome patients. *Sleep*. 1999;22:225–229.
51. Otake K, Delaive K, Walld R, Manfreda J, Kryger MH. Cardiovascular medication use in patients with undiagnosed obstructive sleep apnoea. *Thorax*. 2002;5:417–422.
52. Bahammam A, Delaive K, Ronald J, et al. Health care utilization in males with obstructive sleep apnea syndrome two years after diagnosis and treatment. *Sleep*. 1999;22:740–747.
53. Kapur V, Blough DK, Sandblom RE, et al. The medical cost of undiagnosed sleep apnea. *Sleep*. 1999;22:749–755.
54. American Academy of Sleep Medicine Task Force. Sleep-related breathing disorders in adults: Recommendations for syndrome definition and measurement techniques in clinical research. *Sleep*. 1999;22:667–689.
55. ATS/ACCP/AASM Taskforce Steering Committee. Executive summary on the systematic review and practice parameters for portable monitoring in the investigation of suspected sleep apnea in adults. *Am J Respir Crit Care Med*. 2004;169:1160–1163.
56. Cost justification for diagnosis and treatment of obstructive sleep apnea: Position statement of the American Academy of Sleep Medicine. *Sleep*. 2000;23:1017–1018.
57. Terán-Santos J, Jiménez-Gómez A, Cordero-Guevara J. The association between sleep apnea and the risk of traffic accidents: Cooperative Group Burgos-Santander. *N Engl J Med*. 1999;340:847–851.
58. Krieger J, McNicholas WT, Levy P, et al. Public health and medicolegal implications of sleep apnoea. *Eur Respir J* 2002;20:1594–1609.
59. George CF. Reduction in motor vehicle collisions following treatment of sleep apnoea with nasal CPAP. *Thorax*. 2001;56:508–512.
60. Institute of Medicine. *Sleep Disorders and Sleep Deprivation: An Unmet Public Health Problem*. Washington DC: The National Academies Press; 2006.
61. Perger E, Aron-Wisnewsky J, Arnulf I, Oppert JM, Redolfi S. Diagnostic approach to sleep disordered-breathing among patients with grade III obesity. *Sleep Med* 2021;82:18–22.
62. Wearn J, Akpa B, Mokhlesi B. Adherence to positive airway pressure therapy in obesity hypoventilation syndrome. *Sleep Med Clin*. 2021;16:43–59.
63. Carmona-Pírez J, Poblador-Plou B, Ioakeim-Skoufa I, et al. Multimorbidity clusters in patients with chronic obstructive airway diseases in the EpiChron Cohort. *Sci Rep*. 2021;11:4784.
64. Nattusami L, Hadda V, Khilnani GC, et al. Co-existing obstructive sleep apnea among patients with chronic obstructive pulmonary disease. *Lung India*. 2021;38:12–17.
65. Scrutinio D, Guida P, Aliani M, et al. Age and comorbidities are crucial predictors of mortality in severe obstructive sleep apnoea syndrome. *Eur J Intern Med*. 2021;90:71–76.
66. Nanda A, Wasan AN. Asthma in Adults. *Med Clin North Am*. 2020;104:95–108.
67. Kim DH, Kim B, Han K, Kim SW. The relationship between metabolic syndrome and obstructive sleep apnea syndrome: a nationwide population-based study. *Sci Rep*. 2021;11:8751.
68. Pérez-Martínez P, Mikhailidis DP, Athyros VG, et al. Lifestyle recommendations for the prevention and management of metabolic syndrome: An international panel recommendation. *Nutr Rev*. 2017;75:307–326.
69. MacKintosh EW, Chen ML, Benditt JO. Lifetime care of Duchenne muscular dystrophy. *Sleep Med Clin*. 2020;15:485–495.
70. Mahoney CJ, Ahmed RM, Huynh W, et al. Pathophysiology and treatment of non-motor dysfunction in amyotrophic lateral sclerosis. *CNS Drugs*. 2021;35:483–505.
71. Boentert M, Glatz C, Helmle C, Okegwo A, Young P. Prevalence of sleep apnoea and capnographic detection of nocturnal hypoventilation in amyotrophic lateral sclerosis. *J Neurol Neurosurg Psychiatry*. 2018;89:418–424.
72. Longinetti E, Fang F. Epidemiology of amyotrophic lateral sclerosis: An update of recent literature. *Curr Opin Neurol*. 2019;32:771–776.

Chapter 6

Positive Pressure Treatment of Obstructive Sleep Apnea

Helena Schotland, Matthew Wilson, and Abdullah Arjomand

From 1836 to 1837, Charles Dickens serially published *The Posthumous Papers of the Pickwick Club*,[1] where he introduced readers to a cast of characters, including Joe, the fat boy. Although earlier descriptions of obstructive sleep apnea (OSA) date back to the time of Dionysius,[2] Dickens was credited with the most colorful description of OSA. Joe was a "fat and red-faced boy, in a state of somnolency."[1p38] From the ancient era to the Dickensian era to the 1970s, weight loss was the only known treatment for OSA. Tracheostomy was subsequently utilized to bypass the upper airway obstruction seen in OSA.[3,4] Tracheostomy was seen as a potentially life-saving, but Draconian treatment, with many patients declining therapy.

In 1968, Colin Sullivan, then a young medical student, discovered his mother dead in bed. Overweight, she had had a history of snoring, fatigue, angina, and dyspnea. Dr. Sullivan later began studying the control of respiration during sleep. In 1979, he had an idea for stabilizing the upper airway in sleep apnea using positive pressure and tested his first human patient (who had previously declined tracheostomy) with a nasal continuous positive airway pressure (CPAP) device in 1980.[5] The device consisted of a vacuum cleaner blower motor attached to a wide-bore tube with mechanical resistance at the distal end. The apparatus was secured to the patient's nostrils using soft plastic tubing and rapid-setting silicone rubber. The experiment was a rousing success. The data from this patient and 4 others were published in *The Lancet* by Sullivan and colleagues in their historic paper in 1981 describing the ability of the noninvasive CPAP device to maintain patency of the upper airway and effectively treat OSA.[6] Over time, the device became a part of routine clinical treatment and remains the main treatment modality for OSA today.

The purpose of this chapter is to discuss the utility of positive airway pressure (PAP) therapy for treatment of OSA in adults—including CPAP, bilevel PAP (BPAP), and auto-titrating PAP (APAP).

SEVERITY

Once OSA has been diagnosed by a polysomnogram (PSG) or home sleep apnea test, it is important to determine the severity of disease. This is most commonly done using the apnea hypopnea index (AHI). OSA severity can range from mild (AHI ≥5 events/hour but <15 events/hour), moderate (AHI ≥15 events/hour but <30 events/hour), or severe (AHI ≥30 events/hour).

There is high-quality evidence that PAP therapy is effective in reducing the severity of OSA. Specifically, there are 3 systematic reviews showing the benefit of PAP in OSA using AHI as a clinical endpoint. Gay et al. reviewed 11 randomized controlled trials (RCTs) that compared CPAP to placebo, conservative management, or positional therapy.[7] This systematic review concluded that CPAP was superior to placebo, conservative management, and positional therapy as demonstrated on PSG several weeks or months after treatment. Giles et al. reviewed 8 RCTs that compared CPAP to a control intervention (sham CPAP, conservative measures, no intervention, or placebo tablet).[8] Seven of the examined RCTs (parallel and partial crossover studies) showed a significant mean difference in AHI of −17 events/hour with CPAP therapy. One RCT (crossover study) demonstrated a difference in AHI of −9 events/hour with CPAP therapy. Patil et al. reviewed 11 RCTs that compared CPAP to a control intervention (sham CPAP, conservative measures, no intervention, sham surgery, placebo tablet, or nasal dilator strips).[9] A meta-analysis of these RCTs showed a significant mean difference in AHI of −23 events/hour with CPAP therapy. Another meta-analysis of these RCTs demonstrated a significant mean difference in AHI of −29 events/hour before and after CPAP therapy.[9]

In addition to showing that PAP therapy reduces the severity of OSA as measured by AHI, these reviews provide strong evidence that PAP is both effective and safe. An American Academy of Sleep Medicine (AASM) clinical practice guideline on PAP treatment of OSA endorsed good practice statements including recommending treatment of OSA with PAP therapy.[10] Thus, all OSA patients should be offered PAP therapy.

SLEEPINESS

The Epworth Sleepiness Scale (ESS) is a validated questionnaire that subjectively measures excessive daytime sleepiness, a common complaint among patients with untreated or undertreated OSA.[11] ESS scores range from 0 to 24, with a score of ≥10 suggesting significant daytime somnolence and a score of ≥16 suggesting severe daytime somnolence. The Maintenance of Wakefulness Test (MWT) is a tool that objectively quantifies daytime somnolence. The MWT measures the ability to remain awake in soporific circumstances.[12] Excessive sleepiness during the day can have dangerous consequences, and patients may suffer impaired performance at work and are more likely to have motor vehicle accidents.[13]

Given the long history of CPAP therapy for OSA, there is a significant amount of high-quality evidence demonstrating the effectiveness of PAP to reduce sleepiness. Of the studies discussed in the following, 3 were systematic reviews with 1a level of evidence (systematic reviews with homogeneity of RCTs) and 1 was an RCT with 1b level of evidence (individual RCT with a narrow confidence interval). The clinical endpoint for all 4 studies was daytime sleepiness.

Marshal et al. reviewed 7 RCTs comparing CPAP to placebo or conservative management.[14] This meta-analysis demonstrated significant reduction in subjective sleepiness (ESS) by 1.2 points and improved objective daytime wakefulness (MWT) by 2.1 minutes. McDaid et al. reviewed 48 studies comparing CPAP versus alternatives (placebo, mandibular advancement device, no treatment).[15] This review concluded that CPAP significantly reduced ESS scores compared to control (mean difference: −2.7; 95% confidence intervals [CI]: −3.45, −1.96). Neikrug et al. conducted an RCT involving 38 patients with Parkinson's disease who received PAP for 6 weeks versus placebo for 3 weeks followed by PAP for 3 weeks[16] and concluded that 3 weeks of therapeutic CPAP resulted in overall decreases in daytime sleepiness (p = 0.011). Patil et al. performed a meta-analysis on 38 RCTs comparing PAP versus no PAP[9] and concluded that there was clinically significant improvement in sleepiness with the use of PAP to treat adults with OSA as compared with no treatment. In summary, PAP therapy is highly effective in reducing daytime sleepiness as measured by ESS and MWT among patients with OSA.

MORTALITY

It is now widely recognized that OSA is associated with increased morbidity and mortality due to the adverse effects on the cardiovascular system. While PAP therapy can improve both the severity of OSA and daytime sleepiness, there is uncertainty about a mortality benefit from the current scientific literature.

The 3 studies discussed in the following provide mixed evidence of a mortality benefit using PAP for OSA. Sánchez-de-la-Torre et al. conducted an RCT that enrolled 1264 patients randomized to CPAP treatment plus usual care versus usual care alone.[17] The clinical endpoint was cardiovascular mortality and all-cause mortality, and the level of evidence was 1b. This RCT concluded there was no significant benefit with CPAP therapy for cardiovascular mortality (hazard ratio 0.83) or all-cause mortality (hazard ratio 0.82). Patil et al. performed 2 systematic reviews of 4 RCTs comparing CPAP to no CPAP and 9 non-randomized trials comparing PAP versus control conditions.[9] The clinical endpoint was all-cause mortality for both reviews and the level of evidence was 1a and 2a (systematic reviews with homogeneity of cohort studies), respectively. These reviews concluded that CPAP therapy did not reduce all-cause mortality (risk ratio 0.96); however, there was significant variability in CPAP adherence. A meta-analysis of non-randomized trials demonstrated a clinically significant reduction in all-cause mortality (risk ratio 0.4). Huang et al. performed an RCT involving 83 patients randomized to CPAP versus no therapy.[18] The clinical endpoint was severe cardiovascular and cerebrovascular events (including death), and the level of evidence was 1b. This RCT concluded there was a non-significant trend toward lower severe cardiovascular and cerebrovascular events, with 1 death in the control group. In summary, there is no conclusive evidence showing a clear mortality reduction with PAP therapy for OSA.

CARDIOVASCULAR DISEASE/HYPERTENSION

OSA is a risk factor for several important cardiovascular disorders, most notably stroke and hypertension.[19] Mansukhani et al. performed a meta-analysis evaluating the ability of PAP to reduce major adverse cardiovascular events among patients with OSA.[20] This study evaluated 10 RCTs involving a total of 7266 patients. CPAP was used in all studies with the exception of 1 trial that used adaptive servo-ventilation as the intervention. The primary endpoint of this meta-analysis was a composite endpoint of major adverse cardiovascular events defined as cardiovascular death, nonfatal acute coronary syndrome, nonfatal stroke, or hospitalization for unstable angina. There was no significant association of PAP with major adverse cardiovascular events with relative risk 0.77 (95% CI: 0.53–1.13) and $p = 0.19$. Javaheri et al. examined the effect of PAP therapy to reduce blood pressure using data from the Apnea Positive Pressure Long-term Efficacy Study (APPLES), a randomized, sham-controlled double-blinded study designed to assess the impact of CPAP on neurocognition[21]; 1,101 patients with OSA were included in this analysis, and blood pressure recordings from baseline, 2 months, and 6 months were analyzed. The largest reduction was 2.4 mmHg in the morning systolic pressure that occurred at 2 months in the CPAP arm as compared to an approximately 0.5 mmHg reduction in the sham group (CPAP effect: −1.9 mmHg; $p = 0.008$). At 6 months, the difference between groups decreased and was no longer statistically significant (CPAP effect: −0.9 mmHg; $p = 0.12$). In summary, among patients with OSA there is minimal lowering of blood pressure, and there is no convincing evidence that PAP therapy reduces major adverse cardiovascular events.

QUALITY OF LIFE

Patients with untreated OSA often report symptoms that include gasping, arousals, unrefreshing sleep, excessive daytime sleepiness, sleep fragmentation, dry mouth, and morning headaches. Snoring, a common sign of obstructive sleep apnea, is often unnoticed by patients until reported by bed partners, roommates, or family members. While the snoring may not be bothersome to patients, it can interfere with the sleep of those nearby and consequently cause interpersonal conflict. Frequently, patients must sleep in separate rooms from their partners due to their loud habitual snoring. Increased arousals from untreated OSA may lead to heightened motor activity that disturbs the bed partner's sleep and can be so pronounced that it is mistaken for rapid eye movement (REM) behavior disorder. In addition, untreated OSA can contribute to periodic limb movements and non-rapid eye movement (NREM) parasomnias that can disrupt the bed partner's sleep.

Tools used to assess the effect of OSA on sleep-related quality of life (QOL) include the Calgary Sleep Apnea Quality of Life Index (SAQLI), which consists of 40 questions across 5 domains,[22] and the Functional Outcomes of Sleep Questionnaire (FOSQ), which consists of questions regarding the degree of difficulty in completing 30 different tasks divided among 5 domains.[23] Many other non-OSA QOL measurement instruments exist.

CPAP has been shown to improve sleep-related QOL in patients with OSA, a fact supported by decades of RCTs, systematic reviews,[24] and the recent AASM Clinical Practice Guideline.[10] Some of the literature suggests that QOL improvements are more likely to be seen in patients with more than 4 hours of nightly adherence.[25] While impairment of QOL has not been found to be directly proportional to OSA severity,[26,27] some literature suggests that CPAP may be more likely to improve QOL in those with moderate or severe OSA.[25] The improvement in QOL also can extend to the bed partners of OSA treated with CPAP.[27,28] QOL outcomes are similar when comparing treatment with PAP therapy following in-laboratory titration and direct initiation of APAP therapy (without a laboratory-based study) using both global (non-OSA-specific QOL) and sleep-specific QOL.[9]

The current AASM Clinical Practice Guideline published in 2019 gives a conditional recommendation[10] for PAP use for patients with OSA with impaired sleep QOL, noting that meta-analyses do not demonstrate clinically significant improvement of global QOL, but conclude that based on OSA-specific QOL improvement with CPAP therapy, as evidenced by improvement in SAQLI and FOSQ scores, "in adult patients with OSA and impaired sleep-related QOL, the benefits of PAP therapy compared to no PAP therapy likely outweigh the potential harms and burdens."[10]

NEUROCOGNITIVE EFFECTS

OSA can adversely affect neurocognitive domains, including daytime sleepiness, attention and vigilance, learning and memory, motor skills, and executive function.[29] Individual studies have found improvements in specific neurocognitive domains such as verbal memory and executive function[30] or psychomotor and cognitive processing speed.[31] However, a meta-analysis of 9 RCTs evaluating the effect of treatment of OSA with CPAP for at least 1 month found that overall neurocognitive function was not improved.[9]

BILEVEL PAP (BPAP)

BPAP functions by providing an inspiratory positive airway pressure and a lower expiratory positive airway pressure during sleep. It was developed by Mark Sanders and Nancy Kern, who demonstrated in their landmark paper in 1990 that effective OSA treatment with BPAP could be achieved with a lower pressure setting than that needed with CPAP.[32] BPAP is frequently used when OSA patients require higher pressure settings than can be achieved with CPAP.

As an initial treatment for OSA, BPAP has not been shown to be superior to CPAP therapy. A recent practice guideline commissioned by the AASM reviewed meta-analyses[9] of four RCTs[7,33–35] and did not show significant differences in efficacy, adherence, or self-reported sleepiness with BPAP versus CPAP. The meta-analysis of 2 RCTs[7,35] demonstrated a non-significant reduction of 2.2 events/hour for residual AHI in BPAP compared to CPAP. The meta-analysis of 4 RCTs[7,33–35] showed a mean adherence in the BPAP group of only 0.08 hours less than the CPAP group. Finally, a meta-analysis of 3 RCTs[7,33,35] revealed no significant difference in Epworth Sleepiness Scale scores between BPAP and CPAP groups.

BPAP may be beneficial for patients who have previously struggled with CPAP adherence. A retrospective study[36] evaluated data from a PAP telemonitoring database on 1496 patients who were non-adherent to CPAP therapy. With a change to BPAP therapy, there was an increase in mean usage of 0.9 hours/day (p <0.001). A small prospective study[37] evaluated subjects with OSA who were previously intolerant to CPAP therapy (average use <4 hours/night). With initiation of BPAP therapy, there was an increase in mean daily use (increase of 1.7 + 1.7 hours/day) compared to CPAP (increase of 1.1 + 2.1 hours/day) following an intervention to address mask fit, nasal or oropharyngeal dryness, rhinitis or nasal congestion, and education and counseling regarding OSA. Another small prospective study[38] also evaluated subjects with OSA who were previously intolerant to high CPAP settings (>15 cm H_2O) and found increased BPAP use (7 hours/night) versus CPAP use (2.5 hours/night) at 6 weeks (p = 0.028). Together, these studies suggest that BPAP may be beneficial for patients who have previously struggled with CPAP adherence, although more investigation is needed to further clarify this issue.

AUTO-TITRATING PAP

By 1993, APAP devices were being used to deliver variable CPAP pressure settings to OSA patients.[39] Later, auto-adjusting algorithms were developed for BPAP devices (auto-BPAP). The development of algorithms analyzing snoring, airflow limitation, and obstruction allowed PAP pressures to be adjusted during sleep at home. APAP devices are used for a variety of indications. APAP is most commonly utilized in place of in-laboratory PAP titration PSG. Other reasons include states with significant weight fluctuations (as seen with bariatric surgery and pregnancy), incomplete in-laboratory PAP titration studies, fixed PAP pressure intolerance, use of alcohol or sedative-hypnotic agents, and body position or sleep stage changes. The use of APAP may be disadvantageous when it results in sleep disruption due to pressure fluctuations or the development of treatment-emergent central sleep apnea. Recent meta-analyses[9] demonstrated no significant difference in OSA severity, adherence, QOL, sleepiness, neurocognitive function, or side effects between APAP and CPAP. This study did not determine a consistent pattern of patient preference for APAP versus CPAP and recommended that patients with OSA discuss their individual needs for a particular device with their sleep medicine provider.

ADHERENCE

A major barrier to the effective treatment of obstructive sleep apnea remains adherence to PAP therapy. An analysis examining quoted PAP adherence rates from 82 studies ranging over a time span of 20 years (1994–2015) found a mean average nightly use of 4.6 hours and a "non-adherence rate" (with optimal adherence defined in this review as 7.0 hours of use per night) of 34%.[40] This study initially demonstrated no significant improvement in PAP adherence rates over this 20-year period, and that patients tended to over-report their nightly usage when compared to objective data.

Poor adherence can be due to a host of factors ranging from psychosocial barriers (unstable housing, inability to afford PAP devices or PAP supplies), comfort issues/side effects from PAP therapy, or patient-specific factors (forgetting to use PAP, poor "buy-in" to treatment). When addressing patient non-adherence to PAP therapy, it is essential to identify the underlying barriers to adherence. The availability of educational resources for patients regarding PAP use may have a positive impact on adherence rates.[9] Additionally, behavioral interventions, such as cognitive behavioral therapy or motivational enhancement therapy, and peer support groups may likewise improve PAP adherence.[41] Remote monitoring and telemedicine have been utilized to assess PAP use and have been shown to have a beneficial effect on PAP adherence rates, although telemonitoring is not yet a universal option for patients or sleep medicine providers.[41] Web-based proprietary CPAP patient engagement applications which utilize coaching and support services have also led to improved CPAP adherence.[41] Mask discomfort is a common cause of non-adherence, with some sources stating that a nasal mask offers adherence benefit over an oronasal mask,[42] while others suggest that there is no clear overall adherence benefit to any particular mask style.[9] Mask refitting, including switching mask styles, can be effective in improving patient comfort and consequently consistent PAP usage. Overall, it is currently felt that a nasal mask should be the first choice for most patients[42] with possible advantages in leak rates, residual event rates, and airway patency. An oronasal mask may still be a preferred choice for certain patients for comfort and fit reasons or because of oral air leak or nasal congestion precluding the use of a nasal mask.

A meta-analysis of 10 RCTs did not find a clinically significant difference in adherence in patients with OSA treated with APAP versus a PAP titration study.[9] Patient-specific factors may still lead to adherence differences between initiation of treatment with APAP when compared to PAP titration. For example, some patients may find PAP titration cost-prohibitive, or may live in a remote area without convenient access to a sleep laboratory. Conversely, some patients may have better adherence following a PAP titration study as this allows an opportunity to find a comfortable, well-fitting mask and an optimal pressure setting under the supervision of sleep technicians. Adherence was likewise found to be no different with BPAP when compared to CPAP overall.[9] It should be noted that at higher pressures, BPAP may be better tolerated than CPAP as the pressure support leads to more comfortable exhalation, which could lead to adherence differences on a case-by-case basis.

ADVERSE EVENTS/SIDE EFFECTS

Common causes of discomfort with PAP therapy include discomfort with the mask interface and headgear, dry mouth, air leak, aerophagia, pressure intolerance, and claustrophobia. While rarely dangerous and often easily addressed, providers must be vigilant in addressing these symptoms, as they can lead to PAP non-adherence. The overall side-effect profiles of CPAP versus APAP are similar.[9]

Discomfort with the mask interface can often be addressed by the durable medical equipment companies, which can refit patients with a more comfortable mask. If a patient has a prior history of mask discomfort, choosing to perform an in-laboratory PAP titration, as opposed to using APAP, allows the patient to try multiple mask styles and sizes in a controlled environment.

Dry mouth can be caused by a number of factors. Air flowing through the oropharynx can cause uncomfortable drying of the mucous membranes. In patients with nasal masks, opening of the mouth can cause air venting and worsen dry mouth, which can be addressed with use of a chin strap. The majority of modern PAP machines use heated humidification, and it is important to counsel patients to fill the humidifier reservoirs nightly and adjust the humidification settings for peak comfort. Use of heated tubing can minimize condensation of water in the PAP tubing and lead to optimal delivery of humidified air.

To address the problem of air leak, it is important to first localize the leak. Leak can originate from the machine itself, the interface of tubing and the machine, the tubing itself, the interface of the tubing and the mask, from the mask itself, or, most frequently, from a compromise of the seal between the mask and the face. In addition to changing the tubing, headgear, mask, and mask cushion at regular intervals, it is important that the patient is comfortable adjusting and securing the mask to the face to minimize leak and maximize comfort.

Aerophagia occurs when air from the PAP machine enters the gastrointestinal tract, which can in turn lead to abdominal bloating, belching, and flatulence. Contributing factors to aerophagia include use of high PAP pressures and positioning that decreases the airflow resistance to the upper GI tract. Consequently, aerophagia is best treated by using the lowest effective PAP pressures, PAP with a modified pressure profile, or BPAP in conjunction with optimal positional therapy.

Pressure intolerance is a broad term that encapsulates discomfort as a result of subjectively elevated PAP pressures. Patients may describe pressure intolerance as dyspnea, difficulty with exhalation, a "smothering" sensation, or merely a sensation of "too much pressure." It is important for clinicians to differentiate dyspnea from pressure intolerance from dyspnea due to other medical causes, such as cardiopulmonary disease. Care should be given to use the minimum effective PAP pressures to prevent pressure intolerance. The use of lateral positional therapy often allows for the use of lower pressures. With pressure intolerance affecting adherence, clinical judgment should be used to weigh the risks and benefits of lowering pressure settings below the minimum effective pressure. PAP with a modified pressure profile and BPAP can also be utilized for patients with pressure intolerance.

Claustrophobia with mask use is a complicated entity with psychological and physical contributors. Patients may have had traumatic experiences in the past that predispose them to claustrophobia. Sometimes, use of a lower-profile interface, such as nasal pillows, can be sufficient to address this symptom. Otherwise, gradual desensitization to the offending stimuli should be recommended, generally starting while the patient is awake and out of bed, and eventually advancing to use of PAP during sleep.

Treatment of OSA with PAP therapy can precipitate central sleep apnea (CSA). PAP therapy is not advised for patients with a significant burden of CSA on their baseline sleep study. Some patients, however, may have no CSA risk factors and baseline study showing pure OSA, yet still develop treatment-emergent CSA. This should be suspected in patients started on APAP who fail to respond to therapy, have worsening of their symptoms once therapy is started, or whose PAP-generated data are suggestive of CSA. Likewise, patients on non-auto-adjusting PAP therapy, regardless of duration of treatment or risk factors, may develop treatment-emergent CSA. These patients should undergo an in-laboratory PAP titration study to evaluate treatment-emergent CSA and to determine appropriate PAP settings for treatment of sleep-disordered breathing.

Rare, but potentially harmful, adverse events stemming from PAP use include pneumocephaly, intraocular hypertension, and pulmonary barotrauma. Pneumonia risk is increased in OSA patients, perhaps more prominently in those undergoing treatment with PAP therapy.[43] It is important that PAP therapy be used with caution in patients at risk for aspiration, as PAP use may increase risk of pneumonia in these patients. It is likewise important that PAP equipment be cleaned regularly, and the humidifier water reservoir be cleaned and refilled consistently, as Legionnaires' disease has been associated with PAP use in case studies.[44] Lastly, it is important to carefully address nonspecific symptoms such as headache, nausea, chest discomfort, and dyspnea. These symptoms may be secondary to PAP therapy, or possibly represent a more concerning condition such as coronary artery disease.

Over 40 years have elapsed since Colin Sullivan applied CPAP therapy to his first human subject. CPAP, BPAP, and APAP have all been widely utilized for the care of OSA patients with great success. Other treatment options for OSA have come and gone over the years, but nothing has yet supplanted the crucial role of PAP therapy.

REFERENCES

1. Dickens C. *The Posthumous Papers of the Pickwick Club*. London: Chapman and Hall; 1837.
2. Dring T. *Aelianus C: Various History: Book IX*. London: Printed for Thomas Dring at the George in Fleetstreet near St. Dunstan's Church; 1666.
3. Coccagna G, Mantovani M, Brignani F, et al. Tracheostomy in hypersomnia with periodic breathing. *Bull Physiopathol Respir (Nancy)*. 1972;8(5):1217–1227.
4. Motta J, Guilleminault C, Schroeder JS, et al. Tracheostomy and hemodynamic changes in sleep-inducing apnea. *Ann Intern Med*. 1978;89(4):454–458.
5. Sullivan CE. Nasal positive airway pressure and sleep apnea: Reflections on an experimental method that became a therapy. *Am J Respir Crit Care Med*. 2018;198(5):581–587.
6. Sullivan CE, Issa FG, Berthon-Jones M, et al. Reversal of obstructive sleep apnoea by continuous positive airway pressure applied through the nares. *Lancet*. 1981;1(8225):862–865.
7. Gay P, Weaver T, Loube D, et al. Evaluation of positive airway pressure treatment for sleep related breathing disorders in adults. *Sleep*. 2006;29(3):381–401.
8. Giles TL, Lasserson TJ, Smith BJ, et al. Continuous positive airways pressure for obstructive sleep apnoea in adults. *Cochrane Database Syst Rev*. 2006;3:CD001106.
9. Patil SP, Ayappa IA, Caples SM, et al. Treatment of adult obstructive sleep apnea with positive airway pressure: An American Academy of Sleep Medicine systematic review, meta-analysis, and GRADE assessment. *J Clin Sleep Med*. 2019;15(2):301–334.
10. Patil SP, Ayappa IA, Caples SM, et al. Treatment of adult obstructive sleep apnea with positive airway pressure: An American Academy of Sleep Medicine clinical practice guideline. *J Clin Sleep Med*. 2019;15(2):335–343.
11. Johns MW. A new method for measuring daytime sleepiness: The Epworth sleepiness scale. *Sleep*. 1991;14(6):540–545.
12. Mitler MM, Gujavarty KS, Browman CP. Maintenance of wakefulness test: A polysomnographic technique for evaluation treatment efficacy in patients with excessive somnolence. *Electroencephalogr Clin Neurophysiol*. 1982;53(6):658–661.

13. Spicuzza L, Caruso D, Di Maria G. Obstructive sleep apnoea syndrome and its management. *Ther Adv Chronic Dis*. 2015;6(5):273–285.
14. Marshall NS, Barnes, M, Travier N, et al. Continuous positive airway pressure reduces daytime sleepiness in mild to moderate obstructive sleep apnoea: A meta-analysis. *Thorax*. 2006;61(5):430–434.
15. McDaid C, Duree KH, Griffin SC, et al. A systematic review of continuous positive airway pressure for obstructive sleep apnoea-hypopnoea syndrome. *Sleep Med Rev*. 2009;13(6):427–436.
16. Neikrug AB, Liu L, Avanzino JA, et al. Continuous positive airway pressure improves sleep and daytime sleepiness in patients with Parkinson disease and sleep apnea. *Sleep*. 2014;37(1):177–185.
17. Sánchez-de-la-Torre M, Sánchez-de-la-Torre A, Bertran S, et al. Effect of obstructive sleep apnoea and its treatment with continuous positive airway pressure on the prevalence of cardiovascular events in patients with acute coronary syndrome (ISAACC study): A randomised controlled trial. *Lancet Respir Med*. 2020;8(4):359–367.
18. Huang Z, Liu Z, Luo Q, et al. Long-term effects of continuous positive airway pressure on blood pressure and prognosis in hypertensive patients with coronary heart disease and obstructive sleep apnea: A randomized controlled trial. *Am J Hypertens*. 2015;28(3):300–306.
19. Lavie P, Pro: Sleep apnea causes cardiovascular disease. *Am J Respir Crit Care Med*. 2004;169(2):147–148; discussion 150.
20. Mansukhani MP, Somers VK, Shafazand S. PAP and cardiovascular events in adults with sleep apnea: Is PAP useful? *J Clin Sleep Med*. 2017;13(12):1487–1489.
21. Javaheri S, Gottlieb DJ, Quan SF. Effects of continuous positive airway pressure on blood pressure in obstructive sleep apnea patients: The Apnea Positive Pressure Long-term Efficacy Study (APPLES). *J Sleep Res*. 2020.;29(2):e12943.
22. Flemons WW, Reimer MA. Development of a disease-specific health-related quality of life questionnaire for sleep apnea. *Am J Respir Crit Care Med*. 1998;158(2):494–503.
23. Weaver TE, Laizner AM, Evans LK, et al. An instrument to measure functional status outcomes for disorders of excessive sleepiness. *Sleep*. 1997;20(10):835–843.
24. Moyer CA, Sonnad SS, Garetz SL, et al. Quality of life in obstructive sleep apnea: A systematic review of the literature. *Sleep Med*. 2001;2(6):477–491.
25. Batool-Anwar S, Goodwin JL, Kushida CA, et al. Impact of continuous positive airway pressure (CPAP) on quality of life in patients with obstructive sleep apnea (OSA). *J Sleep Res*. 2016;25(6):731–738.
26. Dutt N, Janmeja AK, Mohapatra PR, et al. Quality of life impairment in patients of obstructive sleep apnea and its relation with the severity of disease. *Lung India*. 2013;30(4):289–294.
27. Coman AC, Borzan C, Vesa CS, et al. Obstructive sleep apnea syndrome and the quality of life. *Clujul Med*. 2016;89(3):390–395.
28. Parish JM, Lyng PJ. Quality of life in bed partners of patients with obstructive sleep apnea or hypopnea after treatment with continuous positive airway pressure. *Chest*. 2003;124(3):942–947.
29. Seda G, Han TS. Effect of obstructive sleep apnea on neurocognitive performance. *Sleep Med Clin*. 2020;15(1):77–85.
30. Antic NA, Catcheside P, Buchan C, et al. The effect of CPAP in normalizing daytime sleepiness, quality of life, and neurocognitive function in patients with moderate to severe OSA. *Sleep*. 2011;34(1):111–119.
31. Richards KC, Gooneratne N, Dicicco B, et al. CPAP Adherence may slow 1-year cognitive decline in older adults with mild cognitive impairment and apnea. *J Am Geriatr Soc*. 2019;67(3):558–564.
32. Sanders MH, Kern N. Obstructive sleep apnea treated by independently adjusted inspiratory and expiratory positive airway pressures via nasal mask: Physiologic and clinical implications. *Chest*. 1990;98(2):317–324.
33. Powell ED, Gay PC, Ojile JM, et al. A pilot study assessing adherence to auto-bilevel following a poor initial encounter with CPAP. *J Clin Sleep Med*. 2012;8(1):43–47.
34. Reeves-Hoché MK, Hudgel DW, Meck R, et al. Continuous versus bilevel positive airway pressure for obstructive sleep apnea. *Am J Respir Crit Care Med*. 1995;151(2 Pt 1):443–449.
35. Blau A, Minx M, Peter JG, et al. Auto bi-level pressure relief-PAP is as effective as CPAP in OSA patients: A pilot study. *Sleep Breath*. 2012;16(3):773–779.
36. Benjafield AV, Pepin JD, Valentine K, et al. Compliance after switching from CPAP to bilevel for patients with non-compliant OSA: big data analysis. *BMJ Open Respir Res*. 2019;6(1):e000380.
37. Ballard RD, Gay PC, Strollo PJ. Interventions to improve compliance in sleep apnea patients previously non-compliant with continuous positive airway pressure. *J Clin Sleep Med*. 2007;3(7):706–712.
38. Ishak A, Ramsay M, Hart N, et al. BPAP is an effective second-line therapy for obese patients with OSA failing regular CPAP: A prospective observational cohort study. *Respirology*. 2020;25(4):443–448.
39. Berthon-Jones M. Feasibility of a self-setting CPAP machine. *Sleep*. 1993;16(8 Suppl):S120–S121; discussion S121–S123.
40. Rotenberg BW, Murariu S, Pang KP. Trends in CPAP adherence over twenty years of data collection: A flattened curve. *J Otolaryngol Head Neck Surg*. 2016;45(1):43.
41. Bakker JP, Weaver TE, Parthasarathy S, et al. Adherence to CPAP: What should we be aiming for and how can we get there? *Chest*. 2019;155(6):1272–1287.
42. Genta, PR, Kaminska M, Edwards BA, et al. The importance of mask selection on continuous positive airway pressure outcomes for obstructive sleep apnea: An official American Thoracic Society workshop report. *Ann Am Thorac Soc*. 2020;17(10):1177–1185.
43. Su VY, Liu C, Wang H, et al. Sleep apnea and risk of pneumonia: A nationwide population-based study. *CMAJ*. 2014;186(6):415–421.
44. Stolk JM, Russcher A, van Elzakker EPM, et al. [Legionella pneumonia after the use of CPAP equipment]. *Ned Tijdschr Geneeskd*. 2016;160:A9855.

Chapter 7

Oral Appliance Therapy for Obstructive Sleep Apnea

Gail Demko and Mitchell Levine

INTRODUCTION

There is an increasing role for knowledgeable dentists in the management of sleep-related breathing disorders, in particular, the use of oral appliance therapy (OAT) to manage obstructive sleep apnea (OSA). OAT encompasses 2 significant iterations of removable devices: the mandibular repositioning device (MRD), which is typically tooth retained and moves and maintains the mandible in an advanced position; and the tongue retaining device (TRD). These appliances alter upper airway (UA) shape, size, and dynamics through a variety of anatomical modifications. Phenotypic considerations, its role in adjunctive therapy, as well as the acknowledgment of improving positive and negative predictors of OAT success, can serve to increase effectiveness of the MRD. Lastly, there may be an expanding role for the dentist and other dental specialists to participate in the care of pediatric obstructive sleep apnea (POSA). The use of orthodontic therapies, growth modification, and other dental interventions are included.

HISTORY OF OAT

With the single exception of Pierre Robin's 1923[1] article on the use of a monobloc mandibular advancement appliance to treat severely retrognathic adolescents with UA obstruction, the inception of successful oral appliance therapy (OAT) for the treatment of OSA was coincident with that of continuous positive airway pressure (CPAP).[2] The initial iteration was the tongue retaining device (TRD), based on a technique for opening the airway during chloroform anesthesia.[3] The TRD was developed in the late 1970s by Charles Samelson; he and Rosalind Cartwright published a case series of 14 subjects using a custom-made soft ethylene vinyl acetate TRD which effectively held the body of the tongue forward by suction[4] (Figure 7.1). The all-male cohort achieved a drop in apnea index (AI) from 55.6 to 27.2; outcomes reported as comparable with uvulopalatopharyngoplasty (UPPP) and tracheostomy."[4p]

Subsequently, Meier-Ewert, a Germany neurologist, postulated that the jaw thrust

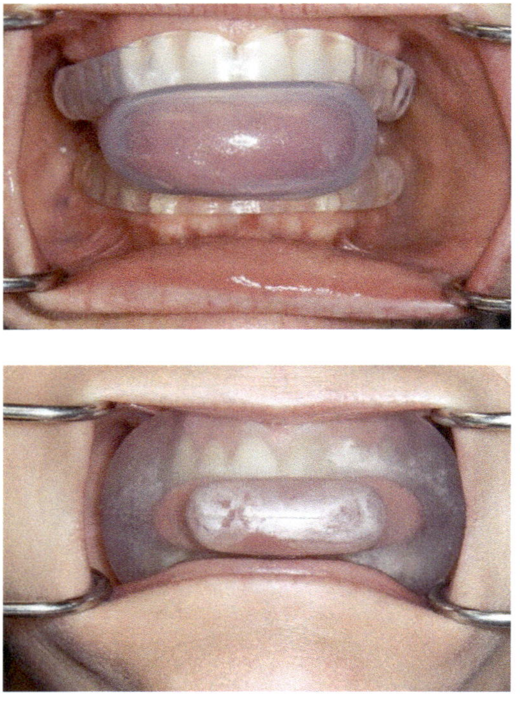

Figure 7.1. Top: Custom made tongue retaining device Bottom: Prefabricated tongue retaining device Courtesy of Nancy Addy, DDS

maneuver (known in Europe as the Esmarch-Heiberg maneuver) might be valuable in maintaining the airway.[5,6] Meier-Ewart consulted his dentist, Heinrich Shäfer, who fabricated a one-piece (monobloc) acrylic resin device oral which would mimic this maneuver.[7] Coincidently, a letter to the editor of the *New England Journal of Medicine* was published by Soll and George, describing successful independent treatment of a patient with severe OSA using a modified orthodontic device.[8] These appliances remain the basis of all present-day oral appliances (OAs) in design and action.

ORAL APPLIANCE TYPES, DESIGNS, CUSTOMIZATION

The most commonly used type of OA is the MRD. Today, with limited availability and sparse supporting data, a custom TRD is infrequently prescribed, and prefabricated TRDs are more readily available. TRD use is often relegated to patients who do not meet criteria for the more effective MRD.[9]

The U.S. Food and Drug Administration (FDA) has approved over 200 iterations of MRDs.[10] They vary by design, prefabricated versus personally customized, adjustability (monobloc vs. bibloc), as well as by the various methods of maintaining the mandibular position and amount of separation of the incisors. Some allow placement of an objective compliance monitor.[11] Others have additional mechanisms which are purported to act as nasal dilators, palatal expanders, and other adjunctive mechanisms.[11,12]

Prefabricated versus Custom Fitted

OAs are available either as a prefabricated, often thermoplastic, version, while others are custom fabricated. Prefabricated thermoplastic MRDs account for a large percentage of OAs cleared by the FDA and, in 2017, were granted over the counter (OTC) status for the treatment of snoring.[13] With a hard exterior and thermoplastic lining that softens when placed in hot water, the lining is impressed as the patient bites into it. (Figure 7.2 A, B, C). Outcomes, adherence, and comfort are variable, depending on factors such as design of the thermoplastic MRD, the severity of OSA, and the expertise of the person fitting the appliance—all of which is complicated by the lack of consensus on a definition of success.[14] In studies where patients fit their own device, the final number of those reaching an AHI <5 was 17%–29% and attrition rates were high, with 33%–78 % discontinuing therapy within 3 months.,[14-16] In studies where the oral appliance was fit in the office of an otolaryngologist, the ability to control mild OSA (AHI <5) was 24% with the thermoplastic OA, but 64% with a custom OAm; patient preference was highly in favor of the custom OAm.[17-19] Adherence, using PAP criteria, was 58.5% at 2 months.[20] When the thermoplastic MRD was fitted by a dentist with knowledge of OAT, the device becomes a custom-fitted thermoplastic device, and outcomes and adherence improve even in those with more severe OSA.[21-24] While thermoplastic appliances can be fit to most patients, their use is limited by the variability of tooth position, arch form, and jaw size.[25]

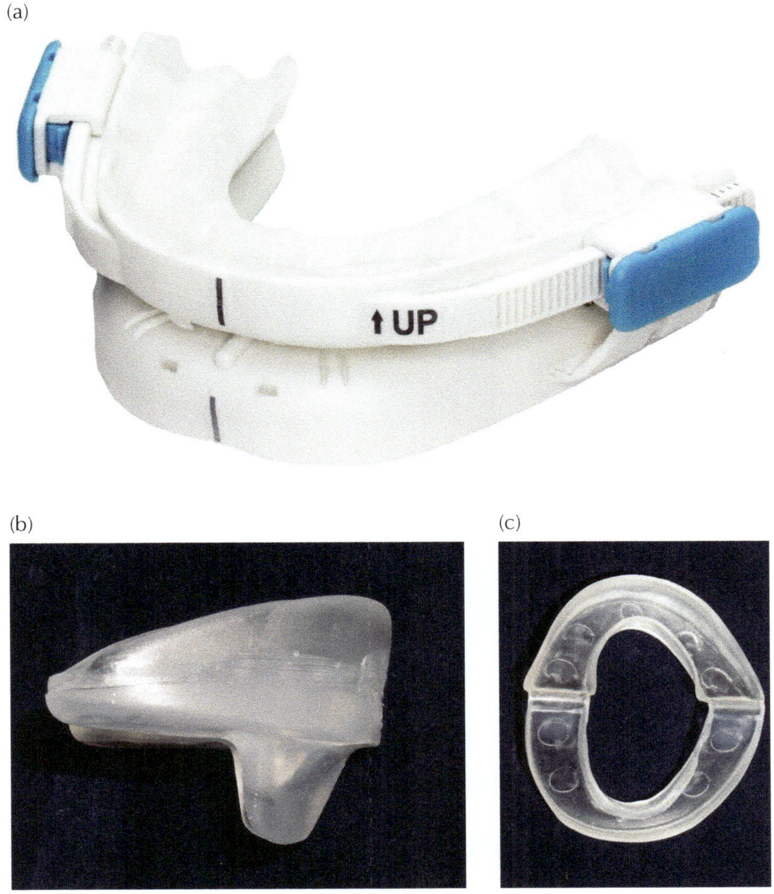

Figure 7.2. A Bibloc Prefabricated Thermoacrylic oral appliance(Courtesy of NewSom and www. Newmed.Fr. B) Two different types of Monobloc Prefabricated Thermoacrylic oral appliances

Custom-fabricated adjustable MRDs are considered the standard of care[26] (Figure 7.3, A, B, C & D). They are made by a dental laboratory from impressions/scans made in the dental office, and with a dental prescription that may alter the design based on the patient's pretreatment occlusion, range of motion, and dental situation. Materials vary from nylon printed, to polycarbonate, hard acrylic, or cast metal. A standardized gauge is required to ascertain the mandibular protrusive range of each patient on a linear scale. Most studies report the optimal mandibular position as a percentage of that person's individual protrusive range. These ranges can vary from 0 to 20 mm, and a 50% advancement in one patient may be very different from 50% advancement in another. Custom-fabricated MRDs are better fitting as well as more comfortable, retentive, and effective than prefabricated OAs.[17,27] Patients not only prefer custom-fabricated MRDs, they also are more adherent to therapy.[28]

Monobloc versus Bibloc Appliances

Monobloc MRDs are one piece and allow no adjustment of mandibular position. Multiple studies have shown monobloc OAs to be effective in reducing AHI and resolving patient symptoms, and they are well accepted by patients.[29,30] The inability to optimize mandibular position with a monobloc OA may limit the use of this style of device to those with mild OSA.[31,32]

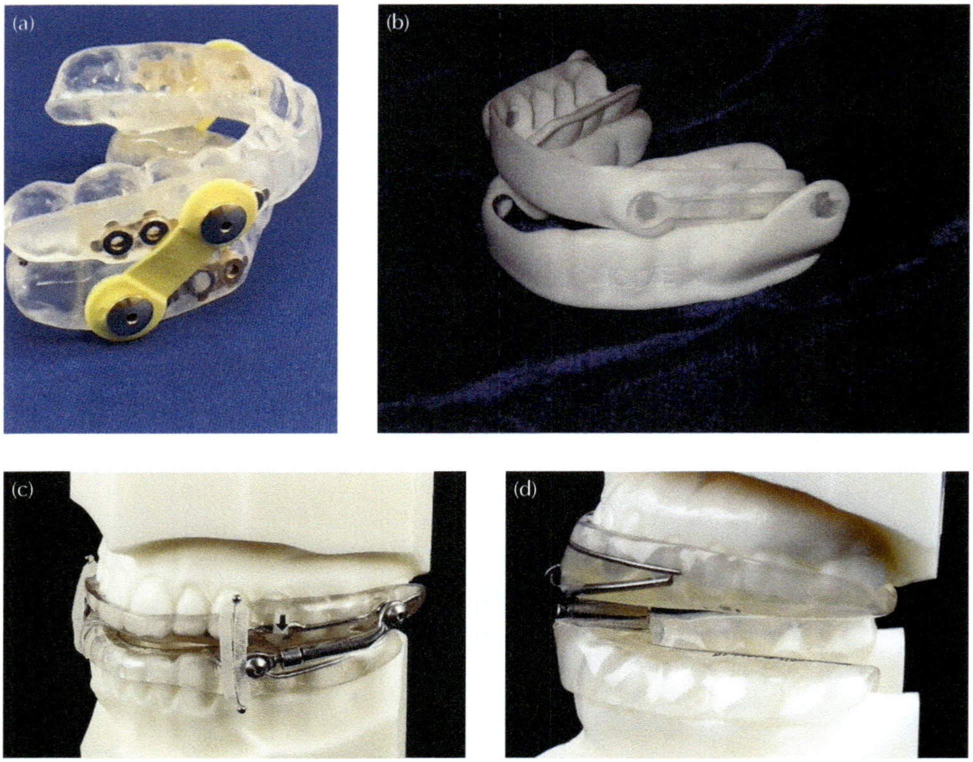

Figure 7.3. Four types of Custom made adjustable Bibloc oral appliances displaying various materials, hardware designs and contours.

A: Courtesy of Robert Rogers, DDS. C&D: Courtesy of Great Lakes Orthodontic Laboratories, Tonawanda, NY

Bibloc MRDs consist of 2 separate segments; each retained on a dental arch. The intersegment adjustment device can be elastic/silicon straps, a metal threaded contrivance, hooks and bars or even various ratchet mechanisms that allow for alteration of mandibular position in both a horizontal and vertical dimension. The ability to adjust the oral appliance is important since the exact mandibular position required for effective treatment is individually unique. While there is a dose-response relationship between mandibular position and airway opening, this nonlinear relationship is based on the design of the MRD and the unique response of that patient.[33–36] Mandibular advancement is required for success of all MRDs, but conflicting data about vertical opening are common since research rarely takes into account the underlying craniofacial presentation of the patient. Studies strongly support the importance of the need for mandibular protrusion, but understanding of the degree of interincisal opening, referred to as "vertical," is ongoing.[37–40]

Similar to PAP, no single mandibular position is effective in every instance of OAT. To achieve the optimal mandibular position requires "titration" or "calibration" of the mandibular position. This results in both improved subjective and functional outcomes.[41–43] Gradually advancing the mandible allows the patient to subjectively determine the balance between symptomatic improvement and discomfort or other unwanted side effects.[44] Ma found that, in an Asian population, the dose-dependent relationship between mandibular protrusion was asymptotic and AHI improvement was linear only until 70% of maximal mandibular protrusion. The position of optimal mandibular advancement also varied with the severity of OSA. "The target protrusion for patients with mild, moderate, and severe OSA was 3.5

± 1.8 mm (38.6 ± 19.4% maximal mandibular protrusion), 5.8 ± 1.9 mm (62.9 ± 18.8% maximal mandibular protrusion), and 5.9 ± 2.2 mm (68.8 ± 15.6% maximal mandibular protrusion), respectively."[45p] Titration during sleep testing has been shown to provide optimal outcomes in terms of AHI reduction, but studies have yet to tie this drop in AHI to medical and functional outcomes.[41,43,44] Re-evaluation by the treating physician is required to determine adequate patient response.

SCREENING PATIENTS FOR OAT

Dentists providing OAT may develop a systemized screening protocol to determine patient suitability for the oral device. A dental evaluation, including a temporomandibular joint (TMJ) and periodontal assessment, are needed to determine the feasibility of OAT and the pretreatment status of the dentition. Dental contraindications may include widespread decay, worn teeth that provide no mechanical retention, or severe periodontal involvement. Periodontal disease is the most common cause for loss of supporting bone and may preclude the practicality of OAT.[46] Amelioration of dental issues may allow for patients who are initially unsuited for therapy to become eligible for OAT.[47] Conventional dental radiographs (panoramic and/or periapical) are required as part of the dental evaluation. There is no need for further dental imaging, including, but not limited to, cephalometric radiographs, sonography, CBCT or magnetic resonance imaging (MRI). None of these imaging modalities has been shown to predict success or failure of OAT or to determine a successful mandibular position for construction of an appliance.[48–52] TMJ dysfunction (TMD) is also not necessarily a contraindication to OAT, unless there is acute disease, pathology, or the presence of severe symptoms which may limit mandibular movement.[53] Some pretreatment jaw sounds, such as clicking, may resolve with OAT. Patients must be able to open their mouths wide enough to allow placement of the oral appliance (>1 cm) while also demonstrating an adequate range of mandibular motion.[25] Patients should have at least 8 healthy teeth per arch, and multi-rooted posterior teeth are considered superior to incisors for retention. Fewer than 8 teeth may provide adequate device retention, but the forces generated from an active device will concentrate over reduced root surface with an increased likelihood of occlusal changes to the dentition. Osseo-integrated dental implants can be excellent for device retention, and the long-term stability of dental implants, even in the face of heavy forces, makes OAT possible in completely edentulous patients.[54]

Dentists require specific knowledge of OAT[55] and are expected to manage patient concerns about comfort with device alteration, support adherence, and determination of the appliance's subjective therapeutic position.[56] Communication with the referring physician should include an initial letter to verify that the patient has been evaluated and the suitability, or lack thereof, for OAT. Additional correspondence should be considered at the time of device placement and when the patient is ready to return to the physician for follow-up evaluation. Periodic recall is suggested on a 6–12-month schedule, for as long as the patient is using the OA. A lack of adherence to therapy should be reported to the referring physician in a timely manner.[57]

PURPORTED METHODS OF ACTIONS OF MRDS

The exact action of mandibular advancement remains elusive. The various suppositions may be interrelated and include alteration in the airway anatomy and possibly neuromuscular control. While many theories have been posited and explored, there remains no consensus.

Anatomical changes of the UA with MRDs have been accepted for more than 30 years.[58] Improvement in UA size has been verified by lateral cephalometry, 3-D MRI, computed tomography (CT) imaging, acoustic reflection, and nasendoscopy.[59–63] The anterior wall of the velopharynx decreases in curvature, allowing for improved airway dynamics,[64] with reduced airflow velocity as well as airway pressure predominantly retropalatally and at the epiglottic tip.[65,66] While all segments of the UA show an increase in size, predominantly in a lateral dimension, these alterations in size and shape vary between responders to MRD and non-responders. Even in patients successful with OAT, the UA shows inconsistent increase in the area of the velopharynx, oropharynx, and hypopharynx, and changes in UA geometry alone do not significantly correlate with treatment response.[67] Direct impact on UA anatomy is thought to be related to stabilization of the mandible in both a forward and relatively closed position. Mandibular advancement alters the position of the tongue via the genioglossus muscle attachment to the genial tubercles on the inner aspect of the anterior mandible. This results in forward movement of the tongue and is thought to prevent relapse of the tongue during sleep. Responders to MRD tend to show anterior displacement of the tongue and a decrease in its length.[68] There is anterior movement of the entire tongue in those with a low AHI, rather than the antero-posterior elongation seen in non-responders.[69] Alteration in tongue position secondarily impacts the palatoglossal and palatopharyngeal arches lateral to the soft palate, and contiguous soft tissue of the UA. Attachments of the hyoid musculature to the mandible result in forward and cephalad movement of the hyoid.[70] Brown hypothesizes that mandibular attachment of the buccinator muscle impacts the lateral dimension of the UA, most likely via the pterygomandibular raphé (PMR), an aponeurotic connection between the buccinator muscle and superior pharyngeal constrictor.[69] Absence of the PMR (36% of people) allows further advancement of the mandible, a greater increase in midline antero-posterior airway diameter, a lower post-treatment AHI, and increased success with OAT.[71,72] Anatomic alterations are also impacted by the subject's head position and level of consciousness.[73–75] Stabilization of the mandible, with reduced mouth opening, impacts the tendency for posterior rotation of the mandible and tongue relapse.[76,77] Jugé and his colleagues looked at the impact of mandibular advancement, in awake patients, on inspiratory tongue movement. They concluded that rather than the MRD resulting in only anatomical changes, there is a complex interaction between anatomical and inspiratory dilatory function which influences an individual's response to OAT.[78] The impact of tongue movement appears to have both a direct and indirect influence on the UA size with individual variability.

Understanding of the neuromuscular impact of mandibular advancement is limited and has predominantly been carried out in animal studies, normal humans, or awake subjects with OSA.[79–82] Responders to MRD have a trend for more activity in the temporalis, masseter, and submandibular muscles than non-responders at both baseline and when the OA is in place.[83] The increase in genioglossus EMG appears significant during wakefulness, but data in sleeping patients are confounded by lack of direct genioglossus EMG measurement.[84,85] In studies during sleep, Kurtlemas et al. found that the resting EMG amplitudes in the submental muscles increased significantly with MRD use in both those with mild OSA and those with moderate OSA. However, the mean EMG amplitude was lower in those with moderate OSA than those with mild OSA, demonstrating a difference in the pattern of EMG activation between the two groups.[86] In subjects with severe OSA, researchers found that while Pcrit improved with mandibular advancement in a dose-dependent manner in responders, non-responders improved Pcrit more with lesser advancement; this improvement with less protrusion was inadequate to effectively improve AHI. The study reported that neither the number of flow arousals nor genioglossus responsiveness changed with mandibular advancement. Bamagoos went on to say that, in this group of severe sleep apneics, there was no difference in pharyngeal muscle effectiveness between MRD responders and non-responders. This may indicate a physiologic difference between subjects with more severe OSA from those with mild OSA. Alteration in neuromuscular activity provided by mandibular advancement may have only a small impact on OSA.[85]

Since mandibular advancement predominantly impacts anatomy, non-anatomical traits related to OSA are thought to be the major impediment to a positive outcome. Research in this area seeks to evaluate the interaction of OAT and non-anatomic phenotypes during natural sleep. Edwards and his colleagues stated: While considering that "there may be a synergistic effect of OA therapy and dilator muscles, manifest as a greater ability of for the upper-airway muscles to dilate and restore flow with reduction in mechanical load on OA therapy . . . we found no change in UA gain. . . . The magnitude of muscle compensation between active and passive conditions was similar on OAT and do [*sic*] not appear to have substantial impact on OSA pathophysiology through improving dilator muscle effectiveness."[87p] In order to predict efficacy requires understanding exactly how the MRD impacts the pathophysiology of the OSA—a relationship that remains very complex.[87]

COMPARATIVE OUTCOMES

MRD versus MRD or No Treatment

The earliest outcome studies of oral appliance intervention were done at a time prior to stratification of OSA severity[88] and concluded that an MRD can be a viable treatment alternative for many patients with OSA stressing the need for a team approach for management of the patients with OSA.[89] By 1996, most studies of MRD effectiveness included only primary snorers, or those with mild-moderate OSA.[58,90–92] There was general control of bothersome snoring, but the response was more variable in those diagnosed with OSA.[93] Vezina compared 2 MRDs with different propulsion mechanisms to see if the method of mandibular advancement impacted side effects. After 2 years, he found no difference in compliance, satisfaction, or objective and subjective efficacy.[94] No single custom MRD has yet been shown to be superior in long-term clinical outcomes such as AHI, RDI, oxygen saturation, or subjective sleepiness; and, other than bulk, preference for a specific MRD has not been elucidated.[95,96] For those patients who respond positively to OAT, the reduction in blood pressure (BP) remains statistically significant for up to 3 years.[97–100] When compared to no treatment, MRDs have been shown to effectively treat the majority of patients with mild to moderate OSA and 25%–46% of those with severe OSA.[11,43,101]

MRD versus Placebo

Comparison of MRD with a placebo device commonly uses a sham OA or an inactive MRD.[102–104] Marklund et al., in a randomized, placebo-controlled trial evaluating improvements in daytime sleepiness and quality of life (QOL) realized a post-treatment AHI <5 in 49% of a trial group and 11% in the control group. Snoring and symptoms of restless legs were also statistically less frequent in patients using the active treatment. When compared with the placebo, there was no improvement in daytime sleepiness. QOL was assessed with the Short-form 36-Item Health Survey (SF-36) and the Functional Outcomes of Sleep Questionnaire (FOSQ), neither of which showed a significant between-group difference.[105] While there are individual studies with contradictory findings,[106] most studies have supported Marklund's findings.[107] Andrén et al. looked at 24-hour mean systolic BP and found a stronger BP reduction in the group using the active MRD. After excluding patients with normal baseline ambulatory BP and patients with a baseline AHI ≤15, they found a 24-hour mean systolic BP reduction of 4.4 mmHg (95% CI: 0.1 to 8.7; $p = 0.044$).[108]

MRD versus UPPP

Uvulopalatopharyngoplasty (UPPP) was an early comparator with OAT. In 1999, Wilhelmsson and colleagues published on 95 sleep apneics with subjective daytime sleepiness and an apnea index (AI) >5. Randomization resulted in 49 patients in the MRD group and 47 in the UPPP group. In this study, OAT provided a better outcome than surgery. Normalization (AI <5 and AHI <10) occurred in 78% of those with an MRD and in 51% of those who underwent UPPP.[109] Additional studies completed on this sample found that subjective daytime sleepiness was similar in both groups regardless of treatment. QOL domains of Vitality and Sleep were comparable post-treatment, but the domain of Contentment was statistically better in the surgical group.[110] A later study also showed efficacy of the MRD and improved polysomnographic (PSG) variables remained steady over 4 years, though adherence to OAT had declined to 62%.[111]

MRD versus PAP

A 2010 metanalysis of 8 studies comparing OAT to PAP found that PSG improvements favored PAP with AHI of −7.7 events/hr, $p < 0.001$. Minimum oxygen saturation remained lower with an MRD (−3.5%) and arousals were more common than with PAP. There was no statistically significant difference in sleep efficiency or time in rapid-eye movement (REM) sleep, nor was there any difference in objective sleepiness as measured with the ESS. Neither intervention was superior in FOSQ, Sleep Apnea Quality of Life Index (SAQLI), or neurocognitive tests.[112] More recent studies have supported these findings, and it may be that there is no difference beyond a placebo effect.[113] Additional studies have found no difference between MRD and PAP in other functional outcomes, including: driving performance, subjective sleep quality, nocturia, psychological distress, and on the Pittsburgh Sleep Quality Index (PSQi).[114–117] Sutherland proposed that higher adherence to OAT may explain the comparable functional outcomes between PAP and MRD.[118] Unlike PAP, no dose-response studies have been done of OA adherence and functional outcomes.[119,120]

When compared to MRD, PAP is consistently superior in improving PSG outcomes, but other objective outcomes are less consistent. Several studies have found improved BP recordings with MRD,[121,122] while others found no difference in outcomes with either treatment.[109,116] In studies of moderate to severe OSA, a subgroup with preexisting hypertension (HTN) had a significant reduction in 24-hour diastolic BP only with PAP.[123] Anandam evaluated the cardiovascular mortality in patients with severe OSA who were treated with either PAP or MRD. There were 42 patients who had a fatal cardiovascular event over a median follow-up of 79 months (76–88 months). The non-apneic group had the lowest cardiovascular death rate (0.28 per 100 person-years) followed by the PAP-treated (0.56 per 100 person-years) and the MRD-treated group (0.61 per 100 person-years). The highest cardiovascular mortality rate was observed in the untreated group (2.1 per 100 person-years). There was no difference in cardiovascular death rate between those treated with PAP and MRD, despite a significantly higher residual AHI in those with an MRD (16.3 ± 5.1/h vs. 4.5 ± 2.3/h; p <0.001). (Anandam) A recent study by Ou found an MRD was not inferior to CPAP for reducing 24-hour mean arterial P in participants with hypertension and increased cardiovascular risk. (Ou Yi-Hui) Both PAP and MRD have been shown to improve other markers of daytimes cardiac function when measuring heart rate variability (HRV), continuous blood pressure and baroreceptor sensitivity in a group with predominantly mild-moderate OSA.[124] In a study of severe apneics treated with MRD, Gagnadoux found no improvement in endothelial function.[128] A randomized controlled study by Silva et al. evaluated the impact of PAP and MRD on dyslipidemia over a 1-year period. While PAP adherence was lower, PAP was still more effective in reducing total cholesterol and low-density lipoprotein cholesterol. In contrast with other studies, they found no statistical difference in insulin metabolism (HbA1C, Insulin (mg/dL)), HOMA B, or uric acid between the 2 treatments.[125,126] "Studies assessing the effect of OAT on circulating cardiovascular biomarkers, endothelial function and arterial stiffness, generally involved small numbers of patients and were heterogeneous and inconclusive."[127p]

SIDE EFFECTS OF OAT

While the mean side effect score is the same regardless of PAP use or OAT, the majority of side-effects with OAT relate to their design similarities with orthodontic devices.[42] OAT typically requires life-time adherence with resultant orthodontic forces directed to the dentition and supporting structures. Patients may report short-term subjective side effects, while objective side effects are often unnoticed.[129,130]

Short-term side effects are normally related to the fit of the device on the dentition and forces exerted by mandibular advancement. At any point in therapy, a patient may express concerns regarding device fit and/or retention and, based on the complaint, the dentist may need to adjust the fit chairside, or in rare cases, consider laboratory techniques to appropriately correct the fit. Device design is an important consideration because, by nature, MRDs can be bulky and may cause soft tissue irritation; they may also impede full mouth closure, resulting in obvious saliva on the pillowcase in the morning or complaints of dry mouth.[128] Patients may experience a gag reaction to the MRD, a feeling of being "constrained," or even an allergic reaction to one of the components. While these are rare occurrences, the providing dentist must be aware of the possibility that these can occur and be prepared to manage them. Patient reassurance and the management of these side effects will help to improve MRD adherence.

Both the dentition and supporting periodontal structures, as well as the TMJ, are subject to orthopedic forces by the MRD. The teeth may experience initial discomfort as pressure from the MRD causes mild edema in the surrounding periodontal ligament. Commonly, the discomfort resolves after removal of the MRD each morning. In a similar fashion, facial muscle tenderness or a transient edematous response in the TMJ may occur with the MRD in place as the mandibular condyle experiences a mild displacement within the glenoid fossa of the temporal bone. Upon device removal, most patients will experience a normal anatomical repositioning of the condyle without incident. Some patients may experience protracted difficulty with normal seating of the mandible; the dentist can address this with palliative care, jaw-stretching exercises, verification of mandibular position during treatment, or alteration of the MRD calibration sequence.[129] It is rare that transient pain interferes with continued OA use.[53]

Over time, there may be long-term side effects related to the orthodontic forces created by the MRD, resulting in permanent tooth movement. This has been noted as early as 6 months, and tooth movement is known to continue, with decreasing severity, for up to 18 years. (Minagi) The magnitude of occlusal changes is not related to the number of teeth, but to the frequency of MRD use and the amount of mandibular advancement.[28,131] The maxillary incisors tend to displace toward the palate, while the mandibular incisors tend to move labially. Protective factors against occlusal changes include higher body mass index (BMI) and an initial deep bite.[28] As patients are rarely aware of alterations in tooth positions, the dentist must maintain strict follow-up and inform the patient if occlusal changes are noted.[132] With proper support and care, dental side-effects do not lead to discontinuing therapy.[133]

PREDICTORS OF OA SUCCESS

The major concern when using oral appliances in the treatment of OSA rests mostly on the clinical inability to determine who will respond favorably to therapy. The various anthropometric variations, respiratory endotypes, design of the MRD, and lack of standardized procedures all impact success with mandibular advancement, as do idiosyncratic anatomical variations in patients.[134] Anthropometric data, easily gathered in a clinical setting, have been shown in some studies to correlate with MRD success. These include low BMI, female sex, lower neck/waist circumference, and younger age, as well as a shorter soft palate.[135] These data are unsupported in other studies, and there appears to be significant racial disparity.[136–139] Other morphological features, such as Mallampati score or pretreatment retroglossal space, do not appear predictive,[140] and combinations of craniofacial characteristics and anthropometric findings have been proposed with little success.[141] Predictive craniofacial characteristics as assessed from cephalometric radiographs, including the cranial base angle, hyoid position, and retrognathic mandible or retracted maxilla, have been correlated with MRD success in many studies; however, the data are inconsistent and no prognostic findings were found that reliably discriminated between poor and good responders.[48] A scoping review of these same features reported no AHI changes for any given trait, and therefore "the majority of the anatomical features for good vs. limited responders may be considered *generalized indicators* of AHI reduction."[134] Other imaging techniques which evaluate the size and shape of the airway or area of narrowing, such as CT and acoustic reflectometry, were also found to be poorly predictive.[51,142–146]

Prefabricated thermoplastic MRDs have been put forth as one alternative to discern whether custom devices will positively impact outcomes.[147,148] Early iterations of thermoplastic MRDs were often bulky and poorly retentive and resulted in a lack of compliance with uncertain effectiveness.[149] More recent versions of these prefabricated devices are thinner, less bulky, and appear to be more retentive.[150] Trzepizur did a real-life observational study in which patients received a thermoplastic MRD, advanced the mandible to a position of subjective improvement or maximum comfort and, after 6 months, were offered the option of a custom-made MRD. Only a small percentage of the subjects (40/111) went on to long-term care with an MRD. A high side-effect rate, ineffective outcome, intolerance of the thermoplastic OA, and preference for an alternative treatment option were all found to impact continued treatment. While there was a high positive predictive value (86%), there was a low negative predictive value (46%).[151] Still, there is little evidence to support or refute the benefit of these trial devices as either predictors of success of a future custom OA, or the ability of the trial device to determine an appropriate therapeutic position for a custom OA. With simple, inexpensive clinically available predictors being unreliable and lacking robust sensitivity, specificity, or consistent cut-off values, there is a trend toward more elaborate strategies to predict OAT outcomes.[152]

Evaluation of actual pharyngeal function was hoped to improve prediction models, and nasopharyngoscopy is a common, clinically based, technique.[153] Sutherland et al. concluded that "qualitative assessment of awake nasopharyngoscopy appears useful for assessing the effect of mandibular advancement on UA collapsibility. However, it is not sensitive enough to predict oral appliance outcome."[154p] This moved researchers to evaluate the functioning airway during sleep-like conditions. Drug-induced sleep endoscopy (DISE) has engendered significant literature aimed at predicting OAT outcomes. Potential limitations to DISE include alteration in neuromuscular function related to use of local anesthetic in the nose, the impact of sedation on the collapsibility of the UA, failure to induce REM sleep, inability to exactly mimic the mandibular position created by the OA with manual manipulation, and the lack of globally agreed-upon protocols for scoring, dosimetry, and sedation administration.[155–160]

PSG parameters have been evaluated as indicators of OA success with contradictory results. Patients with high AHI, REM dominance, or no positional dominance are thought to be less likely to achieve adequate treatment with OAT than those with less severe disease or supine OSA.[112,161–165] Other studies do not support these data or find them unreliable in ruling out non-responders.[135] Recent advances comparing anatomic variations noted during normal sleep with PSG findings have led to a new area of exploration.[87] Using data that are available on a laboratory-based PSG, researchers have looked at respiratory endotypes that may predict MRD response. These data look not only at anatomic variables, but various respiratory and physiologic phenotypes.[135,166–169] The evaluation of arousal threshold, Pcrit, and loop gain from available PSG data has indicated that OAT is most likely to be effective in patients with mild anatomic compromise, moderate pharyngeal collapsibility, and a higher arousal threshold.[87,170,171]

Remote-controlled mechanical positioning (RCMP) of the mandible during sleep testing is thought to mimic the titration of an oral appliance in a single night. Optimization of mandibular position is most consistent when a custom-fitted MRD is titrated during PSG, and using this technique, 41.5% of patients with *severe* OSA can achieve an AHI <5.[172] Various forms of mechanical titration have been developed, which can be carried out without causing arousals.[44,173] Titration can be done during in-laboratory PSG or in a home setting.[174] Sutherland et al. found that the diagnostic characteristics of the RCMP had a sensitivity of 81.8%, specificity of 92.9%, positive predictive value of 90%, and negative predictive value of 86.7% (n = 3 were misclassified).[175] Other studies showed comparable outcomes, except for a negative predictive value of 72%.[176] One major advancement of the RCMP compared to titration of the custom-fitted OA during PSG is that the patient need not be awakened to alter mandibular position.[177] Follow-up testing, with the MRD in place, remains required to verify the effectiveness of the determined mandibular position.

ADHERENCE TO OAT

Objective adherence data, using temperature microsensors, are relatively recent in the field of OAT.[178,179] All previous studies gathered subjective adherence data from sleep diaries and questionnaires. Subjective reports of compliance with OAT were higher than objective findings with PAP, and this difference was thought to explain why there was little difference in outcomes when comparing the 2 treatment options.[72,114,148,180] Subsequent studies comparing subjective reports of compliance with objective data, subjective reports were found to have less than a 30-minute difference in use of either MRD or PAP.[179] More importantly, after 1-year, objective compliance between the OAT and PAP does not appear to be dissimilar.[116,181] Xu found that while the overall use of therapy was not statistically different, the *pattern* of use was. In a randomized, multi-centric study with different MRDs versus PAP, the MRD was used fewer nights (4.4 ± 2.9 vs. PAP 4.7 ± 1.6) but for more hours (6.4 ± 1.9 vs. PAP 5.7 ± 1.2), resulting in comparable utilization of treatment option.[120]

Adherence to OAT decreases with time; the curve representing patients who discontinue therapy is steepest in the first year of use, then appears to flatten. Studies reported 1-year dropouts to be 9.8%–55% of subjects.[2,182,183] Similar to PAP, use in the first week appears to predict long-term use.[5] One factor related to adherence is obviously ineffective therapy. The severity of OSA may be a factor, and failure of therapy is expected to be highest in severe OSA.[184] While some studies have shown adherence highest in those with mild-moderate disease,[121,185] others found superior adherence in those with severe OSA, and 57.7% of patients with severe OSA continued use 44.30 ± 17.3 months after placement.[12,186] Attali found dropout rates were higher among females (65% vs. 35%) and those who were obese (40% vs. 21%), and obese patients were withdrawn for lack of success more than non-obese (44% vs. 19%).[187] Despite a third of patients being inadequately treated with mandibular advancement as defined by less than 50% reduction in AHI, only 22% of patients give insufficient efficacy as a reason for discontinuing therapy.[188] Other factors that correlate with poor adherence are side effects such as a dry mouth, discomfort,[189] a type D "distressed" personality,[190] daily smoking,[191] and those who feel OAs are bothersome to use.[9,128]

Those who continue to use OAT long term are often younger and more concerned about the negative side effects of untreated OSA.[192] Veterans with post-traumatic stress disorder (PTSD) were found to be more compliant with OAT than PAP, using their MRD 5.66 $\pm$ 2.43 hr/night versus 3.4 $\pm$ 2.48 hr/night for PAP.[117] Long-term adherence studies show those who continue to use their appliance are satisfied with the treatment, and 93.7% of continuing users used the MRD more than 4 nights per week at 5 years.[14] Occlusal changes which occur after years of OAT or a return of symptoms may increase the dropout rate. Personalized appliance design and customization can impact the number and severity of side effects and can thus help improve compliance.[37] Long-term follow-up of all patients with OAT by a dentist experienced in this field is important since, as with orthodontic appliances, it is likely that the relationship between the clinician and patient plays a key role in patient adherence to OAT.[193]

ADJUNCTIVE THERAPY

"Oral appliances (OAs) are becoming increasingly recognized not only as an alternative to but also possibly as an adjunct treatment modality for OSA."[28p] Some MRDs have added attachments and extensions that are purported to improve AHI reduction. One such device has flexible buttons that sit in the labial vestibule under the upper lip proximal to the lateral aspect of the nares. While FDA-cleared as nasal dilators, no studies have yet shown improved outcomes with the added attachment.[11] With 50%–60% of patients presenting with supine-dependent OSA,[194] Dieltjens et al. looked at combining OA with a chest-worn sleep-position trainer (SPT) to reduce the time the patient spent sleeping supine. The OA alone significantly reduced the overall AHI from 20.8 at baseline to 11.0, and with SPT alone the AHI was reduced to 11.1. However, when the therapies were combined, the resulting median AHI was 5.7, significantly lower than either treatment individually.[195]

Investigators evaluating the adjunctive benefit of MRD in patients who exhibited limited improvement with uvulopalatopharyngoplasty (UPPP) alone,[196,197] or in those who had undergone a combination of UPPP and genial advancement surgery, found an improved reduction in AHI and higher SaO_2 nadir.[198] MRDs have also been used in conjunction with hypoglossal nerve stimulation (HGNS) which may provide an additive improvement in AHI.[199,200] Studies that look at OAT as rescue therapy were limited in scope, but imply that OAT can provide adjunctive benefit in instances of incomplete/inadequate post-surgical resolution of OSA.

The major area of adjunctive therapy has looked at PAP and MRD, a combination that is shown to improve treatment of PAP-intolerant patients with the potential for further reduction in AHI and daytime symptoms.[201,202] Concomitant use of APAP and OAT found no significant improvement in AHI, but compliance with therapy increased 23.1% with combination therapy.[203] Tong found that combination

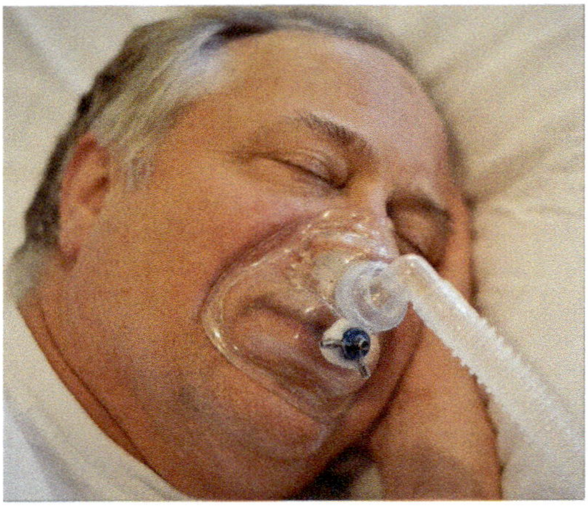

Figure 7.4. Example of interface for integrated PAP and OAT. Courtesy of Ron Prehn, DDS

therapy allowed a decrease in therapeutic PAP requirements by 35%–45% and minimized epiglottic pressure swings. In patients requiring an oro-nasal mask for PAP delivery, there is a subset of mandibular deficient patients who will experience suboptimal resolution due to the need for high effective pressure (Peff). In these patients, addition of an OA to stabilize the mandible can result in a lower Peff requirement.[204] Custom-fitted nasal pillows or masks hybridized with an OA which can be used in patients with severe claustrophobia, allergy to mask straps, or monotherapy failure[205] (Figure 7.4). Overall, oral appliance therapy should not be considered only as a monotherapy, but as one that may improve outcomes with other treatments.

ORTHODONTIC, MYOFUNCTIONAL THERAPY AND OTHER DENTAL APPROACHES TO PEDIATRIC OBSTRUCTIVE SLEEP APNEA (POSA)

The role of orthodontics, pediatric or adult, and the management of sleep-disordered breathing (SDB) remains an enigma, with a lack of robust evidentiary support. There is significant bias noted in much of the literature, with retrospective reviews, small sample sizes, and lack of controls each confounding the evidence. Physicians treating SDB should be familiar with normative pediatric facial growth and how orthodontic therapy may assist those with facial growth disturbances secondary to nasopharyngeal obstruction. In children, rapid maxillary expansion and mandibular advancement devices have been suggested to affect dimensional UA changes,[206–209] while introducing postural effects of the orofacial musculature. In the face of uncertain conviction, is the nature by which tooth extractions in orthodontics may impact the airway[210] or the path by which sleep bruxism may be associated with SRBDs.[211] Moreover, there is increasing interest in the possible role that tethered oral tissues and myofunctional therapy may play in the treatment of SRBDs in both children and adults.[212]

While an exhaustive review of normative facial growth is beyond the scope of this chapter, an understanding of growth concepts of the nasomaxillary complex and the mandible is warranted. The literature suggests numerous risk factors, including insufficient transverse maxillary development (crossbites), mandibular retrognathia, excess vertical growth with or without open bite, and inferior positioning of the hyoid bone as being associated with POSA.[213–217] Despite this finding, Pliska[218] reports that the prevalence of crossbite and overjet (maxillary protrusion) in a pediatric cohort suspected of sleep breathing concerns was no different than in the general population.

In relation to the cranial base, normative growth of the nasomaxillary complex and mandible is essentially downward and forward, away from the cranial base. This displacement provides both a sagittal and a vertical component to facial growth. As the nasomaxillary complex and the mandible translate away from the cranial base, it is the development of the alveolar processes and the teeth which provide the basis for vertical facial growth. Finally, there is sutural and periosteal growth in the maxilla and a combination of periosteal and cartilaginous growth within the mandible which provide for width development of the facial complex. Certain components of facial growth and bone remodeling may be in response to the developing nasopharyngeal airway, as suggested by Moss's functional matrix hypothesis.[219] Some have associated a shorter cranial base length (CBL)[220] with pediatric SDB, implying that shorter cranial base growth may fail to provide the desired forward translation of the nose and maxilla, resulting in a retrusion of the entire craniofacial skeleton and a smaller UA. In contrast, a systematic review of SDB and CBL found that neither an association nor lack thereof could be supported or refuted, citing high bias and low study quality.[221] Others have posited that maxillary retrusion may be a source of SDB, which may be mollified by orthopedic advancement of the maxilla, thus enlarging the pharyngeal airway.[222] Lee et al.,[223] in a systematic review of 3-D pharyngeal airway changes following expansion and protraction, conclude that the nasal passage airway volume above the palatal plane increase(s) significantly, though there was no significant difference in the airway volume below the palatal plane. These findings may call into question the potential benefit of airway enlargement in the child staving off adult-onset OSA.

Important aspects of facial growth and development are associated with the presence of lymphoid tissue within the nasopharynx. The literature is replete with the putative role of adeno-tonsillar hypertrophy in POSA.[224–226] The adenoids and tonsils follow a unique differential growth trajectory, which is different from the neural, visceral, or genital systems.[227,228] Scammon's composite curves assess growth as a percentage of total gain of these tissue systems from birth to 20 years of age. Unlike the other tissue systems, lymphoid tissue curve shows a relatively steep ascent, reaching 100% by age 8–10 and increasing to 180% around age 13–14, and then begins to involute and return to 100% by age 20. Some authors[229] posit that mouth-breathing may be a trigger for lymph enlargement and may be the genesis of excess vertical facial growth, narrow arches, and crossbites associated with POSA.

The normal course of untreated POSA may best be understood in context to the Scammon growth curve for lymph tissue. The resolution of untreated POSA in the non-syndromic population is the range of 60%–91%[230–232] and may be attributed to several aging phenomena. The involution of the tonsil and adenoid tissue both contribute to reducing of the site of nasopharyngeal collapse, and this results in a relative increase in size of the airway. Also, the forward displacement of the craniofacial skeleton and the normative lengthening of the oropharyngeal airway contribute to an absolute increase in airway dimensions. Normative pediatric airway dimensions have been described by Masoud,[233] and there does not appear to be an association with pharyngeal airway dimension and the collapsibility of the airway. A study by Schendel shows that both the minimal cross-sectional area of the airway and overall volume of the airway increase with aging up until age 30.[234] Studies which fail to include controls, or those remiss in accounting for the effects of normative growth, introduce bias and may embellish the true therapeutic effect of orthodontic intervention.

The present literature focuses on the use of orthopedic/orthodontic expansion of the jaws, with emphasis on the widening the maxilla in children. Additionally, mandibular advancement or functional devices have been implemented to encourage a retrognathic mandible to assume a more anterior or forward position. Maxillary orthopedic expansion and, in certain instances, mandibular orthodontic expansion are indicated when either one or both jaws are narrow or lack transverse coordination. Expansion of the maxilla and the resulting increase in arch perimeter are said to encourage a more forward or anterior position of the tongue. As the tongue comes forward, the base of the tongue moves out from the oropharyngeal (OP) airway and into the oral cavity, resulting in a relative increase in the OP volume. As well, the raising of the tongue has been associated with elevation of the hyoid bone, reducing the distance between the hyoid bone and the mandibular plane.[235]

Bony dimensional changes in the nose and maxilla and a reduction in nasal resistance have been attributed to maxillary expansion. An overall 12% increase in nasomaxillary volume has been seen following expansion, though less than a third of the total expansion is witnessed in the nasal vault itself.[236] Additionally, there may be some improvement in nasal septal deviation following expansion which might reduce resistance, though systematic reviews remain inconclusive.[237] Maxillary expansion has been shown to also increase nasal valve area, contributing to a reduction in nasal resistance.[238]

Rapid maxillary expansion (RME) is an orthodontic procedure in which an adjustable device increases the width of the maxilla and the nasal skeleton. The device typically exerts forces in the range of 1.18 N/mm with each millimeter of activation.[239] The forces may be delivered to the teeth or directly to the bone, dependent upon the device utilized. The intent is to open the maxillary midline suture to address crossbites of a skeletal or dental nature and, as it may relate to SDB, to make the maxilla wider regardless of the presence of crossbites. In prospective observational study of 31 children with OSA and maxillary constriction, the authors found that following a 4-month trial of RME, the AHI was reduced from 12.2 to less than 1.[240] In a quasi-longitudinal observational RME study of pediatric subjects presenting with assorted malocclusions (some with crossbites), the AHI changed differently according to the type of malocclusion. The AHI diminished more in subjects with deep and retrusive bite than in those with crossbite (6.7 ± 8.4 vs. 1.0 ± 1.0 and 4.3 ± 2.1 vs. 2.5 ± 2.2) as noted before therapy and then after 6 months and then 12 months following orthodontic therapy.[241] In contrast, a retrospective observational trial in which 45 pediatric OSA subjects without any crossbites were managed with expansion of both jaws found that one-third of the subjects had greater AHI following expansion and that only in the severe pretreatment subjects was there a statistically significant reduction in AHI.[242] A meta-analysis of 9 RME studies of low to moderate quality found that AHI values underwent a mean reduction of 5.79 events/hour; an increase in mean oxygen saturation of 2.54 % and concluded that RME may be efficient for treating slight or moderate sleep apnea hypopnea syndrome and may be effective adjunct therapy to adenotonsillectomy in severe cases of children with maxillary constriction.[243] Yet, an umbrella review of 10 systematic reviews of RME effects on the UA revealed that 80% of the reviews were of low to critically low rating and finds that while more studies measuring breathing function as related to the UA are needed, RME is an auxiliary method and should only be used when orthodontically indicated.[244]

The association of mandibular retrognathia with POSA is widely noted in the literature,[245–247] yet there is little evidence suggesting causality. The hypothesis is that a small or more posterior placed mandible may impact the pharyngeal airway, contributing to POSA. The use of a mandibular advancement device (MAD) in a growing child *may* help to normalize this sagittal discrepancy, balance the soft tissue profile, harmonize orofacial musculature, and concomitantly increase the pharyngeal volume, which may in turn lead to a reduction in the AHI and ameliorate the symptomology associated with POSA. Nazarali et al. completed a systematic review of 4 highly risked-bias articles and concluded that MAD may result in improvements in AHI scores, though complete normalization of AHI scores was not obtained.[248] In a randomized crossover trial of OSA diagnosed children aged 8–12 years, subjects were randomized to MAD or sham with a washout period. MAD reduced AHI events by 0.6 events per hour and improved O_2 saturation by 3.4 percentage points.[249] A meta-analysis based on 2 high-quality RCTs on mandibular advancement devices demonstrated a mean difference of AHI −1.75 events for the experimental group as compared to the control group.[250] The authors concluded that MAD can be effective for mild to severe patients before the end of the pubertal peak. It is important for the reader to understand that a MAD does not effectively grow the mandible more than the jaws' genetic potential and that these devices bring about an A/P change in mandibular position which will likely mirror otherwise normative growth.

Orthodontic therapy in adults to manage OSA may chiefly be relegated to surgical approaches at reducing skeletal discrepancies. Maxillomandibular advancement (MMA) has been employed to address A/P skeletal discrepancies with good success. Yet, a recent meta-analysis reviewed the maintenance of AHI improvement post-MMA in the intermediate (1 to <4 years), long (4 to <8 years) and very long term (≥8 years). Investigators found that subjects were able to maintain AHI improvement consistent with a diagnosis of mild OSA (a reduction in AHI from a mean 48.3 events/hour (95% CI: 42.1–54.5) pre-MMA to 8.4 (95% CI: 5.6–11.2) in the intermediate term and a reduction in AHI, from a mean 65.8 events/hour (95% CI: 58.8–72.8) pre-MMA to 7.7 (95% CI: 5.9–9.5) in the long term), yet subjects evaluated in the very long-term time frame experienced a reduction in AHI from a mean 53.2 events/hour (95% CI: 45–61.4) pre-MMA to 23.1 (95% CI: 16.3–29.9), which is consistent with a diagnosis of OSA in the moderate to severe range.[251]

Surgically assisted rapid palatal expansion (SARPE) of the maxilla may be utilized to address a width discrepancy in adults. Advances with mini-implant screw-assisted rapid palatal expansion (MARPE) has facilitated non-surgical expansion of the adult maxilla. In a study of 14 adults (mean age 22.7 +/− 3.3 years), investigators demonstrated that MARPE increased both the volume and the cross-sectional area of the nasal cavity and the effect was maintained 1 year post-expansion. Changes in nasal volume have been associated with a decrease in nasal resistance, and MARPE may improve breathing in young adults with maxillary constriction.[252]

The extraction of permanent teeth may be one course of orthodontic therapy in children and adults. When 4 premolars are removed to address crowding of the dentition or to affect soft-tissue profile changes, dependent upon anchorage considerations, there may be an accompanying reduction in arch perimeter. Some dentists have expressed concern that the reduction in arch perimeter could bring about a change in the positional posture of the tongue, with the tongue moving in a posterior direction and affecting the pharyngeal airway dimensions.[253] A systematic review characterized the effect on the pharyngeal airway according to the indications for tooth extraction. The indications for extraction included subjects with over or underbite (A/P) discrepancies, crowding, and unspecified reasons. Those patients who presented with A/P issues and crowding had 4 first premolars extracted and experienced a significant decrease in UA dimension. Subjects who presented with crowding alone and had 4 premolars extracted experienced an increase in the UA dimension. In the group with nonspecific extraction, all patients were adolescents and an increase in UA volume was realized after orthodontic treatment. While certain indications for extraction may result in a smaller pharyngeal airway, no relationship between UA dimensions and respiratory function has been shown, and there is no evidence that a narrowed pharyngeal airway is at increased risk for collapse.[254]

Investigators have also considered the relationship between bruxism and OSA. Bruxism is a repetitive jaw-muscle activity characterized by clenching or grinding of the teeth and/or by bracing or thrusting of the mandible which may occur during sleep (sleep bruxism, SB), or wakefulness (awake bruxism AB).[255] A study involving 1042 subjects who completed a questionnaire and a PSG found that, based on the questionnaire alone, the prevalence was 12.5%. When considering the PSG alone, the prevalence was 7.4%, yet when the questionnaire and PSG were combined, the prevalence dropped to 5.5%.[256] A systematic review seeking to discern an association between SB and OSA describes an inconclusive relationship. Findings that support an association between SB and OSA conclude that SB may be a protective response to respiratory events; that most episodes of SB occur shortly after an obstructive event or are secondary to arousals associated with an obstructive event; and there may be a correlation between the frequency of SB and obstructive events. The investigators also found non-supportive conclusions regarding any association with OSA, including that obstructive events are related to nonspecific SB activity consistent with body movements and arousals related to disturbed sleep patterns, that SB episodes do not necessarily occur at the termination of an obstructive event, and that patients with OSA do not experience more SB events as compared to a control sample.[257] It does seem clear that SB and SDB coexist and may share some common risk factors, but causality is not supported by the evidence.

Airway obstruction may lead to muscle hypotonia and may be associated with excess vertical growth of the face, and there is renewed interest in role of oral myofunctional therapy (OMFT) and the management of OSA. OMFT is a combination of isotonic and isometric exercise[258] directed at the tongue and associated oral/pharyngeal structures to strengthen the intrinsic muscles, improve lip posture, and improve spatial positioning of the tongue at rest. A meta-analysis which considered 11 studies (9 adult and 2 children) found a 50% reduction in the AHI in the adult sample and was characterized by a net change from 24.5 ± 14.3/hour to 12.3 ± 11.8/hour in the AHI. Lowest oxygen saturations improved from 83.9% ± 6.0% to 86.6% ± 7.3%, while PSG snoring decreased from 14.05% ± 4.89% to 3.87% ± 4.12% of total sleep time. The pediatric sample of 14 patients showed a reduction in AHI of 62% following OMFT.[259] Despite these findings, investigators note that the effective benefits of OMFT only remain for as long as the subject maintains the practice and that many patients become noncompliant over time.[260]

Additional interest has centered on the possibility that tethered oral tissues may lead to unfavorable facial growth resulting in growth discrepancies which may be associated with

SDB. A tethered mandibular lingual frenum, often referred to as ankyloglossia, has been implicated in some speech articulation errors and may contribute to latching challenges for the newborn. Some investigators have attributed a short frenum to restricted maxillary transverse growth and concomitant POSA. A retrospective study[261] of children with both POSA and short lingual frenum utilized maxillary expansion, AT, and lingual frenectomy as mixed therapeutics to reduce the AHI. While the AHI was reduced and oxygen levels improved, it should be noted that the subjects were growing and were afforded multiple therapies, making it difficult to attribute any single modality as particularly therapeutic. A study evaluating school-aged children with short lingual frenulum found that there was increased risk for positive correlation to a sleep screening questionnaire (Sleep Clinical Record).[262] In 2020, the American Academy of Otolaryngology–Head and Neck Surgery released consensus positions on controversies associated with tethered tissues and concluded that in some communities, infants and children are being overdiagnosed with ankyloglossia, that a significant number of children are having unnecessary surgery on the lingual frenulum, and that ankyloglossia does not cause sleep apnea.[263]

While there is a great deal of interest and excitement in the role that orthodontics and adjunctive oral therapies might play in the management of SDB, there is a lack of consensus on the efficacy of these approaches. Studies tend to be retrospective in nature, of short-term duration, and are often limited by small sample size. Systematic reviews draw inconclusive results, as there is frequently high heterogeneity among the studies, few RCT, and concerns regarding statistical bias. As is often the case, more higher quality studies are needed to help the clinician discern where benefit may exist in an effort to separate the wheat from the chaff.

SUMMARY

Oral appliances present with many different designs, and adjustable custom-made OA is considered optimal. Advancement of the mandible results in enlargement of the UA via connections between bony insertions of the tongue, suprahyoid and buccinator muscles, and associated soft tissues.

Mandibular advancement improves the anatomy of the UA predominantly in the lateral dimension, reduces the curve of the airway, and decreases Pcrit. Stabilizing the mandible in an advanced position prevents airway compromise during sleep. Impact, other than anatomical, is as yet unproven.

Compared to PAP, MRDs are less effective in reduction of AHI, but cardiovascular mortality, many functional outcomes, and BP reduction is comparable, which implies that some, as yet unknown commonality is impacted. While MRD provides dependable treatment for most patients with mild to moderate OSA as a first-line therapy, multiples studies show good results in many with severe OSA. Provision of OAs in this latter group remains limited by the present inability to predict who will be inadequately treated despite high adherence rates. Adjunctive therapy, combining MRDs with other treatment modalities, can provide improved adherence and outcomes.

Diagnosis of OSA and attendant follow-up is performed by a qualified physician. Selection of which patient is dentally qualified, the oral appliance design and device follow-up are performed by a dentist experienced in treatment of patients with OSA. Improving comfort of the MRD and addressing various patient issues will lead to improved adherence to treatment. The possibility of long-term craniofacial changes also requires continuing dental follow-up. Interdisciplinary collaboration and communication allow for improved personalization of treatment and improved patient outcomes.

The role of pediatric orthodontics in nonsyndromic patients is not well understood. Numerous studies point to the value of expansion in the growing child with OSA, yet the putative mechanism is hardly understood. Research shows that some cohorts see a benefit in airway volume, while others see no change or even a reduction. What we do know is that normative growth must play some role in moderating OSA in children. In general, females and cohorts with an AHI of less than 5 tend to resolve without any interceptive care. The CHAT multicenter trial also finds that 46% of subjects randomized to watchful waiting rather than early AT will normalize PSG findings and reported symptomology. MRDs may play a role in reducing AHI in POSA, though the net change in AHI is often only in the single digits. MRDs may play a more supportive role in airway maintenance until growth provides a more definitive resolution. Adult orthodontics frequently require adjunctive surgery to physically modify the site of flow limitation and the site of collapse in the course of OSA management. In all instances, a physician and dentist should collaborate to establish both a treatment plan and define treatment success.

REFERENCES

1. Robin P. La chute de la base de la langue considérèe comme une nouvelle cause de gêne dans la respiration naso-phayngienne. *Bull Acad Med.* 1923 Jan;LXXXIX(2)#1, 3rd series:37–41.
2. Sullivan C, Berthon-Jones M, Issa F, Eves L. Reversal of obstructive sleep apnoea by continuous positive airway pressure applied through the nares. *Lancet.* 1981;317(8225):862–865.
3. Esmarch V. *Handbuch der Kriegschirurgischen Technik. Eine gekronte Preisschrift.* Carl Rumpler; 1877:112–125.
4. Cartwright RD, Samelson CF. The effects of a nonsurgical treatment for obstructive sleep apnea: The tongue-retaining device. *JAMA.* 1982;248(6):705–709.
5. Kappeler O. *Anaesthetica.* F. Enke;1880:125–126.
6. Defalque RJ, Wright AJ. Who invented the "jaw thrust"? *Anesthesiology.* 2003;99(6):1463–1464.
7. Schwarting S. Meier-Ewert Award of the German Society of Dental Sleep Medicine. *Sleep Breath.* 2006;10:57–61.
8. Soll BA, George PT. Treatment of obstructive sleep apnea with a nocturnal airway-patency appliance. *N Engl J Med.* 1985;313(6):386.
9. Sutherland K, Deane SA, Chan AS, et al. Comparative effects of two oral appliances on upper airway structure in obstructive sleep apnea. *Sleep.* 2011;34(4):469–477.
10. https://www.accessdata.fda.gov/scripts/cdrh/cfdocs/cfPMN/pmn.cfm; LRK and LQZ.
11. Shrivastava D, Bixby JK, Livornese DS, Urena F, Bixby MJ, Jain V. Efficacy of oral appliance therapy in the treatment of severe OSA in CPAP-resistant cases. *Sleep Vigil.* 2018;2(2):119–125.
12. Singh GD, Cress SE. Biomimetic oral appliance therapy in adults with mild to moderate obstructive sleep apnea using combined maxillo-mandibular correction. *J Sleep Disord Manag.* 2017;3(1):014.
13. https://www.accessdata.fda.gov/scripts/cdrh/cfdocs/cfpmn/pmn.cfm?start_search=1&Center=&Panel=&ProductCode=plc&KNumber=&Applicant=&DeviceName=&Type=&ThirdPartyReviewed=&ClinicalTrials=&Decision=&DecisionDateFrom=&DecisionDateTo=12%2F19%2F2019&IVDProducts=&Redact510K=&CombinationProducts=&ZNumber=&PAGENUM=25.
14. Sutherland K, Dalci O. Fake it till you custom-make it: A non-inferior thermoplastic mandibular advancement device? 2019.
15. Soh L, Han HJ, Yue Y, Tay JY, Hao Y, Toh ST. Evaluation of prefabricated adjustable thermoplastic mandibular advancement devices (PAT-MADs) for obstructive sleep apnea: An Asian experience. *Sleep Med.* 202075:96–102.
16. Tsuda H, Almeida FR, Masumi SI, Lowe AA. Side effects of boil and bite type oral appliance therapy in sleep apnea patients. *Sleep Breath.* 2010;14(3):227–232.
17. Johal A, Haria P, Manek S, Joury E, Riha R. Ready-made versus custom-made mandibular repositioning devices in sleep apnea: A randomized clinical trial. *J Clin Sleep Med.* 2017;13(2):175–182.
18. Friedman M, Hamilton C, Samuelson CG, et al. Compliance and efficacy of titratable thermoplastic versus custom mandibular advancement devices. *Otolaryngol Head Neck Surg.* 2012;147(2):379–386.
19. Banhiran W, Assanasen P, Nopmaneejumrudlers C, et al. Adjustable thermoplastic oral appliance versus positive airway pressure for obstructive sleep apnea. *Laryngoscope.* 2018;128(2):516–522.
20. Friedman M, Pulver T, Wilson MN, et al. Otolaryngology office-based treatment of obstructive sleep apnea-hypopnea syndrome with titratable and nontitratable thermoplastic mandibular advancement devices. *Otolaryngol Head Neck Surg.* 2010;143(1):78–84.
21. Gagnadoux F, Nguyen XL, Le Vaillant M, et al. Comparison of titrable thermoplastic versus custom-made mandibular advancement device for the treatment of obstructive sleep apnoea. *Respir Med.* 2017;131:35–42.
22. Quinnell TG, Bennett M, Jordan J, et al. A cross-over randomised controlled trial of oral mandibular advancement devices for obstructive sleep apnoea-hypopnoea (TOMADO). *Thorax.* 2014;69(10):938–945.
23. Marty M, Lacaze O, Arreto CD, et al. Snoring and obstructive sleep apnea: Objective efficacy and impact of a chairside fabricated mandibular advancement device. *J Prosthodontics.* 2017;26(5):381–386.
24. Makihara E, Kawano T, Miyajima R, Masumi SI, Enciso R, Clark GT. Assessment of oral appliance for obstructive sleep apnea patients. *Clin Exper Dent Res.* 2016;2(2):155–161.
25. Clark GT. Mandibular advancement devices and sleep disordered breathing. *Sleep Med Rev.* 1998;2(3):163–174.
26. Scherr SC, Dort LC, Almeida FR, et al. Definition of an effective oral appliance for the treatment of obstructive sleep apnea and snoring: A report of the American Academy of Dental Sleep Medicine. *J Dent Sleep Med.* 2014;1(1):39–50.
27. Bataller A, Cabrera JA, Garcia M, Castillo JJ, Mayoral P. Cam synthesis applied to the design of a customized mandibular advancement device for the treatment of obstructive sleep apnea. *Mech Mach Theory.* 2018;123:153–165.
28. Hamoda MM, Kohzuka Y, Almeida FR. Oral appliances for the management of OSA: An updated review of the literature. *Chest.* 2018;153(2):544–553.
29. Al-Dharrab A. A randomized cross over study comparing the efficacy of two mandibular advancement appliances in the treatment of mild-moderate obstructive sleep apnea. *CRANIO®.* 2017;35(6):379–384.

30. Isacsson G, Nohlert E, Fransson AM, et al. Use of bibloc and monobloc oral appliances in obstructive sleep apnoea: A multicentre, randomized, blinded, parallel-group equivalence trial. *Eur J Orthodontics*. 2019;41(1):80–88.
31. Lettieri CJ, Paolino N, Eliasson AH, Shah AA, Holley AB. Comparison of adjustable and fixed oral appliances for the treatment of obstructive sleep apnea. *J Clin Sleep Med*. 2011;7(5):439–445.
32. Suga H, Mishima K, Nakano H, et al. Different therapeutic mechanisms of rigid and semi-rigid mandibular repositioning devices in obstructive sleep apnea syndrome. *J Cranio-Maxillofac Surg*. 2014;42(8):1650–1654.
33. Kato J, Isono S, Tanaka A, et al. Dose-dependent effects of mandibular advancement on pharyngeal mechanics and nocturnal oxygenation in patients with sleep-disordered breathing. *Chest*. 2000;117(4):1065–1072.
34. Ahrens A, McGrath C, Hägg,U. A systematic review of the efficacy of oral appliance design in the management of obstructive sleep apnoea. *Eur J Orthodontics*. 2011;33(3):318–324.
35. Patel M. Matching oral appliance designs to obstructive sleep apnea patients. *Sleep Rev*. 2017;18(1):18–21.
36. Balevi B. There is no one mandibular advancement device design that fits all for the management of obstructive sleep apnea. *J Am Dent Assoc*. 2014;145(3):280–282.
37. Pitsis AJ, Darendeliler MA, Gotsopoulos H, Petocz P, Cistulli PA. Effect of vertical dimension on efficacy of oral appliance therapy in obstructive sleep apnea. *Am J Resp Crit Care Med*. 2002;166(6):860–864.
38. Milano F, Mutinelli S, Sutherland K, et al. Influence of vertical mouth opening on oral appliance treatment outcome in positional obstructive sleep apnea. *J Dent Sleep Med*. 2018;5(1):17–23.
39. Barbero M, Flores-Mir C, Blanco JC, et al. Tridimensional upper airway assessment in male patients with OSA using oral advancement devices modifying their vertical dimension. *J Clin Sleep Med*. 2020;16(10):1721–1729.
40. García M, Cabrera JA, Bataller A, Vila J, Mayoral P. Mandibular movement analysis by means of a kinematic model applied to the design of oral appliances for the treatment of obstructive sleep apnea. *Sleep Med*. 2020;73:29–37.
41. Almeida FR, Parker JA, Hodges JS, Lowe AA, Ferguson KA. Effect of a titration polysomnogram on treatment success with a mandibular repositioning appliance. *J Clin Sleep Med*. 2009;5(3):198–204.
42. Gagnadoux F, Fleury B, Vielle B, et al. Titrated mandibular advancement versus positive airway pressure for sleep apnoea. *Eur Resp J*. 2009;34(4):914–920.
43. Pételle B, Vincent G, Gagnadoux F, Rakotonanahary D, Meyer B, Fleury B. One-night mandibular advancement titration for obstructive sleep apnea syndrome: A pilot study. *Am J Resp Crit Care Med*. 2002;165(8):1150–1153.
44. Narahara-Eno Y, Fukuda T, Taga H, Nakayama H, Inoue Y, Tsuiki S. Gradual reduction in the STOP score in patients with obstructive sleep apnea undergoing oral appliance therapy. *J Prosthodont Res*. 2021; : . JPR_D_20_00118.
45. Ma Y, Yu M, Gao X. The effect of gradually increased mandibular advancement on the efficacy of an oral appliance in the treatment of obstructive sleep apnea. *J Clin Sleep Med*. 2020;16(8):1369–1376.
46. Petit FX, Pépin JL, Bettega G, Sadek H, Raphaël B, Lévy P. Mandibular advancement devices: Rate of contraindications in 100 consecutive obstructive sleep apnea patients. *Am J Resp Crit Care Med*. 2002;166(3):274–278.
47. Sheats R, Essick G, Grosdidier J, et al. Identifying the appropriate therapeutic position of an oral appliance. *J Dent Sleep Med*. 2020;7(4): .
48. Alessandri-Bonetti G, Ippolito DR, Bartolucci ML, D'anto V, Incerti-Parenti S. Cephalometric predictors of treatment outcome with mandibular advancement devices in adult patients with obstructive sleep apnea: A systematic review. *Korean J Orthodont*. 2015;45(6):308–321.
49. Guarda-Nardini L, Manfredini D, Mion M, Heir G, Marchese-Ragona R. Anatomically based outcome predictors of treatment for obstructive sleep apnea with intraoral splint devices: A systematic review of cephalometric studies. *J Clin Sleep Med*. 2015;11(11):1327–1334.
50. Sutherland K, Almeida FR, de Chazal P, Cistulli PA. Prediction in obstructive sleep apnoea: Diagnosis, comorbidity risk, and treatment outcomes. *Expert Rev Resp Med*. 2018;12(4):293–307.
51. Petri N, Christensen IJ, Svanholt P, Sonnesen L, Wildschiødtz G, Berg S. Mandibular advancement device therapy for obstructive sleep apnea: A prospective study on predictors of treatment success. *Sleep Med*. 2019;54:187–194.
52. Friedman M, Shnowske K, Hamilton C, et al. Mandibular advancement for obstructive sleep apnea: Relating outcomes to anatomy. *JAMA Otolaryngol Head Neck Surg*. 2014;140(1):46–51.
53. Doff MH, Veldhuis SK, Hoekema A, et al. Long-term oral appliance therapy in obstructive sleep apnea syndrome: A controlled study on temporomandibular side effects. *Clin Oral Invest*. 2012;16(3):689–697.
54. Hoekema A, De Vries F, Heydenrijk K, Stegenga B. Implant-retained oral appliances: A novel treatment for edentulous patients with obstructive sleep apnea–hypopnea syndrome. *Clinical Oral Implants Res*. 2007;18(3):383–387.
55. Morgan T, Montaghue J, Melzer V, et al. Factors impacting mandibular-repositioning-device therapy at one-month. [Abstract]. *Sleep Breath*. 2007;13:301–312.
56. Ramar K, Dort LC, Katz SG, et al. Clinical practice guideline for the treatment of obstructive sleep apnea and snoring with oral appliance therapy: An update for 2015: an American Academy of Sleep Medicine and American Academy of Dental Sleep Medicine clinical practice guideline. *J Clin Sleep Med*. 2015;11(7):773–827.
57. Levine M, Bennett K, Cantwell M, Postol K, Schwartz D. Dental sleep medicine standards for screening, treating, and managing adults with sleep-related breathing disorders. *J Dent Sleep Med*. 2018;5(3): .
58. Schmidt-Nowara WW, Meade TE, Hays MB. Treatment of snoring and obstructive sleep apnea with a dental orthosis. *Chest*. 1991;99(6):1378–1385.
59. Smith SD. A three-dimensional airway assessment for the treatment of snoring and/or sleep apnea with jaw repositioning intraoral appliances: A case study. *J Craniomandib Pract*. 1996;14(4):332–342.

60. Doff MHJ, Hoekema A, Pruim GJ, Van Der Hoeven JH, De Bont LGM, Stegenga B. Effects of a mandibular advancement device on the upper airway morphology: A cephalometric analysis. *J Oral Rehabil*. 2009;36(5):330–337.
61. Iwasaki T, Takemoto Y, Inada E, et al. Three-dimensional cone-beam computed tomography analysis of enlargement of the pharyngeal airway by the Herbst appliance. *Am J Orthodont Dentofac Orthop*. 2014;146(6):776–785.
62. Sanner BM, Heise M, Knoben B, et al. MRI of the pharynx and treatment efficacy of a mandibular advancement device in obstructive sleep apnoea syndrome. *Eur Respir J*. 2002;20(1):143–150.
63. Viviano JS. Acoustic reflection: Review and clinical applications for sleep-disordered breathing. *Sleep Breath*. 2002;6(3):129–149.
64. Tsuiki S, Lowe AA, Almeida FR, Kawahata N, Fleetham JA. Effects of mandibular advancement on airway curvature and obstructive sleep apnoea severity. *Eur Respir J*. 2004;23(2):263–268.
65. Suga H, Iwasaki T, Mishima K, Nakano H, Ueyama Y, Yamasaki Y. Evaluation of the effect of oral appliance treatment on upper-airway ventilation conditions in obstructive sleep apnea using computational fluid dynamics. *CRANIO®*. 2019; :1–9.
66. Martínez A, Muñiz AL, Soudah E, et al. Physiological and geometrical effects in the upper airways with and without mandibular advance device for sleep apnea treatment. *Sci Rep*. 2020;10(1):1–9.
67. Zhao M, Barber T, Cistulli P, Sutherland K, Rosengarten G. Computational fluid dynamics for the assessment of upper airway response to oral appliance treatment in obstructive sleep apnea. *J Biomechanics*. 2013;46(1):142–150.
68. Ogawa T, Long J, Sutherland K, Chan AS, Sasaki K, Cistulli PA. Effect of mandibular advancement splint treatment on tongue shape in obstructive sleep apnea. *Sleep Breath*. 2015;19(3):857–863.
69. Brown EC, Cheng S, McKenzie DK, Butler JE, Gandevia SC, Bilston LE. Tongue and lateral upper airway movement with mandibular advancement. *Sleep*. 2013;36(3):397–404.
70. Chan AS, Sutherland K, Schwab RJ, et al. The effect of mandibular advancement on upper airway structure in obstructive sleep apnoea. *Thorax*. 2010;65(8):726–732.
71. Shimada K, Gasser RF. Morphology of the pterygomandibular raphe in human fetuses and adults. *Anat Rec*. 1989;224(1):117–122.
72. Brown EC, Jugé L, Knapman FL, et al. Mandibular advancement splint response is associated with the pterygomandibular raphe. *Sleep*. 2020; : .
73. Isono S, Tanaka A, Sho Y, Konno AI, Nishino T. Advancement of the mandible improves velopharyngeal airway patency. *J Applied Physiol*. 1995;79(6):2132–2138.
74. Gale DJ, Sawyer RH, Woodcock A, Stone P, Thompson R, O'Brien K. Do oral appliances enlarge the airway in patients with obstructive sleep apnoea? A prospective computerized tomographic study. *Eur J Orthodont*. 2000;22(2):159–168.
75. Neelapu BC, Kharbanda OP, Sardana HK, et al. Craniofacial and upper airway morphology in adult obstructive sleep apnea patients: A systematic review and meta-analysis of cephalometric studies. *Sleep Med Rev*. 2017;31:79–90.
76. Lowe AA, Sjöholm TT, Ryan CF, Fleetham JA, Ferguson KA, Remmers JE. Treatment, airway and compliance effects of a titratable oral appliance. *Sleep*. 2000;23:S172–S178.
77. Amatoury J, Kairaitis K, Wheatley JR, Bilston LE, Amis TC. Peripharyngeal tissue deformation, stress distributions, and hyoid bone movement in response to mandibular advancement. *J Appl Physiol*. 2015;118(3):282–291.
78. Jugé L, Yeung J, Knapman FL, et al. Influence of mandibular advancement on tongue dilatory movement during wakefulness and how this is related to oral appliance therapy outcome for obstructive sleep apnoea. *Sleep*. 2020; : . doi:10.1093/sleep/zsaa196.
79. Liu CY, Lu HY, Dong FS, et al. Effects of a mandibular advancement device on genioglossus in obstructive sleep apnoea hypopnea syndrome. *Eur J Orthodont*. 2015;37(3):290–296.
80. Tsuiki S, Ono T, Kuroda T. Mandibular advancement modulates respiratory-related genioglossus electromyographic activity. *Sleep Breath*. 2000;4(2):53–57.
81. Matsuda M, Ogawa T, Sitalaksmi RM, et al. Effect of mandibular position achieved using an oral appliance on genioglossus activity in healthy adults during sleep. *Head Face Med*. 2019;15(1):1–7.
82. Johal A, Gill G, Ferman A, McLaughlin K. The effect of mandibular advancement appliances on awake upper airway and masticatory muscle activity in patients with obstructive sleep apnoea. *Clin Physiol Funct Imaging*. 2007;27(1):47–53.
83. Ma SYL, Whittle T, Descallar J, et al. Association between resting jaw muscle electromyographic activity and mandibular advancement splint outcome in patients with obstructive sleep apnea. *Am J Orthodont Dentofac Orthop*. 2013;144(3):357–367.
84. Yoshida K. Effect of a prosthetic appliance for treatment of sleep apnea syndrome on masticatory and tongue muscle activity. *J Prosthet Dentistry*. 1998;79(5):537–544.
85. Bamagoos AA, Cistulli PA, Sutherland K, et al. Dose-dependent effects of mandibular advancement on upper airway collapsibility and muscle function in obstructive sleep apnea. *Sleep*, 2019;42(6):zsz049.
86. Kurtulmus H, Cotert S, Bilgen C, On AY, Boyacioglu H. The effect of a mandibular advancement splint on electromyographic activity of the submental and masseter muscles in patients with obstructive sleep apnea. *Int J Prosthodont*. 2009;22(6): .
87. Edwards BA, Andara C, Landry S, et al. Upper-airway collapsibility and loop gain predict the response to oral appliance therapy in patients with obstructive sleep apnea. *Am J Resp Crit Care Med*. 2016;194(11):1413–1422.
88. Meier-Ewert K, Brosig B. Treatment of Sleep Apnea by Prosthetic Mandibular Advancement. In: *Sleep Related Disorders and Internal Diseases*. Springer; 1987:341–345.
89. Bonham PE, Currier GF, Orr WC, Othman J, Nanda RS. The effect of a modified functional appliance on obstructive sleep apnea. *Am J Orthodont Dentofac Orthop*. 1988;94(5):384–392.
90. Menn SJ, Loube DI, Morgan TD, Mitler MM, Berger JS, Erman MK. The mandibular repositioning device: Role in the treatment of obstructive sleep apnea. *Sleep*. 1996;19(10):794–800.

91. Eveloff SE, Rosenberg CL, Carlisle CC, Millman RP. Efficacy of a Herbst mandibular advancement device in obstructive sleep apnea. *Am J Resp Crit Care Med*, 1994;149(4):905–909.
92. Clark GT, Arand D, Chung E, Tong D. Effect of anterior mandibular positioning on obstructive sleep apnea. *Am Rev Resp Dis*. 1993;147:624–624.
93. Schmidt-Nowara W, Lowe A, Wiegand L, Cartwright R, Perez-Guerra F, Menn S. Oral appliances for the treatment of snoring and obstructive sleep apnea: a review. *Sleep*. 1995;18(6):501–510.
94. Vezina JP, Blumen MB, Buchet I, Hausser-Hauw C, Chabolle F. Does propulsion mechanism influence the long-term side effects of oral appliances in the treatment of sleep-disordered breathing? *Chest*, 2011;140(5):1184–1191.
95. Bishop B, Verrett R, Girvan T. A randomized crossover study comparing two mandibular repositioning appliances for treatment of obstructive sleep apnea. *Sleep Breath*. 2014;18(1):125–131.
96. Gauthier L, Laberge L, Beaudry M, Laforte M, Rompré PH, Lavigne GJ. Efficacy of two mandibular advancement appliances in the management of snoring and mild-moderate sleep apnea: A cross-over randomized study. *Sleep Med*. 2009;10(3):329–336.
97. Yoshida K. Effect on blood pressure of oral appliance therapy for sleep apnea syndrome. *Int J Prosthodont*. 2006;19(1): .
98. Otsuka R, De Almeida FR, Lowe AA, Linden W, Ryan F. The effect of oral appliance therapy on blood pressure in patients with obstructive sleep apnea. *Sleep Breath*. 2006;10(1):29–36.
99. Gotsopoulos H, Kelly JJ, Cistulli PA. Oral appliance therapy reduces blood pressure in obstructive sleep apnea: A randomized, controlled trial. *Sleep*. 2004;27(5):934–941.
100. Andrén A, Sjöquist M, Tegelberg Å. Effects on blood pressure after treatment of obstructive sleep apnoea with a mandibular advancement appliance: A three-year follow-up. *J Oral Rehabil*. 2009;36(10):719–725.
101. Haviv Y, Bachar G, Aframian DJ, Almoznino G, Michaeli E, Benoliel R. A 2-year mean follow-up of oral appliance therapy for severe obstructive sleep apnea: A cohort study. *Oral Dis*. 2015;21(3):386–392.
102. Dal-Fabbro C, Garbuio S, D'Almeida V, Cintra FD, Tufik S, Bittencourt L. Mandibular advancement device and CPAP upon cardiovascular parameters in OSA. *Sleep Breath*. 2014;18(4):749–759.
103. Hans MG, Nelson S, Luks VG, Baek SJ. Comparison of two dental devices for treatment of obstructive sleep apnea syndrome (OSAS). *Am J Orthodont Dentofac Orthop*. 1997;111(5):562–570.
104. Durán-Cantolla J, Crovetto-Martínez R, Alkhraisat MH, et al. Efficacy of mandibular advancement device in the treatment of obstructive sleep apnea syndrome: A randomized controlled crossover clinical trial. *Med Oral Patol Oral Cirug Bucal*. 2015;20(5):e605.
105. Marklund M, Carlberg B, Forsgren L, Olsson T, Stenlund H, Franklin KA. Oral appliance therapy in patients with daytime sleepiness and snoring or mild to moderate sleep apnea: A randomized clinical trial. *JAMA Intern Med*. 2015;175(8):1278–1285.
106. Naismith SL, Winter VR, Hickie IB, Cistulli PA. Effect of oral appliance therapy on neurobehavioral functioning in obstructive sleep apnea: A randomized controlled trial. *J Clin Sleep Med*. 2005;1(04):374–380.
107. Gagnadoux F, Pepin JL, Vielle B, et al. Impact of mandibular advancement therapy on endothelial function in severe obstructive sleep apnea. *Am J Resp Crit Care Med*. 2017;195(9):1244–1252.
108. Andrén A, Hedberg P, Walker-Engström ML, Wahlén P, Tegelberg Å. Effects of treatment with oral appliance on 24-h blood pressure in patients with obstructive sleep apnea and hypertension: A randomized clinical trial. *Sleep Breath*. 2013;17(2):705–712.
109. Wilhelmsson B, Tegelberg Å, Walker-Engström ML, et al. A prospective randomized study of a dental appliance compared with uvulopalatopharyngoplasty in the treatment of obstructive sleep apnoea. *Acta Oto-laryngol*. 1999;119(4):503–509.
110. Walker-Engström ML, Wilhelmsson B, Tegelberg Å, Dimenäs E, Ringqvist I. Quality of life assessment of treatment with dental appliance or UPPP in patients with mild to moderate obstructive sleep apnea. *J Sleep Res*. 2000;9:303–308.
111. Walker-Engström ML, Tegelberg Å, Wilhelmsson B, Ringqvist I. 4-year follow-up of treatment with dental appliance or uvulopalatopharyngoplasty in patients with obstructive sleep apnea: A randomized study. *Chest*. 2002;121(3):739–746.
112. Agency for Healthcare Research and Quality. Diagnosis and treatment of obstructive sleep apnea in adults. 2011 Jul. https://effectivehealthcare.ahrq.gov/sites/default/files/pdf/sleep-apnea_research.pdf.
113. Nikolopoulou M, Byraki A, Ahlberg J, et al. Oral appliance therapy versus nasal continuous positive airway pressure in obstructive sleep apnoea syndrome: A randomised, placebo-controlled trial on self-reported symptoms of common sleep disorders and sleep-related problems. *J Oral Rehabil*. 2017;44(6):452–460.
114. Phillips CL, Grunstein RR, Darendeliler MA, et al. Health outcomes of continuous positive airway pressure versus oral appliance treatment for obstructive sleep apnea: a randomized controlled trial. *Am J Resp Crit Care Med*, 2013;187(8):879–887.
115. Aarab G, Nikolopoulou M, Ahlberg J, et al. Oral appliance therapy versus nasal continuous positive airway pressure in obstructive sleep apnea: A randomized, placebo-controlled trial on psychological distress. *Clin Oral Invest*. 2017;21(7):2371–2378.
116. Yamamoto U, Nishizaka M, Tsuda H, Tsutsui H, Ando SI. Crossover comparison between CPAP and mandibular advancement device with adherence monitor about the effects on endothelial function, blood pressure and symptoms in patients with obstructive sleep apnea. *Heart Vessels*. 2019;34(10):1692–1702.
117. El-Solh AA, Homish GG, Ditursi G, et al. A randomized crossover trial evaluating continuous positive airway pressure versus mandibular advancement device on health outcomes in veterans with posttraumatic stress disorder. *J Clin Sleep Med*. 2017;13(11):1327–1335.
118. Sutherland K, Phillips CL, Cistulli PA. Efficacy versus effectiveness in the treatment of obstructive sleep apnea: CPAP and oral appliances. *J Dent Sleep Med*. 2015;2(4):175–181.

119. Weaver TE, Menno DM, Bron M, Crosby RD, Morris S, Mathias SD. Determination of thresholds for minimally important difference and clinically important response on the functional outcomes of sleep questionnaire short version in adults with narcolepsy or obstructive sleep apnea. *Sleep Breath*. ; :1–9.
120. Xu L, Xie D, Griffin KS, et al. Objective adherence to dental device versus positive airway pressure treatment in adults with obstructive sleep apnea. *J Sleep Res*. 2020; :e13240.
121. Barnes M, McEvoy RD, Banks S, et al. Efficacy of positive airway pressure and oral appliance in mild to moderate obstructive sleep apnea. *Am J Resp Crit Care Med*, 2004;170(6):656–664.
122. Lam B, Sam K, Mok WY, et al. Randomised study of three non-surgical treatments in mild to moderate obstructive sleep apnoea. *Thorax*. 2007;62(4):354–359.
123. Dissanayake HU, Sutherland K, Phillips CL, Grunstein RR, Mihailidou AS, Cistulli PA. Comparative effects of CPAP and mandibular advancement splint therapy on blood pressure variability in moderate to severe obstructive sleep apnoea. *Sleep Med*. 2021; : .
124. Glos M, Penzel T, Schoebel C, et al. Comparison of effects of OSA treatment by MAD and by CPAP on cardiac autonomic function during daytime. *Sleep Breath*. 2016;20(2):635–646.
125. D Silva LO-E, Guimarães TM, Pontes G, et al. The effects of continuous positive airway pressure and mandibular advancement therapy on metabolic outcomes of patients with mild obstructive sleep apnea: A randomized controlled study. *Sleep Breath*. ; :1–9.
126. Galic T, Bozic J, Ivkovic N, Gunjaca G, Ticinovic TK, Dogas Z. Effects of mandibular advancement device treatment on arterial stiffness and glucose metabolism in patients with mild to moderate obstructive sleep apnea: A prospective 1 year study. *Sleep Breath*. 2016;20(1):69–77.
127. De Vries, G. E., Wijkstra, PJ, Houwerzijl EJ, Kerstjens HA, Hoekema A. Cardiovascular effects of oral appliance therapy in obstructive sleep apnea: A systematic review and meta-analysis. *Sleep Med Rev*. 2018;40:55–68.
128. Nishigawa K, Hayama R, Matsuka Y. Complications causing patients to discontinue using oral appliances for treatment of obstructive sleep apnea. *J Prosthodont Res*. 2017;61(2):133–138.
129. Sheats RD, Schell TG, Blanton AO, et al. Management of side effects of oral appliance therapy for sleep-disordered breathing. *J Dent Sleep Med*. 2017;4(4):111–125.
130. Marklund M, Franklin KA, Persson M. Orthodontic side-effects of mandibular advancement devices during treatment of snoring and sleep apnoea. *Eur J Orthodont*. 2001;23(2):135–144.
131. Bartolucci ML, Bortolotti F, Martina S, Corazza G, Michelotti A, Alessandri-Bonetti G. Dental and skeletal long-term side effects of mandibular advancement devices in obstructive sleep apnea patients: A systematic review with meta-regression analysis. *Eur J Orthodont*. 2019;41(1):89–100.
132. Martins ODFM, Chaves CM Jr, Rossi RRP, Cunali PA, Dal-Fabbro C, Bittencourt L. Side effects of mandibular advancement splints for the treatment of snoring and obstructive sleep apnea: A systematic review. *Dent Press J Orthodont*. 2018;23(4):45–54.
133. Hammond RJ, Gotsopoulos H, Shen G, Petocz P, Cistulli PA, Darendeliler MA. A follow-up study of dental and skeletal changes associated with mandibular advancement splint use in obstructive sleep apnea. *Am J Orthodont Dentofac Orthop*. 2007;132(6):806–814.
134. Haskell BS, Voor MJ, Roberts AM. A consideration of factors affecting palliative oral appliance effectiveness for obstructive sleep apnea: a scoping review. *J Clin Sleep Med*. 2020; :jcsm-9018.
135. Chen H, Eckert DJ, van der Stelt PF, et al. Phenotypes of responders to mandibular advancement device therapy in obstructive sleep apnea patients: A systematic review and meta-analysis. *Sleep Med Rev*. 2020;49:101229.
136. Ng ATM, Darendeliler MA, Petocz P, Cistulli PA. Cephalometry and prediction of oral appliance treatment outcome. *Sleep Breath*. 2012;16(1):47–58.
137. Sutherland K, Takaya H, Qian J, Petocz P, Ng AT, Cistulli PA. Oral appliance treatment response and polysomnographic phenotypes of obstructive sleep apnea. *J Clin Sleep Med*. 2015;11(8):861–868.
138. Tsuiki S, Ito E, Isono S, et al. Oropharyngeal crowding and obesity as predictors of oral appliance treatment response to moderate obstructive sleep apnea. *Chest*. 2013;144(2):558–563.
139. Cunha TCA, Guimaraes TDM, Schultz TCB, et al. Predictors of success for mandibular repositioning appliance in obstructive sleep apnea syndrome. *Brazil Oral Res*. 2017;31: .
140. Suzuki K, Nakata S, Tagaya M, et al. Prediction of oral appliance treatment outcome in obstructive sleep apnoea syndrome: a preliminary study. *B-ENT*. 2014;10(3):185–191.
141. Chan ASL, Lee RWW, Srinivasan VK, Darendeliler MA, Grunstein RR, Cistulli PA. Nasopharyngoscopic evaluation of oral appliance therapy for obstructive sleep apnoea. *Eur Resp J*. 2010;35(4):836–842.
142. Shen HL, Wen YW, Chen NH, Liao YF. Craniofacial morphologic predictors of oral appliance outcomes in patients with obstructive sleep apnea. *J Am Dent Assoc*. 2012;143(11):1209–1217.
143. Gurani SF, Di Carlo G, Cattaneo PM, Thorn JJ, Pinholt EM. Effect of head and tongue posture on the pharyngeal airway dimensions and morphology in three-dimensional imaging: A systematic review. *J Oral Maxillofac Res*. 2016;7(1): .
144. Mostafiz W, Dalci O, Sutherland K, et al. Influence of oral and craniofacial dimensions on mandibular advancement splint treatment outcome in patients with obstructive sleep apnea. *Chest*. 2011;139(6):1331–1339.
145. Zimmerman JN, Lee J, Pliska BT. Reliability of upper pharyngeal airway assessment using dental CBCT: A systematic review. *Eur J Orthodont*. 2017;39(5):489–496.
146. Kendzerska T, Grewal M, Ryan CM. Utility of acoustic pharyngometry for the diagnosis of obstructive sleep apnea. *Ann Am Thorac Soc*. 2016;13(11):2019–2026.
147. García NM, Blaya F, Urquijo EL, Heras ES, D'Amato R. Oral appliance for obstructive sleep apnea:

Prototyping and optimization of the mandibular protrusion device. *J Med Systems*. 2019;43(5):1–9.
148. Sharples L, Glover M, Clutterbuck-James A, et al. Clinical effectiveness and cost-effectiveness results from the randomised controlled Trial of Oral Mandibular Advancement Devices for Obstructive sleep apnoea-hypopnoea (TOMADO) and long-term economic analysis of oral devices and continuous positive airway pressure. *Health Technol Assess (Winchester, England)*. 2014;18(67):1.
149. Vanderveken OM, Devolder A, Marklund M, et al. Comparison of a custom-made and a thermoplastic oral appliance for the treatment of mild sleep apnea. *Am J Resp Crit Care Med*. 2008;*178*(2):197–202.
150. Vanderveken OM, Van de Heyning P, Braem MJ. Retention of mandibular advancement devices in the treatment of obstructive sleep apnea: an in vitro pilot study. *Sleep Breath*. 2014;18(2):313–318.
151. Trzepizur W, Adrian B, Le Vaillant M, Meslier N, Kün-Darbois JD, Gagnadoux F. Predicting treatment response to mandibular advancement therapy using a titratable thermoplastic device. *Clin Oral Invest*. 2021; :1–9.
152. Okuno K, Pliska BT, Hamoda M, Lowe AA, Almeida FR. Prediction of oral appliance treatment outcomes in obstructive sleep apnea: A systematic review. *Sleep Med Rev*. 2016;30:25–33.
153. Van de Perck E, Op de Beeck S, Dieltjens M, et al. The relationship between specific nasopharyngoscopic features and treatment deterioration with mandibular advancement devices: a prospective study. *J Clin Sleep Med*. 2020;*16*(7):1189–1198.
154. Sutherland K, Chan AS, Ngiam J, Darendeliler MA, Cistulli PA. Qualitative assessment of awake nasopharyngoscopy for prediction of oral appliance treatment response in obstructive sleep apnoea. *Sleep Breath*. 2018;22(4):1029–1036.
155. Johal A, Hector MP, Battagel JM, Kotecha BT. Impact of sleep nasendoscopy on the outcome of mandibular advancement splint therapy in subjects with sleep-related breathing disorders. *J Laryngol Otol*. 2007;121(7):668.
156. Kellner P, Herzog B, Plößl S, et al. Depth-dependent changes of obstruction patterns under increasing sedation during drug-induced sedation endoscopy: Results of a German monocentric clinical trial. *Sleep Breath*. 2016;20(3):1035–1043.
157. Vanderveken OM, Vroegop AV, van de Heyning PH, Braem MJ. Drug-induced sleep endoscopy completed with a simulation bite approach for the prediction of the outcome of treatment of obstructive sleep apnea with mandibular repositioning appliances. *Oper Tech Otolaryngol Head Neck Surg*. 2011;22(2):175–182.
158. Vanderveken OM. The global and evident need to increase the validity and uniformity when performing drug-induced sleep endoscopy. *Sleep Breath*. 2018;22(1):191–192.
159. Kastoer C, Benoist LBL, Dieltjens M, et al. Comparison of upper airway collapse patterns and its clinical significance: Drug-induced sleep endoscopy in patients without obstructive sleep apnea, positional and non-positional obstructive sleep apnea. *Sleep Breath*. 2018;22(4):939–948.
160. Murabito P, Serra A, Zappia M, et al. Comparison of genioglossus muscle activity and efficiency of dexmedetomidine or propofol during drug-induced sleep endoscopy in patients with obstructive sleep apnea/hypopnea syndrome. *Eur Rev Med Pharmacol Sci*, 2019;23(1):389–396.
161. Chung JW, Enciso R, Levendowski DJ, Morgan TD, Westbrook PR, Clark GT. Treatment outcomes of mandibular advancement devices in positional and nonpositional OSA patients. *Oral Surg Oral Med Oral Pathol Oral Radiol Endodontol*. 2010;109(5):724–731.
162. Lee CH, Jung HJ, Lee WH, et al. The effect of positional dependency on outcomes of treatment with a mandibular advancement device. *Arch Otolaryngol Head Neck Surg*. 2012;138(5):479–483.
163. Marklund M, Persson M, Franklin KA. Treatment success with a mandibular advancement device is related to supine-dependent sleep apnea. *Chest*. 1998;114(6):1630–1635.
164. Liu Y, Lowe AA, Orthodont D, Fleetham JA, Park YC. Cephalometric and physiologic predictors of the efficacy of an adjustable oral appliance for treating obstructive sleep apnea. *Am J Orthodont Dentofac Orthop*. 2001;120(6):639–647.
165. Marklund M, Stenlund H, Franklin KA. Mandibular advancement devices in 630 men and women with obstructive sleep apnea and snoring: T2004olerability and predictors of treatment success. *Chest*, 2004;125(4):1270–1278.
166. Azarbarzin A, Marques M, Sands SA, et al. Predicting epiglottic collapse in patients with obstructive sleep apnoea. *Eur Resp J*. 2017;50(3): .
167. Edwards BA, Eckert DJ, McSharry DG, et al. Clinical predictors of the respiratory arousal threshold in patients with obstructive sleep apnea. *Am J Resp Crit Care Med*, 2014;190(11):1293–1300.
168. Sands SA, Terrill PI, Edwards BA, et al. Quantifying the arousal threshold using polysomnography in obstructive sleep apnea. *Sleep*. 2018;41(1):zsx183.
169. Wellman A, Edwards BA, Sands SA, et al. A simplified method for determining phenotypic traits in patients with obstructive sleep apnea. *J Appl Physiol*. 2013;114(7):911–922.
170. Genta PR, Schorr F, Edwards BA, Wellman A, Lorenzi-Filho G. Discriminating the severity of pharyngeal collapsibility in men using anthropometric and polysomnographic indices. *J Clin Sleep Med*. 2020;16(9):1531–1537.
171. Bamagoos AA, Cistulli PA, Sutherland K, et al. Polysomnographic endotyping to select patients with obstructive sleep apnea for oral appliances. *Ann Am Thorac Soc*. 2019;16(11):1422–1431.
172. Holley AB, Lettieri CJ, Shah AA. Efficacy of an adjustable oral appliance and comparison with continuous positive airway pressure for the treatment of obstructive sleep apnea syndrome. *Chest*. 2011;140(6):1511–1516.
173. Dort LC, Hadjuk E, Remmers JE. Mandibular advancement and obstructive sleep apnoea: a method for determining effective mandibular protrusion. *Eur Resp J*. 2006;27(5):1003–1009.
174. Brugarolas R, Valero-Sarmiento JM, Bozkurt A, Essick GK. Auto-adjusting mandibular repositioning device for in-home use. In: *2016 38th Annual*

International Conference of the IEEE Engineering in Medicine and Biology Society (EMBC). IEEE; 2016 Aug:4296–4299.

175. Sutherland K, Ngiam J, Cistulli PA. Performance of remotely controlled mandibular protrusion sleep studies for prediction of oral appliance treatment response. *J Clin Sleep Med*. 2017;13(3):411–417.
176. Remmers JE, Topor Z, Grosse J, et al. A feedback-controlled mandibular positioner identifies individuals with sleep apnea who will respond to oral appliance therapy. *J Clin Sleep Med*. 2017;13(7):871–880.
177. Kastoer C, Dieltjens M, Oorts E, et al. The use of remotely controlled mandibular positioner as a predictive screening tool for mandibular advancement device therapy in patients with obstructive sleep apnea through single-night progressive titration of the mandible: A systematic review. *J Clin Sleep Med*. 2016;12(10):1411–1421.
178. Kirshenblatt S, Chen H, Dieltjens M, Pliska B, Almeida FR. Accuracy of thermosensitive microsensors intended to monitor patient use of removable oral appliances. *J Can Dent Assoc*. 2018;84(i2):1488–2159.
179. Dieltjens M, Braem MJ, Vroegop AV, et al. Objectively measured vs self-reported compliance during oral appliance therapy for sleep-disordered breathing. *Chest*. 2013;144(5):1495–1502.
180. Lai H, Huang W, Chen W, Wang D. Effectiveness of continuous positive airway pressure versus mandibular advancement device in severe obstructive sleep apnea patients with mandibular retrognathia: A prospective clinical trial. *Ear Nose Throat J*. 2020; :0145561320969251.
181. de Vries GE, Hoekema A, Claessen JQ, et al. Long-term objective adherence to mandibular advancement device therapy versus continuous positive airway pressure in patients with moderate obstructive sleep apnea. *J Clin Sleep Med*. 2019;15(11):1655–1663.
182. de Almeida FR, Lowe AA, Tsuiki S, et al. Long-term compliance and side effects of oral appliances used for the treatment of snoring and obstructive sleep apnea syndrome. *J Clin Sleep Med*. 2005;1(02):143–152.
183. Saglam-Aydinatay B, Taner T. Oral appliance therapy in obstructive sleep apnea: Long-term adherence and patients' experiences. *Med Oral Patol Oral Cirug Bucal*. 2018;23(1):e72.
184. Petri N, Svanholt P, Solow B, Wildschiødtz G, Winkel P. Mandibular advancement appliance for obstructive sleep apnoea: Results of a randomised placebo controlled trial using parallel group design. *J Sleep Res*. 2008;17(2):221–229.
185. Berg LM, Ankjell TKS, Trovik TA. Self-reported sleep quality with mandibular advancement device or continuous positive airway pressure: A randomized clinical trial on patients with mild and moderate obstructive sleep apnea. *J Dent Sleep Med*. 2020;7(2): .
186. Haviv Y, Zini A, Almoznino G, Keshet N, Sharav Y, Aframian DJ. Assessment of interfering factors in non-adherence to oral appliance therapy in severe sleep apnea. *Oral Dis*. 2017;23(5):629–635.
187. Attali V, Vecchierini MF, Collet JM, et al. Efficacy and tolerability of a custom-made Narval mandibular repositioning device for the treatment of obstructive sleep apnea: ORCADES study 2-year follow-up data. *Sleep Med*. 2019;63:64–74.
188. Haviv Y. Adherence to oral appliance therapy in severe sleep apnea. *J Sleep Disord Ther*. 2015;5:6(Suppl):29.
189. Mullane S, Loke W. Influence of short-term side effects on oral sleep appliance compliance among CPAP-intolerant patients: An objective monitoring of compliance. *J Oral Rehabil*. 2019;*46*(8):715–722.
190. Dieltjens M, Vanderveken OM, Van den Bosch D, et al. Impact of type D personality on adherence to oral appliance therapy for sleep-disordered breathing. *Sleep Breath*. 2013;17(3):985–991.
191. Pahkala R, Suominen AL. Adherence to oral appliance treatment and its determinants in obstructive sleep apnoea patients. *Eur J Orthodont*. 2021; : .
192. Murphy S, Maerz R, Sheets V, et al. Adherence and side effects among patients treated with oral appliance therapy for obstructive sleep apnea. *J Dent Sleep Med*. 2020;7(1): .
193. Sutherland K, Dalci O, Cistulli PA. What do we know about adherence to oral appliances? *Sleep Med Clin*. 2021;16(1):145–154.
194. Cartwright, R. D. (1984). Effect of sleep position on sleep apnea severity. *Sleep*, 1984;7(2):110–114.
195. Dieltjens M, Vroegop AV, Verbruggen AE, et al. A promising concept of combination therapy for positional obstructive sleep apnea. *Sleep Breath*. 2015;19(2):637–644.
196. Millman RP, Rosenberg CL, Carlisle CC, Kramer NR, Kahn DM, Bonitati AE. The efficacy of oral appliances in the treatment of persistent sleep apnea after uvulopalatopharyngoplasty. *Chest*. 1998;113(4):992–996.
197. Yang D, Zhou HF, Xie Y. Efficacy of uvulopalatopharyngoplasty combined with oral appliance in treatment of obstructive sleep apnea–hypopnea syndrome. *Irish J Med Sci (1971–)*. 2015;184(2):329–334.
198. Luo H, Tang X, Xiong Y, Meng L, Yi H, Yin S. Efficacy and mechanism of mandibular advancement devices for persistent sleep apnea after surgery: a prospective study. *J Otolaryngol Head Neck Surg*. 2016;45(1):1–8.
199. Lee JJ, Sahu N, Rogers R, Soose RJ. Severe obstructive sleep apnea treated with combination hypoglossal nerve stimulation and oral appliance therapy. *J Dent Sleep Med*. 2015;2:185–186.
200. Oliven R, Tov N, Odeh M, et al. Interacting effects of genioglossus stimulation and mandibular advancement in sleep apnea. *J Appl Physiol*. 2009;106(5):1668–1673.
201. El-Solh AA, Moitheennazima B, Akinnusi ME, Churder PM, Lafornara AM. Combined oral appliance and positive airway pressure therapy for obstructive sleep apnea: A pilot study. *Sleep Breath*. 2011;15(2):203–208.
202. De Vries GE, Doff MHJ, Hoekema A, Kerstjens HA, Wijkstra PJ. Continuous positive airway pressure and oral appliance hybrid therapy in obstructive sleep apnea: Patient comfort, compliance, and preference: A pilot study. *J Dent Sleep Med*. 2016;3(1):6.
203. Premaraj TS, Stadiem J, Premaraj SA, Davies CR, Dennis M, Harrington JJ. Continuous positive airway pressure-mandibular advancement device combination

therapy for moderate-to-severe obstructive sleep apnea: A preliminary study. *Eur J Dent*. 2021; : .
204. Kaminska M, Montpetit A, Mathieu A, Jobin V, Morisson F, Mayer P. Higher effective oronasal versus nasal continuous positive airway pressure in obstructive sleep apnea: Effect of mandibular stabilization. *Can Resp J*. 2014;21(4):234–238.
205. Prehn RS, Swick T. A descriptive report of combination therapy (custom face mask for CPAP integrated with a mandibular advancement splint) for long-term treatment of OSA with literature review. *J Dent Sleep Med*. 2017;4(2):29–36.
206. (Baratieri, Alves, Souza, Araújo, & Maia, 2011)
207. (Chang, et al., 2013)
208. (El & Palomo, 2014)
209. (Noller, 2018)
210. (Hu, 2015)
211. (Hosoya, et al., 2014)
212. (Huang, 2015)
213. (Vieira, et al., 2014)
214. (Yashmin, 2018)
215. (Gungor, 2013)
216. (Pahkala, 2019)
217. (AlHammad, 2015)
218. (Pliska, 2017)
219. (Moss, 1968)
220. (Pisacane, 2019;6(4))
221. (Abtahi, 2018)
222. (Quo, 2019)
223. (Lee, 2017)
224. (Oh & Lee, 2013)
225. (Tagaya, et al., 2012)
226. (Lin & Koltai, 2012)
227. (Scammon, 1930)
228. (Fujii, 2017)
229. (Huang & Guilleminault, 2013)
230. (Spilsbury, 2015)
231. (Goodwin, Vasquez, Silva, & Quan, 2010)
232. (Bixler, 2016)
233. (Masoud, et al., 2020)
234. (Schendel, Jacobson, & Khalessi, 2012)
235. (Phoenix, Valiathan, Nelson, Strohl, & Hans, 2011)
236. (Bouserhal, 2014)
237. (Aziz, Ansari, Lagravère, Major, & Flores-Mir, 2015)
238. (De Felippe, 2008)
239. (Cohen-Levy, 2013)
240. (Pirelli, 2004)
241. (Pia Villa, 2007)
242. (Quo, Hyunh, & Guilleminault, 2017)
243. (Sanchez-sucar, 2019)
244. (Gianoni-Capenakas, 2020;7(4))
245. (Capan, Kılıçoğlu, Kiyan, & Ersu, 2013)
246. (Kawashima, et al., 2000)
247. (Johns, Strollo, Buckley, & Constantino, 1998)
248. (Nazarali, 2015)
249. (Idris, 2018)
250. (Yanyan, 2019)
251. (Camacho, 2019)
252. (Kim, 2018)
253. (Wang, 2012)
254. (Zhiai Hu, 2015)
255. (Lobbezoo F, 2013)
256. (Maluly M, 2013)
257. (da Costa Lopes, 2020)
258. (Guimaraes, 2009)
259. (Camacho M. e., 2015)
260. (Guilleminault, 2013)
261. (Yu-Shu Huang, 2015)
262. (Villa, Evangelisti, Barreto, Cecili, & Kaditis, 2020)
263. (Messner, 2020)

Chapter 8

Surgical Therapy for Obstructive Sleep Apnea

Susan L. Garetz and Paul T. Hoff

ADULT OSA SURGERY

Conservative therapy is recommended as the first line-treatment for adults diagnosed with obstructive sleep apnea (OSA). Recent innovations in both identification of the site of airway obstruction and surgical techniques have made surgery for OSA an increasingly viable option for those patients unable to tolerate conservative treatment modalities. The surgical treatment of OSA falls within a number of disciplines, including otolaryngology, oral-maxillofacial surgery, and bariatric surgery. Close collaboration between sleep medicine physicians and surgeons improves the ability to provide appropriate and individualized care for patients with OSA.

Evaluation for Surgical Candidacy

Successful surgery requires both a comprehensive sleep surgery–directed examination to establish the individual's OSA phenotype and an understanding of underlying patient factors that may influence outcomes. Surgical treatment of OSA carries attendant risk, ranging from short-term, expected consequences, such as pain, dehydration, and weight loss, to devastating long-term complications. Careful patient selection is incumbent upon the surgeon in order to avoid long-term, impactful side effects.

HISTORY

The patient's overall medical history, including anticoagulation status, comorbidities, body mass index (BMI), and American Society of Anesthesia (ASA) class assessing overall patient health and risk for anesthesia and surgery should be documented. Patient's swallowing function should be assessed prior to surgical intervention. Assessment of mental well-being and previous psychiatric diagnoses is also recommended. A thorough sleep history should be obtained. The most recent polysomnogram (PSG), including tested positive airway pressure (PAP) settings if used, should be reviewed, as well as reasons for failure of conservative treatment measures.

PHYSICAL EXAM

Unlike pediatric patients, who frequently present with adeno-tonsillar hypertrophy as the primary cause of obstruction, the adult OSA phenotype is highly variable. The physical examination can be categorized as: (1) standard examination done without the need for specialized equipment; or (2) comprehensive examination requiring the use of specialized instruments and/or sedation, typically performed by an otolaryngologist/sleep surgeon. The patient history and physical exam information can be consolidated in a patient data sheet (Figure 8.1).

Standard Examination

The standard examination begins with an assessment of basic body habitus including BMI and neck circumference as well as the patient's facial skeletal profile. The nasal examination can be performed with either an otoscope or a nasal speculum. The septum, turbinates, and nasal valve area should be examined and the presence of masses such as polyps documented. The oral cavity examination can be performed with a tongue depressor and an otoscope or alternative light source. Condition of the dentition should be documented, as well as class of dental occlusion and inter-incisor opening distance. The configuration of the hard palate (high arched vs. broad) is a measure of oral crowding and should be noted. The most important component of the oral cavity examination is the relationship between the oral tongue and the palate using the Friedman tongue classification (FTP) system:[1]

FTP 1: Able to see the entire uvula and tonsils
FTP 2a: Able to see entire uvula and part of the tonsils
FTP 2b: Able to see entire soft palate to the base of the uvula without being able to see the entire uvula or the tonsils
FTP 3: Able to see some of the soft palate
FTP 4: Able to only see the hard palate.

The oropharyngeal examination includes the soft palate, tongue posterior to the circumvallate papillae, lateral pharyngeal walls, and tonsil size using the Brodsky system size 0 (absent) to size 4 (touching in the midline) as shown in Figure 8.1. The length of the palate and uvula, presence of medialization of the posterior palatal arch, and any evidence of cleft palate or sub-mucous cleft such as a bifid uvula should be documented.

Specialized Examination

Endoscopic Evaluation

Specialized instrumentation is required to examine the nasopharynx, base of tongue (BOT,) and the larynx. The BOT plays a significant role in most patients with moderate to severe OSA. Endoscopic evaluation can be used to visualize these areas of obstruction but does have limitations, as it does not assess the patient's airway during sleep when neuromuscular tone is decreased. During endoscopy the entire airway is visualized. Adenoid hypertrophy is rare in adults, but occasionally an obstructing nasopharyngeal cyst or polyp will be encountered. The endoscopic dimensions of the soft and hard palate (velum) can be characterized as oblique, intermediate, and vertical.[2] The slope of the tongue base can be characterized as vertical (A), mixed (B), or horizontal (C).[3] The size of the lingual tonsils (0–4) is documented.[4] Large lingual tonsils are not common but play a significant role in OSA when present. Laryngeal abnormalities in vocal cord mobility, polyps, or inflammation secondary to acid reflux can be observed. The epiglottis can play a significant role in OSA and PAP noncompliance, although epiglottic prolapse is rarely seen during the awake examination. In addition, the sub-glottis can be visualized, allowing the examiner to rule out subglottic stenosis.

Imaging

The lateral cephalogram is used for the analysis of facial skeletal anatomy. It provides a number of measurements that can be helpful when considering surgical alternatives involving the skeletal framework. The mandibular-hyoid plane (MHP) is the vertical distance between the body of the mandible and the anterior superior edge of the hyoid and represents an elongated retro-lingual space. The patient's skeletal class (relative orientation of the maxilla to the mandible) can also be determined.

MICHIGAN MEDICINE OSA SURG DATA FORM

Patient Name: ______________________________
Date: ______________________________
Examiner: ______________________________

Height (cm)__________
Weight (kg)__________
BMI (m2/kg) __________
Collar size (cm)__________

Physical Examination:

Brodsky Tonsil Size

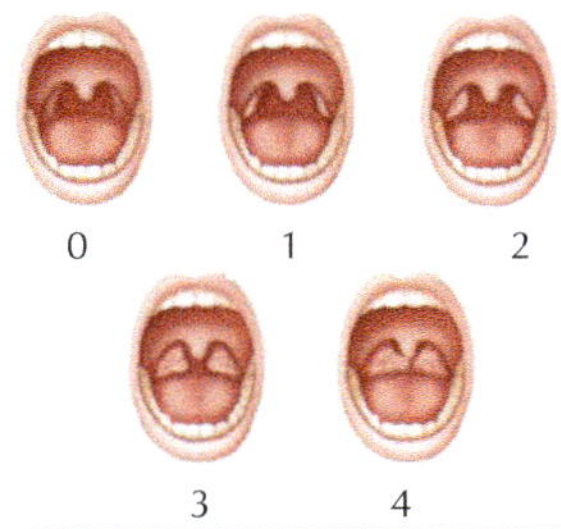

Friedman Tongue Position

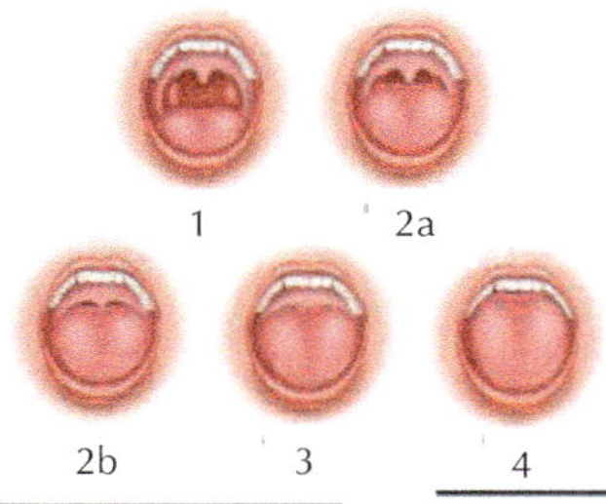

Moore Classification

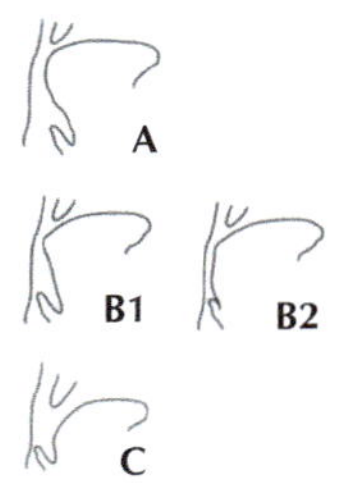

	Friedman Palate Position	Tonsil Size	BMI
Stage I	1	3, 4	<40
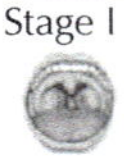	2	3, 4	<40
Stage II	1, 2	1, 2	<40
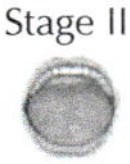	3, 4	3, 4	<40
Stage III	3	0, 1, 2	<40
	4	0, 1, 2	<40
Stage IV	1, 2, 3, 4	0, 1, 2, 3, 4	>40

All patients with significant craniofacial or other anatomic deformities.

BMI = Body Mass Index.

VOTE classification system

Level	Direction: A-P	Lateral	Concentric
Velum			
Oropharynx			
Tongue base			
Epiglottis			

DISE Date_______ VOTE score _______

Sleep Study Data:

Date of Study: __________
Home Study: **Y N** | Monitored Study: **Y N**
AHI: ______________
Min Sa02: ______________
Hypopnea Index: __________
Apnea Index: ____________
ODI:________________
PAP: **Y N**
Prior PAP: **Y N**
Epworth scale: ____________
Snoring scale: ____________
Other: ________________

Physical Exam:

Handedness: **R L**
Nose ____________________
Oral Cavity____________________
Oropharynx ____________________
Flexible Laryngoscopy:
Woodson phenotype (1, 2, 3)
Moore Class (A, B1, B2, C)
Lingual Tonsil Size (0–4)_____
Laryngoscopy view (1, 2a, 2b, 3)
Angle Class (1, 2, 3)______________
Skeletal Class ________________
Dentition __________________

Comorbidities:

HTN CAD BMI Insomnia Anticoagulants
DM CVD Psych Other: ____________

Impression:

Plan:

Figure 8.1. Example of clinic form used to consolidate data of adult patients being evaluated for OSA surgery.Brodsky tonsil size drawing based on text description.[88]

Friedman Tongue Position diagram reproduced with permission from: Friedman M, Friedman Tongue Position and the Staging of Obstructive Sleep Apnea/Hypopnea Syndrome. In: Scheidt S, Clansey N, eds. *Sleep Apnea and Snoring: Surgical and Non-Surgical Therapy*. Elsevier; 2009.[89]

Moore classification diagram reproduced with permission from: Moore KE, C. Phillips. A practical method for describing patterns of tongue-base narrowing (modification of Fujita) in awake adult patients with obstructive sleep apnea. *J Oral Maxillofac Surg* 2002;60(3):252–260.[3]

Friedman Clinical Staging System diagram reproduced with permission from: Friedman M, Ibrahim H, Joseph NJ. Staging of obstructive sleep apnea/hypopnea syndrome: A guide to appropriate treatment. *Laryngoscope* 2004;114(3):454–459.[8]

Cine magnetic resonance imaging (MRI) is a method to assess dynamic collapse of the airway during sedation and is described in more detail in the pediatric surgery section later in this chapter.

Drug-induced sleep endoscopy (DISE)
Drug-induced sleep endoscopy (DISE) is a stand-alone, sedated examination of the upper airway that compliments the traditional office examination and is used to assess the dynamic collapse of the airway. DISE provides the surgeon information about the direction and degree of collapse at defined segments of the collapsible airway. The VOTE system has become the most widely utilized DISE classification system for adult OSA patients and describes the extent and orientation of obstruction at the velum, oropharynx, tongue base, and epiglottis.[5] Absolute indications for DISE in adults prior to surgical intervention include craniofacial anomalies, physical exam discordant with history or other testing and consideration for neuro stimulation surgery. Relative indications include revision surgery or moderate-severe OSA. DISE has been shown to change surgical decision-making in up to 50% of cases[6] and in some circumstances is a predictor of surgical outcomes.[6,7]

Patient Selection

The patient's OSA phenotype will determine the surgical treatment options. In general, phenotype can be broken down into 3 domains: soft tissue, skeletal framework, and neuromuscular tone. Additionally, BMI is often the most important determinant of surgical success or failure; patients with a significantly elevated BMI (over 40) are not candidates for most upper airway surgical procedures.

Several physical exam characteristics help direct the choice of surgical procedure. The Friedman staging system uses a combination of BMI, tonsil size, and relative tongue position to ascertain chances of success with oral-pharyngeal soft tissue surgery.[8] The presence of a medialized posterior palatal arch may contribute to less predictable surgical outcomes due to instability of the lateral wall of the pharynx. Patients with a vertical phenotype are poor candidates for traditional palatal surgery and require shortening of the hard palate or maxillary advancement.[9] Moore Class C is considered more favorable for BOT and neuro-stimulation procedures, especially in the setting of lingual tonsil hypertrophy, as the tongue base slopes forward, creating a wide vallecular.[3] Another important morphologic characteristic is the patient's skeletal profile; patients with retrognathia are poor candidates for soft tissue surgery and may be best served by orthognathic surgery or neuro-stimulation.

SURGICAL TREATMENTS FOR OSA

We are in a golden age of surgical treatment for OSA. The combination of diagnostic tools, improved patient selection, and surgical advancements have provided patients with more reliable and less morbid treatment options than were previously available. Surgical treatment can range from nasal surgery to improve PAP or mandibular advancing appliance (MAD) adherence to tracheostomy for severe refractory OSA. In between lie a variety of procedures addressing the soft tissue of the palate, pharyngeal walls, and tongue base, as well as the skeletal framework of the maxilla and mandible. This information is summarized in Table 8.1 at the end of the chapter. The most recent advances address the issue of neuromuscular tone and its impact on OSA.

Nasal Surgery

Nasal obstruction plays an important role in snoring and respiratory event related arousals, but little evidence has shown a correlation between nasal obstruction and OSA.[10,11] Nasal surgery is primarily used to improve compliance with PAP or MAD. In addition, correction of nasal obstruction can improve subjective sleep and markedly reduce snoring. Minimally invasive surgical treatment, including reduction of inferior turbinate hypertrophy, or stabilization of the nasal valve using radiofrequency technology, can be performed in the office setting. More invasive procedures such as septoplasty and functional septorhinoplasty are performed under anesthesia. Risks can include bleeding, septal perforation, cosmetic deformity, and scarring.

Table 8.1 **Current Surgical Techniques, Indications, and Outcomes for Adult OSA**

Type of Surgery	Area of Obstruction	Recommended Criteria	Outcomes – landmark studies
Tonsillectomy	Oropharynx	BMI <40 Tonsil size 3–4 FTP 1–2 Friedman stage 1	80% success rate (Sher criteria). Large tonsils (size 3 and 4) in adults are a predictor of surgical success in the setting of a BMI under 40 and small oral tongue.[8]
Multilevel TORS tongue base resection with pharyngoplasty	Tongue base/ oropharynx	Lin criteria: BMI <30 AHI 15–60 DISE no lateral collapse velopharynx	Surgical success in 86% of patients.[82] Meta-analysis: 67% success rate with a 23% cure rate.[83]
TORS in isolation	BOT–lingual tonsillectomy	BMI <35 Lingual tonsils size 3–4	56% reduction in AHI[84]
Coblation™ tongue base resection with lateral pharyngoplasty	Tongue base and oropharynx	BMI<30 AHI >15 FTP 3	72% surgical response AHI <15[20]
Coblation™ BOT isolated	Tongue base	Moderate to severe OSA BMI <30	52% Surgical success rate[85]
UPPP isolated	Velum	BMI<40 FTP 1–2 Tonsil size 3–4 Friedman Stage 1	UPPP achieved a 49% reduction in AHI as well as significant improvement in subjective measures of QOL.[86]
Lateral pharyngoplasty isolated	Oropharynx	Lateral collapse	77% reduction in AHI[12]
Trans-palatal advancement pharyngoplasty	Oropharynx	Vertical phenotype	65% reduction AHI[9]
Hypoglossal nerve stimulation (HGNS)	Multilevel collapse	BMI<32 AHI 15–65 CAI <25%	72% reduction in AHI at 1 year and a 63% responder rate at 5 years[29,31]
Hyoid suspension	Epiglottis and hypopharynx	Primary epiglottic collapse	43% reduction in AHI in isolation[24]
Hyoid suspension and pharyngoplasty	Hypopharynx and oropharynx	MPH >25 mm Multilevel obstruction: palate, lateral wall, BOT, epiglottis	67% reduction[87]
Bariatric surgery	N/A	BMI >40 BMI >35 with one obesity-related comorbidity	75% of patients had improvement in their sleep apnea. AHI reduced by 38.2 events/hour[34]
Maxillary-mandibular advancement	Multilevel collapse	BMI <35 AHI <60	Rates of surgical success and cure were 85.5% and 38.5%. Similar results with ESS and nadir oxygen saturation.[28]
Tracheostomy	N/A	Life-threatening Fails to meet criteria for alternative treatment	100% effective

Palatal Surgery

During the early years of sleep apnea surgery, uvulopharyngopalatoplasty (UPPP) was the most commonly performed procedure. Variable success rates which decreased over time and complications including prolonged hospital stay, pharyngeal stenosis, velopharyngeal insufficiency (VPI), and aspiration or globus sensation ultimately limited the utility of this procedure.

More recently procedures, such as UPPP, which involve excision of midline palate structures have been largely replaced by techniques using repositioning of tissue and conservation of midline structures. Michel Cahali was the first to describe repositioning of pharyngeal tissue laterally as an alternative to UPPP.[12] Lateral pharyngoplasty (LP) repositions pharyngeal tissue to the sides, securing the muscular tissue to rigid anchor points (the pterygo-mandibular raphe and pterygoid hamulus). A variety of other modifications to the pharyngoplasty technique have been described.[13–16] These techniques can all create significant enlargement of the retro-palatal airway space and have been accompanied by both a marked improvement in surgical outcomes and a decrease in postoperative VPI.

Tongue Base Reduction Procedures

Patients with moderate to severe OSA often have significant obstruction due to the BOT and/or lingual tonsil hypertrophy. Friedman tongue positions 3 and 4 have been associated with tongue base hypertrophy and flexible laryngoscopy can confirm the presence of lymphoid hypertrophy[4] or muscular hypertrophy using the Moore classification.[3] Fujita was the first to recognize multilevel obstruction in OSA; he introduced CO_2 laser partial glossectomy for the treatment of OSA, often in combination with UPPP.[17] Due to the high morbidity of this procedure, it was not widely adopted. A number of techniques have since been introduced with the goal of either minimizing morbidity by utilizing radiofrequency ablation (RFA) and cold ablation (Coblation™) or improving success through a trans-cervical excision of tissue from the tongue base.[18–21] In 2010, Vicini and colleagues introduced transoral robotic surgery (TORS) for the removal of both lymphoid and muscular tissue from the BOT.[22] TORS was routinely performed as a multilevel procedure, combined with pharyngoplasty.

Successful treatment of the tongue base using ablative techniques is highly dependent on BMI; elevated BMI greater than 30 kg/m^2 is associated with poor surgical outcomes. All tongue base procedures, including partial glossectomy and lingual tonsillectomy, particularly when combined with palate surgery, can result in significant short- and long-term morbidity, including taste disturbance, dysphagia, and foreign body sensation.[23]

Supraglottoplasty, Thyro-Hyoidpexy, and Mandibulo-Hyoidpexy

Drug-induced sleep endoscopy (DISE) may demonstrate prolapse of the epiglottis or collapse of the lateral pharyngeal walls.

Supraglottoplasty is indicated in cases of primary epiglottic collapse and involves either direct resection of the upper third of the epiglottis or adhesion of the epiglottis to the tongue base by removing mucosa or suturing the epiglottis to the tongue base (pexy). Supraglottoplasty may result in chronic aspiration as a result of extensive adhesion of the epiglottis to the tongue base or due to restriction of epiglottic inversion during the pharyngeal phase of swallowing. It is important with both tongue base and laryngeal procedures to assess swallowing function before surgery with validated surveys such as the Dysphagia Handicap Index or the MD Anderson Dysphagia Index. Extra precautions should be used in elderly patients in whom swallowing function may already be compromised.

Many patients with supraglottic, lateral wall, and BOT prolapse also have cephalomentric elongation of the hyoid to mandibular plane (>2.5cm) and retro-displacement of the hyoid bone on physical examination. Hyoid suspension can address these deficiencies. Anterior traction on the hyo-epiglottic ligament lifts the epiglottis and opens the airway. Two techniques have evolved: the thyro-hyoidpexy (THP) and the mandibulo-hyoidpexy (MHP). The THP moves the hyoid bone anteriorly and inferiorly approximating the thyroid cartilage. The MHP moves the hyoid bone anteriorly and superiorly in the direction of the mentum. In isolation, THP and MHP will result in success in less than 50% of patients[24]; many patients with multilevel collapse of the palate and BOT will undergo a combination of hyoid and palatal surgery. Complications can include fracture of the hyoid bone, submental edema or seroma, and transient dysphagia.

Skeletal Surgery

Skeletal framework surgery is reserved for patients with significant deficiencies in skeletal anatomy, often manifested as retrognathia, mid-face hypoplasia, or high arched palate. Retrognathia presents a significant challenge. Soft tissue surgery alone cannot correct the posterior displacement of the tongue present in this condition. In addition, retrognathia results in significant cosmetic deformity, which in men is often camouflaged with a beard.

LEFORT 1 OSTEOTOMY, MAXILLARY EXPANSION, AND TRANS-PALATAL ADVANCEMENT

Patients with maxillary hypoplasia or an elongated hard palate require skeletal framework surgery in the form of Lefort 1 osteotomy or trans-palatal advancement.[9] If the maxillary hypoplasia is associated with dental occlusal abnormalities or cosmetic deformity, Lefort 1 osteotomy is favored. The procedure is performed through a trans-oral incision; the tooth-bearing segment of the maxilla and hard palate is separated from the superior maxilla and the mobilized segment is advanced to correct cosmetic deformity, while simultaneously opening the retro-palatal airway. Orthodontics are necessary following Lefort 1 procedures.

Patients with a high arched palate can benefit from lateral expansion of the maxilla. Rapid maxillary expansion is commonly performed in the pediatric population, but similar results can be accomplished in adults with limited ostetomies. Distraction osteogenisis maxillary expansion (DOME) improves both the oral and oropharyngeal airway, and also markedly improves the nasal airway.[25]

Trans-palatal advancement (TPA) is reserved for those patients who demonstrate a vertical palatal phenotype based on endoscopic evaluation. TPA is performed through a trans-oral incision and results in 1 cm shortening of the hard palate and widening of the retro-palatal space. An oronasal fistula can occur, especially in patients with a high arched palate or tobacco use.

MAXILLARY-MANDIBULAR ADVANCEMENT

Maxillary-mandibular advancement was pioneered by Riley and Powell in the 1980s as the second stage of the well-known Stanford protocol.[26] Advancement is performed through a trans-oral approach. Osteotomies are performed through the maxilla (Lefort 1) and the body of the mandible posterior to the inferior alveolar nerve. The degree of advancement is greater in OSA surgery than is typical in orthognathic surgery, and the procedure is thus generally performed by oro-maxillofacial surgeons with specialized training in sleep surgery. Maxillary-mandibular advancement has a high success rate and has long been considered the most reliable surgical treatment for OSA, with the exception of tracheostomy.[27] Maxillary-mandibular advancement can improve cosmetic deformity in patients with skeletal deficiencies but can cause deformity in patients who present with a normal mandibular profile. In addition, the procedure can result in facial hypoesthesia in the region of the mental nerve and often results in malocclusion. Patients must remain on a soft diet and in soft rubber band restraints for 6 weeks after surgery.[28]

Hypoglossal Nerve Stimulation

Neuro-stimulation of the hypoglossal nerve (HGNS) was introduced in 2014 with the STAR trial and has rapidly been accepted as a reliable treatment for patients with moderate to severe OSA.[29] Upper airway simulation Patients who are intolerant of conservative therapy must meet strict inclusion criteria in order to qualify for the procedure. The stimulator device can be implanted in many patients with OSA who may not be candidates for traditional pharyngeal surgery. The procedure is performed through 2 small incisions in the neck and chest; postoperative pain is minimal, patients can be discharged on the same day of surgery, and anticoagulants can be resumed within days of surgery if needed. There is an average reduction in apnea hypopnea index (AHI) of 80%.[30] The long-term outcomes of the HGNS have been studied extensively. Five-year outcomes data from the STAR trial confirm a durable response, including adherence to therapy, as well as improvement in subjective (Epworth Sleepiness Scale [ESS], snoring) and objective outcomes (AHI and ODI).[31]

The device was previously not compatible with MRI scans of the shoulders, torso, and hips postoperatively, but the newer Inspire device is now MRI compatible with full body 1.5 T MRIs. A careful inventory of the patient's occupational duties and hobbies is important to ensure proper patient selection. Short-term risks include hypoglossal neuropraxia, lower lip weakness, and pneumothorax; long-term risks include device failure or failure to tolerate the device at any setting. In addition, battery life is 10–11 years, which for many patients will mean one or more battery replacement procedures during their lifetime.[32]

Multilevel Surgery

Multilevel procedures, involving surgical correction of 1 or more areas of possible obstruction, has been a common practice. Although success rates are often good, the option of staging procedures is likely preferable for safety reasons. However, many patients may insist on having all potential sites of collapse addressed at one time. Ultimately, this decision at the discretion of the surgeon, based on whether the added morbidity of multilevel surgery is worth the incremental improvement in outcome. Combined multilevel surgery may also result in circumferential scarring of the oropharynx; it is critical that the surgeon avoid this problem by preserving a bridge of normal mucosa between the tonsillar fossa and the vallecula.

Bariatric Surgery

Obesity is the major contributing factor in over 50% of adult patients with OSA.[33] The majority of standard surgical options for the treatment of OSA are contraindicated or considerably less successful in patients with morbid obesity. Bariatric surgery is therefore becoming an increasingly utilized modality for obese patients with OSA who are unable to tolerate conservative therapy, The National Institutes of Health (NIH) consensus panel guidelines state that bariatric surgery is appropriate for all patients with BMI >40 kg/m^2 and for patients with BMI 35–40 kg/m^2 with associated comorbid conditions.

Several large meta-analyses have shown bariatric surgery to be successful in reducing the severity of OSA postoperatively. An analysis of almost 14 000 patients demonstrated that 75% of the patients had some improvement in their OSA.[34] Another meta-analysis showed that gastric bypass was the most successful in improving or resolving OSA, with 94.8% of patients undergoing resolution.[35]

Although complication rates and mortality for bariatric surgery have improved considerably, this remains a relatively high-risk group for surgical intervention. The NIH longitudinal assessment of bariatric surgery (LABS) consortium reported a 30-day follow-up of 2458 participants undergoing bariatric surgery. A serious complication occurred in 4.1% of all patients, including blood clots, need for additional surgery or prolonged hospital stay, and the mortality rate was 0.3%.[36] Longer-term complications include intestinal obstruction, marginal ulcer, ventral hernia, gallstones, and metabolic complications including nephrolithiasis and hypoglycemia. Mineral and vitamin deficiencies as well as weight regain are also commonly reported.[37]

Surgical Success Measurements

Surgical success has historically been defined as >50% reduction of AHI and an AHI <20 events/hr.[38] The surgical sleep literature has relied on this definition for over 30 years, which has led to considerable concern in the sleep medicine community, where patients considered a surgical success may still have significant residual OSA. There is now an effort among sleep surgeons to define success in terms of both objective and subjective response to surgical therapy—for example, measuring surgical response as an AHI <15 events/hr and an ESS <10.

Treatment Algorithms

The sleep surgeon has a large armamentarium of procedures to deploy. In order to best utilize these procedures, integration of a patient's physical characteristics, medical comorbidities, social dynamics, parasomnias, and in some cases psychiatric disorders, must all be considered. A surgical algorithm can be helpful to build a framework upon which to build a treatment plan (Figures 8.2 and 8.3).

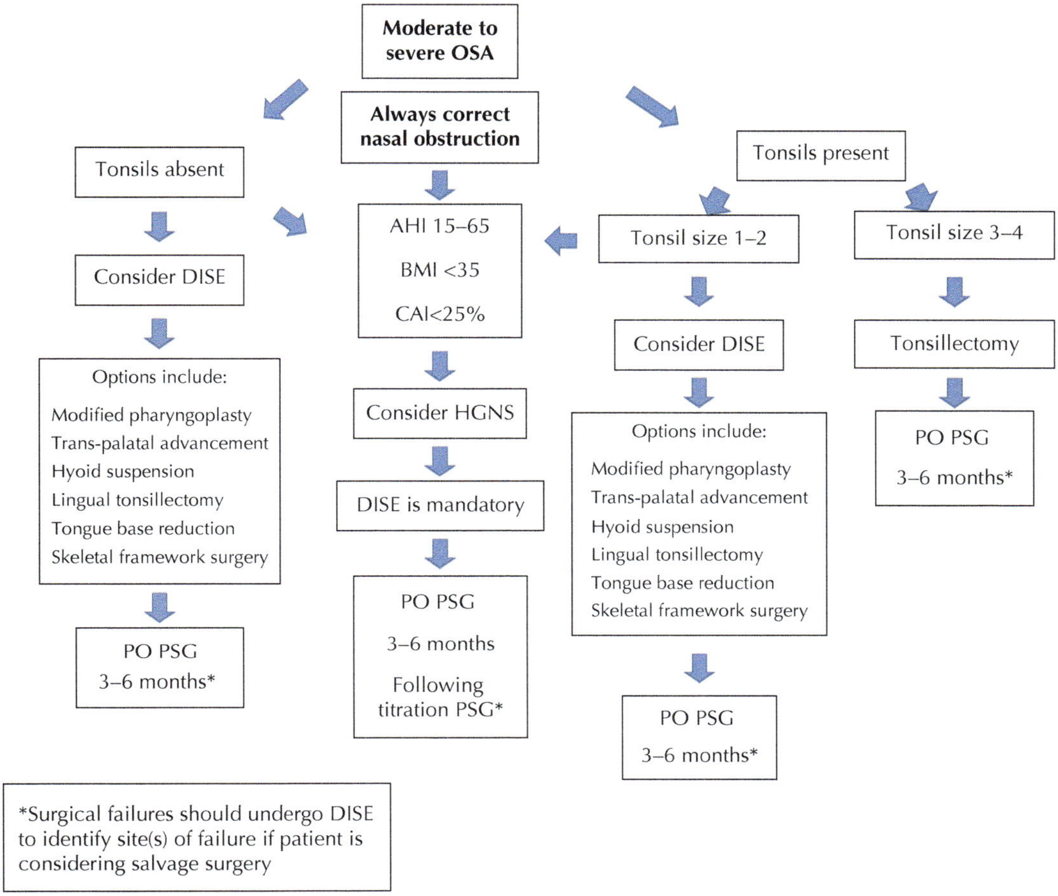

Figure 8.2. Adult moderate to severe OSA treatment algorithm. *Surgical failures should undergo DISE to identify site(s) of failure if patient is considering salvage surgery.

Conclusion

Proper selection of patients seeking a surgical alternative to conservative therapy for OSA remains a challenge. Improvements in diagnostic techniques and the understanding of OSA phenotypes have improved patient selection. The standardization of DISE has provided a tremendous benefit in our understanding of dynamic collapse patterns of the airway. A wide variety of surgical treatment options can now be tailored to a patient's unique anatomic phenotype. The advent of neuromuscular stimulation is a welcome addition to the surgical armamentarium. Surgical salvage, particularly with HGNS, now rivals best outcomes with PAP therapy. Moreover, sleep surgeons have revised their definition of surgical success to parameters more in keeping with the sleep medicine literature; success will no longer be defined by the traditional criteria (AHI < 20 events/hr and a 50% reduction in AHI), but rather by definitions more aligned with meaningful clinical metrics.

SURGERY FOR PEDIATRIC SLEEP-DISORDERED BREATHING

In contrast to the conservative therapies initially recommended for adults with OSA, surgical intervention in the form of adenotonsillecomy (AT) is considered the first-line treatment for obstructive sleep-disordered breathing (SDB) in otherwise healthy children. The term SDB instead of OSA is often used in reference to pediatric patients because a PSG is required for the diagnosis of OSA and that study is not

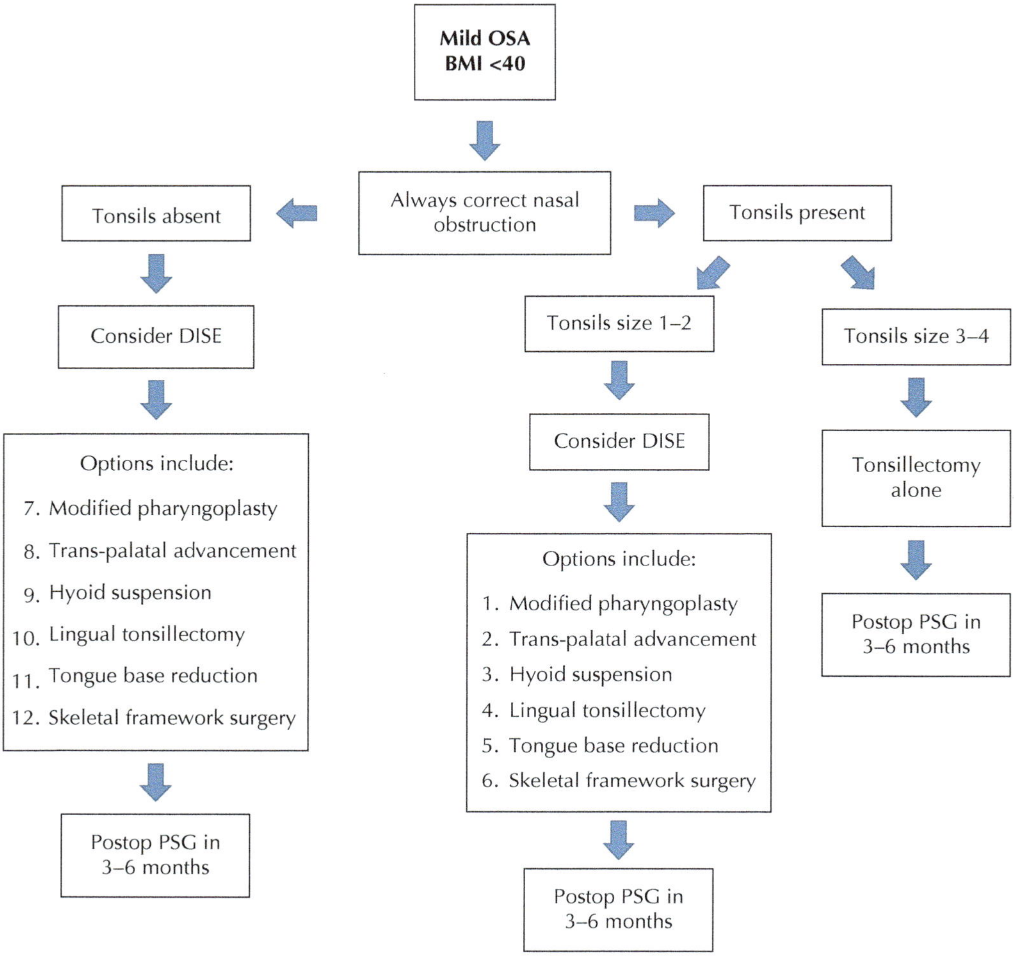

Figure 8.3. Adult mild OSA treatment algorithm.

routinely performed in otherwise healthy children prior to surgical intervention. As with adults, recent advancements in both diagnostic and surgical techniques have expanded the options for surgical treatment of SDB in children. Populations of children with significant risk for multilevel obstruction are therefore increasingly likely to undergo more detailed initial evaluations to determine specific sites of obstruction with a goal of determining an optimal individualized surgical recommendation. A detailed algorithm for pediatric SDB is noted in Figure 8.4.

Adenotonsillectomy (AT)

Guidelines from both the American Academy of Pediatrics (AAP) and the American Academy of Otolaryngology-Head and Neck Surgery (AAO-HNS) recommend AT as first-line therapy for otherwise healthy children over 2 years of age with moderate or severe OSA and adenotonsillar hypertrophy.[39,40] Adenotonsillectomy may also be used as initial therapy for children with multifactorial OSA, including contributions from obesity, if appreciable adenotonsillar tissue is present.

PREOPERATIVE ASSESSMENT FOR AT

The decision to initiate any surgical treatment for SDB in children is made on a case-by-case basis. Important considerations include severity of symptoms, the child's age, PSG abnormalities, and any underlying medical issues or complications related to OSA. In addition to a comprehensive general and sleep history, a detailed physical exam should be performed including growth curves, BMI, labored breathing patterns, facial skeletal morphology, mouth breathing, nasal turbinate hypertrophy, tonsillar size, palatal configuration (including length, width, and height), and tongue size and position. Any symptoms of unusual bleeding or bruising in the patient or family should be elicited. If PSG was not already performed for diagnostic purposes, it is recommended as part of preoperative planning for patients with conditions that increase the risk for respiratory complications, including severe obesity, trisomy 21, craniofacial abnormalities, neuromuscular disorders, sickle cell disease, or mucopolysaccharidoses. Children with these disorders also require additional evaluation and disease-specific management. Relative contraindications to AT include minimal or absent adenotonsillar tissue, submucous cleft palate, a bleeding disorder that cannot be adequately controlled for surgery, or other underlying disorders that render the patient medically unstable for surgery.

AT SURGICAL TECHNIQUES

A variety of instruments have been devised for the removal of tonsillar and adenoid tissue. Traditionally, the most common approach has been extracapsular (complete) tonsillectomy, which includes removal of the entire palatine tonsil and the surrounding fascia or capsule. Intracapsular (partial) tonsillectomy or tonsillotomy is now increasingly being used for the treatment of obstructive SDB in children and consists of debulking the obstructing portions of the tonsil tissue.[41,42] However, tonsillotomy also may be associated with a greater risk of tonsillar regrowth, which occasionally requires revision surgery.

During adenoidectomy, the obstructing portions of adenoid tissue are removed from the nasopharynx with the use of ether sharp curettes (sharp or cold dissection), electrocautery, Coblation™, or microdebrider. The procedure is generally done trans-orally after retraction of the soft palate, taking care to avoid trauma to the undersurface of the palate or Eustachian tube orifices. Occasionally, tissue removal via a trans-nasal approach also may be necessary.

COMPLICATIONS OF AT

The vast majority of children will have throat pain, otalgia, halitosis, and odynophagia for up to 2 weeks after adenotonsillar surgery until the tonsillar fossae are fully mucosalized. Transient nausea and vomiting are not uncommon, sometimes requiring admission or readmission for dehydration.[43] Post-tonsillectomy bleeding can occur either within 24 hours (termed early, or primary hemorrhage) or at any subsequent time (termed delayed or secondary hemorrhage). Primary hemorrhage typically ranges from 0.2% to 2.2% and secondary hemorrhage between 0.1% and 3%.[44] Postoperative respiratory complications are also frequent after AT and can range from transient laryngospasm or mild desaturation to life-threatening airway obstruction or pulmonary edema. OSA is an important risk factor for developing postoperative respiratory complications, particularly if the OSA is severe.[45] Other risk factors include cardiac morbidity (due to the OSA or other factors), obesity, craniofacial or neuromuscular disorders, history of seizures, asthma, or prematurity, or recent upper respiratory infections.[46] Children with any of these risk factors should be carefully observed for respiratory complications during the postoperative period and admitted for observation as indicated.

SUCCESS RATES FOR PEDIATRIC AT

Most otherwise healthy children with obstructive SDB and adenotonsillar hypertrophy will derive some benefit from AT, as measured by improvement in PSG parameters and symptoms. Reported PSG outcomes after AT vary considerably, with reported success rates ranging from 27% to 80%, depending on study design and PSG criteria used to define success.[47–50] A randomized trial (Childhood Adenotonsillectomy Trial [CHAT]) compared the outcomes of AT with those of watchful waiting in children with PSG documented mild-moderate OSA.[50] At 7 month's follow-up, 79% of children treated with adenotonsillectomy had normalization of PSG findings, compared with 46% of the control group. In a meta-analysis including over 1000 children who underwent tonsillectomy for OSA, 59% had complete normalization of PSG parameters, defined by AHI <1. The resolution rate was 39% in patients with severe obesity or severe OSA, compared with 74% in uncomplicated patients.[49] However, a retrospective multisite study demonstrated that only 27% of children had resolution of OSA using the same criteria.[47] This discrepancy may be partially explained by the study population, which had a higher prevalence of risk factors associated with residual disease, including older age, obesity, or more severe OSA at baseline (AHI >5). Improvement in symptomatic outcomes has also been demonstrated for many children after AT. There is moderately good evidence that AT improves quality of life for children with OSA.[47,50–52] Adenotonsillectomy may also improve cognitive function and behavior in children with OSA, although the evidence for this is somewhat weaker.[53,54]

RISK FACTORS FOR PERSISTENT OSA AFTER AT

A substantial proportion of children undergoing AT have persistent disease. Recurrence of OSA can also be seen long after AT, even when initial resolution of disease is achieved.[55] In a prospective longitudinal study of 135 children undergoing AT for documented OSA, a worsening of postoperative AHI was seen in 68% of children during the 36-month follow-up period.[56] The likelihood of persistent disease is significantly increased in the setting of obesity, more severe baseline OSA, craniofacial anomalies, Trisomy 21, Prader-Willi syndrome, hypotonia, or mucopolysaccharidoses.[57–61]

INDICATIONS FOR POST-AT POLYSOMNOGRAPHY

A clinical re-evaluation of all children several months after AT is recommended to determine whether snoring and other symptoms of SDB have resolved. For those with persistent symptoms or concerns, repeat PSG is recommended. In children with higher risk of persistent disease, such as those with severe obesity or craniofacial syndromes, a postoperative PSG should be considered even in the absence of snoring or other symptoms.[39]

Management of Patients with Residual OSA After AT or at High Risk for Multilevel Obstruction

Patients with clinically significant OSA after AT should be further evaluated to determine the site(s) of obstruction and to guide further interventions.

DIAGNOSTIC PROCEDURES

Evaluation beyond a standard physical examination is generally required to determine areas of concern for obstruction in children with persistent OSA after AT.

Flexible Nasolaryngoscopy

Flexible fiber-optic nasolaryngoscopy can generally be done in the office without sedation. It is often used as a first step in evaluating children with residual disease and may identify nasopharyngeal stenosis, lingual tonsillar hypertrophy, or laryngomalacia.

Drug-Induced Sleep Endoscopy (DISE)

DISE is increasingly used to evaluate sites of airway collapse prior to surgical intervention in children anatomically predisposed to multilevel collapse, or in those with persistent OSA after AT.[62–68] As described previously, this procedure assesses the entire airway using a flexible fiber-optic laryngoscope during anesthetically simulated sleep with preservation of spontaneous respiration. DISE evaluates the extent and orientation of obstruction at 4–5 anatomical sites of potential collapse (adenoids, palate or velum, lateral pharyngeal wall, tongue base, and epiglottis). In a study of 56 children with either persistent OSA following AT or infant OSA, DISE-directed surgery led to significant improvements in the AHI.[65] Increasing evidence supports the use of DISE prior to surgical intervention for children considered at high risk for persistence disease after AT due either to syndromes (trisomy 21, craniofacial conditions, or neuromuscular disorders with hypotonia) or factors such as age >7 years, small tonsils, obesity, or severe baseline OSA. In a group of 62 surgically naive children whose type of surgical intervention was determined by DISE, an intervention other than AT was performed in 58% of the patients. DISE-directed surgery was successful in reducing the total number of obstructive respiratory events in 79% of subjects in this high-risk group.[69]

Magnetic Resonance Imaging (MRI)

Cine MRI is done under sedation and allows for 3-dimensional analysis of the upper airway. This technique is useful for surgical planning in children in whom multiple sites of obstruction are suspected due to obesity, craniofacial syndromes, or neuromuscular disorders, or in children with persistent OSA after AT.[70,71] In a group of 27 patients with trisomy 21 and persistent OSA after adenotonsillectomy, cine MRI identified multiple sites of anatomical collapse, including glossoptosis and recurrent adenoid tissue, hypopharyngeal collapse, lingual tonsillar hypertrophy), and macroglossia.[72]

Pediatric Surgical Procedures Beyond AT

A variety of surgical procedures have been developed to treat OSA in children without significant tonsillar hypertrophy, with residual disease after AT, or with known multilevel obstruction.

TONGUE BASE REDUCTION PROCEDURES

Airway obstruction at the level of the base of tongue is increasingly recognized as a cause of persistent OSA after AT, especially in children with obesity, trisomy 21, and craniofacial or neuromuscular disorders. Previous methods to reduce tongue tissue, primarily with the use of lasers, were limited by morbidity and were not widely performed.[17] More recently, endoscopic-assisted Coblation™ lingual tonsillectomy has emerged as a safe and effective technique to treat tongue base collapse in children with OSA and large lingual tonsils. A systematic review identified a total of 6 studies addressing the use of lingual tonsillectomy for persistent OSA after AT.[73] Rates of OSA resolution ranged between 57% and 88%, although in 3 of the studies additional sites of obstruction were noted and supplemental surgical procedures were performed.

HYPOGLOSSAL NERVE STIMULATION (HGNS)

HGNS employs an implantable device to deliver electrical impulses to branches of the hypoglossal nerve in response to the respiratory cycle, resulting in protrusion of the tongue base musculature. As described previously, this procedure is increasingly used to alleviate BOT obstruction in adults but has not yet been extensively studied in the pediatric population. In a case series of 20 non-obese children with trisomy 21 and severe OSA after AT, HGNS resulted in significant improvement in OSA, with a median reduction in AHI of 85% 2 months postoperatively.[74] The device was well tolerated, with 2 complications requiring minor revision surgery and no long-term complications.

EXPANSION AND LATERAL PHARYNGOPLASTY

In some children, OSA is associated with collapse of the lateral pharyngeal wall.[68,71] Surgical procedures to correct this problem include expansion sphincter pharyngoplasty (ESP) or lateral pharyngoplasty. In ESP, the palatopharyngeus muscle in the lateral pharyngeal wall is rotated and sutured superiorly and laterally to create lateral wall tension. A complete or partial uvulectomy is then performed.[15] The outcomes of ESP were reported for a group of 25 children with severe OSA and lateral pharyngeal wall collapse identified on DISE who underwent modified ESP with AT, and compared with 25 AHI-matched children who underwent only AT.[75] The AHI after surgery was lower in both groups. Cure (defined by AHI <1 event/hr) was seen in 64% of children treated with modified ESP, compared with 8% in the group undergoing AT alone.

Lateral pharyngoplasty (suturing of the tonsillar pillars) after AT may also address lateral pharyngeal wall collapse and provide better control of OSA. In a prospective controlled study, 24 children with OSA underwent either AT with suturing of the tonsillar pillars or the control treatment of AT alone.[76] The AHI improved by 79.9% in the intervention group, compared with 42.6% in the control group. Complete resolution of OSA (defined by AHI <1) was seen in 50% of the children in the intervention group, compared with 16.7% in the control group.

SUPRAGLOTTOPLASTY

Supraglottoplasty is moderately effective for treating children with laryngomalacia and OSA. A systematic review examining studies of supraglottoplasty in children with persistent OSA after AT identified 4 studies reporting on 77 children.[77] The pooled mean AHI improved from 12.1 to 4.4 events/hr after surgery. In another systematic review and meta-analysis, a subgroup of children with sleep-exclusive laryngomalacia had improvement of mean AHI from 14.0 to 3.3 events/hr. Only 10.5% of children had resolution of OSA, defined as an AHI <1/hr. In the subgroup of children with congenital laryngomalacia, the mean AHI improved from 20.4 to 4.0 and oxygen saturation nadir also improved, while 26.5% had resolution of their OSA.[73]

RAPID MAXILLARY EXPANSION (RME)

Patients with high-arched and/or narrow hard palates (transverse maxillary deficiency) are at higher risk for OSA and can often be addressed by rapid expansion of the palate. Because their palatal suture is not yet fused, RME can be accomplished in children without the need for surgical intervention by using specialized orthodontic appliances containing expansion screws. The screws are turned at regular intervals, producing a transverse widening. A meta-analysis including 17 studies and over 300 children showed a decrease in AHI from a mean of 8.9 to 2.7 events/hr, representing a 70% reduction. In the 90 patients for whom it could be determined, the cure rate (AHI <1) was approximately 25%.[78]

MANDIBULAR DISTRACTION OSTEOGENESIS

Mandibular distraction osteogenesis had been used successfully to address severe OSA due to mandibular hypoplasia (micrognathia) in infants and children. The mandible is divided bilaterally, and internal or external distraction devices are placed on each side. The distraction devices are then used to move the mandible forward at a rate of 1–2 mm/day until the desired advancement is achieved. Outcomes of mandibular distraction osteogenesis were examined in a meta-analysis that included 74 articles and a total of 711 patients with a variety of craniofacial anomalies including Pierre Robin sequence and Treacher Collins syndrome.[79] Successful treatment of airway obstruction (defined as either tracheotomy avoidance or decannulation, avoidance of CPAP, or significant improvement or absence of OSA symptoms) was observed in 89% of

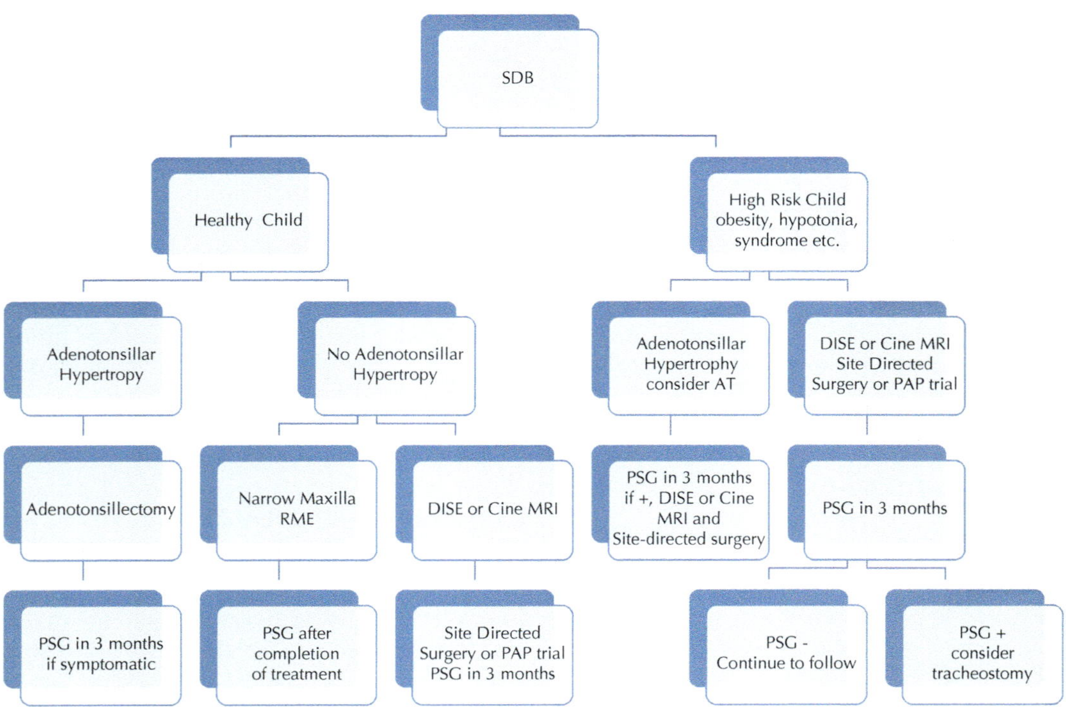

Figure 8.4. Pediatric OSA treatment algorithm.

children. Analysis was complicated by the fact that a variety of outcome measures were included and specific PSG values were not provided. Of note, a 23.8% complication rate was seen, most often in the form of infection, abscess, open bite deformity, nerve injuries, or hypertrophic scarring. These data suggest that distraction osteogenesis can be considered as a treatment for severe OSA in selected patients with mandibular hypoplasia but that the high complication rate mandates careful consideration when contemplating the procedure.

TRACHEOSTOMY

Tracheostomy can be considered in children with persistent severe OSA despite surgical intervention, especially if they are intolerant of CPAP therapy. It can also be considered as a first-line treatment in children with severe OSA and airway obstruction who are not considered appropriate candidates for other surgical procedures. Although tracheostomy is an effective treatment for OSA and airway obstruction, it is associated with complications in as many as 43%–77% of children, including bleeding, tracheoesophageal fistula, accidental decannulation, or tube occlusion.[80,81]

Conclusion

As with adults, recent innovations in both diagnostic modalities and surgical techniques have increased the available options for surgical treatment of children with SDB. These advances have been especially helpful in the treatment of children with residual disease after AT, as well as those populations at high risk for severe refractory disease due to hypotonia, skeletal deformities, and/or multilevel obstruction.

REFERENCES

1. Friedman M, Ibrahim H, Bass L. Clinical staging for sleep-disordered breathing. *Otolaryngol Head Neck Surg*. Jul 2002;127(1):13–21. doi:10.1067/mhn.2002.126477
2. Woodson BT. A method to describe the pharyngeal airway. *Laryngoscope*. May 2015;125(5):1233–1238. doi:10.1002/lary.24972
3. Moore KE, Phillips C. A practical method for describing patterns of tongue-base narrowing (modification of Fujita) in awake adult patients with obstructive sleep apnea. *J Oral Maxillofac Surg*. Mar 2002;60(3):252–260; discussion 260–261. doi:10.1053/joms.2002.30567
4. Friedman M, Yalamanchali S, Gorelick G, Joseph NJ, Hwang MS. A standardized lingual tonsil grading system: interexaminer agreement. *Otolaryngol Head Neck Surg*. Apr 2015;152(4):667–672. doi:10.1177/0194599815568970
5. Kezirian EJ, Hohenhorst W, de Vries N. Drug-induced sleep endoscopy: the VOTE classification. *Eur Arch Otorhinolaryngol*. Aug 2011;268(8):1233–1236. doi:10.1007/s00405-011-1633-8
6. Vanderveken OM, Maurer JT, Hohenhorst W, et al. Evaluation of drug-induced sleep endoscopy as a patient selection tool for implanted upper airway stimulation for obstructive sleep apnea. *J Clin Sleep Med*. May 15 2013;9(5):433–438. doi:10.5664/jcsm.2658
7. Ong AA, Murphey AW, Nguyen SA, et al. Efficacy of upper airway stimulation on collapse patterns observed during drug-Induced sedation endoscopy. *Otolaryngol Head Neck Surg*. May 2016;154(5):970–977. doi:10.1177/0194599816636835
8. Friedman M, Ibrahim H, Joseph NJ. Staging of obstructive sleep apnea/hypopnea syndrome: a guide to appropriate treatment. *Laryngoscope*. Mar 2004;114(3):454–459. doi:10.1097/00005537-200403000-00013
9. Woodson BT, Toohill RJ. Transpalatal advancement pharyngoplasty for obstructive sleep apnea. *Laryngoscope*. Mar 1993;103(3):269–276. doi:10.1288/00005537-199303000-00006
10. Young T, Finn L, Kim H. Nasal obstruction as a risk factor for sleep-disordered breathing. The University of Wisconsin Sleep and Respiratory Research Group. *J Allergy Clin Immunol*. Feb 1997;99(2):S757–762. doi:10.1016/s0091-6749(97)70124-6
11. Young T, Finn L, Palta M. Chronic nasal congestion at night is a risk factor for snoring in a population-based cohort study. *Arch Intern Med*. Jun 25 2001;161(12):1514–1519. doi:10.1001/archinte.161.12.1514
12. Cahali MB. Lateral pharyngoplasty: a new treatment for obstructive sleep apnea hypopnea syndrome. *Laryngoscope*. Nov 2003;113(11):1961–1968. doi:10.1097/00005537-200311000-00020
13. Li HY, Lee LA. Relocation pharyngoplasty for obstructive sleep apnea. *Laryngoscope*. Dec 2009;119(12):2472–2477. doi:10.1002/lary.20634
14. MacKay SG, Carney AS, Woods C, et al. Modified uvulopalatopharyngoplasty and coblation channeling of the tongue for obstructive sleep apnea: a multi-centre Australian trial. *J Clin Sleep Med*. Feb 1 2013;9(2):117–124. doi:10.5664/jcsm.2402
15. Pang KP, Woodson BT. Expansion sphincter pharyngoplasty: a new technique for the treatment of obstructive sleep apnea. *Otolaryngol Head Neck Surg*. Jul 2007;137(1):110–114. doi:10.1016/j.otohns.2007.03.014
16. Vicini C, Hendawy E, Campanini A, et al. Barbed reposition pharyngoplasty (BRP) for OSAHS: a feasibility, safety, efficacy and teachability pilot study. "We are on the giant's shoulders". *Eur Arch Otorhinolaryngol*. Oct 2015;272(10):3065–3070. doi:10.1007/s00405-015-3628-3
17. Fujita S, Woodson BT, Clark JL, Wittig R. Laser midline glossectomy as a treatment for obstructive sleep

apnea. *Laryngoscope*. Aug 1991;101(8):805–809. doi:10.1288/00005537-199108000-00001
18. Chabolle F, Wagner I, Blumen MB, Sequert C, Fleury B, De Dieuleveult T. Tongue base reduction with hyoepiglottoplasty: a treatment for severe obstructive sleep apnea. *Laryngoscope*. Aug 1999;109(8):1273–1280. doi:10.1097/00005537-199908000-00017
19. Gunawardena I, Robinson S, MacKay S, et al. Submucosal lingualplasty for adult obstructive sleep apnea. *Otolaryngol Head Neck Surg*. Jan 2013;148(1):157–165. doi:10.1177/0194599812461750
20. Li HY, Lee LA, Kezirian EJ. Coblation endoscopic lingual lightening (CELL) for obstructive sleep apnea. *Eur Arch Otorhinolaryngol*. Jan 2016;273(1):231–236. doi:10.1007/s00405-014-3475-7
21. Li KK, Powell NB, Riley RW, Guilleminault C. Temperature-controlled radiofrequency tongue base reduction for sleep-disordered breathing: Long-term outcomes. *Otolaryngol Head Neck Surg*. Sep 2002;127(3):230–234. doi:10.1067/mhn.2002.126900
22. Vicini C, Montevecchi F, Campanini A, et al. Clinical outcomes and complications associated with TORS for OSAHS: a benchmark for evaluating an emerging surgical technology in a targeted application for benign disease. *ORL J Otorhinolaryngol Relat Spec*. 2014;76(2):63–69. doi:10.1159/000360768
23. Hoff PT, D'Agostino MA, Thaler ER. Transoral robotic surgery in benign diseases including obstructive sleep apnea: Safety and feasibility. *Laryngoscope*. May 2015;125(5):1249–1253. doi:10.1002/lary.25026
24. Ong AA, Buttram J, Nguyen SA, Platter D, Abidin MR, Gillespie MB. Hyoid myotomy and suspension without simultaneous palate or tongue base surgery for obstructive sleep apnea. *World J Otorhinolaryngol Head Neck Surg*. Jun 2017;3(2):110–114. doi:10.1016/j.wjorl.2017.05.008
25. Liu SY-C, Guilleminault C, Huon L-K, Yoon A. Distraction osteogenesis maxillary expansion (DOME) for adult obstructive sleep apnea patients with high arched palate. *Otolaryngology–Head and Neck Surgery*. 2017;157(2):345–348. doi:10.1177/0194599817707168
26. Riley RW, Powell NB, Guilleminault C, Nino-Murcia G. Maxillary, mandibular, and hyoid advancement: an alternative to tracheostomy in obstructive sleep apnea syndrome. *Otolaryngol Head Neck Surg*. Jun 1986;94(5):584–588. doi:10.1177/019459988609400509
27. Riley RW, Powell NB, Guilleminault C. Obstructive sleep apnea syndrome: A review of 306 consecutively treated surgical patients. *Otolaryngol Head Neck Surg*. Feb 1993;108(2):117–125. doi:10.1177/019459989310800203
28. Zaghi S, Holty JE, Certal V, et al. Maxillomandibular Advancement for Treatment of Obstructive Sleep Apnea: A Meta-analysis. *JAMA Otolaryngol Head Neck Surg*. Jan 2016;142(1):58–66. doi:10.1001/jamaoto.2015.2678
29. Strollo PJ, Jr., Soose RJ, Maurer JT, et al. Upper-airway stimulation for obstructive sleep apnea. *N Engl J Med*. Jan 9 2014;370(2):139–149. doi:10.1056/NEJMoa1308659
30. Thaler E, Schwab R, Maurer J, et al. Results of the ADHERE upper airway stimulation registry and predictors of therapy efficacy. *Laryngoscope*. May 2020;130(5):1333–1338. doi:10.1002/lary.28286
31. Woodson BT, Strohl KP, Soose RJ, et al. Upper Airway Stimulation for Obstructive Sleep Apnea: 5-Year Outcomes. *Otolaryngol Head Neck Surg*. Jul 2018;159(1):194–202. doi:10.1177/0194599818762383
32. Bellamkonda N, Shiba T, Mendelsohn AH. Adverse Events in Hypoglossal Nerve Stimulator Implantation: 5-Year Analysis of the FDA MAUDE Database. *Otolaryngol Head Neck Surg*. Feb 2021;164(2):443–447. doi:10.1177/0194599820960069
33. Young T, Peppard PE, Taheri S. Excess weight and sleep-disordered breathing. *J Appl Physiol (1985)*. Oct 2005;99(4):1592–1599. doi:10.1152/japplphysiol.00587.2005
34. Sarkhosh K, Switzer NJ, El-Hadi M, Birch DW, Shi X, Karmali S. The impact of bariatric surgery on obstructive sleep apnea: a systematic review. *Obes Surg*. Mar 2013;23(3):414–423. doi:10.1007/s11695-012-0862-2
35. Buchwald H, Avidor Y, Braunwald E, et al. Bariatric surgery: a systematic review and meta-analysis. *JAMA*. Oct 13 2004;292(14):1724–1737. doi:10.1001/jama.292.14.1724
36. Longitudinal Assessment of Bariatric Surgery Consortium, Flum DR, Belle SH, et al. Perioperative safety in the longitudinal assessment of bariatric surgery. *N Engl J Med*. Jul 30 2009;361(5):445–454. doi:10.1056/NEJMoa0901836
37. Wolfe BM, Kvach E, Eckel RH. Treatment of Obesity: Weight Loss and Bariatric Surgery. *Circ Res*. May 27 2016;118(11):1844–1855. doi:10.1161/CIRCRESAHA.116.307591
38. Sher AE, Schechtman KB, Piccirillo JF. The efficacy of surgical modifications of the upper airway in adults with obstructive sleep apnea syndrome. *Sleep*. Feb 1996;19(2):156–177. doi:10.1093/sleep/19.2.156
39. Marcus CL, Brooks LJ, Draper KA, et al. Diagnosis and management of childhood obstructive sleep apnea syndrome. *Pediatrics*. Sep 2012;130(3):e714–755. doi:10.1542/peds.2012-1672
40. Mitchell RB, Archer SM, Ishman SL, et al. Clinical Practice Guideline: Tonsillectomy in Children (Update)-Executive Summary. *Otolaryngol Head Neck Surg*. Feb 2019;160(2):187–205. doi:10.1177/0194599818807917
41. Burton MJ, Doree C. Coblation versus other surgical techniques for tonsillectomy. *The Cochrane Database of Systematic Reviews*. 2007;(3):CD004619. doi:10.1002/14651858.CD004619.pub2
42. Mösges R, Hellmich M, Allekotte S, Albrecht K, Böhm M. Hemorrhage rate after coblation tonsillectomy: a meta-analysis of published trials. *European archives of oto-rhino-laryngology: official journal of the European Federation of Oto-Rhino-Laryngological Societies (EUFOS): affiliated with the German Society for Oto-Rhino-Laryngology - Head and Neck Surgery*. 2011;268(6):807–816. doi:10.1007/s00405-011-1535-9
43. Johnson LB, Elluru RG, Myer CM. Complications of adenotonsillectomy. *The Laryngoscope*. 2002;112(8 Pt 2 Suppl 100):35–36. doi:10.1002/lary.5541121413

44. Windfuhr JP, Chen YS, Remmert S. Hemorrhage following tonsillectomy and adenoidectomy in 15,218 patients. *Otolaryngol Head Neck Surg*. Feb 2005;132(2):281–286. doi:10.1016/j.otohns.2004.09.007
45. De Luca Canto G, Pacheco-Pereira C, Aydinoz S, et al. Adenotonsillectomy Complications: A Meta-analysis. *Pediatrics*. Oct 2015;136(4):702–718. doi:10.1542/peds.2015-1283
46. Leong AC, Davis JP. Morbidity after adenotonsillectomy for paediatric obstructive sleep apnoea syndrome: waking up to a pragmatic approach. *J Laryngol Otol*. Sep 2007;121(9):809–817. doi:10.1017/S0022215107008900
47. Bhattacharjee R, Kheirandish-Gozal L, Spruyt K, et al. Adenotonsillectomy outcomes in treatment of obstructive sleep apnea in children: a multicenter retrospective study. *Am J Respir Crit Care Med*. Sep 1 2010;182(5):676–683. doi:10.1164/rccm.200912-1930OC
48. Brietzke SE, Gallagher D. The effectiveness of tonsillectomy and adenoidectomy in the treatment of pediatric obstructive sleep apnea/hypopnea syndrome: a meta-analysis. *Otolaryngol Head Neck Surg*. Jun 2006;134(6):979–984. doi:10.1016/j.otohns.2006.02.033
49. Friedman M, Wilson M, Lin HC, Chang HW. Updated systematic review of tonsillectomy and adenoidectomy for treatment of pediatric obstructive sleep apnea/hypopnea syndrome. *Otolaryngol Head Neck Surg*. Jun 2009;140(6):800–808. doi:10.1016/j.otohns.2009.01.043
50. Marcus CL, Moore RH, Rosen CL, et al. A randomized trial of adenotonsillectomy for childhood sleep apnea. *N Engl J Med*. Jun 20 2013;368(25):2366–2376. doi:10.1056/NEJMoa1215881
51. Garetz SL, Mitchell RB, Parker PD, et al. Quality of life and obstructive sleep apnea symptoms after pediatric adenotonsillectomy. *Pediatrics*. Feb 2015;135(2):e477–486. doi:10.1542/peds.2014-0620
52. Venekamp RP, Hearne BJ, Chandrasekharan D, Blackshaw H, Lim J, Schilder AG. Tonsillectomy or adenotonsillectomy versus non-surgical management for obstructive sleep-disordered breathing in children. *Cochrane Database Syst Rev*. Oct 14 2015;(10):CD011165. doi:10.1002/14651858.CD011165.pub2
53. Avior G, Fishman G, Leor A, Sivan Y, Kaysar N, Derowe A. The effect of tonsillectomy and adenoidectomy on inattention and impulsivity as measured by the Test of Variables of Attention (TOVA) in children with obstructive sleep apnea syndrome. *Otolaryngol Head Neck Surg*. Oct 2004;131(4):367–371. doi:10.1016/j.otohns.2004.04.015
54. Chervin RD, Ruzicka DL, Giordani BJ, et al. Sleep-disordered breathing, behavior, and cognition in children before and after adenotonsillectomy. *Pediatrics*. Apr 2006;117(4):e769–778. doi:10.1542/peds.2005-1837
55. Amin R, Anthony L, Somers V, et al. Growth velocity predicts recurrence of sleep-disordered breathing 1 year after adenotonsillectomy. *Am J Respir Crit Care Med*. Mar 15 2008;177(6):654–659. doi:10.1164/rccm.200710-1610OC
56. Huang YS, Guilleminault C, Lee LA, Lin CH, Hwang FM. Treatment outcomes of adenotonsillectomy for children with obstructive sleep apnea: a prospective longitudinal study. *Sleep*. Jan 1 2014;37(1):71–76. doi:10.5665/sleep.3310
57. Costa DJ, Mitchell R. Adenotonsillectomy for obstructive sleep apnea in obese children: a meta-analysis. *Otolaryngol Head Neck Surg*. Apr 2009;140(4):455–460. doi:10.1016/j.otohns.2008.12.038
58. Gonuldas B, Yilmaz T, Sivri HS, et al. Mucopolysaccharidosis: Otolaryngologic findings, obstructive sleep apnea and accumulation of glucosaminoglycans in lymphatic tissue of the upper airway. *Int J Pediatr Otorhinolaryngol*. Jun 2014;78(6):944–949. doi:10.1016/j.ijporl.2014.03.021
59. Imanguli M, Ulualp SO. Risk factors for residual obstructive sleep apnea after adenotonsillectomy in children. *Laryngoscope*. Nov 2016;126(11):2624–2629. doi:10.1002/lary.25979
60. Lee CH, Hsu WC, Ko JY, Yeh TH, Lin MT, Kang KT. Adenotonsillectomy for the Treatment of Obstructive Sleep Apnea in Children with Prader-Willi Syndrome: A Meta-analysis. *Otolaryngol Head Neck Surg*. Feb 2020;162(2):168–176. doi:10.1177/0194599819893115
61. Shete MM, Stocks RM, Sebelik ME, Schoumacher RA. Effects of adeno-tonsillectomy on polysomnography patterns in Down syndrome children with obstructive sleep apnea: a comparative study with children without Down syndrome. *Int J Pediatr Otorhinolaryngol*. Mar 2010;74(3):241–244. doi:10.1016/j.ijporl.2009.11.006
62. Boudewyns A, Verhulst S, Maris M, Saldien V, Van de Heyning P. Drug-induced sedation endoscopy in pediatric obstructive sleep apnea syndrome. *Sleep Med*. Dec 2014;15(12):1526–1531. doi:10.1016/j.sleep.2014.06.016
63. Chan DK, Liming BJ, Horn DL, Parikh SR. A new scoring system for upper airway pediatric sleep endoscopy. *JAMA Otolaryngol Head Neck Surg*. Jul 2014;140(7):595–602. doi:10.1001/jamaoto.2014.612
64. Durr ML, Meyer AK, Kezirian EJ, Rosbe KW. Drug-induced sleep endoscopy in persistent pediatric sleep-disordered breathing after adenotonsillectomy. *Arch Otolaryngol Head Neck Surg*. Jul 2012;138(7):638–643. doi:10.1001/archoto.2012.1067
65. He S, Peddireddy NS, Smith DF, et al. Outcomes of Drug-Induced Sleep Endoscopy-Directed Surgery for Pediatric Obstructive Sleep Apnea. *Otolaryngol Head Neck Surg*. Mar 2018;158(3):559–565. doi:10.1177/0194599817740332
66. Lam DJ, Weaver EM, Macarthur CJ, et al. Assessment of pediatric obstructive sleep apnea using a drug-induced sleep endoscopy rating scale. *Laryngoscope*. Jun 2016;126(6):1492–498. doi:10.1002/lary.25842
67. Truong MT, Woo VG, Koltai PJ. Sleep endoscopy as a diagnostic tool in pediatric obstructive sleep apnea. *Int J Pediatr Otorhinolaryngol*. May 2012;76(5):722–727. doi:10.1016/j.ijporl.2012.02.028
68. Ulualp SO, Szmuk P. Drug-induced sleep endoscopy for upper airway evaluation in children with obstructive sleep apnea. *Laryngoscope*. Jan 2013;123(1):292–297. doi:10.1002/lary.23832
69. Kirkham E, Ma CC, Filipek N, et al. Polysomnography outcomes of sleep endoscopy-directed intervention in surgically naive children at risk for persistent obstructive sleep apnea. *Sleep Breath*. Sep 2020;24(3):1143–1150. doi:10.1007/s11325-019-02006-y

70. Isaiah A, Kiss E, Olomu P, Koral K, Mitchell RB. Characterization of upper airway obstruction using cine MRI in children with residual obstructive sleep apnea after adenotonsillectomy. *Sleep Med.* Oct 2018;50:79–86. doi:10.1016/j.sleep.2017.10.006
71. Shott SR, Donnelly LF. Cine magnetic resonance imaging: evaluation of persistent airway obstruction after tonsil and adenoidectomy in children with Down syndrome. *Laryngoscope.* Oct 2004;114(10):1724–1729. doi:10.1097/00005537-200410000-00009
72. Donnelly LF, Shott SR, LaRose CR, Chini BA, Amin RS. Causes of persistent obstructive sleep apnea despite previous tonsillectomy and adenoidectomy in children with down syndrome as depicted on static and dynamic cine MRI. *AJR Am J Roentgenol.* Jul 2004;183(1):175–181. doi:10.2214/ajr.183.1.1830175
73. Manickam PV, Shott SR, Boss EF, et al. Systematic review of site of obstruction identification and non-CPAP treatment options for children with persistent pediatric obstructive sleep apnea. *Laryngoscope.* Feb 2016;126(2):491–500. doi:10.1002/lary.25459
74. Caloway CL, Diercks GR, Keamy D, et al. Update on hypoglossal nerve stimulation in children with down syndrome and obstructive sleep apnea. *Laryngoscope.* Apr 2020;130(4):E263–E267. doi:10.1002/lary.28138
75. Ulualp SO. Modified expansion sphincter pharyngoplasty for treatment of children with obstructive sleep apnea. *JAMA Otolaryngol Head Neck Surg.* Sep 2014;140(9):817–822. doi:10.1001/jamaoto.2014.1329
76. Chiu PH, Ramar K, Chen KC, et al. Can pillar suturing promote efficacy of adenotonsillectomy for pediatric OSAS? A prospective randomized controlled trial. *Laryngoscope.* Oct 2013;123(10):2573–2577. doi:10.1002/lary.24011
77. Camacho M, Dunn B, Torre C, et al. Supraglottoplasty for laryngomalacia with obstructive sleep apnea: A systematic review and meta-analysis. *Laryngoscope.* May 2016;126(5):1246–1255. doi:10.1002/lary.25827
78. Camacho M, Chang ET, Song SA, et al. Rapid maxillary expansion for pediatric obstructive sleep apnea: A systematic review and meta-analysis. *Laryngoscope.* Jul 2017;127(7):1712–1719. doi:10.1002/lary.26352
79. Tahiri Y, Viezel-Mathieu A, Aldekhayel S, Lee J, Gilardino M. The effectiveness of mandibular distraction in improving airway obstruction in the pediatric population. *Plast Reconstr Surg.* Mar 2014;133(3):352e–359e. doi:10.1097/01.prs.0000438049.29258.a8
80. Carr MM, Poje CP, Kingston L, Kielma D, Heard C. Complications in pediatric tracheostomies. *Laryngoscope.* Nov 2001;111(11 Pt 1):1925–1928. doi:10.1097/00005537-200111000-00010
81. Mahadevan M, Barber C, Salkeld L, Douglas G, Mills N. Pediatric tracheotomy: 17 year review. *Int J Pediatr Otorhinolaryngol.* Dec 2007;71(12):1829–1835. doi:10.1016/j.ijporl.2007.08.007
82. Lin HS, Rowley JA, Folbe AJ, Yoo GH, Badr MS, Chen W. Transoral robotic surgery for treatment of obstructive sleep apnea: factors predicting surgical response. *Laryngoscope.* Apr 2015;125(4):1013–1020. doi:10.1002/lary.24970
83. Meccariello G, Cammaroto G, Montevecchi F, et al. Transoral robotic surgery for the management of obstructive sleep apnea: a systematic review and meta-analysis. *Eur Arch Otorhinolaryngol.* Feb 2017;274(2):647–653. doi:10.1007/s00405-016-4113-3
84. Lin HS, Rowley JA, Badr MS, et al. Transoral robotic surgery for treatment of obstructive sleep apnea-hypopnea syndrome. *Laryngoscope.* Jul 2013;123(7):1811–1816. doi:10.1002/lary.23913
85. Suslu AE, Katar O, Jafarov S, Ozer S, Onerci M. Results of coblation midline glossectomy for obstructive sleep apnea. *Auris Nasus Larynx.* Nov 24 2020. doi:10.1016/j.anl.2020.11.002
86. Stuck BA, Ravesloot MJL, Eschenhagen T, de Vet HCW, Sommer JU. Uvulopalatopharyngoplasty with or without tonsillectomy in the treatment of adult obstructive sleep apnea - A systematic review. *Sleep Med.* Oct 2018;50:152–165. doi:10.1016/j.sleep.2018.05.004
87. Canzi P, Berardi A, Tinelli C, et al. Thirteen Years of Hyoid Suspension Experience in Multilevel OSAHS Surgery: The Short-Term Results of a Bicentric Study. *Int J Otolaryngol.* 2013;2013:263043. doi:10.1155/2013/263043
88. Brodsky L. Modern assessment of tonsils and adenoids. *Pediatr Clin North Am.* Dec 1989;36(6):1551–1569. doi:10.1016/s0031-3955(16)36806-7
89. Friedman M. *Sleep apnea and snoring: surgical and non-surgical therapy.* Saunders/Elsevier; 2009.

Chapter 9

Medical Treatments of Obstructive Sleep Apnea

Sasikanth Gorantla and Sarah Zallek

The mainstay of treatment for obstructive sleep apnea (OSA) continues to be positive airway pressure (PAP). When used consistently, it is highly effective. Developments in PAP technology and interfaces have made PAP therapy increasingly comfortable since its introduction in 1981. Adherence to treatment varies considerably, however, leaving many patients partially or not at all treated.

Several alternatives to PAP therapy are available. The options appropriate for any individual depend on several factors, including sleep apnea severity and other characteristics. This chapter will focus on positional therapy, nasal dilators, weight loss, and medications as alternatives to PAP therapy. Surgical treatments and oral appliances are addressed in other chapters in this volume.

WEIGHT LOSS

According to the Centers for Disease Control and Prevention 2017–2018 health statistics, 42.4% of adults in the United States are obese (body mass index [BMI] ≥30 kg/m^2), a significant increase from 30.5% in 1999–2000.[9] The association between OSA and obesity—a possible causal relationship—has been widely reported.[1] The exact pathophysiological mechanisms by which obesity causes OSA is not well understood.

The association between OSA and weight has been demonstrated in a few population-based cohort studies. A longitudinal population-based cohort study conducted from 1989 to 2000 with 690 randomly selected subjects in Wisconsin provided critical insights into OSA and body weight relationship. Forty-one percent of adult OSA cases and 58% of moderate to severe OSA cases were attributed to obesity. A 10% weight gain predicted a 32% increase in apnea hypopnea index (AHI) and a 6-fold increase in the odds of moderate to severe OSA, and a 10% weight loss predicted a 26% reduction in AHI.[1]

The OSA and weight relationship is not uniform across all age groups. The Cleveland Family study—another large epidemiological study with 1149 participants—revealed that the obesity and OSA association decreases with age, and becomes negligible after age 60 years.[2] Moreover, gender has also been shown to mediate the effect of weight on OSA. In the Cleveland Family Study, OSA incidence is equally distributed among men and women after age 50 years; the male predominance pattern disappeared with age.[2] Furthermore, the association between sleep-disordered breathing (SDB) and weight was more noticeable in men than women in the Sleep Heart Health Study.[3] SDB progressed over time, even in a setting of stable weight. These population-based studies provided key insights into the intricate relationship between OSA, weight, and gender.

Weight is a modifiable risk factor for OSA, but weight loss is an underutilized strategy in OSA treatment. Obesity results from a complex interplay between genetic and environmental variables.[4] Weight loss is not an easy task to accomplish, and it frequently needs a multidisciplinary approach.

Surgical interventions have shown superior long-term weight loss and reduction in AHI compared to nonsurgical weight loss options.[5] In a 2014 meta-analysis by Ashrafian et al., bariatric surgery demonstrated a greater pooled reduction in BMI and AHI of 14 kg/m^2 (11.91, 16.44) and 29/hr (22.41, 36.74), respectively, when compared with nonsurgical weight loss interventions (BMI reduction of 3.1 kg/m^2 [2.42, 3.79] and AHI reduction of 11/hr [7.81, 14.98]); 19 surgical studies (n = 525) and 20 nonsurgical (n = 825) were included in the meta-analysis.[6]

Bariatric surgery, however, is associated with an increased risk of additional GI surgeries, nutritional deficiencies, and GI ulcers.[5] Maintaining weight loss is challenging in patients who do not want to pursue surgical options. Contrary to the hypothesis that treatment of OSA leads to weight loss, OSA treatment with continuous positive airway pressure (CPAP) was associated with a weight gain of 0.35 ± 5.01 kg in a large multi-center randomized controlled trial (RCT).[7] The authors point to evidence for the mechanism as a reduction in energy expenditure (EE) during sleep without a compensatory increase in EE or decrease in energy intake during wake. This was attributed to a possible increase in muscle mass and the reduction in appetite-suppressing inflammatory cytokines.

In addition to bariatric surgery, medications can also facilitate weight loss. The therapeutic role of weight-loss medications for OSA has been investigated in a few RCTs. Liraglutide, a glucagon like peptide –1 (GLP-1) analog, at 3 mg dose was investigated in a double-blinded RCT; obese OSA subjects without diabetes were included in the study. A mean AHI and weight reduction of –6.1 (–11.0 to –1.2, p = 0.0150) and –4.2% (–5.2 to –3.1%, p < 0.0001) was noted after 32 weeks, respectively.[8] In 2024, the U.S. FDA approved tirzepatide for treating moderate to severe OSA in adults with obesity. A phase III randomized controlled trial showed significant reductions in apnea-hypopnea index (AHI) with tirzepatide compared to placebo: –20.0 events/hour (95% CI, –25.8 to –14.2; p < 0.001) in patients not using PAP therapy and –23.8 events/hour (95% CI, –29.6 to –17.9; p < 0.001) in those using CPAP prior to study enrolment.[78]

Another double-blinded RCT investigated zonisamide, a carbonic anhydrase inhibitor, in 42 OSA patients; subjects were allotted to zonisamide, CPAP, or placebo. The CPAP arm served as the control. After 4 weeks, zonisamide resulted in a 33% ± 39% mean reduction in AHI (p = 0.02) Of note, weight gain was noted with CPAP after 20 weeks in the extension phase of the study. Zonisamide was associated with weight loss as expected (–2.7 ± 3.0 kg vs. 2.3 ± 2.0 kg, p <0.001).[9] At 24 weeks, CPAP and zonisamide reduced AHI by 61% and 13% (p = 0.001), respectively. Zonisamide, like acetazolamide, can also improve OSA by lowering loop gain and stabilizing ventilatory control in OSA patients.

A phase 2 RCT that evaluated the effect of 15 mg of phentermine and 92 mg of topiramate demonstrated a mean AHI reduction of –16.6 events per hour (95% CI: –25.0, –8.2) (p = 0.0084) at week 28.[10] A significant weight loss of 10.8 kg (–13.5, –8.0) was noted with topiramate and phentermine combination when compared to placebo 4.7 kg (–7.2, –2.2) (p = 0.0006). As expected, a positive correlation was seen between percent weight loss and AHI reduction in all 3 studies. The results of these studies support a potential adjunct role for weight-loss medications in OSA management. Weight-loss medications seem to have a place in OSA treatment.

POSITIONAL THERAPY

In some, but not all, cases of OSA, body position during sleep may significantly impact the severity of the sleep-disordered breathing. In those cases, therapy to alter the sleeping position may reduce or eliminate OSA.

Positional Obstructive Sleep Apnea

In more than half of patients, OSA is worse in the supine position; upper airway collapsibility increases in supine sleep. Apneic events while supine are more severe (longer and associated with greater oxygen desaturation) than those occurring in the lateral positions.[11] Several criteria have been proposed to define positional OSA, though there are currently no universally accepted criteria.

In 1984, Cartwright first described the positional difference in apnea severity in a study of 30 men with OSA. Of the 24 whose sleep position varied through the night of recording, 14 (58%) had positional apnea, defined as a supine AHI ≥ twice the non-supine AHI. The difference between supine and non-supine AHI inversely correlated with obesity; thinner patients were more likely to have positional obstructive sleep apnea (POSA).[12] POSA may be more common in Asian populations.[13,14]

In a 1998 study to evaluate treatment with a mandibular advancement device, Marklund defined supine-dependent sleep apnea as an AHI ≥10 and a non-supine AHI of <10.[15] Further, in 2005 and 2010, respectively, Mador and Permut used the Cartwright criteria of 50% AHI reduction in the non-supine position with the additional condition that the non-supine AHI be <5.[16,17]

In an effort to identify suitable candidates for positional therapy, Frank proposed a new classification system, by consensus, in 2015; the Amsterdam Positional OSA Classification (APOC) requires the patient to be diagnosed with OSA according to the American Academy of Sleep Medicine (AASM) criteria, to spend greater than 10% of their total sleep time (TST) in both their best and worst sleeping positions (BSP, WSP, respectively).[18] Further study confirmed the inverse relationship between BMI and POSA, as Cartwright had originally noted.

Barnes summed this up by saying there are 2 generally accepted definitions of supine OSA.[19] Supine-predominant OSA is characterized by a total AHI >5, with the supine frequency of events occurring at least twice the frequency of non-supine events. This accounts for about 60% of patients with OSA. Supine-isolated OSA is characterized by a non-supine AHI <5, and the supine AHI is at least twice the frequency of non-supine events. Approximately 32% of OSA patients who present to sleep clinics have supine-isolated sleep apnea. Regardless of naming conventions and criteria for inclusion in subtypes, positional apnea is very common.

Treatment of Positional OSA (POSA) with Positional Therapy

Positional therapy (PT) aims to prevent supine sleep, and therefore reduce apnea severity by eliminating the position in which apnea is often most severe. It may be used as a sole treatment modality in patients with apnea predominantly in the supine position, or as adjunctive therapy with other modalities. In some patients who refuse all other treatment modalities, it may be a last resort to treating OSA at least in part, rather than not treating it at all.

PT was most recently reviewed by Omobomi and Quan in 2018.[20] At the time of publication, the U.S. Food and Drug Administration (FDA) had cleared 3 PT devices for clinical use: the Zzoma, Night Shift Sleep Positioner, and SONA Pillow. Since that time a fourth device, NightBalance, has been cleared.

The Zzoma consists of an adjustable belt worn around the upper torso, with a non-compressible foam wedge situated at the back to prevent supine sleep. Two sleep position trainers (SPT) vibrate when the wearer turns supine; the Night Shift Sleep Positioner is worn around the neck or chest, and the NightBalance is worn around the chest. The SONA Pillow is a shaped pillow designed to encourage non-supine sleep. Market availability of specific products changes over time. Several other products are commercially available but have not been cleared for use by the FDA.

In addition to the many forms of commercially available PT devices, self-constructed apparatuses have long been used to prevent supine sleep. The Tennis Ball Technique (TBT) involves one or more tennis balls positioned in the back of a T-shirt, pajama top, or strap-on device. Many variations of TBT apparatus have been tried. A row of 3 tennis balls arranged horizontally across the upper back might be more likely to prevent supine sleep than just 1, and a snug fit of the T-shirt might prevent shifting of the tennis balls to the side.

Effectiveness and Adherence

As with any treatment, PT is only effective if a patient uses it. Adherence to treatment varies, but the following studies suggest that long-standing continued use is uncommon.

In a meta-analysis of 3 prospective cohort studies and 4 RCTs on the efficacy of vibrating SPTs, Ravesloot reported that these devices, on the whole, are quite effective. Supine sleep was reduced by 83.8%, from 40.1% ± 17.2% to 6.5% ± 10.8%. AHI improved 53.6%, from a mean of 21.8 ± 7.2 to 9.9 ± 10.6.[21] Unlike other positioning devices, vibrating devices have the capacity to record and store sleeping-position data.

Long-term adherence to a chest-worn, vibrating sleep position trainer (SPT) after a several-day training period, with >4 hours of nightly use, was 64.4% at 6 months among those still using the device (46.9% when drop-outs were taken into consideration). Supine sleep was reduced from 21% to 3% of total sleep time with the device, and this finding was maintained over the 6-month follow-up period.[22]

In a retrospective study by de Vries, patients chose either a commercially available device (Werkmeister SnurkStop) or constructed their own device using tennis balls or other stiff material. All options mimicked TBT. Both the SnurkStop and self-made constructions were equally effective in reducing time spent supine and AHI, and improving daytime sleepiness (Epworth Sleepiness Scale [ESS] score). Adherence to treatment was high in the first few weeks, but declined to 35% after about 1 year.[23]

Oksenberg reported 19 of 50 patients (38%) were still using TBT after 6 months.[24] Bignold surveyed patients using a standardized TBT device manufactured according to a pattern previously shown by Gordon to reduce supine sleep time: a single tennis ball positioned mid-back, with a belt around the torso and straps over each shoulder.[25,26] Of 67 survey respondents (follow-up time 2.5 ± 1 years), only 4 (6%) reported regular use of the device, 9 (13.4%) claimed to have learned to sleep supine without the device, and 54 (80.6%) had ceased to use the device. In all, fewer than 10% of patients reported continued use by 30 months after prescription. Reasons for discontinuation included the tennis ball moving around, no improvement in sleep quality of daytime sleepiness, ineffectiveness at preventing supine sleep, and discomfort.

Bidarian-Moniri and others studied the effect of a mattress and pillow facilitating prone positioning on 27 patients, 15 with positional OSA (POSA) and 12 patients with non-POSA. It was very effective, reducing time spent supine (from median time 142 to <1 minute), and the median AHI decreased from 23 to 7.[27]

In a study of a chest-worn SPT and mandibular repositioning device, Dieltjens found the combination of both to be more effective than either modality alone. Both AHI and arousals were lower with combination therapy than either modality alone.[28]

Benoist and others compared PT and oral appliance therapy (OAT) in patients with POSA defined as supine AHI at least twice as high as non-supine AHI. PT and OAT were equally effective at reducing the median AHI in patients with POSA.[29]

PT may provide effective adjunctive treatment for some patients with OSA that is difficult to treat in the supine position. In a 2021 study, 191 of 272 OSA patients with AHI ≥15 were successfully titrated with CPAP, and 27 with bilevel PAP, in the supine position (AHI <10). The remaining 54, in whom titration in the supine position was unacceptable, were all successfully titrated in the lateral position, using a combination of PAP and PT.[30]

Cost of PT varies significantly among devices, including self-made constructions, but in general it is lower than most alternative device options. Although there is little published on this subject, Ramos reported the cost of PT was about 30% of the cost of CPAP.[31]

NASAL DILATORS

Internal (NoZovent) and external (Breathe Right Strips) nasal dilators have demonstrated improved nasal breathing and have been pursued as possible treatment for OSA.

A systematic review of the international literature by Camacho published in 2016 found no significant change in AHI, lowest oxygen saturation, or snoring index in OSA patients when using nasal dilators. Sub-analysis found the apnea index was slightly reduced with internal nasal dilators (decrease by 4.87 events/hr). Only minimal change in apnea index was found with the use of external nasal dilators (increase by 0.64 events/hr).[32] The inability to objectively monitor treatment efficacy is a limitation of this less commonly used OSA treatment modality.

PHARMACOTHERAPY

Pharmacotherapy for OSA remains the holy grail of sleep medicine. The first clinical trial that evaluated the efficacy of medications on OSA was published in 1982. Naloxone was investigated in 4 subjects with OSA but the results were uninterpretable because of sleep architecture disruption.[31,33] Later that year, Brownell et al. published the effect of protriptyline on OSA in the *New England Journal of Medicine*.[34] The quest for OSA pharmacotherapeutic options continued and expanded over the years with unsuccessful attempts. Over the last 4 decades, approximately 60 RCTs have been conducted to analyze the effect of medications on OSA. The failure to advance OSA pharmacological research is partly due to a relatively slow-paced accumulation of knowledge on OSA pathophysiological mechanisms.

A systematic review and meta-analysis from 2019 identified 58 RCTs with 44 medications, either monotherapy or in combination. There are only 7 medications (acetazolamide, mirtazapine, paroxetine, protriptyline, donepezil, ondansetron, and theophylline) with more than one RCT; only acetazolamide showed a small effect among these medications. Out of 51 RCTs that were included in the network meta-analysis, only 9 medications (tramazoline, liraglutide, spironolactone/furosemide, acetazolamide, dronabinol, zonisamide, phentermine, spironolactone, and ondansetron/fluoxetine) showed significant OSA severity reduction—as measured by AHI—compared to placebo. Most of these clinical trials were designed as proof-of-concept studies. None of these medications was investigated extensively in a multi-center phase III trials to determine their efficacy and safety. The possibility of type 2 error—false negative results—due to inadequate sample size is another noticeable limitation in a majority of studies. It is also worth highlighting the sampling bias introduced into these studies. Subjects with mild to moderate OSA were included in a significant proportion of these RCTs; the same sample characteristic was associated with greater medication response. Theoretically, some of the existing medications or their combinations may improve OSA, but their role as an adjunct pharmacotherapeutic intervention is not yet supported by robust evidence.

Several unique endotypes—probable pathophysiological mechanism responsible for airway obstruction during sleep—have been identified, prompting researchers to conduct RCTs with medications targeting the proposed pathophysiology. OSA endotypes are broadly categorized into anatomical and non-anatomical subtypes. Anatomical endotypes are characterized by upper airway abnormalities such as tonsillar hypertrophy (particularly in pediatric patients), crowded airway, and abnormal adipose tissue distribution in the neck due to obesity; these factors are believed to facilitate airway collapsibility during sleep. Non-anatomical characteristics have been shown to play a substantial role in OSA pathogenicity, contradicting the notion that OSA is predominantly an anatomical problem. These non-anatomical endotypes are grouped into 3 distinct pathophysiological categories: (1) dilator muscle dysfunction/impaired pharyngeal tone, resulting in reduced ability to maintain airway patency; (2) low arousal threshold; and (3) increased loop gain, causing hypersensitive ventilatory drive. OSA can be predominantly due to a single endotype or a complex interplay of more than 1 endotype; robust diagnostic tools to determine OSA endotypes accurately are yet to be developed. Table 9.1 lists medications studied on the basis of endotype.

In addition to endotypes, phenotypes are also relevant in the management of OSA. OSA phenotype knowledge may not contribute to drug development, but it can be used to prioritize or escalate treatment needs in "high-risk" phenotypes. The existing body of literature classifies OSA into 3 major phenotypes based on clinical presentation: "minimal symptoms," "disturbed sleep," and "excessive sleepiness" subgroups.[35] This classification of phenotypes, however, is incomplete and requires more research and external validation.[35] Medications aimed at "symptomatic" phenotypes do not seem to address the core pathophysiological mechanisms. However, phenotypic categorization

Table 9.1 **Medications Investigated for OSA, Based on Proposed Target Pathophysiological Mechanisms**

Improving Pharyngeal Muscle Tone	Enhancing Ventilatory Control Instability	Increasing Arousal Threshold	Increasing Upper Airway Diameter
Paroxetine	Theophylline	Trazodone	Fluticasone
Protriptyline	Acetazolamide	Zopiclone	Xylometazoline
Mirtazapine	Naloxone	Eszopiclone	Mometasone/desloratadine
Fluoxetine	Naltrexone	Temazepam	Tramazoline/dexamethasone
Physostigmine	Aminophylline	Tiagabine	Montelukast
Flumazenil	Sabeluzole		Spironolactone/furosemide
Ondansetron	Almitrine		
Desipramine	Doxapram		
Donepezil*	AR-R15896AR/NMDA receptor antagonist		
Salmeterol	Dronabinol		
Medroxy progesterone	Buspirone		
Atomoxetine	Sulthiame		
Oxybutynin			
Reboxetine			

* May act by both increasing muscle tone and stabilizing ventilatory drive.

appears to have a prognostic value in assessing cardiovascular benefits from various treatment options. A large multicentered trial with 2717 subjects with "minimal sleepiness" phenotype failed to demonstrate cardiovascular protection with PAP therapy, but CPAP significantly reduced snoring and daytime sleepiness.[36] Furthermore, the consequences of untreated OSA do not seem to be shared equally among all phenotypes. The "sleepiness" phenotype of OSA was shown to be associated with significant cardiovascular risk.[37]

Medications Proposed to Improve Sleep-Related Hypotonia of Airway Dilator Muscles

The role of serotonin on airway patency was initially reported in animal studies in the early 1990s. In vitro, neonatal rat hypoglossal motor neuron slices showed increased excitation with serotonin.[38] This finding was further investigated in an animal model of sleep-disordered breathing (English bulldog); systemic administration of serotonin precursors showed significant reduction in upper airway dilator muscle activity and upper airway cross-sectional area.[39] These results from animal studies provided a rationale to conduct clinical trials with medications that alter serotonergic neuronal activity.

Antidepressants (protriptyline, desipramine, fluoxetine, mirtazapine, and paroxetine) that antagonize serotonin, norepinephrine, and to some extent acetylcholine receptors, hypothesized to enhance airway muscle tone, have been investigated as potential OSA treatment agents. Mirtazapine, paroxetine, and protriptyline were used in more than 1 RCT; the pooled reduction in oxygen desaturation index did not reach statistical significance.[33] Low-dose mirtazapine, a tetracyclic antidepressant, showed increased genioglossus activity in rat model[40] but failed to demonstrate the same effect on OSA in humans.[41] Paroxetine did not improve OSA (75.2 ± 5.5 vs. placebo: 73.7 ± 6.9 events/hr) in 8 men with severe sleep-disordered breathing, but it enhanced genioglossus activity to some extent as measured by peak inspiratory and tonic electromyography values.[42] Protriptyline, a tricyclic antidepressant, was used in 3 clinical trials in 1980s. In addition to tolerance issues due to anticholinergic side effects, it did not show much benefit in terms of reducing apnea desaturation index.[33] Furthermore, the rationale for its use in OSA clinical trials is based on serotonin hypothesis derived from animal studies. The improvement in oxygenation during sleep was partly due to rapid eye movement (REM) sleep suppression with nortriptyline.[34]

Desipramine was investigated as a potential airway muscle tone–enhancing medication in a randomized placebo controlled trial with 14 OSA subjects.[43] Overall, there was no evidence of AHI reduction, but the post hoc subgroup analysis revealed significant reduction in AHI for patients with minimal upper airway response at baseline.[43] Similarly, protriptyline—another tricyclic antidepressant—was evaluated in 3 RCTs with sample size ranging from 14 to 45. The pooled medication effect calculated in the meta-analysis did not demonstrate significant AHI reduction.[33]

This hypothesis that acetylcholine (ACh) influences ventilatory drive, particularly during REM sleep,[44] has led to the investigation of cholinergic medications on OSA. A single dose of donepezil 10 mg at night did not improve OSA in an RCT with 41 OSA patients.[45] A month of donepezil treatment, however, improved OSA in an RCT (AHI improved by 4.5 ± 6.7), but sleep efficiency was reduced significantly. A 3-month treatment of donepezil in patients with Alzheimer disease showed significant improvement in OSA (AHI 20.0 ± 15.9 vs. 9.9 ± 11.5). Only 11 subjects were included in the last 2 studies that demonstrated beneficial effect of donepezil. Another RCT in Thailand with a larger sample size failed to demonstrate the efficacy of donepezil on OSA.[46] Gaisl et al. conducted a meta-analysis of donepezil RCTs, and it reiterated the lack of efficacy on OSA severity.[33] Thus far, the evidence argues against the use of donepezil for the treatment of OSA. Physostigmine (known to modify ACh levels) infusion reduced AHI by 13.6 (95% CI: 2.2–25.1) in a double-blinded crossover placebo controlled trial (n = 10). The AHI reduction was predominantly noticed in REM sleep.[47] Salmeterol (sympathomimetic) and medroxy progesterone did not show improvement in OSA metrics.[33]

Medications Proposed to Stabilize Ventilatory Control

Over-sensitive brainstem respiratory centers/chemo receptors—due to high loop gain—interrupt dilator muscle activation, creating a more collapsible airway.[48] Interestingly, upper airway surgery fails to improve OSA in patients with high loop gain endotype.

Pharmacological interventions that target ventilator drive have been investigated. Acetazolamide gained popularity as a potential therapeutic intervention because of its ability to lower loop gain. One of the early studies, in 1988, demonstrated beneficial effect of acetazolamide 250 mg 4 times a day dosage on OSA (50 ± 26 vs. 26 ± 20/h) (p = 0.03).[49] Another study with an experimental design used twice daily acetazolamide 500 mg in 13 CPAP-treated OSA patients; AHI improved by 51% and loop gain was reduced by 41% in this study.[50] The pooled effect of these 2 studies showed significant reduction in AHI (−9.6 [−17.7, −1.4]).[33] A recent systematic review and meta-analysis concluded that acetazolamide is not helpful for patients with OSA.[51]

Respiratory stimulants such as theophylline and aminophylline showed minimal improvement in OSA, but substantial impairment in sleep quality was noted.[33] Similar results were noted with other medications (naloxone, naltrexone, almitrine, and doxapram) proposed to alleviate the severity of OSA by stabilizing ventilator drive. N-methyl-D-aspartate (NMDA) receptor antagonists were tested for OSA treatment in a couple of studies. Sabeluzole showed serum concentration dependent improvement in oxygen desaturation index.[52] Another medication with NMDA receptor blockade (AR-R15896AR) did not show significant effect on OSA.[53] Cannabinoid receptor agonist activity was postulated to be a potential target to stabilize breathing in OSA patients. Initial phase 1 study with Dronabinol, a cannabinoid receptor agonist, showed improvement in AHI. The promising results in a phase 1 trial prompted further investigation. A phase II RCT revealed dose-dependent response, and the maximal reduction in AHI (12.9 ± 4.3) (p = .003) and ESS was demonstrated at 10 mg dosage.[54] Buspirone (20 mg), an anti-anxiety medication, was investigated in 1991 for OSA (n = 5) and it reduced AHI (30.8 ± 9.4 to 19.6 ± 10.0) without substantial improvement in oxygenation.[55] A recent RCT with 68 PAP-intolerant subjects showed a 50% reduction of AHI in 40% and 25% of the participants who received sulthiame (a carbonic anhydrase inhibitor) 400 mg and 200 mg dosage when compared with placebo, but no improvement in patient-related outcomes.[56]

Medications Proposed to Enhance Arousal Threshold

Arousal threshold—respiratory stimuli that induce awakening from sleep—has been hypothesized as an important OSA pathophysiological mechanism, but there is no clear consensus. Prior studies offered some explanation on possible underlying mechanisms.[57,58] Negative pressure in the thorax, increased carbon dioxide (CO_2) level, and/or hypoxemia were identified as possible respiratory stimuli that activate genioglossus.[59] Increased genioglossus activity is known to reduce airway collapsibility.[60] In order to recruit genioglossus muscle, the respiratory stimuli have to be accumulated to a certain threshold.[59] Unstable breathing due to frequent arousals—due to low arousal threshold—prevents the accumulation of respiratory stimuli.[61,59] High arousal threshold, via stable breathing pattern, facilitates the buildup of negative intrathoracic pressure and CO_2 that drives genioglossus activity.[59] Increasing the arousal threshold with sedating medications theoretically enables the accumulation of respiratory stimuli that eventually increases dilator muscle recruitment. Impaired/low arousal threshold can be seen in approximately one-third of OSA patients.[58,60]

Sedating medications may alleviate OSA by enhancing arousal threshold. Several RCTs have evaluated the effect of hypnotics (nitrazepam, flurazepam, triazolam, temezepam, zolpidem, zopiclone, eszopiclone, ramelteon, trazodone, daridorexant, and pseudoephedrine + diphenydramine) on OSA.[62] Contrary to the conventional belief, none of the sedating hypnotic medications worsened OSA. Eszopiclone 3 mg (25 ± 6 vs. 14 ± 4 events/hr of sleep; $p < 0.01$) and trazodone 100 mg (38.7 vs. 28.5 events/hr; $p = 0.041$) reduced AHI when compared to placebo.[63,64] Tiagabine, a γ-aminobutyric acid (GABA) reuptake receptor (GAT-1) inhibitor, was investigated to be a potential therapeutic option because of its ability to enhance slow-wave sleep and arousal threshold; OSA severity was not reduced, but slow-wave sleep was increased in the RCT.[65]

Medications Proposed to Increase Airway Diameter

Airway diameter can be increased by reducing nasal congestion and rostral fluids in the neck. Nasal obstruction due to congestion may contribute to sleep-disordered breathing by altering airflow velocity and resistance.[66] Topical intranasal steroids (fluticasone, dexamethasone, mometasone), antihistamines (desloratidine), and decongestants (tramazoline, xylometazoline) were investigated either independently or concomitantly in a few clinical trials. A crossover trial with tramazoline and dexamethasone combination for a week reduced AHI by 21% in patients with normal nasal resistance, and the improvement in OSA is correlated with enhanced nasal breathing.[67] Another RCT with montelukast and fluticasone in patients with mild OSA, without rhinitis, did not show any benefit.[68] Intranasal corticosteroids such as fluticasone and mometasone improved AHI in OSA patients with rhinitis, but the nasal decongestant xylometazoline did not show substantial benefit.[33] Tarantomontemurro et al. conducted an RCT with pseudoephedrine and diphenhydramine on OSA and it did not show any effect on OSA.[69]

Interventions that reduce rostral fluid displacement (furosemide, spironolactone, low salt intake) were investigated in a couple of RCTs; partial improvement of OSA severity was noted in these studies.[70,71]

Miscellaneous and Understudied Endotypes

A topically/nasally applied pharmacological agent (BAY 2253651) that targets and amplifies genioglossus muscle activity failed to show therapeutic benefit in patients with OSA.[72] A proof of concept studies with surfactant (RDI pre 79.7 vs. post 59.6 events/hr) and mineral oil (mean AHI reduction of 10 [6–13; $p = 0.0003$]) demonstrated modest reduction in OSA outcome measures.[33]

NOCTURNAL OXYGEN THERAPY

In a 2013 systematic review and meta-analysis, nocturnal oxygen supplementation was not associated with AHI reduction. Furthermore, oxygen increased the duration of obstructive events.[73] Oxygen supplementation improved AHI in OSA patients with high loop gain when compared to low loop gain, which highlights the value of endotype identification.[74]

A single-blinded randomized crossover study of 20 OSA subjects, 3 mg eszopiclone, and 40% supplemental oxygen in combination significantly reduced AHI (51.9 ± 6.2 vs. 29.5 ± 5.3 events/h; p <0.001) when compared with placebo and sham air intervention. Subjects with more than 50% reduction in AHI in this study had less severe OSA, less collapsible airway, and greater upper airway muscle effectiveness. Reducing loop gain with oxygen supplementation and increasing the arousal threshold with eszopiclone (hypnotics) may serve as an alternative therapeutic intervention, especially in patients without marked anatomical abnormalities.

COMBINATION THERAPIES

It is not known whether the strategies that target multiple subtypes yield meaningful reduction in OSA severity in specific subgroups. A randomized, placebo-controlled, double-blind, crossover study with 80 mg of atomoxetine and 5 mg of oxybutynin showed a median AHI reduction of 63% (34%–86%) and a median AHI reduction of 15.9 (−35.3 to −7.3; p <0.001).[75] Nineteen of 20 subjects showed improved AHI.[75] The promising result from this study is that complete OSA resolution was seen in patients with relatively lower AHI and less severe upper airway collapsibility, suggesting the role of endotype/phenotype in medication response.[76] The drug combination significantly improved upper airway collapsibility measures, breathing stability, and reduced the arousal threshold in OSA patients.[76] A similar study with 4 mg of reboxetine and 5 mg of oxybutynin for a week reduced AHI by 50% in 81% of participants in medication arm versus 13% in placebo arm (p <001).[77] Reboxetine and oxybutynin combination reduced median AHI by 59% versus 6% (p <.001); however, sleepiness as measured by ESS did not improve in this trial.

FUTURE DIRECTIONS

There is a need for additional research focused on determination of OSA endotypes and the development of medications that target specific OSA pathophysiological mechanisms. Successful development of additional effective alternatives to PAP therapy will have significant implications in the treatment of the growing population of patients with OSA.

REFERENCES

1. Peppard PE, Young T, Palta M, Dempsey J, Skatrud J. Longitudinal study of moderate weight change and sleep-disordered breathing. *JAMA*. 2000;284(23):3015–3021. doi:10.1001/jama.284.23.3015.
2. Tishler PV, Larkin EK, Schluchter MD, Redline S. Incidence of sleep-disordered breathing in an urban adult population: The relative importance of risk factors in the development of sleep-disordered breathing. *JAMA*. 2003;289(17):2230–2237. doi:10.1001/jama.289.17.2230.
3. Newman AB, Foster G, Givelber R, Nieto FJ, Redline S, Young T. Progression and regression of sleep-disordered breathing with changes in weight: the Sleep Heart Health Study. *Arch Intern Med*. 2005;165(20):2408–2413. doi:10.1001/archinte.165.20.2408.
4. Evert AB, Franz MJ. Why weight loss maintenance is difficult. *Diabetes Spectr*. 2017;30(3):153–156. doi:10.2337/ds017–0025.
5. Maciejewski ML, Arterburn DE, Van Scoyoc L, et al. Bariatric surgery and long-term durability of weight loss. *JAMA Surg*. 2016;151(11):1046–1055. doi:10.1001/jamasurg.2016.2317.
6. Ashrafian H, Toma T, Rowland SP, et al. Bariatric surgery or non-surgical weight loss for obstructive sleep apnoea? A systematic review and comparison of meta-analyses. *Obes Surg*. 2015;25(7):1239–1250. doi:10.1007/s11695-014-1533-2.
7. Quan SF, Budhiraja R, Clarke DP, et al. Impact of treatment with continuous positive airway pressure (CPAP) on weight in obstructive sleep apnea. *J Clin Sleep Med*. 2013;9(10):989–993. doi:10.5664/jcsm.3064.
8. Blackman A, Foster GD, Zammit G, et al. Effect of liraglutide 3.0 mg in individuals with obesity and moderate or severe obstructive sleep apnea: The SCALE sleep apnea randomized clinical trial. *Int J Obes (Lond)*. 2016;40(8):1310–1319. doi:10.1038/ijo.2016.52.
9. Eskandari D, Zou D, Karimi M, Stenlöf K, Grote L, Hedner J. Zonisamide reduces obstructive sleep apnoea: a randomised placebo-controlled study. *Eur Respir J*. 2014;44(1):140–149. doi:10.1183/09031936.00158413.
10. Winslow DH, Bowden CH, DiDonato KP, McCullough PA. A randomized, double-blind, placebo-controlled study of an oral, extended-release formulation of phentermine/topiramate for the treatment of obstructive sleep apnea in obese adults. *Sleep*. 2012;35(11):1529–1539. doi:10.5665/sleep.2204.
11. Oksenberg A, Khamaysi I, Silverberg DS, Tarasiuk A. Association of body position with severity of apneic events in patients with severe nonpositional obstructive sleep apnea. *Chest*. 2000;118(4):1018–1024. doi:10.1378/chest.118.4.1018.
12. Cartwright RD. Effect of sleep position on sleep apnea severity. Sleep. 1984; 7(2):110–114.

13. Mo J-H, Lee CH, Rhee C-S, Yoon I-Y, Kim J-W. Positional dependency in Asian patients with obstructive sleep apnea and its implication for hypertension. *Arch Otolaryngol Head Neck Surg*. 2011;137(8):786–790. doi:10.1001/archoto.2011.122.
14. Teerapraipruk B, Chirakalwasan N, Simon R, et al. Clinical and polysomnographic data of positional sleep apnea and its predictors. *Sleep Breath*. 2012;16(4):1167–1172. doi:10.1007/s11325-011-0627-5.
15. Marklund M, Persson M, Franklin KA. Treatment success with a mandibular advancement device is related to supine-dependent sleep apnea. *Chest*. 1998;114(6):1630–1635. doi:10.1378/chest.114.6.1630.
16. Mador MJ, Kufel TJ, Magalang UJ, Rajesh SK, Watwe V, Grant BJB. Prevalence of positional sleep apnea in patients undergoing polysomnography. *Chest*. 2005;128(4):2130–2137. doi:10.1378/chest.128.4.2130.
17. Permut I, Diaz-Abad M, Chatila W, et al. Comparison of positional therapy to CPAP in patients with positional obstructive sleep apnea. *J Clin Sleep Med*. 2010;6(3):238–243.
18. Frank MH, Ravesloot MJL, van Maanen JP, Verhagen E, de Lange J, de Vries N. Positional OSA part 1: Towards a clinical classification system for position-dependent obstructive sleep apnoea. *Sleep Breath*. 2015;19(2):473–480. doi:10.1007/s11325-014-1022-9.
19. Barnes H, Edwards BA, Joosten SA, Naughton MT, Hamilton GS, Dabscheck E. Positional modification techniques for supine obstructive sleep apnea: A systematic review and meta-analysis. *Sleep Med Rev*. 2017;36:107–115. doi:10.1016/j.smrv.2016.11.004.
20. Omobomi O, Quan SF. Positional therapy in the management of positional obstructive sleep apnea: A review of the current literature. *Sleep Breath*. 2018;22(2):297–304. doi:10.1007/s11325-017-1561-y.
21. Ravesloot MJL, White D, Heinzer R, Oksenberg A, Pépin J-L. Efficacy of the new generation of devices for positional therapy for patients with positional obstructive sleep apnea: A systematic review of the literature and meta-analysis. *J Clin Sleep Med*. 2017;13(6):813–824. doi:10.5664/jcsm.6622.
22. van Maanen JP, de Vries N. Long-term effectiveness and compliance of positional therapy with the sleep position trainer in the treatment of positional obstructive sleep apnea syndrome. *Sleep*. 2014;37(7):1209–1215. doi:10.5665/sleep.3840.
23. de Vries GE, Hoekema A, Doff MHJ, et al. Usage of positional therapy in adults with obstructive sleep apnea. *J Clin Sleep Med*. 2015;11(2):131–137. doi:10.5664/jcsm.4458.
24. Oksenberg A, Silverberg D, Offenbach D, Arons E. Positional therapy for obstructive sleep apnea patients: A 6-month follow-up study. *Laryngoscope*. 2006;116(11):1995–2000. doi:10.1097/01.mlg.0000237674.66716.a7.
25. Bignold JJ, Deans-Costi G, Goldsworthy MR, et al. Poor long-term patient compliance with the tennis ball technique for treating positional obstructive sleep apnea. *J Clin Sleep Med*. 2009;5(5):428–430.
26. Gordon L, Jackson M, Pierce RJ, Barnes M. Sleep position modification effectively treats positional obstructive sleep apnoea: The Thoracic Society of Australia and New Zealand, Sydney, 2004. *Respirology*. 2004;9S:A72.
27. Bidarian-Moniri A, Nilsson M, Attia J, Ejnell H. Mattress and pillow for prone positioning for treatment of obstructive sleep apnoea. *Acta Otolaryngol*. 2015;135(3):271–276. doi:10.3109/00016489.2014.968674.
28. Dieltjens M, Vroegop AV, Verbruggen AE, et al. A promising concept of combination therapy for positional obstructive sleep apnea. *Sleep Breath*. 2015;19(2):637–644. doi:10.1007/s11325-014-1068-8.
29. Benoist LBL, Verhagen M, Torensma B, van Maanen JP, de Vries N. Positional therapy in patients with residual positional obstructive sleep apnea after upper airway surgery. *Sleep Breath*. 2017;21(2):279–288. doi:10.1007/s11325-016-1397-x.
30. Goyal A, Pakhare A, Subhedar R, Khurana A, Chaudhary P. Combination of positional therapy with positive airway pressure for titration in patients with difficult to treat obstructive sleep apnea. *Sleep Breath*. 2021;25(4):1867–1873. doi:10.1007/s11325-021-02291-6.
31. Ramos FL, Chatila W, Shariff T, et al. Cost effectiveness of incorporating positional therapy into a treatment algorithm for obstructive sleep apnea. *Sleep*. 2015;38(Suppl 1):A442.
32. Camacho M, Malu OO, Kram YA, et al. Nasal dilators (Breathe Right Strips and NoZovent) for snoring and OSA: A systematic review and meta-analysis. *Pulm Med*. 2016;2016:4841310. doi:10.1155/2016/4841310.
33. Gaisl T, Haile SR, Thiel S, Osswald M, Kohler M. Efficacy of pharmacotherapy for OSA in adults: A systematic review and network meta-analysis. *Sleep Med Rev*. 2019;46:74–86. doi:10.1016/j.smrv.2019.04.009.
34. Brownell LG, West P, Sweatman P, Acres JC, Kryger MH. Protriptyline in obstructive sleep apnea: A double-blind trial. *N Engl J Med*. 1982;307(17):1037–1042. doi:10.1056/NEJM198210213071701.
35. Martínez-García MÁ, Labarca G. Sleep apnea phenotypes: Do not forget the external validation. *Sleep*. 2021;44(12):zsab213.
36. McEvoy RD, Antic NA, Heeley E, et al. CPAP for prevention of cardiovascular events in obstructive sleep apnea. *N Engl J Med*. 2016;375(10):919–931. doi:10.1056/NEJMoa1606599.
37. Kim J, Keenan BT, Lim DC, Lee SK, Pack AI, Shin C. Symptom-based subgroups of koreans with obstructive sleep apnea. *J Clin Sleep Med*. 2018;14(3):437–443. doi:10.5664/jcsm.6994.
38. Berger AJ, Bayliss DA, Viana F. Modulation of neonatal rat hypoglossal motoneuron excitability by serotonin. *Neurosci Lett*. 1992;143(1–2):164–168. doi:10.1016/0304-3940(92)90257-8.
39. Veasey SC, Panckeri KA, Hoffman EA, Pack AI, Hendricks JC. The effects of serotonin antagonists in an animal model of sleep-disordered breathing. *Am J Respir Crit Care Med*. 1996;153(2):776–786. doi:10.1164/ajrccm.153.2.8564132.
40. Berry RB, Koch GL, Hayward LF. Low-dose mirtazapine increases genioglossus activity in the anesthetized rat. *Sleep*. 2005;28(1):78–84. doi:10.1093/sleep/28.1.78.
41. Marshall NS, Yee BJ, Desai AV, et al. Two randomized placebo-controlled trials to evaluate the efficacy and tolerability of mirtazapine for the treatment of

obstructive sleep apnea. *Sleep*. 2008;31(6):824–831. doi:10.1093/sleep/31.6.824.
42. Berry RB, Yamaura EM, Gill K, Reist C. Acute effects of paroxetine on genioglossus activity in obstructive sleep apnea. *Sleep*. 1999;22(8):1087–1092. doi:10.1093/sleep/22.8.1087.
43. Taranto-Montemurro L, Edwards BA, Sands SA, et al. Desipramine increases genioglossus activity and reduces upper airway collapsibility during non-REM sleep in healthy subjects. *Am J Respir Crit Care Med*. 2016;194(7):878–885. doi:10.1164/rccm.201511-2172OC.
44. Bellingham MC, Ireland MF. Contribution of cholinergic systems to state-dependent modulation of respiratory control. *Respir Physiol Neurobiol*. 2002;131(1-2):135–144. doi:10.1016/s1569-9048(02)00043-5.
45. Li Y, Owens RL, Sands S, et al. The effect of donepezil on arousal threshold and apnea-hypopnea index: A randomized, double-blind, cross-over study. *Ann Am Thorac Soc*. 2016;13(11):2012–2018. doi:10.1513/AnnalsATS.201605-384OC.
46. Hunchaisri N, Chalermsuwiwattanakan W. Efficacy of donepezil in the treatment of obstructive sleep apnea: A placebo-controlled trial. *J Med Assoc Thai*. 2016;99(Suppl 8):S31–S35.
47. Hedner J, Kraiczi H, Peker Y, Murphy P. Reduction of sleep-disordered breathing after physostigmine. *Am J Respir Crit Care Med*. 2003;168(10):1246–1251. doi:10.1164/rccm.200211-1344OC.
48. Malhotra A, Mesarwi O, Pepin J-L, Owens RL. Endotypes and phenotypes in obstructive sleep apnea. *Curr Opin Pulm Med*. 2020;26(6):609–614. doi:10.1097/MCP.0000000000000724.
49. Whyte KF, Gould GA, Airlie MA, Shapiro CM, Douglas NJ. Role of protriptyline and acetazolamide in the sleep apnea/hypopnea syndrome. *Sleep*. 1988;11(5):463–472. doi:10.1093/sleep/11.5.463.
50. Edwards BA, Sands SA, Eckert DJ, et al. Acetazolamide improves loop gain but not the other physiological traits causing obstructive sleep apnoea. *J Physiol*. 2012;590(5):1199–1211. doi:10.1113/jphysiol.2011.223925.
51. Ni Y-N, Yang H, Thomas RJ. The role of acetazolamide in sleep apnea at sea level: A systematic review and meta-analysis. *J Clin Sleep Med*. 2021;17(6):1295–1304. doi:10.5664/jcsm.9116.
52. Hedner J, Grunstein R, Eriksson B, Ejnell H. A double-blind, randomized trial of sabeluzole: A putative glutamate antagonist in obstructive sleep apnea. *Sleep*. 1996;19(4):287–289. doi:10.1093/sleep/19.4.287.
53. Torvaldsson S, Grote L, Peker Y, Basun H, Hedner J. A randomized placebo-controlled trial of an NMDA receptor antagonist in sleep-disordered breathing. *J Sleep Res*. 2005;14(2):149–155. doi:10.1111/j.1365-2869.2005.00441.x.
54. Carley DW, Prasad B, Reid KJ, et al. Pharmacotherapy of apnea by cannabimimetic enhancement, the PACE Clinical Trial: effects of dronabinol in obstructive sleep apnea. *Sleep*. 2018;41(1):zsx184. doi:10.1093/sleep/zsx184.
55. Mendelson WB, Maczaj M, Holt J. Buspirone administration to sleep apnea patients. *J Clin Psychopharmacol*. 1991;11(1):71–72. doi:10.1097/00004714-199102000-00019.
56. Hedner J, Stenlöf K, Zou D, et al. A randomized controlled trial exploring safety and tolerability of sulthiame in sleep apnea. *Am J Respir Crit Care Med*. 2022 Jun 15;205(12):1461–1469. doi:10.1164/rccm.202109-2043OC.
57. Berry RB, Gleeson K. Respiratory arousal from sleep: Mechanisms and significance. *Sleep*. 1997;20(8):654–675. doi:10.1093/sleep/20.8.654.
58. Edwards BA, Eckert DJ, McSharry DG, et al. Clinical predictors of the respiratory arousal threshold in patients with obstructive sleep apnea. *Am J Respir Crit Care Med*. 2014;190(11):1293–1300. doi:10.1164/rccm.201404-0718OC.
59. Li Y, Orr J, Jen R, et al. Is there a threshold that triggers cortical arousals in obstructive sleep apnea? *Sleep*. 2019;42(6):zsz047. doi:10.1093/sleep/zsz047.
60. Eckert DJ, White DP, Jordan AS, Malhotra A, Wellman A. Defining phenotypic causes of obstructive sleep apnea: Identification of novel therapeutic targets. *Am J Respir Crit Care Med*. 2013;188(8):996–1004. doi:10.1164/rccm.201303-0448OC.
61. Shin W, Jen R, Li Y, Malhotra A. Tailored treatment strategies for obstructive sleep apnea. *Respir Investig*. 2016;54(1):2–7. doi:10.1016/j.resinv.2015.09.007.
62. Carter SG, Eckert DJ. Effects of hypnotics on obstructive sleep apnea endotypes and severity: Novel insights into pathophysiology and treatment. *Sleep Med Rev*. 2021;58:101492. doi:10.1016/j.smrv.2021.101492.
63. Smales ET, Edwards BA, Deyoung PN, et al. Trazodone effects on obstructive sleep apnea and non-REM arousal threshold. *Ann Am Thorac Soc*. 2015;12(5):758–764. doi:10.1513/AnnalsATS.201408-399OC.
64. Eckert DJ, Owens RL, Kehlmann GB, et al. Eszopiclone increases the respiratory arousal threshold and lowers the apnoea/hypopnoea index in obstructive sleep apnoea patients with a low arousal threshold. *Clin Sci (Lond)*. 2011;120(12):505–514. doi:10.1042/CS20100588.
65. Taranto-Montemurro L, Sands SA, Edwards BA, et al. Effects of tiagabine on slow wave sleep and arousal threshold in patients with obstructive sleep apnea. *Sleep*. 2017;40(2):zsw047. doi:10.1093/sleep/zsw047.
66. Awad MI, Kacker A. Nasal obstruction considerations in sleep apnea. *Otolaryngol Clin North Am*. 2018;51(5):1003–1009. doi:10.1016/j.otc.2018.05.012.
67. Koutsourelakis I, Minaritzoglou A, Zakynthinos G, Vagiakis E, Zakynthinos S. The effect of nasal tramazoline with dexamethasone in obstructive sleep apnoea patients. *Eur Respir J*. 2013;42(4):1055–1063. doi:10.1183/09031936.00142312.
68. Smith DF, Sarber KM, Spiceland CP, Ishman SL, Augelli DM, Romaker AM. Effects of medical therapy on mild obstructive sleep apnea in adult patients. *J Clin Sleep Med*. 2019;15(7):979–983. doi:10.5664/jcsm.7876.
69. Taranto-Montemurro L, Sands S, Azarbarzin A, et al. Impact of cold and flu medication on obstructive sleep apnoea and its underlying traits: A pilot randomized controlled trial. *Respirology*. 2021;26(5):485–492. doi:10.1111/resp.14009.
70. Fiori CZ, Martinez D, Montanari CC, et al. Diuretic or sodium-restricted diet for obstructive sleep apnea: A randomized trial. *Sleep*. 2018;41(4):zsy016. doi:10.1093/sleep/zsy016.

71. Yang L, Zhang H, Cai M, et al. Effect of spironolactone on patients with resistant hypertension and obstructive sleep apnea. *Clin Exp Hypertens*. 2016;38(5):464–468. doi:10.3109/10641963.2015.1131290.
72. Gaisl T, Turnbull CD, Weimann G, et al. BAY 2253651 for the treatment of obstructive sleep apnoea: A multicentre, double-blind, randomised controlled trial (SANDMAN). *Eur Respir J*. 2021;58(5):2101937. doi:10.1183/13993003.01937-2021.
73. Mehta V, Vasu TS, Phillips B, Chung F. Obstructive sleep apnea and oxygen therapy: A systematic review of the literature and meta-analysis. *J Clin Sleep Med*. 2013;9(3):271–279. doi:10.5664/jcsm.2500.
74. Wellman A, Malhotra A, Jordan AS, Stevenson KE, Gautam S, White DP. Effect of oxygen in obstructive sleep apnea: Role of loop gain. *Respir Physiol Neurobiol*. 2008;162(2):144–151. doi:10.1016/j.resp.2008.05.019.
75. Taranto-Montemurro L, Messineo L, Sands SA, et al. The combination of atomoxetine and oxybutynin greatly reduces obstructive sleep apnea severity: A randomized, placebo-controlled, double-blind crossover trial. *Am J Respir Crit Care Med*. 2019;199(10):1267–1276. doi:10.1164/rccm.201808-1493OC.
76. Taranto-Montemurro L, Messineo L, Azarbarzin A, et al. Effects of the combination of atomoxetine and oxybutynin on OSA endotypic traits. *Chest*. 2020;157(6):1626–1636. doi:10.1016/j.chest.2020.01.012.
77. Perger E, Taranto Montemurro L, Rosa D, et al. Reboxetine plus oxybutynin for OSA treatment: A 1-week, randomized, placebo-controlled, double-blind crossover trial. *Chest*. 2022;161(1):237–247. doi:10.1016/j.chest.2021.08.080.
78. Malhotra A, Grunstein RR, Fietze I, et al.; SURMOUNT-OSA Investigators. Tirzepatide for the Treatment of Obstructive Sleep Apnea and Obesity. *N Engl J Med*. 2024 Oct 3;391(13):1193–1205. doi:10.1056/NEJMoa2404881. Epub 2024 Jun 21. Erratum in: *N Engl J Med*. 2024 Oct 17;391(15):1464. doi:10.1056/NEJMx240005. PMID: 38912654; PMCID: PMC11598664.

Chapter 10

Hypoventilation in Sleep and Central Sleep Apnea

Neeraj Kaplish, Chandra M. Cherukuri, and Fauziya Hassan

HYPOVENTILATION IN SLEEP

Introduction

The respiratory system is particularly vulnerable in sleep, as conscious control is lost, and minute ventilation is primarily dependent on metabolic pathways and central mediators for sleep. The primary respiratory generators are medullary nuclei which include the dorsal respiratory group (DRG) containing inspiratory neurons and the ventral respiratory group (VRG) which includes inspiratory (pre-Botzinger complex) as well as expiratory neurons with efferents to spinal motor neurons that are critical for respiration.[1] These nuclei, along with other bulbar nuclei, premotor and motor neurons often referred to as central respiratory generator (CRG), are responsible for respiratory drive and rhythm.[2] Sleep results in reduction of functional residual capacity (FRC), increased airway resistance, and altered gas exchange.[3–6] Minute ventilation is reduced in sleep (with a greater reduction in rapid eye movement [REM] sleep than in non-rapid eye movement [NREM] sleep), primarily due to reduction in tidal volume.[7,8] With reduction in minute ventilation during sleep, there is a rise in partial pressure of carbon dioxide ($PaCO_2$) by up to 4 mmHg, which can occur even in normal population, but pathological elevation in $PaCO_2$ (hypercapnia) can occur in patients with comorbidities.[9,10]

Ancillary testing is commonly used by clinicians in evaluation for hypoventilation:

1. An arterial blood gas analysis (ABG) is done to document carbon dioxide (CO_2) elevation for suspected awake hypoventilation or hypercapnia;
2. Elevated serum bicarbonate as a compensatory renal response to elevated CO_2;
3. End tidal CO_2 ($EtCO_2$) and transcutaneous CO_2 ($TcCO_2$) are surrogate measures for $PaCO_2$ during polysomnogram, as ABG is not practical;

Table 10.1 **Scoring Criteria for Sleep Related Hypoventilation in Adult and Pediatric Patient per AASM Scoring Manual**

	CO_2 values in sleep as measured by $EtCO_2$ or $TcCO_2$ in PSG	Duration of CO_2 elevation
Adult Criteria for sleep related hypoventilation	1. 55 mmHg or greater in sleep or 2. Values higher than 10 mmHg sleep when compared to wakefulness with absolute values of 50 mmHg or higher in sleep	≥10 minutes in sleep in PSG
Pediatric Criteria for sleep related hypoventilation	50 mmHg or higher in sleep	25% of total sleep time in PSG

CO_2, carbon dioxide; $EtCO_2$, end-tidal carbon dioxide; $TcCO_2$, transcutaneous carbon dioxide; PSG, polysomnogram.

4. Pulmonary function testing (PFT) can help differentiate between obstructive versus restrictive ventilatory defect;
5. Radiological imaging: chest x-ray, computed tomography (CT) scan of chest, fluoroscopy to detect diaphragmatic paralysis or imaging of spine for deformities such as scoliosis or kyphosis;
6. Maximum inspiratory pressure (MIP) and expiratory pressure (MEP) assessment: these often are quick sensitive tests to assess respiratory strength when administered properly. Values less than 60 cm of water often represent decline in respiratory muscle strength and need for ventilatory support, especially among patients with neuromuscular disorders.

Scoring criteria for hypoventilation in both adults and pediatrics has been standardized in the American Academy of Sleep Medicine (AASM) scoring manual (see Table 10.1). Sleep-related hypoventilation disorders have been categorized in the 3rd edition of the International Classification of Sleep Disorders (ICSD-3) as follows:

- Obesity Hypoventilation Syndrome (OHS)
- Congenital Central Alveolar Hypoventilation Syndrome (CCHS)
- Rapid (Late) Onset Central Hypoventilation with Hypothalamic Dysfunction (ROHHAD) Syndrome
- Idiopathic Central Alveolar Hypoventilation (ICAH)
- Hypoventilation in Sleep due to Medication or Substance
- Hypoventilation in Sleep due to a Medical Disorders such as chest wall or neuromuscular disease.

OBESITY HYPOVENTILATION SYNDROME

Obesity hypoventilation syndrome (OHS) is being commonly recognized due to the increasing prevalence of obesity in the United States and around the world. Prevalence of obesity in the United States has increased from 30.5% (in 1999–2000) to 42.4% (in 2107–2018). Use of *Pickwickian syndrome*[11] as a synonym for OHS does not accurately reflect the underlying co-morbidities associated with the syndrome. Untreated obstructive sleep apnea (OSA) in these patients may also contribute to clinical semiology of hypersomnia, hypoxemia, polycythemia, cor pulmonale, and right heart failure. OHS carries the burden of negative consequences of obesity and hypoventilation on cardiovascular health, shortened life span, and impaired quality of life.[12,13] Prevalence of OHS remains unknown, but an estimated prevalence of 0.4% has been quoted in the United States.[14] Gender difference in OHS are not as striking as with OSA, though diagnosis of OHS is often delayed in women and is associated with a higher pathology burden.[15,16]

Clinical Features

OHS is clinically diagnosed often in an acute care setting with presentation of acute or chronic respiratory failure or upon consultation with a sleep medicine physician or a pulmonologist.[17,18] Often the diagnosis is made in the 5th or 6th decade of life with symptoms of excessive sleepiness, awakenings at night, morning headaches or nausea, mood symptoms, nightmares, enuresis, signs of pulmonary hypertension or cor pulmonale.[19,20]

Pathophysiology

Excessive adipose tissue and its distribution in the chest, abdomen, and neck play a critical role in hypercapnia in OHS. Adiposity often restricts ventilation by respiratory muscles, including the diaphragm. Over a period of time, this contributes to atelectasis, with reduction in lung compliance and increased resistance in the lower respiratory pathways. The additional component of muscle fatigue, due to increased work of breathing, further promotes CO_2 retention. Collectively, all of these result in reduced FRC and tidal volume.[21,22]

Loss of tone in REM sleep affecting striated respiratory muscles, particularly the external intercostal group of muscles, likely worsens hypoventilation. This is postulated to occur early in course of the progression, but over a period of time may result in suppression of components of the CRG, including resistance to leptin, a potent respiratory stimulant.[14,23]

OHS is also tends to be worse in patients with lower extremity edema due to sleeping in a horizontal position. Being in horizontal position leads to a rostral shift of fluids from the legs to the neck region, which can worsen upper airway narrowing.[24] Narrowing of the airway leads to a higher frequency of prolonged apneas and hypopneas, which then causes a rise in $PaCO_2$ levels.[25]

Diagnosis

OHS diagnosis can be made if all of the following criteria are met:

1. Presence of obesity with a body mass index (BMI) ≥30 kg/m^2 or >95th percentile for age and sex for children.
2. Presence of hypoventilation during wakefulness ($PaCO_2$ >45 mmHg) as measured by arterial $PaCO_2$, $EtCO_2$, or $TcCO_2$.
3. Hypoventilation is not primarily due to another etiology such as lung parenchymal or airway disease, pulmonary vascular pathology, chest wall disorder, myxedema, medication or substance, neuromuscular disease.

OSA is common in OHS patients; hence diagnosis of OSA and OHS can be made simultaneously. Patients with suspected OHS should undergo a comprehensive clinical evaluation, followed by pulmonary function tests (in both sitting and supine position if possible), ABGs, appropriate pulmonary imaging, thyroid function tests, and polysomnography with $EtCO_2$ or $TcCO_2$ monitoring. Serum bicarbonate ≥27 mmol/L has been shown to be predictive for OHS with a sensitivity of 92% and specificity of 50%.[26]

Management

It is clear that adiposity plays a key role in pathogenesis in OHS; therefore weight loss should be an important management strategy. Lifestyle modifications with a structured weight loss program consultation should be sought if available. In some cases, weight loss surgery may be an effective step while treating with continuous positive airway pressure (CPAP) in the interval period to minimize the perioperative complications related to comorbid sleep apnea.

Positive airway pressure (PAP) therapy with CPAP or noninvasive ventilation (NIV) should be considered for management for OHS. CPAP may be a better initial PAP modality for an OHS patient among those with comorbid severe OSA, but NIV may be a better alternative for long-term treatment of OHS patients.[27,28] Recently, PAP modalities with more complex algorithms with dynamic inspiratory pressure supports to deliver predetermined tidal volumes with or without expiratory pressure support have become available. These novel modes of NIV need to be better understood, though they offer exciting potential for the management of OHS.

Pharmacotherapy with a respiratory stimulant such as medroxyprogesterone and acetazolamide does not offer significant benefit, and their use must be restricted to patients with OHS who are unable to tolerate PAP therapy. If chosen, close monitoring for worsening upper airway obstruction and sexual dysfunction is warranted.

Aggressive management with supplemental oxygen, loop diuretics, and other pharmacological treatment should be avoided whenever possible during management of

OHS-related complications in inpatient or acute care settings.

CONGENITAL CENTRAL ALVEOLAR HYPOVENTILATION SYNDROME

Congenital central alveolar hypoventilation syndrome (CCHS) is a genetic disorder characterized by lack of central chemoreceptor responsiveness to hypercapnia, and failure of increase in tidal volume. It was previously referred to as "Ondine's curse,"[29] as in German mythology. Disordered breathing in CCHS occurs primarily in sleep, but in more severe cases it is noted in wakefulness as well, characterized by daytime hypoventilation and pauses in breathing. It is a rare disorder with about 1000 cases reported worldwide (though this may be an underestimation) and without gender predisposition. Exact prevalence is unknown, though incidence of CCHS is at 1 in 200,000 live births.[30]

Clinical Features

Symptoms are commonly present in the more severe cases in the first few days after birth, with observations of apneas or shallow breathing in sleep, cyanosis, hypotonia, or feeding abnormalities. Without intervention, which includes mechanical ventilation, death may occur in due to cor pulmonale associated with profound oxygen desaturations due to central apneas and worsening hypoventilation with underlying respiratory failure. In most cases, ventilator support is initially needed during wakefulness and sleep, but depending on the severity of mutation (which is characterized by the number of polyalanine repeats), ventilation may only be required during sleep.

Clinical presentation may also be later in life in milder cases of CCHS (with a lower number of polyalanine repeats), where hypoventilation may be significantly worsened by respiratory infections, respiratory depressant medications, or even pregnancy.[31–36] Close monitoring of daytime CO_2 levels is often warranted to assess for worsening respiratory failure. CCHS, if not treated by appropriate mechanical ventilation, may lead to significant neurocognitive deficits, delay in achievement of developmental milestones, failure to thrive, seizures, or pulmonary hypertension with resultant cor pulmonale.

In addition to hypercapnia, due to failure of migration of neural crest cells, CCHS has been associated with disorders such as life-threatening cardiac arrhythmias. In the neonatal period, patients may develop symptoms of Hirschsprung's disease and later may be diagnosed with neural crest tumors such as neuroblastoma. In addition, there may be an effect on temperature homeostasis and pupillary abnormalities, and patients may show inadequate response to infections.

Pathophysiology

A mutation of paired-like homeobox 2b (*PHOX2B*) gene regulator of ANS maturation, neural crest cell migration and differentiation, on chromosome 4p12.3 is found in 93%–100% of CCHS cases.[33,37–39] *PHOX2B* mutations come in 2 forms: polyalanine repeat expansion mutation (PARM, common) and non-polyalanine repeat expansion mutation (NPARM, uncommon). Patients with NPARM often need 24-hour ventilation and have more comorbidities. *PHOX2B* mutation genotyping can help with the prediction of clinical course and phenotyping CCHS.32 CCHS's association with Hirschsprung's disease suggests that the mutation impacts the neural crest growth, migration, and differentiation. Brain imaging and postmortem studies have shown abnormalities in brain areas that play a key role in the homeostasis of respiration in both sleep and wakefulness.

Diagnosis

The following criteria must be met to make a diagnosis of CCHS:

1. Sleep-related hypoventilation: Polysomnogram with $EtCO_2$ or $TcCO_2$ monitoring to evaluate for hypoventilation and hypoxemia. Central apneas may be present. Hypercapnia during wakefulness may or may not be present depending on the severity of disease present.
2. *PHOX2B mutation* must be present during genetic testing.

Figure 10.1 categorizes clinical features that may suggest an underlying diagnosis of CCHS. In contrast to other forms of sleep-disordered breathing where findings tend to be worse during REM sleep, the hypercapnia in CCHS is worse during NREM sleep without associated arousals or increased tidal volume. This finding can help differentiate hypoventilation secondary to CCHS, as opposed to hypoventilation related to neuromuscular disease, OHS, or Chiari malformation. Pulmonary function testing (PFT), genetic testing, and radiological imaging also help differentiate CCHS-related hypoventilation from other causes of hypoventilation. Lastly, snoring and paradoxical breathing are usually not present in CCHS.

Management

CCHS is a rare disorder with significant comorbidities if not suspected and treated early. Depending on the genotype, it can be fatal; even in milder cases, if the diagnosis if delayed, there may be profound neurocognitive and cardiopulmonary sequelae. Mechanical ventilation is required during sleep, and in the more severe presentation, daytime mechanical ventilation is also required. Care of patients with CCHS requires a complex multidisciplinary team approach with significant involvement of parents and/or caregivers.

Mechanical ventilation is the cornerstone of prolonged survival in CCHS patients and can be administered through tracheotomy or NIV. Ventilation via tracheotomy is considered safer, especially among infants and toddlers who have a long duration of sleep and children who are intolerant to NIV or are at risk for mid-face hypoplasia or aspiration. Diaphragmatic or phrenic nerve pacing (DP) may be another alternative, either in conjunction with positive pressure ventilation or as a stand-alone therapy when positive pressure ventilation is

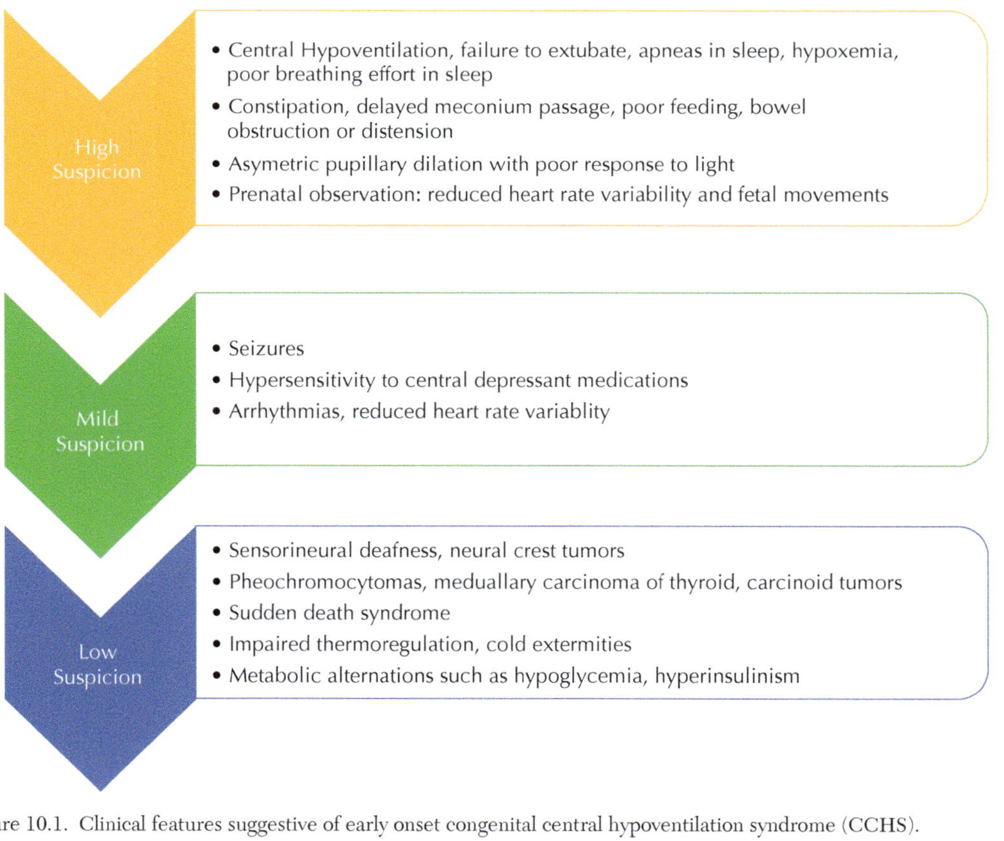

Figure 10.1. Clinical features suggestive of early onset congenital central hypoventilation syndrome (CCHS).

not tolerated. When pacing is used, patients should be monitored closely due to the risk of OSA.[40–42]

CCHS patients, given the risk of associated disorders, may require 72-hour Holter monitoring, echocardiogram, ophthalmologic exams, abdominal ultrasounds (screening for neural crest tumors), polysomnograms to assess the efficacy of invasive and noninvasive mechanical ventilation, or DP, and neurocognitive assessments periodically at various intervals.[34]

RAPID (LATE) ONSET CENTRAL HYPOVENTILATION WITH HYPOTHALAMIC AND AUTONOMIC DYSFUNCTION SYNDROME

Rapid (late) onset central hypoventilation with hypothalamic and autonomic dysfunction syndrome (ROHHAD), a rare syndrome, is defined by rapid weight gain, hormonal dysfunction (primarily hypothalamic), autonomic dysregulation, and centrally mediated hypoventilation. *PHOX2B* testing can help differentiate ROHHAD from late onset CCHS due to an overlap of clinical semiology, since *PHOX2B* mutation is not present in ROHHAD.[43] Prevalence is unknown, and there does not seem to be any gender predomination.

Clinical Features

The most striking feature of ROHHAD is rapid substantial weight gain, in the range of 20–30 pounds over a few months. Clinical presentation often begins around 2–4 years of age, prior to which children are developmentally normal. There is hyperphagia associated with rapid weight gain, followed by autonomic dysfunction manifesting as: ophthalmic disorders (pupillary disturbance, strabismus, upward gaze restriction or opsoclonus), gastrointestinal disorders (constipation or chronic diarrhea), and profound thermal dysregulation (typically hypothermia). Ventilatory dysfunction, depending on the severity of clinical manifestation, can present early or at a later age in the form of hypercapnia, oxygen desaturations during sleep, OSA, and cyanotic spells in wakefulness (see Figure 10.2). Children often fail to show compensatory changes in breathing, such as increase in tidal volume and arousals in response to the hypercapnia. Untreated hypoventilation can be fatal, primarily related to cardiopulmonary arrest. Patients are also at risk for developing neural crest tumors, such

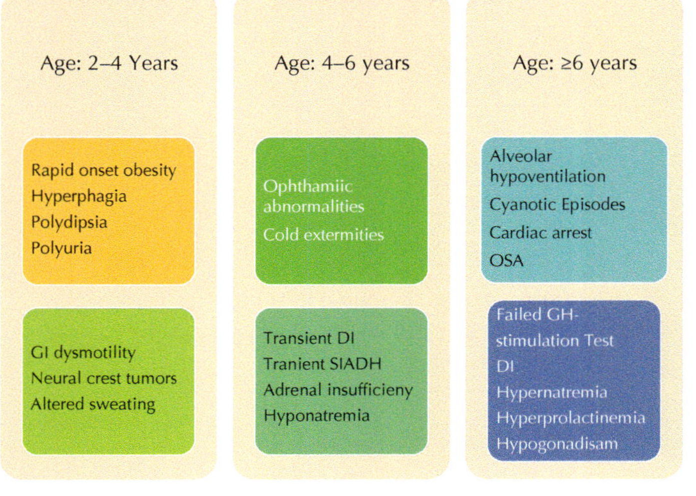

Figure 10.2. The median age of clinical semiology of ROHHAD.

DI: diabetes insipidus; GI: gastro intestinal; SIADH: syndrome of inappropriate antidiuretic hormone; OSA: obstructive sleep apnea; GH: growth hormone.

as ganglioneuroblastoma and ganglioneuroma. Figure 10.2 shows that median age of clinical semiology of ROHHAD.

Laboratory testing to assess hypothalamic function demonstrates hypernatremia or hyponatremia, hyperprolactinemia, hypothyroidism, adrenal insufficiency, or growth hormone deficiency. Neuroimaging with magnetic resonance imaging (MRI), if done, may show abnormalities in the hypothalamus, periaqueductal region, pontine tegmentum, or upper medulla.[44,45]

Diagnosis

All of the following criteria must be met for diagnosis of ROHHAD[43,46,47]:

1. Evidence of alveolar hypoventilation after 2 years of age
2. Evidence for hypothalamic dysfunction with ≥2 of the following findings:
   a. Rapid onset obesity
   b. Hypothalamic endocrinal dysfunction such as hyperprolactinemia, central hypothyroidism, failed growth hormone stimulation test, corticotrophin deficiency, delayed/precocious puberty, or impaired water balance.
   c. Tumors of neural origin
   d. Severe emotional or behavioral disturbance
3. Genetic testing is negative for mutations testing CCHS (*PHOX2B*) and Prader Willi (DNA methylation).
4. The disorder is not explained by another sleep, medical, or neurological disorder or by medication/substance use.

Management

ROHHAD diagnosis is often delayed since respiratory dysfunction may not be the presenting symptom. Recognition of ROHHAD early in its course allows for more appropriate medication, multidisciplinary management of endocrinal disturbance, weight loss interventions, and emotional and behavioral intervention. Respiratory support is invariably required at increasing levels as the disease progresses. Different ventilation modalities are utilized, including NIV, though many patients require mechanical ventilation via tracheostomy. Avoidance of medications that negatively impact ventilation and judicious use of anesthesia when necessary are important given that patients with ROHHAD are at high risk for postoperative complications. Screening for neural crest tumors is needed initially following a diagnosis of ROHHAD and intermittently thereafter as tumors have been identified at different stages of the disorder. It is currently unclear if any specific medical management strategy, including mechanical ventilation, alters the overall life expectancy or disease progression. Mortality rates are high early in life, with cardiac arrest being a common cause.

HYPOVENTILATION IN SLEEP DUE TO NEUROMUSCULAR DISEASE OR CHEST WALL DEFORMITY

About 40% of patients with neuromuscular disease (NMD) have disordered breathing during sleep.[48] With progressive worsening in neuromuscular weakness impacting upper airway muscle tone and chest wall musculature, the frequency of sleep-disordered breathing becomes higher. Hypoventilation is the most common form of sleep-disordered breathing in NMD, though OSA and central sleep apnea (CSA) may also occur.[49–54] Hypoventilation during sleep affects nearly 25% of children and about 9% of adults with NMD.[55,56] Respiratory management is critical in NMD, as higher morbidity and mortality are noted due to muscle fatigue, atelectasis, recurrent pneumonias, mucus plugs in patients with tracheotomies, and chronic respiratory failure.

Pathophysiology

Hypoventilation risk in NMD is due to multiple factors, including:

- Reduction in many PFT variables such as vital capacity (VC), functional residual capacity (FRC), and tidal volume (TV) that becomes prominent in the supine position (primarily related to reduced excursion of the diaphragm)
- Reduced chest wall compliance due to neuromuscular scoliosis and muscle weakness
- REM atonia causing REM-related hypoventilation can be an early feature of more severe

disease, typically occurring with weakness of thoracic respiratory muscles, particularly the external intercostal.
- Reduced ventilatory response secondary to altered chemoreceptor response to hypoxemia or hypercapnia.

OSA may present earlier than hypoventilation in patients with certain NMD such as Duchene muscular dystrophy (DMD), acid maltase deficiency (AMD), and Charcot-Marie-Tooth disease.[57] Postulated causes of OSA in these patients include upper airway hypotonia with weakness of the upper airway dilator muscles (the genioglossus and geniohyoid group of muscles) or pharyngeal neuropathy.[49,58,59] Central apneas with Cheyne Stokes respiration is often seen in congenital muscular dystrophies, glycogen storage disorder, or cervical/higher spinal cord injuries. Central sleep-disordered breathing is likely related to cardiomyopathy, but in spinal cord injuries it may be due to diaphragmatic weakness.

Clinical Features

NMD encompasses disorders that affect the neural axis at different locations: motor neurons/motor nerves, neuromuscular junction, or the muscle. Clinical presentation in NMD may vary due to the localization of neural axis dysfunction; however, they do tend to share semiology of sleep disruption. Patients with NMD have several symptoms and signs of sleep-disordered breathing, including: shallow breathing or apneas in sleep; air hunger (especially in supine sleep); noisy breathing such as snoring or stridor; unrefreshing sleep; frequent arousals; excessive daytime sleepiness; or morning headaches. There is a significant overlap with signs and symptoms of OSA. Comprehensive physical exam may reveal proximal muscle weakness, muscle atrophy, fasciculations, diplopia, inducible muscle weakness with activity followed by recovery with rest, hyperreflexia and bulbar involvement with impaired speech or dysphagia. Clinical or imaging of the spine may reveal skeletal or spinal cord abnormalities. Daytime symptoms of dyspnea, orthopnea, poor cough, facial weakness, and drooling may suggest potential hypoventilation in patients with NMDs.

The following criteria must be met for diagnosis of hypoventilation in sleep due to NMD:

1. Sleep-related hypoventilation is present.
2. Hypoventilation is due to neurological disorder or muscle weakness.
3. Hypoventilation is not primarily due to lung or airway disease, pulmonary vascular pathology, obesity, medication use, CCHS, or ROHHAD.

Sleep disturbance in a patient with an NMD should alert the clinician to assess for hypoventilation during sleep. There are many ancillary tests which help clinicians evaluate and manage NMD. PFT aids in assessment of the severity of respiratory impairment, as there is often a reduction in maximal minute ventilation, VC, or forced VC. Diffusion capacity is generally preserved in these patients. MIP/MEP are reduced and can help with assessment of respiratory impairment and the decision to initiate respiratory support. Diaphragm function can be assessed with electromyography (EMG) or an imaging study such as fluoroscopic sniff test. An ABG assesses for hypercapnia during the daytime, a finding that is suggestive of daytime hypoventilation, which occurs later in the course of the disease process and may not reflect CO_2 levels during sleep.

Diagnostic polysomnography (PSG) can characterize sleep-disordered breathing in patients with NMD who have hypercapnia or hypoxemia in sleep, comorbid OSA or CSA, and/or a disturbance of sleep architecture. Routine screening PSG is recommended in patients with DMD or spinal muscular atrophy to initially diagnose the sleep-disordered breathing and again after treatment to assess the adequacy of ventilatory support.[60,61]

Management

NIV is mainstay therapy that has improved survival in NMD, even in rapidly progressive conditions such as amyotrophic lateral sclerosis.[60–66] With worsening neuromuscular weakness, ventilation via tracheotomy is often needed. Patients with NMD who are initiated on CPAP for OSA should be carefully monitored for development of hypoventilation. Newer NIV devices have been developed with advanced algorithms that deliver target tidal volumes for management of hypoventilation. Effective NIV titration by a trained technologist has been shown to improve sleep quality, improve hypoxemia, and reduce hypopneas.[67,68] NIV titration should be tailored for type of NMD, as the current guidelines for management of DMD suggest that elevation in CO_2 for as low as 2% of sleep time is considered diagnostic for sleep-related hypoventilation.[61] While NIV titration during polysomnography offers benefits, it may not always be feasible to do sleep studies due to limited patient mobility, limited access to tertiary level sleep centers with a respiratory therapist available at bedside, and availability of CO_2 monitoring in the sleep laboratory. Patients receiving NIV should be closely monitored for asynchronous breathing, irregular or auto triggering, and glottic closures. Patients need to be counseled about NIV and monitored closely for development of heart failure or significant bulbar symptoms.[64,69]

Phrenic nerve pacing via stimulation of bilateral phrenic nerves in patients with spinal cord injury benefits quality of life, improves speech, and reduces infections, though it does not clearly improve survival.[70] PSG with EMG and CO_2 monitoring can help ensure that effective stimulation occurs in both wakefulness and sleep (NREM and REM). Pacing has its limitation, as it cannot be done around the clock due to concern for diaphragmatic fatigue, and there is an ongoing risk of untreated upper airway obstruction with increased diaphragmatic activity.[71] Negative pressure ventilation using a cuirass has also been considered for treatment of spinal cord injury, though it can cause upper airway obstruction and deformity to the chest wall.

HYPOVENTILATION IN SLEEP DUE TO MEDICATION OR SUBSTANCE

Hypoventilation in sleep can be caused by chronic use of medications that suppress respiratory drive, even in the absence of underlying conditions such as OHS, NMD, pulmonary or airway disease, and CCHS. Medications often implicated in hypoventilation include sedating medications such as opioids, anesthetics, muscle relaxants, and illicit drugs. Concurrent use of alcohol with these substances may worsen hypercapnia and hypoxemia. Due to the effect on ventilation and atonia due to these medications, OSA and CSA may occur in addition to hypoventilation. Patients with comorbid pulmonary pathology, static or mild NMD, or obesity may be more susceptible to hypercapnia with certain medications.

Pathophysiology

Of all the medications that have an impact on ventilation during sleep, opioids have been closely studied. Opioid-induced ventilatory impairment (OIVI) describes the global negative impact on breathing during sleep.[72] Adverse patient outcomes have been reported in the setting of opioid use during postoperative care. OIVI is related to the inhibitory effects on central respiratory drive, altered arousal effects due to sedation, and inhibition of upper airway dilator muscles. Suppression of respiratory drive is primarily due to opioid impact on the mu-opioid receptors in the pre-Botzinger complex, but there is an effect on kappa-opioid receptors as well. Affinity to these receptors, total dose, and route of administration of opioids can determine the potency of suppression. Ensuing hypercapnia can worsen sedation, which augments the central sedating effects of opioids. Sedation from opioids is mediated due to mu-opioid receptors in hypothalamus and inhibition of hypocretin-arousal network.[73] Sedating medications may enhance the inhibition of genioglossus muscle, the primary dilator of the upper airway.[74,75] Ventilation impairment in sleep due to medications often occurs via more than one pathway and complex circuitry.

Clinical Features

Patients may present at any age with shortness of breath, chest tightness, or excessive fatigue, though some patients are asymptomatic. Presenting complaints include frequent arousals, irregular breathing, or unrefreshing sleep. Impaired concentration and other cognitive dysfunction symptoms can also occur, either due to hypoventilation or direct medication effect. There is no known gender predisposition or familial pattern reported. Detailed history-taking may show onset of symptoms with initiation or increase in the dose of a medication or illicit drug. Lower respiratory rate or ataxic breathing during awake state in a susceptible patient can be a sign for hypoventilation in sleep. Complications in the postoperative period, such as prolonged intubation, respiratory or heart failure, and prolonged hospital stay, may be seen in patients with hypoventilation.

Management

Treatment begins with identification of the medication or substance that is causing clinical symptoms in sleep or wakefulness. ABGs can help with documenting $PaCO_2$ if hypoventilation is present during the day, but often PSG with CO_2 monitoring is needed to diagnose and understand the severity of hypoventilation and hypoxemia in sleep. Counseling, re-evaluating management, and considering alternative medications are warranted once hypoventilation is confirmed. Avoiding sedating medications in these patients, if possible, is best practice.

Monitoring of respiratory rates, level of sedation, and oxygen saturations may be used to monitor for respiratory depression. If long-term use of medication such as an opioid is warranted, doses and route of administration need to be personalized to mitigate OIVI. Since these patients are vulnerable to postoperative complications, oxygen monitoring, supplemental oxygen if needed, and cautious use of opioids or other similar medications are necessary. CPAP or NIV is indicated if medications cannot be discontinued or conservative management is ineffective.

IDIOPATHIC CENTRAL ALVEOLAR HYPOVENTILATION

Idiopathic central alveolar hypoventilation (ICAH) is characterized by hypoventilation, often with hypoxemia in sleep, in the absence of any pulmonary, neuromuscular, severe obesity, CCHS, hypothalamic dysfunction, or chest wall disorders. Exact prevalence is unknown, though true ICAH is likely uncommon. Pathophysiology is unclear, but reduced tidal volume with sustained desaturations is often noted. Due to these findings, a blunted central chemoreceptor response to CO_2 is postulated.[76,77]

The patient can present at any age with morning headaches, tiredness, cognitive issues, unrefreshing sleep or impaired sleep quality, or it can be an incidental finding on PSG or ABG performed for other indications. Diagnostic testing to ascertain etiology is warranted and usually unrevealing except for sequelae of chronic hypoventilation/hypoxemia such as polycythemia, pulmonary hypertension, or cor pulmonale.

PAP therapy with NIV is effective. Supplemental oxygen may be warranted to correct hypoxemia or for management of comorbidities such as pulmonary hypertension. Often comorbidities are managed with multidisciplinary interventions. The patient must be counseled against use of alcohol or other recreational drugs. Medications that can worsen hypoventilation, such as opioids, hypnotics, and benzodiazepines, should be avoided or used judiciously with close monitoring.[78,79]

CENTRAL SLEEP APNEA

Central sleep apnea (CSA) in adults is defined is a decrement of airflow due to lack of ventilatory effort as measured by thoracic of abdominal effort lasting for ≥10 seconds.[80] Decrement in airflow may meet the criteria for an apnea or central hypopnea resulting from reduction of ventilatory effort, primarily due to lack of control of breathing by the medullary pacemaker nuclei. Etiology of central apnea is due to loss of wakefulness drive ventilatory drive or sensitivity to $PaCO_2$ apneic threshold. With sleep onset, when the $PaCO_2$ falls below the patient's individually determined apneic threshold, central apnea is the expected outcome. Central apnea may be more frequent in patients where the $PaCO_2$ oscillations are much wider crossing the apneic threshold.

CSA may or may not be associated with hypercapnia, and it helps clinicians narrow the diagnostic considerations for underlying etiology for CSA (see Table 10.2). An attended in laboratory polysomnogram is recommended to assess for evaluation if there is clinical suspicion for CSA. Home sleep apnea testing is currently not recommended as a primary diagnostic modality for assessment of CSA. Many clinicians, including the authors, consider that frequency of central apneas or hypopnea

Table 10.2 **Classification of CSA based on their CO_2 Levels with Underlying Etiologies Described**

Hypocapnic or Eucapnic CSA	Hypercapnic CSA
1. Physiologic • Sleep onset • Post arousal • With phasic-REM sleep 2. Pathologic • Associated with heart failure • Primary CSA • Treatment emergent CSA • High altitude breathing • CSA with medical disorders such as post stroke or with chronic kidney disease	1. CSA due to medication or substance use 2. Congenital central hypoventilation syndrome 3. Idiopathic central alveolar hypoventilation 4. CSA associated with brain stem lesions 5. CSA in the setting of neuro-muscular or spinal cord/chest wall disorders

CSA, central sleep apnea; REM, rapid eye movement; CO_2, carbon dioxide.

occurring at a frequency of 5 or greater per hour may be significant in an adult patient.

In this chapter, we discuss the following CSA syndromes listed in the 3rd edition of the International Classification of Sleep Disorders (ICSD-3):

- CSA with Cheyne Stokes breathing (CSB)
- Treatment emergent CSA
- CSA due to high altitude breathing
- CSA due to medications or substance use.

CSA with CSB

CSA with CSB is a form of periodic breathing highly prevalent in patients with chronic heart failure (CHF), yet it is often underdiagnosed. CSB is also observed in other medical disorders, such as among patients with stroke or end stage renal disease. The breathing pattern is characterized by periodic crescendo-decrescendo breathing, alternating with central apneas or central hypopneas. The respiratory cycle length is typically more than 40 seconds in duration. An attended PSG is required for definitive diagnosis of CSA with CSB.

It remains unclear if CSA with CSB is simply a manifestation of worsening CHF, a cause of HF progression, or a compensatory mechanism to maintain stroke volume in severe CHF. Detailed analyses of CSA with CSB have been reported to have two patterns, positive or negative. Pattern with end-expiratory lung volume (ERLC) ≥ FRC is termed "positive." A "negative" pattern is when the ERLC < FRC. Negative pattern has been associated with more severe CHF.[81] A diverse body of evidence demonstrates increased morbidity and mortality in the presence of CSB. CSB has been described in both CHF patients with preserved and reduced ejection fraction, regardless of drug treatment. Risk factors for CSB in a patient with CHF are older age, male gender, high BMI, atrial fibrillation, and hypocapnia.

Pathophysiology

Control of breathing has been explained by the loop gain theory. Loop gain (LG) is the engineering term describing a system with negative feedback control by quantitative assessment of its (in)-stability. LG is a product of the controller gain (CG) and the plant gain (PG) and their temporal interaction (time delay). Translated to the control of breathing, the controller gain represents the magnitude of the breathing drive produced by the respiratory center with respect to the $PaCO_2$, the plant gain is the efficiency of the lungs to eliminate CO_2, and time delay is the lung-to-chemoreceptor time (aka circulatory delay). CSB occurs due to increased loop gain, because of increased controller gain, plant gain, and circulatory delay, frequently in combination.

Several factors may increase the CG in patients who have CHF. For example, moderate hypoxemia affects the chemo responsiveness by increasing the chemosensitivity (the intrinsic gain),[82] but also by influencing the upper airway patency. The latter can be altered in patients with OSA. Obstructive events also trigger respiratory-associated arousals with associated hypoxemia and increase in tidal volume due to activation of peripheral chemoreceptors. There is an abrupt change in the apnea threshold (AT) and fluctuations of $PaCO_2$ under and over the AT. Any cause of sleep fragmentation and increased arousals may elicit the same result. This mechanism may be facilitated further by the inadequate decrease of the AT during sleep, in patients with CHF.[83] Pulmonary congestion increases the pulmonary capillary wedge pressure (PCWP) and triggers the reflex, resulting in tachypnea and hyperventilation, followed by hypocapnia and central apnea. PCWP has been correlated with $PaCO_2$ levels, as well as the severity and number of the central apneas.[84] Left ventricle end-diastolic and end-systolic volumes were 2 times higher in patients with CHF and concomitant CSB than in CHF only.[85] The mixing gain is increased by a prolonged arterial circulation time because of pulmonary congestion, ventricular enlargement, and decreased stroke volume. CHF is also associated with increased arterial circulatory time, causing increased circulatory delay and hence increasing the LG. Though the importance of circulatory delay is not equivocally accepted, most of the studies support its leading role.

Clinical Features

Patients with HF often report classic symptoms, such as poor sleep quality with frequent awakenings, paroxysmal nocturnal dyspnea (PND), orthopnea, and frequent urination at night, each of which may be explained by CSA-CSB.[86] Patients with CHF also may report several somatic complaints, such as generalized fatigue, insomnia, and impaired neuropsychologic functions[87]; which closely resemble symptoms seen in patients with OSA. The clinical manifestation of CSA with CSB itself can be ambiguous in some cases, as they lack striking symptoms and complaints. Witnessed apneas and snoring are infrequently reported by the sleep partner. Recognizing this, ICSD-3 does not require clinical symptoms in at-risk patients, such as those with comorbid CHF or atrial fibrillation.

The respiratory characteristics noted on PSG include a crescendo-decrescendo ventilatory pattern (see Figure 10.3). To assess for comorbid hypoventilation, $TcCO_2$ or $EtCO_2$ may be used. The EEG characteristics noted on PSG shows that CSB usually occurs during the transition from wakefulness to NREM 1 and 2 sleep stages. Notably, CSB may is improve with sleep in a non-supine body position,[88] and during slow wave sleep and REM sleep, when the ventilation tends to normalize.[89] Unlike obstructive events, ending with arousals, EEG arousals in CSB occur appear at the peak of the hyperventilation phase of the CSB cycle.

Management

Treatment of CSB aims at improving the cardiac function, quality of life, and life expectancy in these patients. Despite the variety of treatment modalities proposed, it is important to note that, so far, guidelines do not offer a

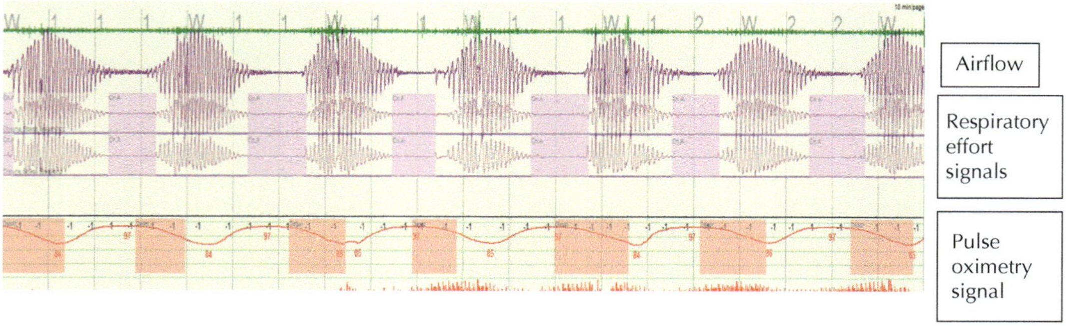

Figure 10.3. An 10-minute epoch showing a periodic breathing pattern with central apneas meeting the criteria for Cheyne Stokes breathing (CSB).

uniform treatment strategy for CSA in patients with CHF.

Optimizing medical therapy for heart failure is the important first step toward CSA treatment in CHF patients, which may include diuretic therapy, angiotensin converting enzyme (ACE) inhibitors, or beta-blockers. Cardiac resynchronization therapy has been shown to increase cardiac pump function and quality of life.[90] Studies have indicated that treatments of heart failure that improve left ventricular ejection fraction (LVEF) can alleviate or resolve CSA (e.g., medical management, mitral valvuloplasty, cardiac resynchronization therapy, or left ventricular assist device and cardiac transplantation), but such interventions do not always lead to complete resolution of the abnormal breathing pattern.[90–92]

CPAP as first-line therapy is based on results of a limited number of small randomized trials which have consistently demonstrated that CPAP decreases the frequency of central apneas in patients with CSA associated with heart failure.[93,94] Nocturnal home oxygen via nasal cannula in patients with CSA related to CHF increases the oxygen supply to the left ventricle and additionally may reduce reflex activation of the peripheral chemoreceptors. Oxygen therapy may suppresses periodic breathing because it blunts the hypoxemic respiratory drive and the consecutive hyperventilation. Oxygen supplementation may be beneficial in patients with poor compliance with noninvasive ventilation.[95,96]

Adaptive servo-ventilation (ASV), despite being effective in improving CSA, may not be the best option in patients with heart failure as indicated by results of the SERVE-HF trial which showed a statistically significant increase in all-cause and cardiovascular mortality in the ASV group.[69] An ongoing study, the ADVENT-HF trial (Effect of Adaptive Servo Ventilation [ASV] on Survival and Hospital Admissions in Heart Failure; NCT01128816), aim to investigate whether the concern raised by SERVE-HF for CSA treatment with ASV represents a class effect or is device-specific. This trial differs from SERVE-HF by including patients with reduced ejection fraction without hypersomnia and using an ASV with a refined algorithm.

Acetazolamide had been used to improve CSA with CHF, and its effect is mediated by respiratory stimulation (controller gain) and diuretic effect (plant gain), leading to significant decrease of the $PaCO_2$, which indicates increased ventilation, reduction in pulmonary congestion and likely lowering of the apneic threshold.[97] Use of this treatment led to a 38% improvement in proportion of sleep time with periodic breathing, improved the quality of sleep, and reduced of daytime sleepiness.[98]

TREATMENT-EMERGENT CENTRAL SLEEP APNEA

Treatment-emergent central sleep apnea (TECSA), previously known as complex sleep apnea, is characterized by the emergence or persistence of central respiratory events during PAP titration for treatment of OSA, after restoration of pharyngeal patency with PAP. Although the disorder is most commonly observed following PAP therapy, TECSA may also be observed following treatment of OSA with tracheostomy and oral mandibular advancement devices (MAD).[99,100]

The ICSD-3 defines treatment-emergent CSA by:

1. ≥5 events per hour of predominantly obstructive respiratory events in the diagnostic PSG; and
2. Significant resolution of obstructive events and emergence or persistence of central events during PAP treatment with a central AHI ≥5 events per hour and ≥50% central events; and
3. The phenomenon must not be better explained by another CSA disorder.

Pathophysiology

Exact mechanisms of TECSA remain unclear, but it is suspected that it involves the relief of inspiratory flow limitation. In some patients with pharyngeal compromise, increasing ventilatory drive with increasing CO_2 may not yield increased airflow due to the prevailing upper airway mechanics (i.e., ineffective muscle responses). This means, the presence of flow limitation can markedly reduce the controller gain (i.e., no rise in airflow for increasing effort). When inspiratory flow limitation is then relieved with treatment, a heightened central receptor chemosensitivity can be unmasked to yield CSA.

Clinical Features

Prevalence may vary from 5% to 20%.[101] Patients may present with persistent apneas or impaired sleep quality despite use of PAP therapy. It is not uncommon for patients to be asymptomatic, and CSA is identified on the PAP-generated reports. Some of the risk factors for development of TECSA include male sex, older age, underlying medical disorders of CAD or CHF. Additionally, split night studies with inadequate time for PAP titration may lead to rushed or aggressive titrations, leading to higher mask leak, and higher arousal index contributing to risk of TECSA (see Figure 10.4).[102]

Management

The 2012 AASM practice parameters for the treatment of CSA syndromes in adults do not specifically address TECSA, as the available evidence was deemed insufficient to warrant a treatment recommendation.[95] In general, management options for TECSA are similar to treatment of CSA.

The majority of the patients with TECSA may resolve with continued CPAP therapy,[102,103] and some studies suggest that ASV treatment may lower the AHI.[104,105] CPAP therapy for 4 weeks is associated with decreased controller gain and widening of the CO_2 reserve. Based on this observation, the authors favor a trial of PAP therapy for 3 months in patients without severe symptoms of untreated sleep apnea and disruption in sleep. However, if symptoms are concerning, then consideration can be given to a retitration study or changing to ASV therapy. ASV devices are designed for elevated loop gain or hypocapnic CSA, providing a higher pressure support (PS) during low flow periods and less PS when the flow is high. ASV is more effective than CPAP or BPAP in reducing AHI, though there is no significant reduction in adherence or sleep-related quality of life measures.[106,107]

CPAP with supplemental oxygen improved AHI in patients with TECSA when compared with CPAP alone.[105] Oxygen supplementation may lower loop gain, change the threshold sensitivity to trigger apnea/hyperpnea pattern, and hence reduce AHI.[96,108] Medications such as acetazolamide or concurrent positional therapy with PAP therapy may be considered on a case-by-case basis as salvage therapy.

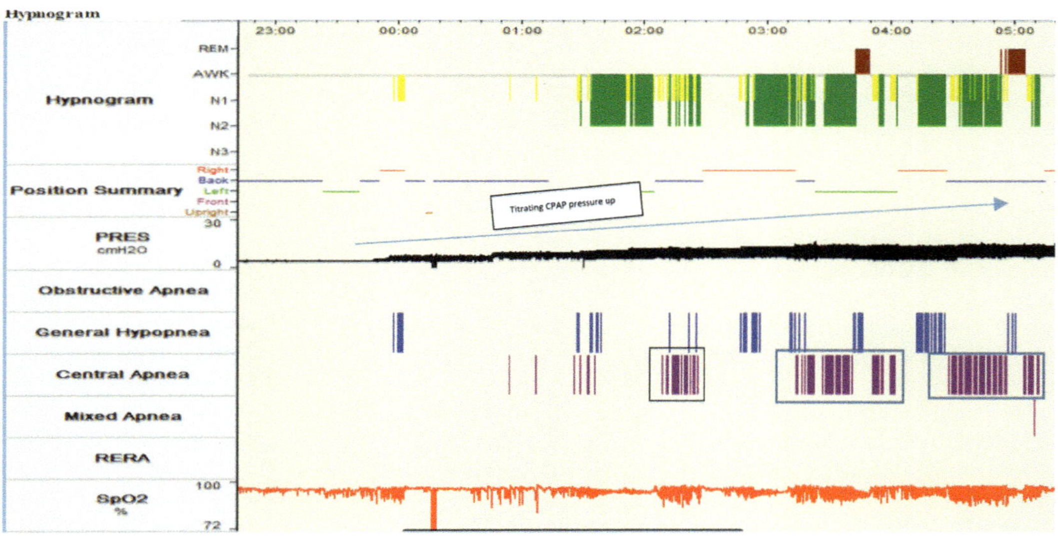

Figure 10.4. Hypnogram showing emergence of central apenas (highlighted in boxes) associated with prominent oxygen desaturations in an elderly male with history of atrial fibrillation and preserved ejection fraction.

CENTRAL SLEEP APNEA DUE TO HIGH-ALTITUDE PERIODIC BREATHING

Periodic breathing is a common response to rising altitude, becoming more common with higher elevations and almost ubiquitous at altitudes >4000 m. High-altitude periodic breathing is characterized by alternating periods of absent respiratory efforts (i.e., CSA) with periods of hyperventilation (hyperpnea) in the absence of other etiologies of periodic breathing (e.g., CHF with Cheyne Stokes breathing or intake of narcotics). Development of CSA due to high altitude will depend not only on altitude itself, but also on speed of ascension, as well as on individual variability to hypoxic responsiveness.

The ICSD-3 defines CSA due to high-altitude periodic breathing as follows:

1. Recent ascent to high altitude
2. Presence of symptoms attributable to high-altitude breathing: sleepiness, sleep onset or maintenance difficulties, non-restorative sleep, waking up with headaches or shortness of breath or witnessed apneas.
3. PSG showing a central AHI ≥5 in NREM sleep
4. Symptoms are not better explained by another sleep, medical, neurological, or medication/substance disorder.

Clinical Features

Emergence of clinical symptoms following recent ascent, especially when associated with sleep disturbance, should raise the suspicion of CSA due to high-altitude breathing. Arousals from sleep increase with rising altitude, which may lead to sleep fragmentation and subsequent complaints of fatigue and excessive daytime sleepiness. Patients may complain of excessive daytime sleepiness, insomnia, gasping awake, morning headaches, and dyspnea. Independent of sex, patients with cardiovascular disease are at increased risk for OSA and CSA at high altitude.[109]

Pathophysiology

Pathophysiologic effects of high altitude are related to changes in barometric pressure and subsequent changes in the ambient pressure of oxygen. As PaO_2 falls due to a low atmospheric pressure (hypobaric hypoxia) upon ascension, ventilation is stimulated, resulting in hypocapnia and respiratory alkalosis. The magnitude of the ventilatory response increases with increasing altitude and progresses over days after ascension. It is this hyperventilation triggered by hypoxia (PaO_2), with subsequent fall in arterial carbon dioxide ($PaCO_2$) below the apneic threshold, which results in central apneas.[110] With breathing cessation, increased $PaCO_2$ will trigger a subsequent hyperventilation period with high tidal volumes, in which the PaO_2 rises and $PaCO_2$ falls to near wakefulness level, perpetuating the respiratory oscillation (periodic breathing). Periodic breathing may still increase in duration and persist in time as a result of the progressive increase in the respiratory control system response to hypoxia and hypercapnia (i.e., a high loop gain). Women stabilize their respiration at high altitude more quickly than do men and demonstrate less proclivity for central apneas. It is thought that women may be protected due to the effect of estrogen and/or progesterone; however, the exact mechanism remains unclear.[111]

Polysomnogram

On polysomnography, central apneas occur during NREM sleep while being largely absent during REM sleep. This is thought to be due to the fact that the primary driver of ventilation during NREM sleep is central receptor chemo-responsiveness, while hypercapnic responsiveness is blunted during REM sleep. Central apneas are generally short (cycles lengths <40 s) in high-altitude periodic breathing, unlike that seen with Cheyne Stokes respiration related to heart failure. Sleep is often disrupted, though overall total sleep time and REM sleep time may be preserved.

Management

In patients with OSA who travel to high altitude (e.g., 2750 m), their home PAP settings may be inadequate to treat their OSA. Although application of PAP is associated with decreased central sleep apnea and hypoxemia that occurs with altitude, baseline PAP settings may be suboptimal to completely resolve OSA, resulting in higher sleep apnea severity and sleep fragmentation.[112]

The physiological adaptations to high altitude, affects oxygen content and oxygen-carrying capacity. Slow ascent can decrease respiratory drive triggered by hypoxia. Therefore, gradual and slow ascending, allowing for subsequent acclimatization are among several interventions to ameliorate the development of sleep-related breathing disorders. Unfortunately, at elevations above 3500–4000 m, acclimatization alone does not restore normal sleep or prevent the development of CSA, leaving very few evidence-based options to treat patients at that altitude. When feasible, however, descending from altitude is always the treatment of choice.

If descending from high altitude is not an option, adjunctive treatment with acetazolamide and/or oxygen has been proven to be an effective measure; however, availability, side effects, and limitations of these interventions should be cautiously considered. Acetazolamide improves sleep apnea at high altitude, by inducing a metabolic acidosis and behaving as a respiratory stimulant.[113] Prophylactic dose of 125–250 mg by mouth twice daily is currently recommended to be started anywhere from 1 to 3 days prior to ascent.[114]

Alternatively, because hypoxia is the main mechanism driving periodic CSA at high altitude, supplementing low-flow oxygen to CPAP may suppress high-altitude periodic CSA in patients with OSA.[115]

CSA DUE TO MEDICATIONS OR SUBSTANCE USE

Similar to hypoventilation due to medications, opioids are often associated with CSA.[116] Widespread use of opioids is being recognized as a health crisis given that many patients are found dead in bed, presumably having died in their sleep. Respiratory depression or cardiac arrhythmias are suspected to be potential etiologies; both of which can be seen with sleep-disordered breathing.[117] A causal relationship between opioids and CSA is highlighted in cases where CSA is resolved following the discontinuation of opioids.[118,119] Discontinuation of opioids, although desirable, may or may not be clinically feasible in many cases. Some of the common opioids—methadone, morphine, oxycodone, fentanyl patch, and suboxone—are all associated with CSA. Studies have reported a direct relationship between dose of opioids and the presence and severity of CSA. CSA was present in 92% of patients who were on morphine equivalent daily dose (MEDD) >200mg/day and 61% in patients with MEDD <200 mg/day.[120] Non-obese patients on opioids had a higher risk for having CSA.[120]

The ICSD-3 defines CSA due to medications or substance use as follows:

1. PSG in a patient on opioids or other respiratory depressants shows a frequency of central apneas or hypopneas ≥5 per hour of sleep and total number of central apneas and hypopneas is >50% of the total number of apneas or hypopneas. In addition, PSG shows absence of CSB.
2. Patient has one or more these symptoms: sleepiness, sleep onset or maintenance difficulties, non-restorative sleep, arousals with shortness of breath, witnessed apneas or snoring.
3. The disorder is due to opioids or other respiratory depressant and cannot be explained by another sleep disorder.

Pathophysiology

Impact of opioids in reducing ventilatory drive is potentiated in sleep, leading to apneas or hypopneas. Prescription opioids have a prominent inhibitory effect on μ-opioid receptors which are present both in CNS and peripherally. The inhibition of μ-opioid receptors in brainstem and carotid body inhibition result in notable changes in many aspects of pulmonary physiology as evidenced by findings on PSG.

Polysomnogram

Different kinds of breathing patterns have been reported to occur in patients with CSA on opioids, including ataxic breathing, Biot respiration, and periodic breathing resembling Cheyne Stokes respiration. Ataxic breathing is characterized by chaotic breathing with irregular tidal volumes with unpredictable pauses. Biot respiration has a similar pattern, though tidal volume is more regular. Bradypnea may be prominent in some patients with lengthy apneas. CO_2 monitoring may show normal or elevated values.

Management

Reduction or gradual discontinuation of opioid therapy may be the most effective strategy if possible in patients with CSA associated with opioids. The CDC published some guidelines for clinicians when prescribing opioids, one of which included using immediate-release over extended-release or longer-acting preparations.[116] PAP modalities are appropriate in patients who remain on chronic opioid management, which include CPAP, BPAP, BPAP with ST, or ASV therapy. Of the PAP modalities, ASV is more likely to suppress the AHI and central apnea index (CAI) when compared with the other PAP modalities.[121–123] ASV may result in reducing sleepiness and improve alertness as well.[121,124]

Summary

CSA or hypoventilation in sleep are much less common than OSA, though either diagnosis should alert a clinician to evaluate for underlying cardiac, neurological, pulmonary, medication, or substance etiologies. Diagnostic workup may be dependent on the pattern of sleep-disordered breathing noted, patient's age, and other known or suspected comorbidities. Effective management and optimal outcomes are typically contingent on establishing the diagnosis and treating the underlying cause, though often PAP therapy (CPAP or NIV) is needed to manage CSA and hypoventilation. Ancillary testing, such as PFTs, toxicology screens, radiological studies, MIP/MEP, or noninvasive CO_2 monitoring, are often helpful diagnostically as well as aiding in long-term management. In cases of ROHHAD, a comprehensive endocrinology workup is needed where patients are monitored for neural crest tumors.

Diagnostic criteria have been clarified in ICSD-3, though there is more to be learned, especially in patients with CSA with CSB where CPAP or oxygen have been ineffective, or in patients at risk for having TECSA so that auto-CPAP therapy can be prescribed more judiciously. NIV can improve survival and sleep in neuromuscular patients, though therapy needs to be monitored more closely in patients once they progress to having bulbar weakness. NIV to treat sleep-related hypoventilation and possible upper airway obstruction may need to be developed, as there is lower minute ventilation and hypotonia of the upper airway. Daytime NIV settings may not be adequate during sleep.

REFERENCES

1. Sowho M, Amatoury J, Kirkness JP, et al. Sleep and respiratory physiology in adults. *Clin Chest Med.* 2014;35(3):469–481.
2. Mitchell GS. Back to the future: Carbon dioxide chemoreceptors in the mammalian brain. *Nat Neurosci.* 2004;**7**(12):1288–1290.
3. Ballard RD, Irvin CG, Martin RJ, et al. Influence of sleep on lung volume in asthmatic patients and normal subjects. *J Appl Physiol (1985).* 1990;68(5):2034–2041.
4. Casey KR, Cantillo KO, Brown LK. Sleep-related hypoventilation/hypoxemic syndromes. *Chest.* 2007;131(6):1936–1948.
5. Hudgel DW, Devadatta P. Decrease in functional residual capacity during sleep in normal humans. *J Appl Physiol Respir Environ Exerc Physiol.* 1984;57(5):1319–1322.
6. Skatrud JB, Dempsey JA. Airway resistance and respiratory muscle function in snorers during NREM sleep. *J Appl Physiol (1985).* 1985;59(2):328–335.
7. Douglas NJ, White DP, Pickett CK, et al. Respiration during sleep in normal man. *Thorax.* 1982;37(11):840–844.
8. Gould GA, Gugger M, Molloy J, et al. Breathing pattern and eye movement density during REM sleep in humans. *Am Rev Respir Dis.* 1988;138(4):874–877.
9. Naifeh KH, Kamiya J. The nature of respiratory changes associated with sleep onset. *Sleep.* 1981;4(1):49–59.
10. Trinder J, Whitworth F, Kay A, et al. Respiratory instability during sleep onset. *J Appl Physiol* (1985). 1992;73(6):2462–2469.
11. Bickelmann AG, Burwell CS, Robin ED, et al. Extreme obesity associated with alveolar hypoventilation: A Pickwickian syndrome. *Am J Med.* 1956;21(5):811–818.
12. Berg G, Delaive K, Manfreda J, et al. The use of health-care resources in obesity-hypoventilation syndrome. *Chest.* 2001;120(2): 377–383.
13. Raebel MA, et al. Health services use and health care costs of obese and nonobese individuals. *Arch Intern Med.* 2004;164(19):2135–2140.
14. Masa JF, Pepin JL, Borel JC, et al. Obesity hypoventilation syndrome. *Eur Respir Rev.* 2019;28(151):1–14.
15. BaHammam, AS, Pandi-Perumal SR, Piper A, et al. Gender differences in patients with obesity hypoventilation syndrome. *J Sleep Res.* 2016;25(4):445–453.
16. Palm A, Midgren B, Janson C, et al. Gender differences in patients starting long-term home mechanical ventilation due to obesity hypoventilation syndrome. *Respir Med.* 2016;110:73–78.

17. Lee WY, Mokhlesi B. Diagnosis and management of obesity hypoventilation syndrome in the ICU. *Crit Care Clin*. 2008;24(3):533–549, vii.
18. Mokhlesi B. Obesity hypoventilation syndrome: A state-of-the-art review. *Respir Care*. 2010;55(10):1347–1362; discussion 1363–1365.
19. Marik PE, Desai H. Characteristics of patients with the "malignant obesity hypoventilation syndrome" admitted to an ICU. *J Intensive Care Med*. 2013;28(2):124–130.
20. Strumpf DA, Millman RP, Hill NS. The management of chronic hypoventilation. *Chest*. 1990;98(2):474–480.
21. Hodgson LE, Murphy PB, Hart N. Respiratory management of the obese patient undergoing surgery. *J Thorac Dis*. 2015;7(5) 943–952.
22. Zavorsky GS, Hoffman SL. Pulmonary gas exchange in the morbidly obese. *Obes Rev*. 2008;9(4):326–339.
23. O'Donnell CP, Schaub CD, Haines AS, et al. Leptin prevents respiratory depression in obesity. *Am J Respir Crit Care Med*. 1999;159(5 Pt 1):1477–1484.
24. White LH, Bradley TD. Role of nocturnal rostral fluid shift in the pathogenesis of obstructive and central sleep apnoea. *J Physiol*. 2013;591(5):1179–1193.
25. Berger KI, Ayappa I, Sorkin B, et al. Postevent ventilation as a function of CO(2) load during respiratory events in obstructive sleep apnea. *J Appl Physiol (1985)*. 2002;93(3):917–924.
26. Mokhlesi B, Tulaimat A, Faibussowitsch I, et al. Obesity hypoventilation syndrome: Prevalence and predictors in patients with obstructive sleep apnea. *Sleep Breath*. 2007;11(2):117–124.
27. de Llano, LP, Castro-Añón O, Castro-Cabana L, et al. Long-term effectiveness of CPAP in patients with severe obesity-hypoventilation syndrome. *Sleep Breath*. 2021;25(2):947–950.
28. Soghier I, Brożek JL, Afshar M, et al. Noninvasive ventilation versus CPAP as initial treatment of obesity hypoventilation syndrome. *Ann Am Thorac Soc*. 2019;16(10):1295–1303.
29. Mellins RB, Balfour Jr, HH, Turino GM, et al. Failure of automatic control of ventilation (Ondine's curse): Report of an infant born with this syndrome and review of the literature. *Medicine (Baltimore)*. 1970;49(6):487–504.
30. Trang H, Dehan M, Beaufils F, et al. The French Congenital Central Hypoventilation Syndrome Registry: General data, phenotype, and genotype. *Chest*. 2005;127(1):72–79.
31. Klaskova E, Drabek, J, Hobzova M, et al. Significant phenotype variability of congenital central hypoventilation syndrome in a family with polyalanine expansion mutation of the PHOX2B gene. *Biomed Pap Med Fac Univ Palacky Olomouc Czech Repub*. 2016;160(4):495–498.
32. Kasi AS, Jurgensen TJ, Yen S, et al. Three-generation family with congenital central hypoventilation syndrome and novel PHOX2B gene non-polyalanine repeat mutation. *J Clin Sleep Med*. 2017;13(7):925–927.
33. Patwari PP, Carroll MS, Rand CM, et al. Congenital central hypoventilation syndrome and the PHOX2B gene: A model of respiratory and autonomic dysregulation. *Respir Physiol Neurobiol*. 2010;173(3):322–335.
34. Weese-Mayer DE, Berry-Kravis EM, Ceccherini I, et al. An official ATS clinical policy statement: Congenital central hypoventilation syndrome: Genetic basis, diagnosis, and management. *Am J Respir Crit Care Med*. 2010;181(6):626–644.
35. Maloney MA, Kun SS, Keens TG, et al. Congenital central hypoventilation syndrome: Diagnosis and management. *Expert Rev Respir Med*. 2018;12(4):283–292.
36. Weese-Mayer DE, Kun SS, Keens TG, et al. Congenital central hypoventilation syndrome from past to future: Model for translational and transitional autonomic medicine. *Pediatr Pulmonol*. 2009;44(6):521–535.
37. Wang TC, Su YN, Lai MC. PHOX2B mutation in a Taiwanese newborn with congenital central hypoventilation syndrome. *Pediatr Neonatol*. 2014;55(1):68–70.
38. Trochet D, O'Brien LM, Gozal D, et al. PHOX2B genotype allows for prediction of tumor risk in congenital central hypoventilation syndrome. *Am J Hum Genet*. 2005;76(3):421–426.
39. Antic NA, Malow BA, Lange N, et al. PHOX2B mutation-confirmed congenital central hypoventilation syndrome: Presentation in adulthood. *Am J Respir Crit Care Med*. 2006;174(8):923–927.
40. Diep B, Wang A, Kun S, et al. Diaphragm pacing without tracheostomy in congenital central hypoventilation syndrome patients. *Respiration*. 2015;89(6):534–538.
41. Wang A, Kun S, Diep B, et al. Obstructive sleep apnea in patients with congenital central hypoventilation syndrome ventilated by diaphragm pacing without tracheostomy. *J Clin Sleep Med*. 2018;14(2):261–264.
42. Dosier LBM, Vaughn BV, Fan Z. Sleep disorders in childhood neurogenetic disorders. *Children (Basel)*. 2017;4(9):1–29.
43. Ize-Ludlow D, Gray JA, Sperling MA, et al. Rapid-onset obesity with hypothalamic dysfunction, hypoventilation, and autonomic dysregulation presenting in childhood. *Pediatrics*. 2007;120(1):e179–e188.
44. Gharial J, Ganesh A, Curtis C, et al. Neuroimaging and pathology findings associated with rapid onset obesity, hypothalamic dysfunction, hypoventilation, and autonomic dysregulation (ROHHAD) syndrome. *J Pediatr Hematol Oncol*. 2021;43(4):e571–e576.
45. Chow C, Fortier MV, Das L, et al. Rapid-onset obesity with hypothalamic dysfunction, hypoventilation, and autonomic dysregulation (ROHHAD) syndrome may have a hypothalamus-periaqueductal gray localization. *Pediatr Neurol*. 2015;52(5):521–525.
46. Ibanez-Mico S, Marcos Oltra AM, Lemauviel S, et al. Rapid-onset obesity with hypothalamic dysregulation, hypoventilation, and autonomic dysregulation (ROHHAD syndrome): A case report and literature review. *Neurologia*. 2017;32(9):616–622.
47. Abaci A, Catli G, Bayram E, et al. A case of rapid-onset obesity with hypothalamic dysfunction, hypoventilation, autonomic dysregulation, and neural crest tumor: ROHHADNET syndrome. *Endocr Pract*. 2013;19(1):e12–e16.
48. Labanowski M, Schmidt-Nowara W, Guilleminault C. Sleep and neuromuscular disease: Frequency of sleep-disordered breathing in a neuromuscular disease clinic population. *Neurology*. 1996;47(5):1173–1180.
49. Aboussouan LS, Mireles-Cabodevila E. Sleep-disordered breathing in neuromuscular disease: Diagnostic and therapeutic challenges. *Chest*. 2017;152(4):880–892.

50. Quera-Salva MA, Guilleminault C, Chevret S, et al. Breathing disorders during sleep in myasthenia gravis. *Ann Neurol*. 1992;31(1):86–92.
51. Dematteis M, Pépin J, Jeanmart M, et al. Charcot-Marie-Tooth disease and sleep apnoea syndrome: A family study. *Lancet*. 2001;357(9252):267–272.
52. Khan Y, Heckmatt JZ. Obstructive apnoeas in Duchenne muscular dystrophy. *Thorax*. 1994;49(2):157–161.
53. Sankari A, Bascom AT, Chowdhuri S, et al. Tetraplegia is a risk factor for central sleep apnea. *J Appl Physiol (1985)*. 2014;116(3):345–353.
54. Arnulf I, Similowski T, Salachas F, et al. Sleep disorders and diaphragmatic function in patients with amyotrophic lateral sclerosis. *Am J Respir Crit Care Med*. 2000;161(3 Pt 1):849–856.
55. Pautrat J, Khirani S, Boulé M, et al. Carbon dioxide levels during polygraphy in children with sleep-disordered breathing. *Sleep Breath*. 2015;19(1):149–157.
56. Ogna A, Quera Salva MA, Prigent H, et al. Nocturnal hypoventilation in neuromuscular disease: Prevalence according to different definitions issued from the literature. *Sleep Breath*. 2016;20(2):575–581.
57. Suresh S, Wales P, Dakin C, et al. Sleep-related breathing disorder in Duchenne muscular dystrophy: Disease spectrum in the paediatric population. *J Paediatr Child Health*. 2005;41(9–10):500–503.
58. Boentert M, Knop K, Schuhmacher C, et al. Sleep disorders in Charcot-Marie-Tooth disease type 1. *J Neurol Neurosurg Psychiatry*. 2014;85(3):319–325.
59. Ragette R, Mellies U, Schwake C, et al. Patterns and predictors of sleep disordered breathing in primary myopathies. *Thorax*. 2002;57(8):724–728.
60. Wang CH, Finkel RS, Bertini ES, et al. Consensus statement for standard of care in spinal muscular atrophy. *J Child Neurol*. 2007;22(8):1027–1049.
61. Birnkrant DJ, Bushby K, Bann CM, et al. Diagnosis and management of Duchenne muscular dystrophy, part 2: Respiratory, cardiac, bone health, and orthopaedic management. *Lancet Neurol*. 2018;17(4):347–361.
62. Kleopa KA, Sherman M, Beal B, et al. Bipap improves survival and rate of pulmonary function decline in patients with ALS. *J Neurol Sci*. 1999;164(1):82–88.
63. Aboussouan LS, Khan SU, Meeker DP, et al. Effect of noninvasive positive-pressure ventilation on survival in amyotrophic lateral sclerosis. *Ann Intern Med*. 1997;127(6):450–453.
64. Bourke, SC, Tomlinson M, Williams TL, et al. Effects of non-invasive ventilation on survival and quality of life in patients with amyotrophic lateral sclerosis: A randomised controlled trial. *Lancet Neurol*. 2006;5(2):140–147.
65. Eagle M, Baudouin SV, Chandler C, et al. Survival in Duchenne muscular dystrophy: Improvements in life expectancy since 1967 and the impact of home nocturnal ventilation. *Neuromuscul Disord*. 2002;12(10):926–929.
66. Castriotta RJ, Murthy JN. Hypoventilation after spinal cord injury. *Semin Respir Crit Care Med*. 2009;30(3):330–338.
67. Crescimanno G, Misuraca A, Purrazella G, et al. Subjective sleep quality in stable neuromuscular patients under non-invasive ventilation. *Sleep Med*. 2014;15(10):1259–1263.
68. Vrijsen B, Buyse B, Belge C, et al. Noninvasive ventilation improves sleep in amyotrophic lateral sclerosis: A prospective polysomnographic study. *J Clin Sleep Med*. 2015;11(5):559–566.
69. Cowie MR, Woehrle H, Wegscheider K, et al. Adaptive servo-ventilation for central sleep apnea in systolic heart failure. *N Engl J Med*. 2015;373(12):1095–1105.
70. Hirschfeld S, Exner G, Luukkaala T, et al. Mechanical ventilation or phrenic nerve stimulation for treatment of spinal cord injury-induced respiratory insufficiency. *Spinal Cord*. 2008;46(11):738–774.
71. McDermott CJ, Bradburn CJ, Maguire C, et al. DiPALS: Diaphragm Pacing in patients with Amyotrophic Lateral Sclerosis: A randomised controlled trial. *Health Technol Assess*. 2016;20(45):1–186.
72. Macintyre PE, Loadsman JA, Scott DA. Opioids, ventilation and acute pain management. *Anaesth Intensive Care*. 2011;39(4):545–558.
73. Li Y, van den Pol AN. Mu-opioid receptor-mediated depression of the hypothalamic hypocretin/orexin arousal system. *J Neurosci*. 2008;28(11):2814–2819.
74. Hajiha M, DuBord M, Liu H, et al. Opioid receptor mechanisms at the hypoglossal motor pool and effects on tongue muscle activity in vivo. *J Physiol*. 2009;587(Pt 11):2677–2692.
75. Hillman DR, Walsh JH, Madison KJ, et al. Evolution of changes in upper airway collapsibility during slow induction of anesthesia with propofol. *Anesthesiology*. 2009;111(1):63–71.
76. D'Alessandro V, Mason T, Pallone MN, et al. Late-onset hypoventilation without PHOX2B mutation or hypothalamic abnormalities. *J Clin Sleep Med*. 2005;1(2):169–172.
77. Hanly PJ. Mechanisms and management of central sleep apnea. *Lung*. 1992;170(1):1–17.
78. American Academy of Sleep Medicine. Idiopathic central alveolar hypoventilation International Classification of Sleep Disorders, 3rd edition. *American Academy of Sleep Medicine*. 2014;4:121–124.
79. Cornips EM, Weber JW, Vles JSH, et al. Pseudo-dermal sinus tract or spinal dermal-sinus-like stalk? *Childs Nerv Syst*. 2011;27(8):1189–1191; author reply 1193.
80. Berry R, Quan SF, Abreu AR, et al. Respiratory Rules for Adults: *The AASM Manual for the Scoring of Sleep and Associated Events: Rules, Terminology and Technical Specifications*. American Academy of Sleep Medicine 2020;Version 2.6:59–60.
81. Perger E, Inami T, Lyons OD, et al. Distinct patterns of hyperpnea during Cheyne-Stokes respiration: Implication for cardiac function in patients with heart failure. *J Clin Sleep Med*. 2017;13(11):1235–1241.
82. Orr JE, Malhotra A, Sands SA. Pathogenesis of central and complex sleep apnoea. *Respirology*. 2017;22(1):43–52.
83. Xie A, Skatrud JB, Puleo DS, et al. Apnea-hypopnea threshold for CO_2 in patients with congestive heart failure. *Am J Respir Crit Care Med*. 2002;165(9):1245–1250.
84. Solin P, Bergin P, Richardson M, et al. Influence of pulmonary capillary wedge pressure on central apnea in heart failure. *Circulation*. 1999;99(12):1574–1579.

85. Tkacova R, Hall MJ, Liu PP, et al. Left ventricular volume in patients with heart failure and Cheyne-Stokes respiration during sleep. Am J Respir Crit Care Med. 1997;156(5):1549–1555.
86. Javaheri S. Sleep disorders in systolic heart failure: A prospective study of 100 male patients: The final report. *Int J Cardiol*. 2006;106(1):21–28.
87. Bitter T, Westerheide N, Hossain SM, et al. Symptoms of sleep apnoea in chronic heart failure: Results from a prospective cohort study in 1,500 patients. *Sleep Breath*. 2012;16(3):781–791.
88. Szollosi I, Roebuck T, Thompson B, et al. Lateral sleeping position reduces severity of central sleep apnea / Cheyne-Stokes respiration. *Sleep*. 2006;29(8):1045–1051.
89. Douglas NJ, White DP, Weil JV, et al. Hypercapnic ventilatory response in sleeping adults. *Am Rev Respir Dis*. 1982;126(5):758–762.
90. Abraham WT, Fisher WG, Smith AL, et al. Cardiac resynchronization in chronic heart failure. *N Engl J Med*. 2002;346(24):1845–1853.
91. Basic K, Fox H, Spießhöfer J, et al. Improvements of central respiratory events, Cheyne-Stokes respiration and oxygenation in patients hospitalized for acute decompensated heart failure. *Sleep Med*. 2016;27–28:15–19.
92. Hagenah G, Zapf A, Schuttert JB. Cheyne-Stokes respiration and prognosis in modern-treated congestive heart failure. *Lung*. 2010;188(4):309–313.
93. Arzt M, Floras JS, Logan AG, et al. Suppression of central sleep apnea by continuous positive airway pressure and transplant-free surviFval in heart failure: A post hoc analysis of the Canadian Continuous Positive Airway Pressure for Patients with Central Sleep Apnea and Heart Failure Trial (CANPAP). *Circulation*. 2007;115(25):3173–3180.
94. Bradley TD, Logan AG, Kimoff RJ, et al. Continuous positive airway pressure for central sleep apnea and heart failure. *N Engl J Med*. 2005;353(19):2025–2033.
95. Aurora RN, Chowdhuri S, Ramar K et al. The treatment of central sleep apnea syndromes in adults: Practice parameters with an evidence-based literature review and meta-analyses. *Sleep*. 2012;35(1):17–40.
96. Nakao YM, Ueshima K, Yasuno S, et al. Effects of nocturnal oxygen therapy in patients with chronic heart failure and central sleep apnea: CHF-HOT study. *Heart Vessels*. 2016;31(2):165–172.
97. DeBacker WA, Verbraecken J, Willemen M, et al. Central apnea index decreases after prolonged treatment with acetazolamide. *Am J Respir Crit Care Med*. 1995;151(1):87–91.
98. Javaheri S. Acetazolamide improves central sleep apnea in heart failure: A double-blind, prospective study. *Am J Respir Crit Care Med*. 2006;173(2):234–237.
99. Guilleminault C, Cummiskey J. Progressive improvement of apnea index and ventilatory response to CO_2 after tracheostomy in obstructive sleep apnea syndrome. *Am Rev Respir Dis*. 1982;126(1):14–20.
100. Kuzniar TJ, Kovacevic-Ristanovic R, Freedom T. Complex sleep apnea unmasked by the use of a mandibular advancement device. *Sleep Breath*. 2011;15(2):249–252.
101. Nigam G, Pathak C, Riaz M. A systematic review on prevalence and risk factors associated with treatment-emergent central sleep apnea. *Ann Thorac Med*. 2016;11(3):202–210.
102. Javaheri S, Smith J, Chung E. The prevalence and natural history of complex sleep apnea. *J Clin Sleep Med*. 2009;5(3):205–211.
103. Kuzniar TJ, Pusalavidyasagar S, Gay PC, et al. Natural course of complex sleep apnea: A retrospective study. *Sleep Breath*. 2008;12(2):135–139.
104. Morgenthaler TI, Gay PC, Gordon N, et al. Adaptive servoventilation versus noninvasive positive pressure ventilation for central, mixed, and complex sleep apnea syndromes. *Sleep*. 2007;30(4):468–475.
105. Allam JS, Olson EJ, Gay PC, et al. Efficacy of adaptive servoventilation in treatment of complex and central sleep apnea syndromes. *ChesKt*. 2007;132(6):1839–1846.
106. Morgenthaler TI, Kuzniar TJ, Wolfe LF, et al. The complex sleep apnea resolution study: A prospective randomized controlled trial of continuous positive airway pressure versus adaptive servoventilation therapy. *Sleep*. 2014;37(5):927–934.
107. Dellweg D, Kerl J, Hoehn E, et al. Randomized controlled trial of noninvasive positive pressure ventilation (NPPV) versus servoventilation in patients with CPAP-induced central sleep apnea (complex sleep apnea). *Sleep*. 2013;36(8):1163–1171.
108. Sakakibara M, Sakata Y, Usui K, et al. Effectiveness of short-term treatment with nocturnal oxygen therapy for central sleep apnea in patients with congestive heart failure. *J Cardiol*. 2005;46(2):53–61.
109. Otero L, Hidalgo P, Gonzalez R, et al. Association of cardiovascular disease and sleep apnea at different altitudes. *High Alt Med Biol*. 2016;17(4):336–341.
110. Smith CA, Chenuel BJ, Henderson KS, et al. The apneic threshold during non-REM sleep in dogs: Sensitivity of carotid body vs. central chemoreceptors. *J Appl Physiol (1985)*. 2007;103(2):578–586.
111. Patz DS, Swihart B, White DP. CPAP pressure requirements for obstructive sleep apnea patients at varying altitudes. *Sleep*. 2010;33(5):715–718.
112. Nishida K, Lanspa MJ, Cloward TV, et al. Effects of positive airway pressure on patients with obstructive sleep apnea during acute ascent to altitude. *Ann Am Thorac Soc*. 2015;12(7):1072–1078.
113. Liu HM, Chiang I-J, Kuo KN, et al. The effect of acetazolamide on sleep apnea at high altitude: A systematic review and meta-analysis. *Ther Adv Respir Dis*. 2017;11(1):20–29.
114. Stadelmann K, Latshang TD, Nussbaumer-Ochsner Y, et al. Impact of acetazolamide and CPAP on cortical activity in obstructive sleep apnea patients. *PLoS One*. 2014;9(4):e93931.
115. Burgess KR, Ainslie PN. Central sleep apnea at high altitude. *Adv Exp Med Biol*. 2016;903:275–283.
116. Dowell D, Haegerich TM, Chou R. CDC guideline for prescribing opioids for chronic pain—United States, 2016. *MMWR Recomm Rep*. 2016;65(1):1–49.
117. Kao D, Bartelson BB, Khatri V, et al. Trends in reporting methadone-associated cardiac arrhythmia, 1997–2011: An analysis of registry data. *Ann Intern Med*. 2013;158(10):735–740.

118. Javaheri S, Patel S. Opioids cause central and complex sleep apnea in humans and reversal with discontinuation: A plea for detoxification. *J Clin Sleep Med.* 2017;13(6):829–833.
119. Davis MJ, Livingston M, Scharf SM. Reversal of central sleep apnea following discontinuation of opioids. *J Clin Sleep Med.* 2012;8(5):579–580.
120. Correa D, Farney RJ, Chung F, et al. Chronic opioid use and central sleep apnea: A review of the prevalence, mechanisms, and perioperative considerations. *Anesth Analg.* 2015;120(6):1273–1285.
121. Cao M, Cordell C, Willes C, et al. A novel adaptive servoventilation (ASVAuto) for the treatment of central sleep apnea associated with chronic use of opioids. *J Clin Sleep Med.* 2014;10(8):855–861.
122. Javaheri S, Harris N, Howard, J, et al. Adaptive servoventilation for treatment of opioid-associated central sleep apnea. *J Clin Sleep Med.* 2014;10(6):637–643.
123. Shapiro CM, Chung SA, Wylie PE, et al. Home-use servo-ventilation therapy in chronic pain patients with central sleep apnea: Initial and 3-month follow-up. *Sleep Breath.* 2015;19(4):1285–1292.
124. Alattar MA, Scharf SM. Opioid-associated central sleep apnea: A case series. *Sleep Breath.* 2009;13(2):201–206.

SECTION III

Abnormal Sleep Patterns

Chapter 11

Health Consequences of Sleep Deprivation

Shelley Hershner

INTRODUCTION

Adequate sleep duration is necessary to support alertness, as well as mental and physical health. Sleep deprivation is increasingly prevalent, with sequelae that impact both public health and an individual's health. It is important to note that sleep deprivation is the volitional curtailment of sleep, rather than the inability to sleep or inadequate opportunity to sleep. Sleep deprivation occurs due to personal and professional obligations, as well as when an individual does not prioritize adequate sleep. Although sleep disorders (e.g., obstructive sleep apnea and insomnia) can result in insufficient sleep, that will not be the focus of this chapter. This chapter will review the epidemiology of sleep deprivation and its adverse consequences.

ADEQUATE SLEEP DURATION

Adequate sleep duration is both individual and age-dependent. The American Academy of Sleep Medicine recommends 7 or more hours of nightly sleep for adults, while the National Sleep Foundation advises that adolescents obtain 8–10 hours of sleep and younger children significantly more (see Figure 11.1).[1,2] Sleep deprivation is present when there is inadequate sleep for that individual. Conceptually, sleep deprivation occurs when there is limited opportunity for sleep, rather than the inability to sleep.[3] Ultimately everyone's sleep requirement is individual, and the best gauge of sufficient sleep is waking refreshed and feeling alert during the day.

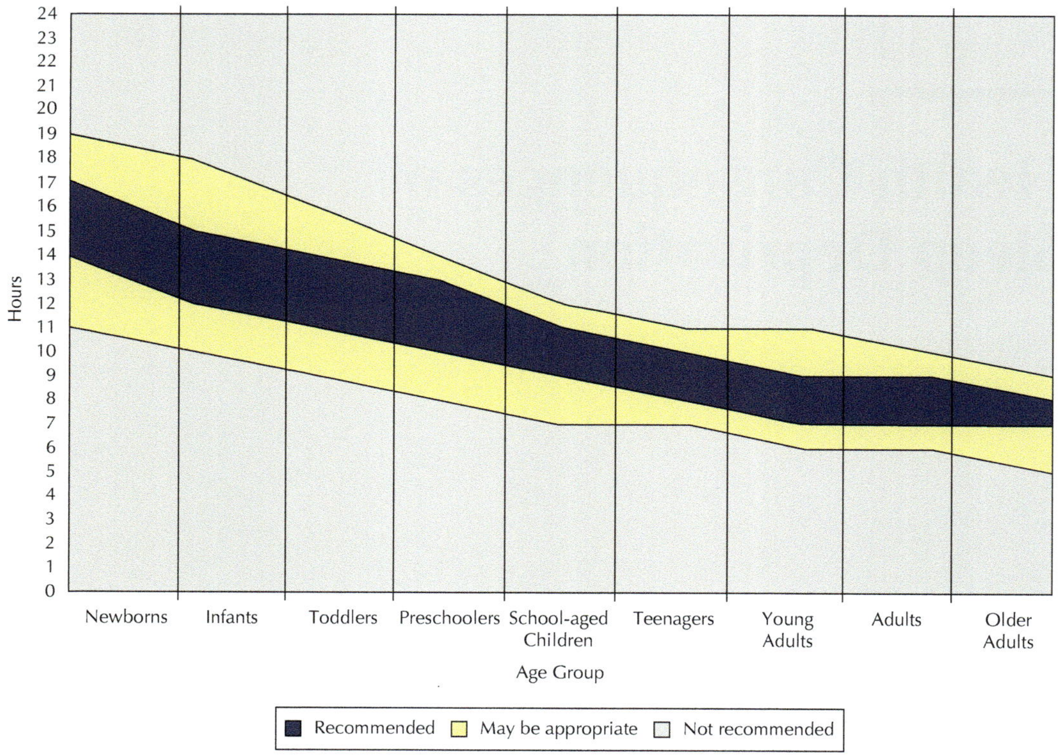

Figure 11.1. Sleep duration recommendations across the life span.

ETIOLOGY

People obtain insufficient sleep due to a multitude of reasons. Society functions on an increasingly busy 24 hours/7 days a week schedule.[4] Many people work varying shifts and long hours. Employees in specific industries, including management, transportation/warehouse, and manufacturing, often experience insufficient sleep.[5] Sleep is truncated as employers expect late and early morning responses to requests and emails.[5] The American Time Use Study showed that "controlling for age, gender, educational attainment, race, income, and the presence of children and partners; time used for monetarily compensated work and work-related activities was consistently associated with sleep time, such that work time increased as sleep time decreased."[6p1090] Additionally, electronic entertainment is ubiquitous. Binge-watching television curtails sleep.[7] In a study among U.S. adults, 28.4% binge-watched television a few times a month. Binge-watching was defined as "watching multiple consecutive episodes of the same television show in one sitting on a screen, be it a television, laptop, computer or tablet computer screen."[p1002] Overall, busy employment and entertainment encourage behaviors other than sleep.

EPIDEMIOLOGY

Sleep deprivation is often divided into acute and chronic partial sleep deprivation. Acute sleep deprivation occurs when a person is kept awake for an entire sleep period. This will result in sustained wakefulness of 24 or more hours. Chronic partial sleep deprivation is when an individual's sleep is restricted, often for multiple days at a time (e.g., 6 hours of nightly sleep for a week).

Estimates of sleep duration by population (e.g., country, state, or geographic region) can be challenging to obtain. Large survey data may be used, but these data require analysis for succinct and accessible reports. Other options include literature on specific populations (e.g., adolescents, college students, the elderly, etc.); however, these data do not apply to the population as a whole. One example of a commonly used large population-based survey in the United States is the Behavioral Risk Factor Surveillance System (BRFSS). The BRFSS is an annual telephone survey of hundreds of thousands of U.S. adults, conducted by the Centers for Disease Control and Prevention (CDC) (http://www.cdc.gov/brfss). Data from the 2014 survey indicate that overall, the prevalence of insufficient sleep (≤6 h) was reported to be 35.1% of the U.S. population.[8] The lowest percentage of adequate sleep was in the southeastern United States and states along the Appalachian Mountains, which per the CDC report "are regions with the highest burdens of obesity and other chronic conditions."[9p140] Consequently, the prevalence of insufficient sleep in this region is especially problematic (see Figure 11.2A and Figure 11.2B).[10]

Multiple factors impact sleep duration, including geographic region, race/ethnicity, and socioeconomic status. In general, gender does not have a major impact on sleep deprivation.[9] In the 2014 BRFSS data, insufficient sleep (≤6 h) was reported by 35.4% of men and 34.8% of women. A lower income is a risk for sleep deprivation. Individuals with an income <$20,000 have a 5.5 greater likelihood of having less than 5 hours of nightly sleep compared to those with an income of family income over $75,000.[11]

Interestingly, the COVID-19 pandemic demonstrated an increase in sleep duration. A prospective observational study using estimated sleep duration data obtained from a smartphone app showed increased sleep duration.[12] Between January 1, 2019, and April 12, 2020, there were 2 871 037 nights from 8218 unique users. The COVID-19 pandemic had a 13.7-minute increase in estimated sleep duration. Significant worldwide geographic variation was observed. Seoul had the smallest increase in sleep duration (12.2 min; 95% confidence interval [CI]: 9.5–14.4 min; p <.001), while New York had the largest (24.5 min; 95% CI: 23.1–25.9 min; p <.001), followed by London (20.8 min; 95% CI: 19.5–22.1 min; p <.001). Another study demonstrated a 44-minute increase in sleep duration during the COVID-19 pandemic.[13] These studies suggest that the COVID-19 pandemic influenced sleep duration, likely through changes in employment, academic, and other obligations.

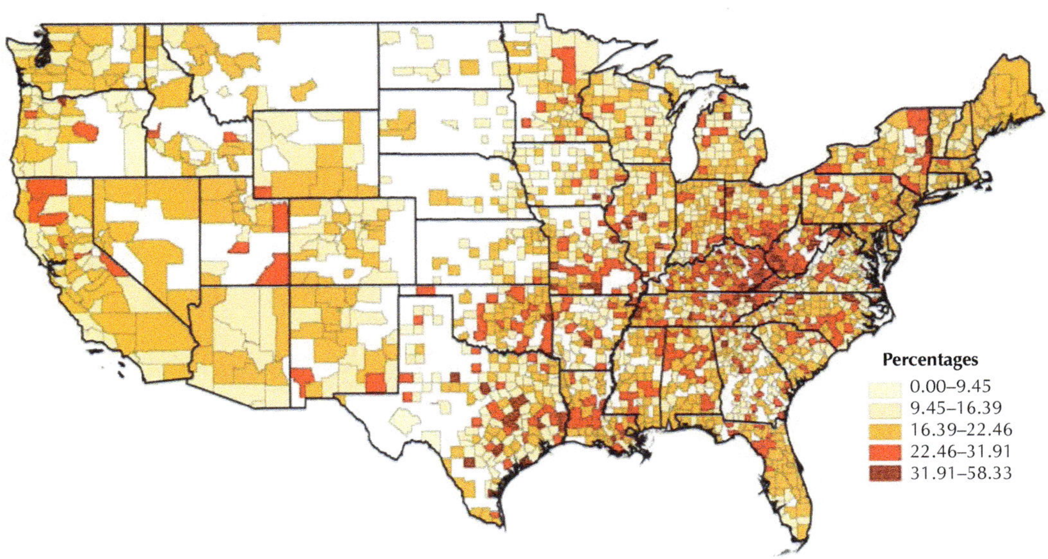

Figure 11.2A. Insufficient sleep by county.

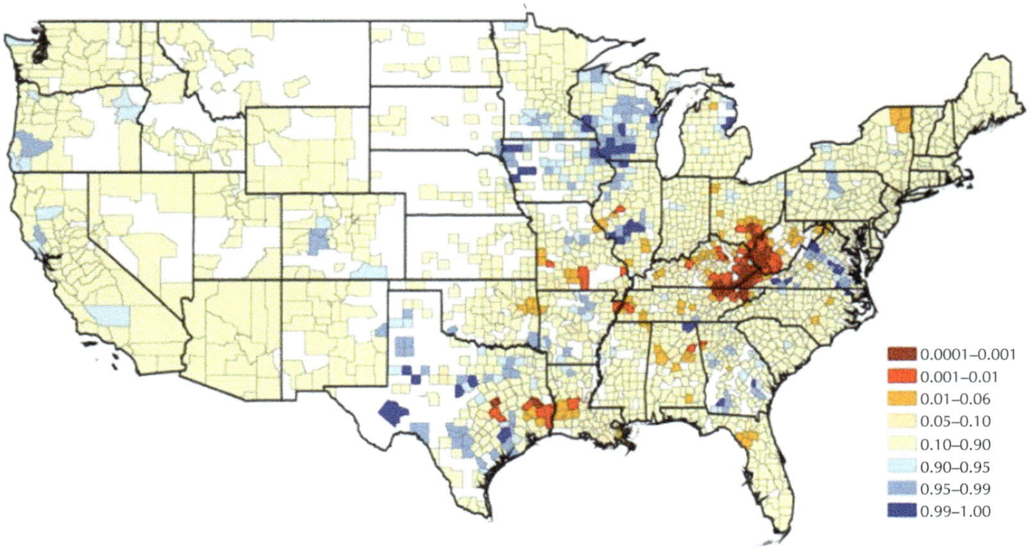

Figure 11.2B. Hotspots and cold spots of insufficient sleep.

ADVERSE HEALTH CONSEQUENCES OF SLEEP DEPRIVATION

The consequences of insufficient sleep are far-reaching, with growing evidence linking chronic sleep restriction to adverse metabolic, cardiovascular, and cognitive outcomes. Epidemiologic and experimental studies have identified associations between short sleep duration and increased risk for obesity, type 2 diabetes, and cardiovascular disease. In parallel, sleep deprivation impairs attention, reaction time, and executive function, contributing to diminished academic performance and reduced workplace safety. The following sections examines the physiologic and neurocognitive effects of sleep deprivation, highlighting its broad impact on individual and public health.

Obesity

The prevalence of obesity among adults in the United States has increased from 33.7% to 39.6% in the past decade.[14] Sleep can have an important role in energy balance and metabolism.[15] Sleep duration, sleep regularity, and circadian rhythms impact weight, dietary intake, and physical activity. Improvement in sleep behaviors may represent a novel, modifiable behavior for weight regulation in children and adults. Short sleep duration (≤5–7 h/day) was associated with obesity, greater adiposity, and larger waist circumferences.[16–19] Sleep duration less than 6 hours has a 12% risk for central obesity.[17] Short sleep duration in preschoolers through teenagers was similarly associated with obesity.[20–22] Insufficient sleep duration among children and adolescents had a 2-fold risk for becoming overweight/obese compared to sufficient sleepers.[23]

The influence of sleep on appetite and weight gain is multifactorial and includes hormonal, circadian, and behavioral changes. Two primary hormones are influenced by sleep duration and impact satiety and hunger. Leptin, the satiety hormone, is released from adipocytes and induces the sensation of fullness.[24] Ghrelin, which is released from the stomach, increases appetite.[25] A foundational study by Spiegel et al. demonstrated that curtailed sleep increased ghrelin and decreased leptin. This study showed that men undergoing intravenous glucose infusion while undergoing 2 nights of sleep restriction (4 h time in bed [TIB]/night) demonstrated a 28% increase in ghrelin and an 18% decrease in leptin levels.[26] Another study among male subjects demonstrated a significant increase in ghrelin following the 3rd night of sleep restriction.[27] The changes in leptin and ghrelin during sleep restriction are not consistent, and this inconsistency may relate to gender. One study found an increase in ghrelin among men, but not women, following sleep restriction.[28]

Sleep deprivation influences weight changes through increased food intake and decreased physical activity. Among adults, sleep restriction was associated with greater calorie consumption, increased portion size, and food impulsivity.[29,30] Men increased caloric intake by 22% after 1 night of sleep restriction.[31] The etiology of these behavioral observations is not known but may be hormonally influenced or related to more opportunity to eat due to a greater time awake. Sleep deprivation decreases physical activity.[32] Sleep restriction reduces subsequent days' moderate to vigorous physical activity.

Circadian timing may influence sleep and obesity. Among 110 participants age 18–22 years, the non-lean subjects consumed most of their calories within 1.1 hours of their dim light melatonin onset.[33] A later bedtime may relate to weight gain.[29,34] In a 4-hour total sleep time protocol, subjects who went to bed later consumed 500 more calories than subjects with the same total sleep time but an earlier bedtime. This shift in food timing was associated with weight gain. Chronotype may influence weight gain. A prospective study in college freshmen found that students characterized as evening types gained more weight over 8 weeks as compared to morning types.[35] Eating later was associated with more weight gain.[36] Late sleepers (sleep midpoint >0530 h) slept less and consumed more calories and fast food items as compared to early midpoint sleepers.[37] Night shift work was associated with weight gain.[38] A meta-analysis showed that night shift workers have an odds ratio of 1.23 for being overweight or obese and an odds ratio of 1.35 for abdominal obesity. Caloric intake was not different between shift workers and day workers. Potential mechanisms for shift work-related obesity may be lower diet quality and decreased physical activity; however, further research is needed.

Interventions that improve sleep may help weight loss. Among women enrolled in a weight-loss program, better sleep quality and duration were associated with greater weight loss.[39] Higher sleep quality scores increased the likelihood of weight loss by 33% (relative risk [RR] 0.67; 95% CI: 0.52–0.86), as did sleeping >7 hour/night. In a weight loss study, an increase in sleep duration by 1 hour decreased fat mass by 0.7 kg.[40] Young children lost weight with improved sleep duration.[41] This study promoted household routines of family meals, adequate sleep duration, limited TV time, and removing the TV from the bedroom. Invention subjects' sleep duration increased, while their body mass index (BMI) decreased. In a randomized clinical trial of 80 adults with short sleep duration, subjects increased their sleep duration to 8.5 hours time in bed; the control group kept their regular sleep patterns.[42] The intervention groups' sleep duration increased by 1.2 hours, with an associated decrease in calories of 270 kilocalories per day. Each 1-hour increase in sleep duration was associated with a decrease in energy intake of approximately 162 kilocalories per day. The control group gained weight while the sleep extension group lost weight. In another randomized controlled trial, sleep extension among short sleepers was not associated with a change in BMI. However, this was a short trial of only 6 weeks.[43] This finding of weight loss in concordance with improved sleep duration is not universal. One study of a weight-loss program demonstrated no difference in weight loss between subjects with adequate sleep as compared to restricted sleep; however, subjects in the sleep restriction group lost a lower percentage of body fat.[44]

Sleep deprivation, night shift work, and a delayed circadian rhythm are associated with weight gain and obesity in children and adults. The influence of sleep deprivation on weight is multifactorial and includes changes in appetite-related hormones, increased caloric intake, and decreased physical activity. The relationship between sleep and weight suggests that sleep interventions may be an essential component of weight loss. Weight-loss interventions should address sleep to augment weight loss.

DIABETES MELLITUS

Diabetes mellitus (T2DM) has increased dramatically over the past 3 decades and is predicted to reach 11% of the global population by 2045.[45] Short (<5–7 hours) sleep duration is associated with T2DM, prediabetes, insulin resistance, and impaired glucose tolerance.[46–48] Sleep duration of 5 hours and less had an odds ratio of 1.47 (95% CI: 1.03–2.09) for the risk of T2DM. Another study demonstrated that individuals with short sleep were 28% more likely to be at risk for T2DM.[49] In another study, unmeasured confounders were thought to explain the relationship with long sleep (>9 hours) and T2DM.[46]

Several proposed mechanisms describe how sleep duration mediates glucose and insulin physiology and pathophysiology. As previously discussed, sleep deprivation results in increased appetite from changes in the appetite-related hormones leptin and ghrelin, with resultant increased consumption of calorie-dense and high-carbohydrate food.[50] This contributes to insulin resistance. Sleep independently can worsen glycemic control.[51] Sleep restriction (5 h/night) for 1 week significantly reduces insulin sensitivity and glucose tolerance. Sleep restriction will increase sympathetic activation, catecholamines, as well serum cortisol levels, especially evening cortisol.[50] Cortisol can increase adiposity and in conjunction with other metabolic avenues increase the likelihood of obesity and insulin resistance.[52] Sleep restriction to 4 hours TIB decreases insulin sensitivity with a 25% reduction in whole-body insulin sensitivity and a 29% reduction in peripheral insulin sensitivity.[53] Sleep deprivation and circadian misalignment can lead to β cell dysfunction and an increase in inflammatory cytokines.[54] In summary, restricted sleep may induce hyperinsulinemia, decrease glucose sensitivity, and stimulate downstream pathways which contribute to pancreatic beta cell failure and lipogenesis, all of which contribute to the development of T2DM.

Little research is available to establish if sleep extension will improve T2DM. In a small study of 16 participants, subjects increased their sleep duration by 44 ± 34 minutes.[55] Sleep extension correlated significantly with improved fasting glucose and insulin sensitivity. Further research is needed to determine if sleep extension can improve T2DM.

CARDIOVASCULAR DISEASE (CVD)

Several studies have found interactions between sleep duration and incident hypertension. The English Longitudinal Study of Ageing followed men and women over the age of 50 years.[56] Sleep duration was by self-report. Short sleep duration was categorized as 5 hours or less of sleep. As compared to subjects sleeping 7–8 hours, men had an adjusted odds ratio of 1.73 (95% CI: 1.08–2.76) and women an adjusted odds ratio of 1.44 (95% CI: 1.00–2.07) for incident hypertension. This relationship was present for subjects under 60 years of age. Other studies support a relationship with sleep duration of 5–6 hours and hypertension.[17,57]

Data on coronary heart disease (CAD) is less clear. Many of the studies that investigate CAD and sleep evaluated obstructive sleep apnea rather than sleep duration.[58] The Nurse's Health Study, a large prospective study of 71617 women, age 45–65, found that ≤5 hours (RR 1.82; 95% CI: 0.34–2.41) of self-reported sleep duration was predictive of incident CAD compared to subjects with 6 and >7 hours of sleep.[59] A study on middle-aged men and women from Germany found a significant relationship between self-reported short sleep (≤5 h) with incident myocardial infarction in women but not men.[60] This longitudinal study followed subjects for a mean of 10 years. This study needs to be interpreted with caution due to the low number of incident cases (295 cases in men and 85 cases among women). Other studies show that sleep disturbances and quality or the combination of short sleep and sleep disturbance may have a greater association with CAD.[61,62] The Whitehall II study, a large longitudinal study of subjects from England, found no gender difference in sleep complaints and incident CAD, nor an association with short sleep duration and CAD.[62] Evidence of an interaction effect between short sleep and disturbed sleep was observed with subjects showing a 1.5 times higher hazard ratio for incident CAD. Subjects with short sleep but without sleep disturbances did not show an association with CAD. A recent study investigated multiple aspects of sleep, including satisfaction, alertness, efficiency, and sleep duration.[63] Among self-reported sleep health dimensions, satisfaction, alertness, and efficiency were independently associated with heart disease, whereas regularity and duration showed no significant associations. Additionally, all-cause mortality is associated with sleep deprivation.[64]

Stroke has an association with sleep deprivation. Short sleepers (<6 hours) had a 2-fold increase for ischemic and hemorrhagic stroke according to the European Prospective Investigation into Cancer and Nutrition

(EPIC)-Potsdam Study.[65] The Women's Health Initiative likewise demonstrated increased stroke risk. This was a prospective study that followed 93 175 postmenopausal women for 7.5 years. Short sleep had a 14% increase in ischemic stroke. Long sleep duration (≥9 hours) had a 70% augmented risk of stroke.[66] Other studies have also found a relationship between long sleep duration and CAD, obesity, stroke.[67] Further research is needed, but the increased risk of stroke among long sleepers is thought to be related to unmeasured factors.[67] Another study found an increased risk of fatal and nonfatal stroke and long sleep duration, but not short sleep duration.[68]

Overall there is support that sleep duration is associated with CVD. In general, short sleep duration may have the strongest support, but as some studies link long sleep duration with CVD, a more accurate viewpoint may be that "extremes of sleep duration" are associated with CVD.

The mechanistic interaction of sleep duration and cardiovascular disease is complex (Figure 11.3). Arterial blood pressure is modulated by the autonomic nervous system and baroreceptors. During healthy sleep, a person's blood pressure decreases by 10%–20%. This is called "dipping."[58] "Non-dipping" is observed in cardiovascular disease. The mechanism is thought to relate to increased sympathetic activity, decreased baroreceptor sensitivity, and a higher baroreflex set-point.[69,70] Baroreflex sensitivity can be considered as a graph of the autonomic nervous system (measured by microneurography) plotted against variable blood pressures.[71] The intercept is baroreflex set-point. In a study of 6 young men, the arterial baroreflex was higher by 12 mmHg after a single night of sleep deprivation.[69]

Inflammation contributes to cardiovascular disease.[72] Sleep deprivation is associated with inflammation. Interleukin 6, C-reactive protein, and tumor necrosis factor are increased in both acute and chronic partial sleep deprivation.[73,74] A potential mechanism for inflammation is that elevated blood pressure causes endothelial shear stresses, which result in the endothelial production of inflammatory mediators.[75] Adiposity also contributes to inflammation cytokines. Insulin resistance contributes to cardiovascular disease. As mentioned previously, short sleep duration contributes to insulin resistance through obesity and endocrine changes.[8] In summary, mechanistically sleep deprivation contributes to CVD in part

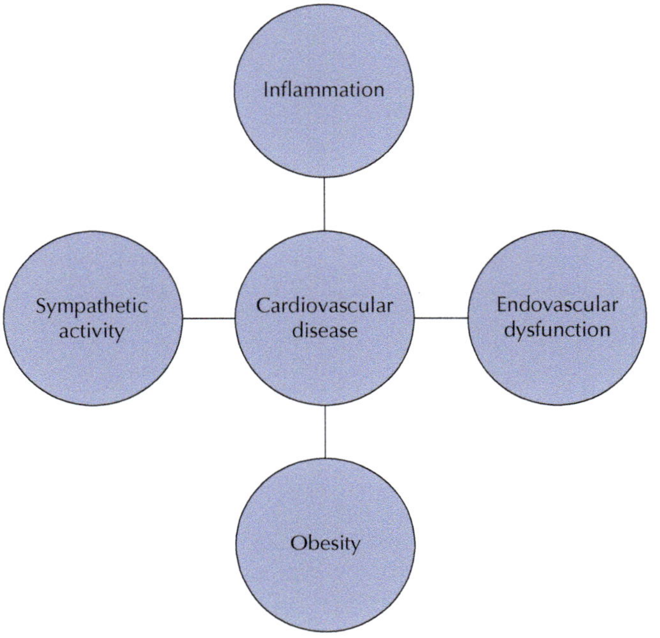

Figure 11.3. Sleep deprivation and cardiovascular disease.

through hypertension, inflammation, and insulin resistance.[76]

IMMUNITY

The goal of this section is to link the immune system with sleep. A barrier to the exploration of immunity and sleep is that many of the studies are cross-sectional. This section will focus on studies from a more controlled environment.[77] In a study investigating the common cold, 153 subjects were inoculated with the rhinovirus.[78] Subjects with <7 hours sleep were 2.94 times more likely to become ill. Sleep efficiency also contributed to infection risk. Subjects with a sleep efficiency of <92% efficiency had an OR of 5.50 to become clinically ill. In another study that also involved the rhinovirus, subjects with actigraphy-assessed shorter sleep duration had a 4-fold increased likelihood of infection.[79]

A host's response to vaccination helps us to better understand the linkage of sleep and immunity. Sleep deprivation, both chronic and partial, impairs antibody response. In a study evaluating the hepatitis B vaccination, chronic partial sleep deprivation was associated with a decreased antibody response.[80] In the study, middle-aged adults had sleep recorded by actigraphy for 6 days prior to their 3rd hepatitis B vaccine injection. Serum antibodies were measured 6 months later. Subjects with a short sleep duration (<6 hours) had a lower antibody response.

Acute sleep deprivation following vaccination may impair immune response. Production of H1N1-specific antibodies for the 2009 H1N1 influenza virus was decreased in men, but not women, among subjects vaccinated for hepatitis B who did not sleep post-vaccination.[81] At 7 weeks, antibody response was equal between both groups. In another study, subjects that slept immediately following vaccination had a nearly 2-fold higher antibody titer to hepatitis A.[82] In another study investigating immunity after the hepatitis A vaccine, subjects that had adequate sleep post-vaccination, as compared to those with prolonged wakefulness, had increased antigen-specific T helper (Th) cell response.[83] A small subset of subjects with acute sleep deprivation following vaccination failed to mount an adequate antibody response to support immunity.[83] Although not measuring sleep duration directly, 23.2% of night-shift workers were non-responders after the 2nd hepatitis B vaccine as compared with 3.5% day-shift workers.[84] After 3 doses, most people did have adequate antibody response. These findings are noteworthy, as healthcare workers may receive their vaccination before their work shift and consequently may have a lower antibody response. Although there are no current studies yet on sleep and the COVID-response, the global COVID-19 pandemic highlights the need to get adequate sleep before and after vaccination, especially among healthcare workers.[85] This population is likely to experience sleep restriction related to work.[85,86]

How sleep can impede antibody response needs further investigation. There is emerging evidence that the circadian rhythm may contribute to immune function and mechanistically, sleep deprivation and the circadian rhythm are intertwined with immune function.[87] Sleep deprivation decreases natural killer cell activity.[88] The immune system also affects sleep and sleep stages. For example, during an infection, inflammatory cytokines can increase the amount of slow-wave sleep.[89] How sleep deprivation interacts with the immune system, host deference, the clock genes merits further elucidation.[90]

NEUROCOGNITIVE EFFECTS

Sleep deprivation affects multiple cognitive domains, which include attention, vigilance, executive function, academic performance, and workplace errors and safety.[91] Research protocols investigate neurocognitive performance function in several ways. Some may operate by teaching participants a simplified task (e.g., visual processing) and then testing the subject following a night of reduced sleep duration.[92] The change in performance is attributed to the influence of sleep duration. Other research algorithms utilize a controlled sleep laboratory environment to help minimize confounders such as work, family, commuting time, light exposure, heat, and so on.[93] More recently, the literature has investigated real-world examples of neurocognitive consequences of insufficient sleep.

Attention, Vigilance, Reaction Time

The psychomotor vigilance test (PVT) is the gold standard measure of behavioral alertness, attention, and vigilance.[94] The test consists of the presentation of a visual stimulus on a screen. The subject quickly presses a button as soon as possible after the visual stimulus. The reaction time measured by the PVT does not involve learning. The PVT shows a slowed reaction time following both acute and chronic partial sleep deprivation. In subjects with acute sleep deprivation, the reaction time was maintained until after approximately 16 hours of wakefulness.[95] A marked slowing in reaction time was observed following 24 hours or more of sustained wakefulness.[96] Simulated driving performance among professional drivers showed a decrease in vigilance and reaction time after 27 hours of sustained wakefulness.

Chronic partial sleep deprivation similarly affects reaction time[97] (see Figure 11.4). Subjects that had time in bed of 3, 5, 7, and 9 hours showed a dose-response curve such that shorter sleep durations had a slower reaction time. Subjects with 3 hours-time in bed had the slowest reaction speed. Other studies support that sleep restriction results in slower reaction times.[98] Subjects underwent sleep restriction for 4 or 6 hours per night for 14 consecutive days. This study also showed a dose-dependent response to sleep restriction. Per Van Dongen et al., "In contrast, subjects in the 4-hour sleep period condition displayed escalating numbers of lapses in behavioral alertness and decreasing cognitive accuracy and speed across the 14 days. The magnitude of changes in performance over days of sleep restriction in the 6-hour sleep period condition was between that observed in the 8 and 4 hour sleep period conditions."[98p120] Chronic partial sleep deprivation of 6 hours or less per night produced cognitive performance deficits equivalent to up to 2 nights of total sleep deprivation. Sleep deprivation will result in attention lapses.[99,100] Simple tasks may be more impacted by sleep deprivation than complex tasks.[91]

Executive Function

Executive function is a more complex construct that involves neurocognitive skills of goal-directed problem-solving, working memory,

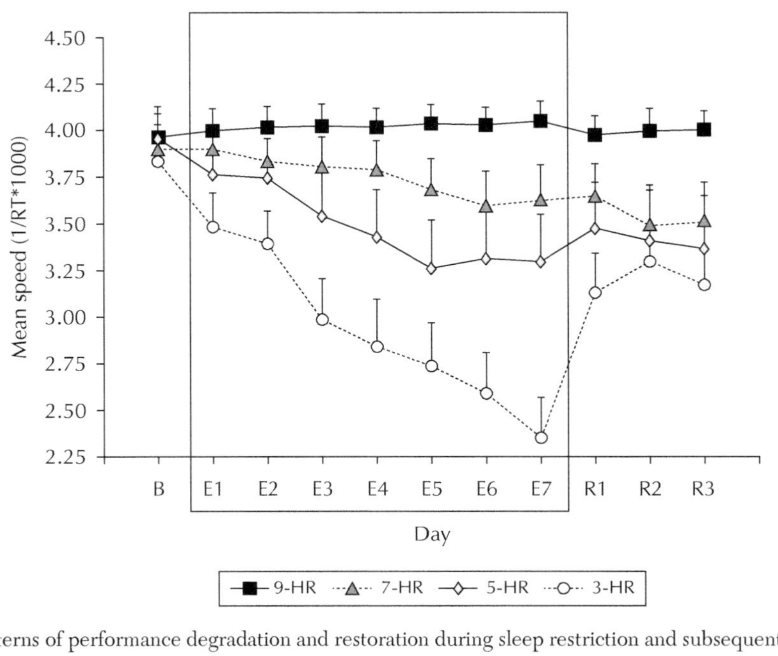

Figure 11.4. Patterns of performance degradation and restoration during sleep restriction and subsequent recovery

and inhibitory control.[101] Executive function allows sustained attention, metal flexibly, switching tasks while suppressing distractors and inhibiting actions.[102] In a large part, executive function depends heavily on the prefrontal cortex.[103] This brain region is sensitive to sleep restriction and shows reduced glucose metabolism following sleep deprivation.[104]

Workplace Errors and Safety

Special focus is warranted on the workplace. Sleep deprivation can result in cognitive impairments which negatively impact workplace errors and safety. Fatigue-related transportation accidents relate in large part to attentional lapses and decreased reaction time.[105,106] Among commercial truck drivers, crashes and near misses occurred most frequently among drivers with 5.8 hours of sleep as compared to drivers with more sleep.[107] Chronic partial sleep deprivation can result in driving performance equivalent to legal intoxication (U.S. standards).[108] In one study, subjects were recruited from the military and transportation industry and underwent 17–19 hours of wakefulness, and in a separate protocol, subjects consumed alcohol until their blood alcohol concentration (BAC) was up to 0.1%. Subjects' reaction time, hand-eye coordination, dual-task, Mackworth clock vigilance tests, and symbol digit were assessed.[108] Sleep deprivation impaired speed in the simple reaction time, dual-task, and Mackworth Clock Vigilance tests. The results demonstrated that performance equivalent to a BAC of 0.05% occurred after 16.9–18.5 hours of wakefulness. Sustained wakefulness between 17.7 and 19.6 hours resulted in performance equivalent to a BAC of 0.1%. In another study, prolonged wakefulness (24+ hr) culminated in reaction times which were slower with worse lateral control of vehicles as compared to subjects who were legally intoxicated.[109] Military pilots had impairments in visual perceptual, complex motor, and psychomotor vigilance (speed and lapses) after 19 hours of wakefulness.[110] Both acute and the more common chronic partial sleep deprivation can impair reaction time, attention, vigilance, and accuracy.

Sleep deprivation in the medical system necessitates particular attention. The death of Libby Zion, an 18-year-old student who died in 1984 in a New York emergency room, was a tragic demonstration that prolonged wakefulness and frequent overnight call among interns and residents increase workplace errors.[111,112] Her death became the impetus to reform medical training as it was thought that resident sleep deprivation contributed to her death. Libby's father wrote in an op-ed originally published, "You don't need kindergarten to know that a resident working a 36-hour shift is in no condition to make any kind of judgment call—forget about life-and-death" (New York Times (1989, May 13). *Doctors know best. The New York Times*, p. 25.). This tragedy became the motivation to change medical education, investigate the impact of sleep duration on medical errors, and enact laws (see Figure 11.5).

Sleep deprivation increases the risk of medical errors. This was demonstrated in a large physician wellness survey which collected data from 11 academic-affiliated medical centers.[113] A physician-related medical error was classified by an affirmative response to "I made a medical error that did result in patient harm," at least once within the last year. Physicians with high sleep-related impairment had a 194% increased odds of self-reported clinically significant medical errors (OR 2.94; 95% CI: 2.22–3.90) as compared to 66% (OR 1.66; 95% CI: 1.22–2.23) in the low sleep-related impairment group.[113] Among interns, each hour of less sleep corresponded to a 27% increase in the odds for reporting medical errors.[114] In a cohort of orthopedic surgical residents, their mean sleep duration was 5.3 hours.[115] Based on the mental effectiveness score, surgical residents were impaired 27% of the time. This level of fatigue was predicted to increase the risk of medical error by 22%. Prolonged wakefulness negatively impacted the technical skills of surgeons in a simulated surgical environment.[116] In the emergency room, sleep deprivation was associated with slower intubation in a simulated clinical scenario.[117]

Medical errors are not the only concern for sleep-deprived medical personnel. In a study among pediatric residents undergoing 24-hour call, riskier clinical decisions correlated to shorter sleep duration.[118] Residents who napped less than an hour during the 24-hour call chose riskier options in the medical decision questionnaire as compared to residents who had at least 3 nights of no-call (with ≥5 hours of sleep.) Medical trainees are at risk of

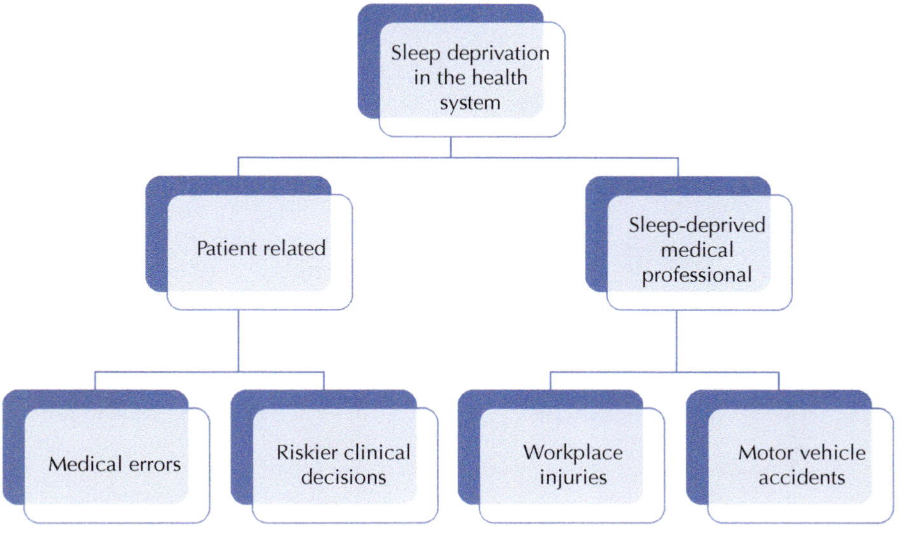

Figure 11.5. Consequences of sleep deprivation in the medical workplace.

workplace injuries. Sleep-deprived residents are more likely to have needle sticks and car accidents.[119,120]

Sleep duration among nurses affects patient safety and medical errors. A study that evaluated data from 2 surveys of nurses found that nurses slept (including naps) an average of 414 minutes on workdays and 497 minutes on nonwork days.[121] Nurses self-reported quality of care and patient safety. Nurses with shorter sleep durations before coming to work reported lower ratings of quality of care and patient safety. An older study found that nurses struggling to stay awake during their shift had a 2-fold increased risk of self-reporting a medical error.[122]

ACADEMIC PERFORMANCE

Most students obtain inadequate sleep.[123,124] Shorter sleep duration is associated with lower grade point averages (GPAs).[124–126] Among university students, those with a GPA <3.0 had the shortest sleep duration.[125] This study demonstrated lower examination scores based on the prior night's sleep duration, although other studies have not replicated this finding.[125,126] One of the first studies on GPA showed adolescents age 13–19 with average grades of Cs went to bed later and obtained 3 hours less sleep per week than higher scoring students (Bs and higher).[127] Other cross-sectional and prospective studies have found variable results of the association of shorter sleep duration and lower academic performance.[124,125] Some of this variability linking GPA and sleep duration may occur as some studies included other sleep measures such as circadian preference and sleep quality. Overall, the data, much of it older, suggest that shorter sleep duration is associated with lower grades, but other sleep measures such as sleep regularity may have a greater impact.[128]

SOLUTIONS FOR IMPROVED SLEEP BEHAVIORS

Improvement in sleep duration may have an impact on both individual health as well as public health. To consider how to improve sleep duration, it is necessary to understand the barriers that prevent adequate sleep. Perceived benefit is a factor for adequate sleep (see Figure 11.6). Many people believe in the importance of sleep to some degree, but responses were variable when asked if inadequate sleep could lead to adverse health consequences.[129] People reported that inadequate sleep could cause sleepiness, decreased energy, and feeling tired. However, most people were

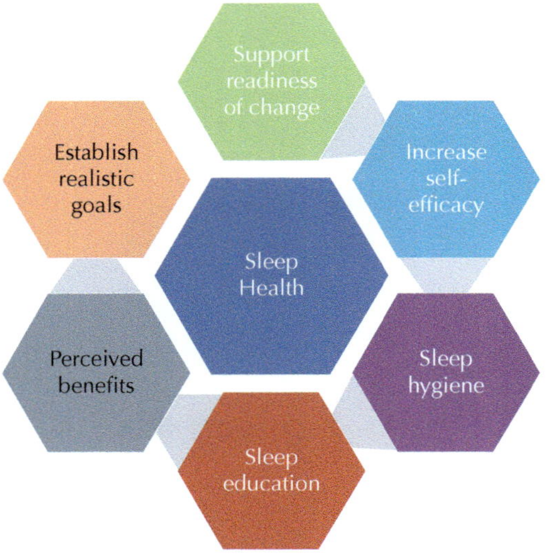

Figure 11.6. Addressing behavior change.

unsure or disagreed that sleep deprivation could contribute to hypertension, diabetes, weight gain, and lower sex drive. A vital part of behavior change is for people to understand the health implications of sleep deprivation.

Work obligations are often reported as one of the main barriers to adequate sleep. However, in a survey of time use, television watching is the most common activity 2 hours before bed.[130] Binge-watching television was a major barrier to sleep.[131] Some TV services have celebrated this finding.[132] For example, the chief executive officer of Netflix, a major provider of television streaming services, was quoted as saying, "You get a show or a movie you're really dying to watch, and you end up staying up late at night, so we actually compete with sleep. . . . And we're winning!"[133] Light from electronic devices results in delayed sleep onset, a later dim light melatonin onset, and daytime sleepiness; therefore electronic use before bed may contribute to sleep deprivation.[134] Many people experience chronic pain. The prevalence of chronic pain increases with age. Chronic pain can reduce sleep duration.[135] Work obligations can interfere with sleep; this is more prevalent among shift workers.[136,137] Longer workdays are associated with shorter sleep.[138] This is by no means an exclusive list of all the factors that contribute to sleep deprivation.

Improvement in sleep behaviors requires addressing the multiple factors that contribute to insufficient sleep. Sleep education interventions should target the relationship of sleep to patient-specific outcomes when possible. For example, if someone is diabetic, highlighting that improved sleep duration may help glycemic control can help encourage behavior change. A major facet of improved sleep duration is to establish realistic goals.[137] It is better to suggest changing sleep duration by 30 minutes rather than a more dramatic change which may not be feasible.[137] Repeated failure to meet goals may lead to frustration, burnout, and giving up. Sleep hygiene is inadequate as a sole intervention but is still a vital aspect of improved sleep habits. Individuals must know the impact of caffeine, naps, and weekend over-sleeping.[139]

Self-efficacy is an important characteristic of behavior change and is a skill set that can be improved.[140] Self-efficacy refers to the perception that a person can improve an intended behavior.[141] There are assessment tools that can evaluate perceived self-efficacy. One example is the Brief Index of Sleep Control.[142] Greater self-control has been shown to increase sleep quality and duration. Higher self-efficacy scores are associated with the perception that subjects are in control of their sleep schedule and that they will make adequate time for sleep. Behavior change can be encouraged by an assessment of the individual's stage of change (see Figure 11.7).[143] Conversations regarding sleep behaviors should target an individual's stage of change.[144] For example, at the precontemplation stage, conversations should focus on the awareness of sleep deprivation. At the preparation stage, conversations should highlight ways to remove barriers and facilitate change. At the action stage, the emphasis should be on specific tools (e.g., meditation apps, etc.). In summary, it is important to utilize interventions that help people improve their sleep duration. These interventions require an understanding of an individual's barriers to adequate sleep. Goals should include concrete and feasible actions steps.

In the workplace, other options exist to improve sleep and mitigate the consequences of sleep deprivation. These workplace options include: (1) scheduling sufficient recovery sleep after a shift; (2) opportunities for naps during work; and (3) adequate pre-work sleep.[145] Other behaviors help promote healthy sleep. A sleep environment that minimizes environmental

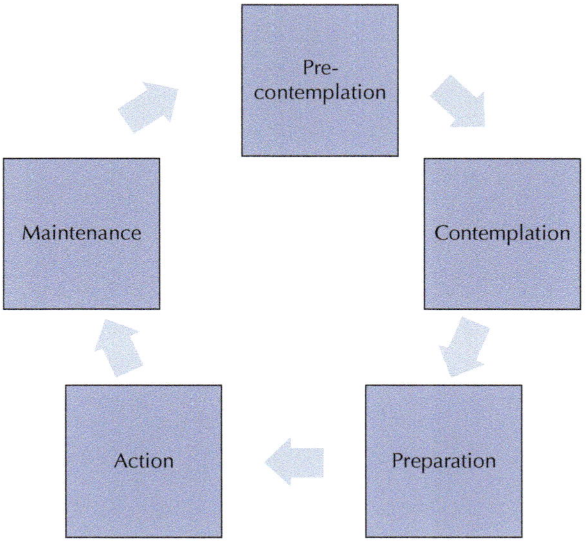

Figure 11.7. Transtheoretical stages of change model.

disruptors (light, noise, temperature, and air quality) improves sleep quality and potentially sleep duration.[146] Exercise and a healthy diet may not directly improve sleep duration but may improve sleep quality.[147] Improvement in work-related safety and morbidity as related to sleep deprivation is complicated and requires further research.

SLEEP AS A HEALTH BEHAVIOR

The social-ecological model is a modification of a model by Grandner et al. that interfaces the individual and society.[64] As stated by Grander, "the core of what the model is describing—sleep exists at the intersection of upstream influences (individual, embedded within social, embedded within societal) and downstream influences that encompass the combination of health outcomes and functioning/performance." This model includes 3 overarching levels: (1) individual; (2) social; (3) societal (see Figure 11.8). At the individual level, factors include a person's beliefs, attitudes, behaviors, physiology, psychology, and health choices.[148] A more global view of sleep as a health behavior occurs at the social level. Here there is an interaction with the individual, but this level includes a broader view of society. These social-level factors include home, family, work, school, neighborhood, religion, and culture. The broadest view is societal-level factors. This includes globalization, 24/7 society, geography, public policy, technology and progress, racism and discrimination, economics, and the natural environment. This framework could be utilized to develop interventions that address individual factors as well as societal factors.

CONCLUSION

The prevalence of sleep deprivation is a substantial, yet unmet public health need. The adverse health consequences of sleep deprivation influence some of the most debilitating contributors to morbidity and mortality. Recognizing the myriad effects of sleep deprivation is the first step toward mitigating the negative consequences of insufficient sleep. Most importantly, the development of solutions that are both practical and feasible is critical. These solutions must focus on both the individual and society. Inventions that educate people, encourage behavior change, and guide policy are needed future steps to ameliorate the negative consequences of sleep deprivation.

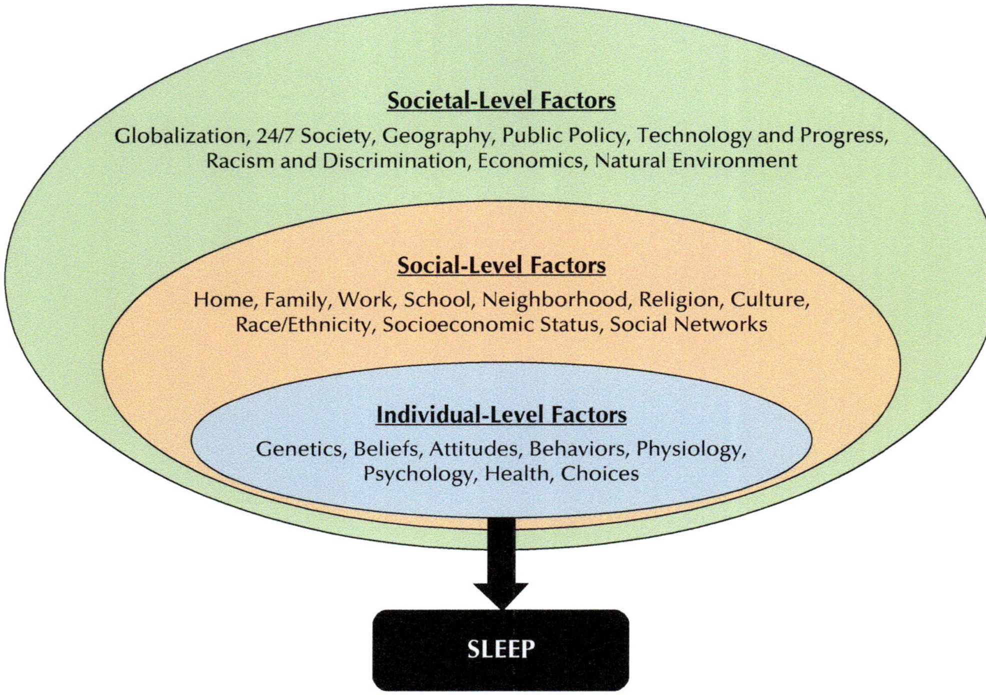

Figure 11.8. Individual, social, and societal influences on sleep.

REFERENCES

1. Paruthi S, Brooks LJ, D'Ambrosio C, et al. Recommended amount of sleep for pediatric populations: A consensus statement of the American Academy of Sleep Medicine. *J Clin Sleep Med.* 2016;12(6):785–786.
2. Hirshkowitz M, Whiton K, Albert SM, et al. National Sleep Foundation's sleep time duration recommendations: Methodology and results summary. *Sleep Health*. 2015;1(1):40–43.
3. American Academy of Sleep Medicine. *International Classification of Sleep Disorders: Diagnostic and Coding Manual*. 3rd ed. American Academy of Sleep Medicine; 2014.
4. Hanson JA, Huecker MR. *Sleep Deprivation*. StatPearls; 2021.
5. Luckhaupt SE, Tak S, Calvert GM. The prevalence of short sleep duration by industry and occupation in the National Health Interview Survey. *Sleep*. 2010;33(2):149–159.
6. Basner M, Fomberstein KM, Razavi FM, et al. American Time Use Survey: Sleep time and its relationship to waking activities. *Sleep*. 2007;30(9):1085–1095.
7. Exelmans L, Van den Bulck J. Binge viewing, sleep, and the role of pre-sleep arousal. *J Clin Sleep Med.* 2017;13(8):1001–1008.
8. Grandner MA, Seixas A, Shetty S, Shenoy S. Sleep duration and diabetes risk: Population trends and potential mechanisms. *Curr Diab Rep*. 2016;16(11):106.
9. Liu Y, Wheaton AG, Chapman DP, Cunningham TJ, Lu H CJ. Prevalence of healthy sleep duration among adults—United States, 2014. *MMWR*. 2016;65(6):140. https://www.cdc.gov/mmwr/volumes/65/wr/mm6506a1.htm.
10. Grandner MA, Smith TE, Jackson N, Jackson T, Burgard S, Branas C. Geographic distribution of insufficient sleep across the United States: A county-level hotspot analysis. *Sleep Health*. 2015;1(3):158–165.
11. Whinnery J, Jackson N, Rattanaumpawan P, Grandner MA. Short and long sleep duration associated with race/ethnicity, sociodemographics, and socioeconomic position. *Sleep*. 2014;37(3):601–611.
12. Robbins R, Affouf M, Weaver MD, et al. Estimated sleep duration before and during the COVID-19 pandemic in major metropolitan areas on different continents: Observational study of smartphone app data. *J Med Internet Res*. 2021;23(2):e20546.
13. Advani I, Gunge D, Banks S, et al. Is increased sleep responsible for reductions in myocardial infarction during the COVID-19 pandemic? *Am J Cardiol.* 2020;131:128–130.
14. Ogden CL, Carroll MD, Lawman HG, et al. Trends in obesity prevalence among children and adolescents in the United States, 1988–1994 through 2013–2014. *JAMA*. 2016;315(21):2292–2299.
15. St-Onge MP. The role of sleep duration in the regulation of energy balance: Effects on energy intakes and expenditure. *J Clin Sleep Med.* 2013;9(1):73–80.
16. Vézina-Im L, Nicklas T, Baranowski T. Associations among sleep, body mass index, waist circumference,

and risk of type 2 diabetes among us childbearing-age women: National Health And Nutrition Examination Survey. *J Womens Health*. 2018;27(11):1400–1407.
17. Deng H-B, Tam T, Zee BC-Y, et al. Short sleep duration increases metabolic impact in healthy adults: A population-based cohort study. *Sleep*. 2017; 40(10):zsx130.
18. Ford ES, Li C, Wheaton AG, Chapman DP, Perry GS, Croft JB. Sleep duration and body mass index and waist circumference among us adults. *Obesity*. 2014;22(2):598–607.
19. Gangwisch JE, Malaspina D, Boden-Albala B, Heymsfield SB. Inadequate sleep as a risk factor for obesity: Analyses of the NHANES I. *Sleep*. 2005;28(10):1289–1296.
20. Chaput J-P, Gray CE, Poitras VJ, et al. Systematic review of the relationships between sleep duration and health indicators in the early years (0–4 years). *BMC Public Health*. 2017;17(5):91–107.
21. Katzmarzyk PT, Barreira TV, Broyles ST, et al. Relationship between lifestyle behaviors and obesity in children ages 9–11: Results from a 12-country study. *Obesity*. 2015;23(8):1696–1702.
22. Halal CSE, Matijasevich A, Howe LD, Santos IS, Barros FC, Nunes ML. Short sleep duration in the first years of life and obesity/overweight at age 4 years: A birth cohort study. *J Pediatr*. 2016;168:99–103.e103.
23. Fatima Y, Doi SA, Mamun AA. Longitudinal impact of sleep on overweight and obesity in children and adolescents: A systematic review and bias-adjusted meta-analysis. *Obes Rev*. 2015;16(2):137–149.
24. Blundell JE, Goodson S, Halford JCG. Regulation of appetite: Role of leptin in signaling systems for drive and satiety. *Int J Obes*. 2001;25(1):S29–S34.
25. Cummings DE. Ghrelin and the short- and long-term regulation of appetite and body weight. *Physiol Behav*. 2006;89(1):71–84.
26. Spiegel K, Tasali E, Penev P, Van Cauter E. Brief communication: Sleep curtailment in healthy young men is associated with decreased leptin levels, elevated ghrelin levels, and increased hunger and appetite. *Ann Intern Med*. 2004;141(11):846–850.
27. Broussard JL, Kilkus JM, Delebecque F, et al. Elevated ghrelin predicts food intake during experimental sleep restriction. *Obesity*. 2016;24(1):132–138.
28. St-Onge MP, O'Keeffe M, Roberts AL, RoyChoudhury A, Laferrere B. Short sleep duration, glucose dysregulation and hormonal regulation of appetite in men and women. *Sleep*. 2012;35(11):1503–1510.
29. Spaeth AM, Dinges DF, Goel N. Effects of experimental sleep restriction on weight gain, caloric intake, and meal timing in healthy adults. *Sleep*. 2013;36(7):981–990.
30. Markwald RR, Melanson EL, Smith MR, et al. Impact of insufficient sleep on total daily energy expenditure, food intake, and weight gain. *PNAS*. 2013;110(14):5695–5700.
31. Brondel L, Romer MA, Nougues PM, Touyarou P, Davenne D. Acute partial sleep deprivation increases food intake in healthy men. *Am J Clin Nutr*. 2010;91(6):1550–1559.
32. Bromley LE, Booth JN III, Kilkus JM, Imperial JG, Penev PD. Sleep restriction decreases the physical activity of adults at risk for type 2 diabetes. *Sleep*. 2012;35(7):977–984.
33. McHill AW, Phillips AJK, Czeisler CA, et al. Later circadian timing of food intake is associated with increased body fat. *Am J Clin Nutr*. 2017;106(5):1213–1219.
34. Spaeth AM, Dinges DF, Goel N. Sex and race differences in caloric intake during sleep restriction in healthy adults. *Am J Clin Nutr*. 2014;100(2):559–566.
35. Culnan E, Kloss JD, Grandner M. A prospective study of weight gain associated with chronotype among college freshmen. *Chronobiol Int*. 2013;30(5):682–690.
36. Allison KC, Goel N. Timing of eating in adults across the weight spectrum: Metabolic factors and potential circadian mechanisms. *Physiol Behav*. 2018;192:158–166.
37. Baron KG, Reid KJ, Kim T, et al. Circadian timing and alignment in healthy adults: Associations with BMI, body fat, caloric intake and physical activity. *Int J Obes*. 2017;41(2):203–209.
38. Sun M, Feng W, Wang F, et al. Meta-analysis on shift work and risks of specific obesity types. *Obes Rev*. 2018;19(1):28–40.
39. Thomson CA, Morrow KL, Flatt SW, et al. Relationship between sleep quality and quantity and weight loss in women participating in a weight-loss intervention trial. *Obesity*. 2012;20(7):1419–1425.
40. Chaput JP, Tremblay A. Sleeping habits predict the magnitude of fat loss in adults exposed to moderate caloric restriction. *Obes Facts*. 2012;5(4):561–566.
41. Haines J, McDonald J, O'Brien A, et al. Healthy habits, happy homes: Randomized trial to improve household routines for obesity prevention among preschool-aged children. *JAMA Pediatr*. 2013;167(11):1072–1079.
42. Tasali E, Wroblewski K, Kahn E, Kilkus J, Schoeller DA. Effect of sleep extension on objectively assessed energy intake among adults with overweight in real-life settings: A randomized clinical trial. *JAMA Intern Med*. 2022;182(4):365–374.
43. Haack M, Serrador J, Cohen D, Simpson N, Meier-Ewert H, Mullington J. Increasing sleep duration to lower beat-to-beat blood pressure: A pilot study. *J Sleep Res*. 2013;22:295–304.
44. Nedeltcheva AV, Kilkus JM, Imperial J, Schoeller DA, Penev PD. Insufficient sleep undermines dietary efforts to reduce adiposity. *Ann Intern Med*. 2010;153(7):435–441.
45. Antza C, Kostopoulos G, Mostafa S, Nirantharakumar K, Tahrani A. The links between sleep duration, obesity and type 2 diabetes mellitus. *J Endocrinol*. 2022;252(2):125–141.
46. Gangwisch JE, Heymsfield SB, Boden-Albala B, et al. Sleep duration as a risk factor for diabetes incidence in a large U.S. sample. *Sleep*. 2007;30(12):1667–1673.
47. Engeda J, Mezuk B, Ratliff S, Ning Y. Association between duration and quality of sleep and the risk of pre-diabetes: Evidence from NHANES. *Diabet Med*. 2013;30(6):676–680.
48. Ford ES, Wheaton AG, Chapman DP, Li C, Perry GS, Croft JB. Associations between self-reported sleep duration and sleeping disorder with concentrations of fasting and 2-h glucose, insulin, and glycosylated hemoglobin among adults without diagnosed diabetes. *J Diabetes*. 2014;6(4):338–350.
49. LeBlanc ES, Smith NX, Nichols GA, Allison MJ, Clarke GN. Insomnia is associated with an increased risk of type 2 diabetes in the clinical setting. *BMJ Open Diabetes Res Care*. 2018;6(1):e000604.
50. Spiegel K, Leproult R, L'Hermite-Balériaux M, Copinschi G, Penev PD, Van Cauter E. Leptin levels are dependent on sleep duration: Relationships

with sympathovagal balance, carbohydrate regulation, cortisol, and thyrotropin. *J Clin Endocrinol Metab*. 2004;89(11):5762–5771.
51. Buxton OM, Pavlova M, Reid EW, Wang W, Simonson DC, Adler GK. Sleep restriction for 1 week reduces insulin sensitivity in healthy men. *Diabetes*. 2010;59(9):2126–2133.
52. Champaneri S, Xu X, Carnethon MR, et al. Diurnal salivary cortisol is associated with body mass index and waist circumference: The Multiethnic Study of Atherosclerosis. *Obesity (Silver Spring)*. 2013;21(1):E56–E63.
53. Rao MN, Neylan TC, Grunfeld C, Mulligan K, Schambelan M, Schwarz J-M. Subchronic sleep restriction causes tissue-specific insulin resistance. *J Clin Endocrinol Metab*. 2015;100(4):1664–1671.
54. Briançon-Marjollet A, Weiszenstein M, Henri M, Thomas A, Godin-Ribuot D, Polak J. The impact of sleep disorders on glucose metabolism: Endocrine and molecular mechanisms. *Diabetol Metab Syndr*. 2015;7(1):25.
55. Leproult R, Deliens G, Gilson M, Peigneux P. Beneficial impact of sleep extension on fasting insulin sensitivity in adults with habitual sleep restriction. *Sleep*. 2015;38:707–715.
56. Jackowska M, Steptoe A. Sleep and future cardiovascular risk: Prospective analysis from the English Longitudinal Study of Ageing. *Sleep Med*. 2015;16(6):768–774.
57. Gangwisch JE, Heymsfield SB, Boden-Albala B, et al. Short sleep duration as a risk factor for hypertension. *Hypertension*. 2006;47(5):833–839.
58. Javaheri S, Omobomi O, Redline S. Insufficient sleep and cardiovascular disease risk. In: Grandner MA, ed. *Sleep and Health*. Academic Press; 2019:203–212.
59. Ayas NT, White DP, Manson JE, et al. A prospective study of sleep duration and coronary heart disease in women. *Arch Intern Med*. 2003;163(2):205–209.
60. Meisinger C, Heier M, Löwel H, Schneider A, Döring A. Sleep duration and sleep complaints and risk of myocardial infarction in middle-aged men and women from the general population: The Monica/Kora Augsburg cohort study. *Sleep*. 2007;30(9):1121–1127.
61. Mallon L, Broman JE, Hetta J. Sleep complaints predict coronary artery disease mortality in males: A 12-year follow-up study of a middle-aged Swedish population. *J Intern Med*. 2002;251(3):207–216.
62. Chandola T, Ferrie JE, Perski A, Akbaraly T, Marmot MG. The effect of short sleep duration on coronary heart disease risk is greatest among those with sleep disturbance: A prospective study from the Whitehall II Cohort. *Sleep*. 2010;33(6):739–744.
63. Lee S, Mu CX, Wallace ML, et al. Sleep health composites are associated with the risk of heart disease across sex and race. *Sci Rep*. 2022;12(1):2023.
64. Grandner MA, Hale L, Moore M, Patel NP. Mortality associated with short sleep duration: The evidence, the possible mechanisms, and the future. *Sleep Med Rev*. 2010;14(3):191–203.
65. Von Ruesten A, Weikert C, Fietze I, Boeing H. Association of sleep duration with chronic diseases in the European Prospective Investigation into Cancer and Nutrition (Epic)-Potsdam Study. *PLoS One*. 2012;7(1):e30972.
66. Chen JC, Brunner RL, Ren H, et al. Sleep duration and risk of ischemic stroke in postmenopausal women. *Stroke*. 2008;39(12):3185–3192.
67. Buxton OM, Marcelli E. Short and long sleep are positively associated with obesity, diabetes, hypertension, and cardiovascular disease among adults in the United States. *Soc Sci Med*. 2010;71(5):1027–1036.
68. He Q, Sun H, Wu X, et al. Sleep duration and risk of stroke: A dose–response meta-analysis of prospective cohort studies. *Sleep Med*. 2017;32:66–74.
69. Ogawa Y, Kanbayashi T, Saito Y, et al. Total sleep deprivation elevates blood pressure through arterial baroreflex resetting: A study with microneurographic technique. *Sleep*. 2003;26(8):986–989.
70. Spiegel K, Leproult R, Van Cauter E. Impact of sleep debt on metabolic and endocrine function. *Lancet*. 1999;354(9188):1435–1439.
71. Mullington JM, Haack M, Toth M, Serrador JM, Meier-Ewert HK. Cardiovascular, inflammatory, and metabolic consequences of sleep deprivation. *Prog Cardiovasc Dis*. 2009;51(4):294–302.
72. Steven S, Frenis K, Oelze M, et al. Vascular inflammation and oxidative stress: Major triggers for cardiovascular disease. *Oxid Med Cell Longev*. 2019;2019:7092151.
73. Shearer WT, Reuben JM, Mullington JM, et al. Soluble TNF-α receptor 1 and IL-6 plasma levels in humans subjected to the sleep deprivation model of spaceflight. *J Allergy Clin Immunol*. 2001;107(1):165–170.
74. Vgontzas AN, Zoumakis E, Bixler EO, et al. Adverse effects of modest sleep restriction on sleepiness, performance, and inflammatory cytokines. *J Clin Endocrinol Metab*. 2004;89(5):2119–2126.
75. Chae CU, Lee RT, Rifai N, Ridker PM. Blood pressure and inflammation in apparently healthy men. *Hypertension*. 2001;38(3):399–403.
76. Ormazabal V, Nair S, Elfeky O, Aguayo C, Salomon C, Zuñiga FA. Association between insulin resistance and the development of cardiovascular disease. *Cardiovasc Diabetol*. 2018;17(1):122.
77. Irwin MR. Why sleep is important for health: A psychoneuroimmunology perspective. *Annu Rev Psychol*. 2015;66(1):143–172.
78. Cohen S, Doyle WJ, Alper CM, Janicki-Deverts D, Turner RB. Sleep habits and susceptibility to the common cold. *Arch Intern Med*. 2009;169(1):62–67.
79. Prather AA, Janicki-Deverts D, Hall MH, Cohen S. Behaviorally assessed sleep and susceptibility to the common cold. *Sleep*. 2015;38(9):1353–1359.
80. Prather AA, Hall M, Fury JM, et al. Sleep and antibody response to hepatitis B vaccination. *Sleep*. 2012;35(8):1063–1069.
81. Benedict C, Brytting M, Markström A, Broman J-E, Schiöth HB. Acute sleep deprivation has no lasting effects on the human antibody titer response following a novel influenza a H1N1 virus vaccination. *BMC Immunol*. 2012;13(1):1–5.
82. Lange T, Perras B, Fehm HL, Born J. Sleep enhances the human antibody response to hepatitis A vaccination. *Psychosom Med*. 2003;65(5):831–835.
83. Lange T, Dimitrov S, Bollinger T, Diekelmann S, Born J. Sleep after vaccination boosts immunological memory. *J Immunol*. 2011;187(1):283–290.
84. Izadi N, Aminian O, Eftekhari S, Piruznia R. Do occupational factors affect the immune response to

Hepatitis B vaccination in healthcare workers? *Arch Clin Infect Dis*. 2020;15(1):e96758.
85. Lammers-van der Holst HM, Lammers GJ, van der Horst GTJ, et al. Understanding the association between sleep, shift work and COVID-19 vaccine immune response efficacy: Protocol of the S-CORE study. *J Sleep Res*. 2022;31(2):e13496.
86. Zhu J, Zhang M, Sanford LD, Tang X. Advice for COVID-19 vaccination: Get some sleep. *Sleep Breath*. 2021;25(4):2287–2288.
87. Haspel JA, Anafi R, Brown MK, et al. Perfect timing: Circadian rhythms, sleep, and immunity: An NIH workshop summary. *JCI Insight*. 2020;5(1):e131487.
88. Irwin M, Mascovich A, Gillin JC, Willoughby R, Pike J, Smith TL. Partial sleep deprivation reduced natural killer cell activity in humans. *Psychosom Med*. 1994:56(6):493–498.
89. Majde JA, Krueger JM. Links between the innate immune system and sleep. *J Allergy Clin Immunol*. 2005;116(6):1188–1198.
90. Besedovsky L, Lange T, Haack M. The sleep-immune crosstalk in health and disease. *Physiol Rev*. 2019;99(3):1325–1380.
91. Lowe CJ, Safati A, Hall PA. The neurocognitive consequences of sleep restriction: A meta-analytic review. *Neurosci Biobehav Rev*. 2017;80:586–604.
92. de Bruin EJ, Van Run C, Staaks J, Meijer AM. Effects of sleep manipulation on cognitive functioning of adolescents: A systematic review. *Sleep Med Rev*. 2017;32:45–57.
93. Dawson D, Sprajcer M, Thomas M. How much sleep do you need? A comprehensive review of fatigue related impairment and the capacity to work or drive safely. *Accid Anal Prev*. 2021;151:105955.
94. Dinges DF, Powell JW. Microcomputer analyses of performance on a portable, simple visual RT task during sustained operations. *Behav Res Methods Instrum Comput*. 1985;17(6):652–655.
95. Cajochen C, Khalsa SBS, Wyatt JK, Czeisler CA, Dijk DJ. EEG and ocular correlates of circadian melatonin phase and human performance decrements during sleep loss. *Am J Physiol Regul Integr Comp Physiol*. 1999;277(3):R640–R649.
96. Jackson ML, Croft RJ, Kennedy GA, Owens K, Howard ME. Cognitive components of simulated driving performance: Sleep loss effects and predictors. *Accid Anal Prev*. 2013;50:438–444.
97. Belenky G, Wesensten NJ, Thorne DR, et al. Patterns of performance degradation and restoration during sleep restriction and subsequent recovery: A sleep dose-response study. *J Sleep Res*. 2003;12(1):1–12.
98. Van Dongen HP, Maislin G, Mullington JM, Dinges DF. The cumulative cost of additional wakefulness: Dose-response effects on neurobehavioral functions and sleep physiology from chronic sleep restriction and total sleep deprivation. *Sleep*. 2003;26(2):117–126.
99. Lim J, Dinges DF. Sleep deprivation and vigilant attention. *Ann N Y Acad Sci*. 2008;1129:305–322.
100. Hudson AN, Van Dongen HPA, Honn KA. Sleep deprivation, vigilant attention, and brain function: A review. *Neuropsychopharmacology*. 2020;45(1):21–30.
101. Carlson SM, Zelazo PD, Faja S. Executive function. In Zelazo, PD, ed. *The Oxford Handbook of Developmental Psychology*. Vol. 1: *Body and Mind*. Oxford University Press; 2013:706–743.
102. Bari A, Robbins TW. Inhibition and impulsivity: Behavioral and neural basis of response control. *Prog Neurobiol*. 2013;108:44–79.
103. Harrison Y, Horne JA. The impact of sleep deprivation on decision making: A review. *J Exp Psychol Appl*. 2000;6(3):236–249.
104. Wu JC, Gillin JC, Buchsbaum MS, et al. Frontal lobe metabolic decreases with sleep deprivation not totally reversed by recovery sleep. *Neuropsychopharmacology*. 2006;31(12):2783–2792.
105. Schwarz JF, Geisler P, Hajak G, et al. The effect of partial sleep deprivation on computer-based measures of fitness to drive. *Sleep Breath*. 2016;20(1):285–292.
106. Philip P, Åkerstedt T. Transport and industrial safety, how are they affected by sleepiness and sleep restriction? *Sleep Med Rev*. 2006;10(5):347–356.
107. Chen GX, Fang Y, Guo F, Hanowski RJ. The influence of daily sleep patterns of commercial truck drivers on driving performance. *Accid Anal Prev*. 2016;91:55–63.
108. Williamson AM, Feyer AM. Moderate sleep deprivation produces impairments in cognitive and motor performance equivalent to legally prescribed levels of alcohol intoxication. *Occup Environ Med*. 2000;57(10):649–655.
109. Lowrie J, Brownlow H. The impact of sleep deprivation and alcohol on driving: A comparative study. *BMC Public Health*. 2020;20(1):980.
110. Russo MB, Kendall AP, Johnson DE, et al. Visual perception, psychomotor performance, and complex motor performance during an overnight air refueling simulated flight. *Aviat Space Environ Med*. 2005;76(7):C92–C103.
111. Mulenga A, Sasangohar F. The impacts of sleep deprivation on medical residents: A scoping review of literature. *Proc Human Factors Ergon Soc Annu Meet*. 2020;64(1):1898–1902.
112. Patel N. Learning lessons. *J Am Coll Cardiol*. 2014;64(25):2802–2804.
113. Trockel MT, Menon NK, Rowe SG, et al. Assessment of physician sleep and wellness, burnout, and clinically significant medical errors. *JAMA Netw Open*. 2020;3(12):e2028111
114. Kalmbach DA, Arnedt JT, Song PX, Guille C, Sen S. Sleep disturbance and short sleep as risk factors for depression and perceived medical errors in first-year residents. *Sleep*. 2017;40(3).
115. McCormick F, Kadzielski J, Landrigan CP, Evans B, Herndon JH, Rubash HE. Surgeon fatigue: A prospective analysis of the incidence, risk, and intervals of predicted fatigue-related impairment in residents. *Arch Surg*. 2012;147(5):430–435.
116. Whelehan DF, McCarrick CA, Ridgway PF. A systematic review of sleep deprivation and technical skill in surgery. *Surgeon*. 2020;18(6):375–384.
117. Smith-Coggins R, Rosekind MR, Buccino KR, Dinges DF, Moser RP. Rotating shiftwork schedules: Can we enhance physician adaptation to night shifts? *Acad Emerg Med*. 1997;4(10):951–961.
118. Aran A, Wasserteil N, Gross I, Mendlovic J, Pollak Y. Medical decisions of pediatric residents turn

riskier after a 24-hour call with no sleep. *Med Decis Making*. 2017;37(1):127–133.
119. Puddester D. Managing and mitigating fatigue in the era of changing resident duty hours. *BMC Med Educ*. 2014;14(Suppl 1):S3–S3.
120. Arnedt JT, Owens J, Crouch M, Stahl J, Carskadon MA. Neurobehavioral performance of residents after heavy night call vs after alcohol ingestion. *JAMA*. 2005;294(9):1025–1033.
121. Stimpfel AW, Fatehi F, Kovner C. Nurses' sleep, work hours, and patient care quality, and safety. *Sleep Health*. 2020;6(3):314–320.
122. Dorrian J, Lamond N, van den Heuvel C, Pincombe J, Rogers AE, Dawson D. A pilot study of the safety implications of Australian nurses' sleep and work hours. *Chronobiol Int*. 2006;23(6):1149–1163.
123. Kroshus E, Wagner J, Wyrick D, et al. Wake up call for collegiate athlete sleep: Narrative review and consensus recommendations from the NCAA Interassociation Task Force on Sleep And Wellness. *Br J Sports Med*. 2019;53(12):731–736.
124. Shochat T, Cohen-Zion M, Tzischinsky O. Functional consequences of inadequate sleep in adolescents: A systematic review. *Sleep Med Rev*. 2014;18(1):75–87.
125. Raley H, Naber J, Cross S, Perlow M. The impact of duration of sleep on academic performance in university students. *Madridge J Nursing*. 2016;1:11–18.
126. Okano K, Kaczmarzyk JR, Dave N, Gabrieli JDE, Grossman JC. Sleep quality, duration, and consistency are associated with better academic performance in college students. *NPJ Sci Learn*. 2019;4(1):16.
127. Wolfson AR, Carskadon MA. Sleep schedules and daytime functioning in adolescents. *Child Dev*. 1998;69(4):875–887.
128. Phillips AJK, Clerx WM, O'Brien CS, et al. Irregular sleep/wake patterns are associated with poorer academic performance and delayed circadian and sleep/wake timing. *Sci Rep*. 2017;7(1):3216.
129. Grandner MA, Jackson N, Gooneratne NS, Patel NP. The development of a questionnaire to assess sleep-related practices, beliefs, and attitudes. *Behav Sleep Med*. 2014;12(2):123–142.
130. Basner M, Dinges DF. Dubious bargain: Trading sleep for Leno and Letterman. *Sleep*. 2009;32(6):747–752.
131. Exelmans L, Van den Bulck J. Bedtime, shuteye time and electronic media: Sleep displacement is a two-step process. *J Sleep Res*. 2017;26(3):364–370.
132. Jindal RD. Is binge-watching competing with sleep? And winning? Comment. *J Clin Sleep Med*. 2020;16:31S–32S.
133. Raphael R. Netflix CEO Reed Hastings: Sleep is our competition. https://www.fastcompany.com/40491939/netflix-ceo-reed-hastings-sleep-is-our-competition. Published 2021. Accessed 1/18/2022.
134. Chang A-M, Aeschbach D, Duffy JF, Czeisler CA. Evening use of light-emitting E-readers negatively affects sleep, circadian timing, and next-morning alertness. *PNAS*. 2015;112(4):1232–1237.
135. Haack M, Simpson N, Sethna N, Kaur S, Mullington J. Sleep deficiency and chronic pain: Potential underlying mechanisms and clinical implications. *Neuropsychopharmacology*. 2020;45(1):205–216.
136. Costa G. Sleep deprivation due to shift work. In: Lotti M, Bleecker ML, eds. *Handbook of Clinical Neurology*. Vol. 131. Elsevier; 2015:437–446.
137. Grandner MA. Obstacles to overcome when improving sleep health at a societal level. In: Grandner MA, ed. *Sleep and Health*. Elsevier; 2019:107–115.
138. Basner M, Spaeth AM, Dinges DF. Sociodemographic characteristics and waking activities and their role in the timing and duration of sleep. *Sleep*. 2014;37(12):1889–1906.
139. Stepanski EJ, Wyatt JK. Use of sleep hygiene in the treatment of insomnia. *Sleep Med Rev*. 2003;7(3):215–225.
140. Bartimote-Aufflick K, Bridgeman A, Walker R, Sharma M, Smith L. The study, evaluation, and improvement of university student self-efficacy. *Stud High Educ*. 2016;41(11):1918–1942.
141. Bandura A. Health promotion by social cognitive means. *Health Educ Behav*. 2004;31(2):143–164.
142. Grandner MA, Olivier K, Gallagher R, et al. Quantifying impact of real-world barriers to sleep: The Brief Index of Sleep Control (BRISC). *Sleep Health*. 2020;6(5):587–593.
143. DiClemente CC, Prochaska JO. Toward a comprehensive, transtheoretical model of change: Stages of change and addictive behaviors. In: Miller WR, Heather N, eds. *Treating Addictive Behaviors*. 2nd ed. Plenum Press; 1998:3–24.
144. Grandner MA. Sleep, health, and society. *Sleep Med Clin*. 2017;12(1):1–22.
145. Rupp TL, Wesensten NJ, Bliese PD, Balkin TJ. Banking sleep: Realization of benefits during subsequent sleep restriction and recovery. *Sleep*. 2009;32(3):311–321.
146. Caddick ZA, Gregory K, Arsintescu L, Flynn-Evans EE. A review of the environmental parameters necessary for an optimal sleep environment. *Build Environ*. 2018;132:11–20.
147. Wunsch K, Kasten N, Fuchs R. The effect of physical activity on sleep quality, well-being, and affect in academic stress periods. *Nat Sci Sleep*. 2017;9:117–126.
148. Grandner MA. Social-ecological model of sleep health. In: Grandner MA, ed. *Sleep and Health*. Academic Press; 2019:45–53.

Chapter 12

The Insomnia Patient

Epidemiology, Symptoms and Signs, and Impact of the Disorder

Gwendolyn C. Carlson and Jennifer L. Martin

PREVALENCE OF INSOMNIA

Insomnia is highly prevalent within the U.S. population, with more than half of U.S. adults reporting difficulty sleeping and 23.2% of U.S adults reporting insomnia symptoms.[1] Not only are insomnia symptoms highly prevalent, insomnia symptoms appear to be increasing. National Health Interview Survey data from 2002 to 2012 revealed that "trouble sleeping" increased from 17.5% (37.5 million adults) to 19.2% (46 million adults).[2] Medical visits related to insomnia in the United States increased by 13% (5.5 million visits) from 1999 to 2019.[3] Similar trends have been observed in Canada, where medical visits related to insomnia have increased by nearly 10% from 2002 to 2015.[4] Globally, the prevalence of insomnia is estimated to be between 10% and 30%, with higher prevalence among various subpopulations and with variability across the lifespan.[5–7]

Prevalence of Insomnia Across Gender and Age Groups

In young children, insomnia has a similar prevalence in boys and girls; however, insomnia is more prevalent in adolescent girls and adult women than in adolescent boys and men. In a cross-sectional study of 700 participants, researchers examined the prevalence of insomnia in children.[8] Results revealed that, among children age 5–7 years, the prevalence of insomnia was 21.9% among boys and 20.8% among girls. For children age 8–10 years, the prevalence was 17.3% among boys and 16.3% among girls, and for children age 11–12 years, the prevalence was 16.7% among boys and 30.6% for girls.[8] A significant interaction between gender and age was observed, with girls endorsing the highest rate of insomnia in late childhood. The overall prevalence of insomnia in children was 19.3%.[8] Insomnia disorder is the most prevalent disorder reported during adolescence.[9,10] Gender differences in rates of insomnia continue into adolescence. Among 16- to 18-year-olds, the prevalence of insomnia is 12.5% among adolescent boys and 23.6% among adolescent girls.[11] This trend continues into adulthood, with 23% of women and 17% of men in the United States experiencing insomnia.[12] Within the working population, insomnia is also more prevalent in women (27.1%) than men (19.7%).[1] Globally, women are 1.4 times more likely to have insomnia than men.[13] Women are also less likely to achieve insomnia remission (46%) than men (52%).[14,15] The higher prevalence of insomnia among women may be better explained by lower remission rates rather than a surge of new cases.

Regarding sexual and gender minority populations, there are mixed findings regarding differential rates of insomnia among heterosexual and sexual-minority men.[16–18] There are some data indicating that insomnia is more prevalent in bisexual women compared to women who identify as heterosexual.[19,20] There is limited research regarding the prevalence of insomnia within the transgender population. One qualitative study, involving 40 in-depth interviews with individuals who identified as transgender or gender nonbinary, found that 35% of participants reported that their gender identity negatively impacted their sleep.[21] Another study found that transgender individuals reported high rates of sleep disturbance, with 79.2% of transgender women and 81.2% of transgender men reporting a Pittsburgh Sleep Quality Index (PSQI) score ≥5,[22] which is indicative of clinically significant sleep disturbance.[23,24] Additional research regarding the prevalence of insomnia in sexual and gender minorities is needed. Stress associated with minority group membership status and experiences of discrimination likely contribute to higher rates of insomnia disorder in gender and sexual-minority groups.

Women also experience insomnia at increasing rates over the course of pregnancy.[25] A meta-analysis of 24 studies, including 15564 participants, revealed that 38.2% of women experience insomnia during pregnancy, with 25.3% experiencing insomnia in the first trimester, 27.2% in the second trimester, and 39.7% in the third trimester.[26] Another study found 60.8 % of women experienced insomnia at 32 weeks of pregnancy, and among these women, 50% still experienced insomnia 2 years postpartum.[27] It is important to assess women's opportunity for sleep following childbirth. Breastfeeding schedules and challenges may also contribute to disturbed sleep among new mothers. Pregnancy, childbirth, and infant/child care appear to have a significant and lasting impact on insomnia symptoms in women.

It is generally accepted that rates of insomnia increase with age across men and women,[28] a trend that can be attributed to the sleep cycle changes, hormonal changes, and increased comorbidities that occur with age.[29,30] It is estimated that up to half of older adults may struggle with insomnia symptoms.[31] In women, menopause has been identified as a precipitant of insomnia symptoms as well. A 10-year study (i.e., Study of Women Across the National [SWAN]), found 46%–48% of menopausal women experience insomnia, compared to 38% of premenopausal women.[32,33] Gender differences between men and women continue into older adulthood. In sample of older adults (65 years or older; men = 2873; women = 3213), women were significantly more likely than their male counterparts to endorse insomnia symptoms.[34] While cross-sectional studies have been fairly consistent in the past, there are some newer studies showing that younger men and middle-aged women may have the highest rates of poor sleep,[35,36] leading to questions about whether prior cross-sectional research may reflect both age-related changes and age cohort differences.

Prevalence of Insomnia Across Racial/Ethnic Groups and Socioeconomic Statuses

Disparities in insomnia have also been found across racial and ethnic groups. Overall, racial and ethnic minorities report greater sleep disturbance than individuals who identify as non-Hispanic white, with ethnic/racial minority group members reporting shorter sleep duration (≤6 hours) and poorer sleep quality than individuals who identify as non-Hispanic white.[37,38] Specifically, being Black/African American has been found to predict shorter duration sleep and disturbed sleep quality.[39,40] Black/African American patients have a 67% increased risk for insomnia disorder and are twice as likely to experience chronic insomnia symptoms (>1 year) compared to non-Hispanic white patients.[41] Another study found that Asian Americans report shorter sleep duration than non-Hispanic white individuals.[42] Insufficient sleep has also been observed in Native Americans, with members of this group reporting the highest level of severe insomnia symptoms compared to other racial/ethnic groups.[43] Conversely, a large study of 159 856 participants across the United States found that non-Hispanic white participants reported more sleep complaints than Hispanic, Black/African American, or Asian participants.[44]

There has been very limited research examining insomnia symptoms in the Hispanic/Latinx population in the United States,[45] and disparities may vary by heritage group.[46] Additional research is needed in this area. Additionally, research suggests that demographic variables may have an interactive effect on insomnia symptoms. In a recent study of older Korean-American immigrants, being employed for wages was associated with better sleep quality, after accounting for demographic and health-related factors.[44] It is important to consider the role of acculturation-related distress and discrimination when examining insomnia symptoms among racial and ethnic minorities. Socioeconomic status has also been shown to contribute to sleep disturbance.[47] In a cultural study of mothers of 10 085 young children across Western and Asian countries, 54.7% of mothers reported poor sleep quality (PSQI >5), and lower socioeconomic status, lower education level, and greater number of children significantly predicted poorer sleep quality.[48] This suggested that fewer resources and greater socioeconomic stressors contribute to the development of insomnia symptoms. This finding is also consistent with studies examining insomnia in the homeless population. The prevalence of insomnia among the U.S. homeless population (42%) is twice as high as in the general population (19%).[49]

COMMON COMORBIDITIES WITH INSOMNIA

Difficulty with sleep can be a symptom of multiple other sleep disorders, medical conditions, and psychiatric conditions. Due to this symptom overlap, insomnia disorder frequently cooccurs with other conditions. Sometimes insomnia may precede and contribute to the development of another condition. Alternatively, insomnia may develop secondary to another condition.

Sleep-Related Comorbidities

Insomnia symptoms are common in other sleep disorders such as circadian rhythm sleep/wake phase disorders, sleep-related breathing disorder (e.g., obstructive sleep apnea [OSA]), restless legs syndrome (RLS), period limb movement disorder, and nightmare disorder.[50,51] For some patients, treatment of the primary disorder leads to resolution of insomnia symptoms; however, it is more common for insomnia symptoms to persist even after other sleep disorders are managed. Given that insomnia often requires independent treatment, clinicians should evaluate insomnia, even when a comorbid sleep disorder has been diagnosed. For example, approximately 39%–55% of OSA patients also report insomnia symptoms, and nearly a third of older patients diagnosed with insomnia disorder are later found to have OSA (apnea hypopnea index [AHI] ≥15)[52] Insomnia is a known risk factor for non-adherence to OSA treatment with continuous positive airway pressure therapy;[53,54] therefore, failure to diagnose insomnia may prevent clinicians from addressing a significant treatment barrier.

In terms of RLS, approximately 30% of individuals with insomnia disorder also report symptoms consistent with RLS, with the comorbidity between RLS and periodic limb movement being upward of 85%.[55,56] In this case, RLS and/or periodic limb movement disorder (PLMD) may prevent patients from achieving insomnia remission with direct treatment, and a combined approach may be needed. There is also a high level of comorbidity between insomnia disorder and nightmare disorder. Compared to nightmares experienced by the general population (2.4%–5.1%),[57,58] individuals with insomnia disorder are significantly more likely to report frequent nightmares (18.3%), with nightmares predicting more severe insomnia symptoms.[59] In some instances, nightmare disorders may play a causal role in the development of chronic insomnia disorder, as individuals with frequent nightmares may develop a pattern of sleep avoidance or negative associations with the sleep environment.

Medical Comorbidities

In addition to sleep disorders, insomnia disorder is more common among individuals with medical comorbidities, with more than 75% of insomnia patients reporting comorbid medical disorders.[60] While insomnia disorder may develop as a result of medical conditions, there is growing evidence that untreated insomnia may also contribute to the development or worsening of common medical conditions. For example, patients with insomnia are 1.28 times more likely to develop type 2 diabetes, 1.53 times more likely to experience coronary heart disease, and 1.34 times to develop chronic kidney disease.[61–63] Not surprisingly, insomnia symptoms are associated with a higher total incidence of cardiovascular disease.[64] Among patients with chronic obstructive pulmonary disease, 27.3% report experiencing insomnia.[65] Chronic pain is a frequent complaint in patients who experience insomnia disorder,[66] with 20% of individuals living with chronic pain reporting one or more insomnia symptoms.[67] Compared to adults without arthritis (16.4%), adults with arthritis (23.1%) are significantly more likely to experience insomnia, excessive daytime sleepiness, and short sleep duration.[68]

Psychiatric Comorbidities

While insomnia disorder increases the risk of developing multiple medical conditions, psychiatric comorbidities occur at an even higher rate among insomnia patients than the previously mentioned medical comorbidities. It is estimated that up to 80% of patients seeking psychiatric care experience insomnia.[69] Conversely, 40% of all insomnia patients also have a psychiatric condition.[70,71] Common psychiatric comorbidities include: anxiety disorders, depressive disorders, bipolar-related disorders, substance use disorders, and trauma- and stress-related disorders, with anxiety and depression disorders being the most frequently cooccurring psychiatric conditions with insomnia disorder.[51,72] Historically, insomnia was conceptualized as purely a symptom when psychiatric illnesses are also present; however, it appears that a bidirectional relationship is more likely. Individuals with insomnia disorder are 3.23 times more likely to experience anxiety and 2.83 times more likely to experience depression.[73] Sleep disturbance is a symptom for both anxiety and depressive disorders and a core feature of bipolar-related disorders.[51] During a manic episode, 69%–99% of patients experience reduced need for sleep, with rates of insomnia varying considerably in patients with a comorbid bipolar-related disorder.[74]

Individuals with insomnia disorder may also use substances to intervene on their sleep. The positive relationship between caffeine and sleep disturbance is well established, as is the positive relationship between nicotine use and sleep disturbance.[75–77] Additionally, 15%–30% of individuals with sleep disturbance endorse alcohol consumption as a sleep-management strategy. Individuals with insomnia are 1.35 times more likely to abuse alcohol compared to those without insomnia.[73] Among patients with alcohol dependence, it is estimated that up to 91% experience insomnia, with insomnia serving as a significant predictor of alcohol relapse among abusers.[78] Within the United States, cannabis is one of the most commonly used recreational drugs[79]; however, the relationship between cannabis and insomnia is only an emerging area of research. One study found that compared to non-daily users, daily cannabis users report more disturbed sleep based on the PSQI and more severe insomnia symptoms based on the Insomnia Severity Index (ISI).[80] This "self-medication" may lead to problematic substance use in the future. One recent study found that women who report using alcohol for sleep are more likely to drink daily, which is a known risk factor for future problematic alcohol use.[81]

The relationship between disturbed sleep and post-traumatic stress disorder (PTSD) is well documented. It is estimated the 35%–61% of individual with PTSD also meet diagnostic criteria for insomnia disorder.[82–84] Other estimates suggested that as many as 90% of PTSD patients experience sleep disturbance,[85] which may be attributed to the re-experiencing symptoms (e.g., nightmares) and hyperarousal symptoms associated with a PTSD diagnosis. Patients who link their insomnia symptoms to a traumatic event experience more severe insomnia symptoms compared to patients who link their insomnia to a non-traumatic event. Patients who endorse traumatic insomnia-precipitating events endorse more severe mental health symptoms than those who endorse non-traumatic insomnia-precipitating events.[86] While insomnia has often been thought of as an outcome of psychiatric conditions, including depression and PTSD, there is a growing body of literature suggesting that insomnia symptoms may precede psychiatric symptoms and may contribute to the subsequent development and severity of these aforementioned psychiatric conditions.[87–89]

Patients with neurodevelopmental and neurocognitive disorders also experience high rates of insomnia. Among children with neurodevelopmental disorders (e.g., autism spectrum disorder and attention deficit hyperactivity disorder), the prevalence of sleep disorders is 50%–95%, with insomnia disorder being the most common comorbidity.[90,91] However, diagnosis of insomnia disorder in children with neurodevelopmental disorders may be complicated by the side effects of medications prescribed to treat underlying neurodevelopmental disorders. There is a need for additional research examining the benefits of insomnia interventions among children with neurocognitive disorders, though early research examining the efficacy of behavioral sleep interventions within this population is promising.[92]

It is estimated that 20%–35% of patients with dementia experience insomnia.[93] Insomnia symptoms within this population can lead to increased risk of falls, which contribute to greater caregiver burden and earlier nursing home placement.[94,95] Some research suggests that insomnia may be a risk factor for neurocognitive disorders,[96] but the relationship is likely bidirectional. Additionally, prevalence rates for both insomnia disorder and neurocognitive disorder increase with age. Similar to neurodevelopmental disorders, it is important to assess how medications may impact sleep patterns and fall risk. Research supports the efficacy of insomnia treatment (i.e., behavioral sleep interventions) among patients with cognitive impairment.[97]

In recent years, there has been an increased research focus on traumatic brain injuries (TBIs) and associated consequences. Insomnia is a common complaint associated with TBIs. It is estimated that 50% of individuals with TBIs experience sleep disturbance.[98] Approximately 30%–50% of these patients report worsening insomnia symptoms following TBIs.[98] Each year in the United States, there are 2.8 million TBIs, most of which are classified as mild TBIs.[99] Surprisingly, mild TBIs are associated with insomnia more than moderate or severe TBIs.[100–102] Understanding the relationship between insomnia disorder and TBIs remains an emerging area of research.

INSOMNIA DISORDER DIAGNOSIS

There are 2 primary diagnostic systems for the identification of clinically significant insomnia symptoms: (1) the American Psychiatric Association's *Diagnostic and Statistical Manual of Mental Disorders*, 5th edition (DSM-5)[51]; and (2) the *International Classification of Sleep Disorders*, 3rd edition (ICSD-3) of the American Academy of Sleep Medicine.[103] Overall, the diagnostic criteria are consistent across these 2 systems, requiring poor sleep with daytime consequences that persists for 3 months and occurs at least 3 times a week. Per the DSM-5, for patients to meet criteria for insomnia disorder, they must report one of the following: difficulty falling asleep, difficulty maintaining sleep, or early morning awakenings (Criterion A). Patients must report significant distress or daytime impairment (Criterion B) and report experiencing sleep disturbance at least 3 nights per week (Criterion C) for at least 3 months (Criterion D). Additionally, participants must have the opportunity to sleep (Criterion E).[51] For instance, some patients may reside in environment in which they cannot sleep (i.e., do not have a place to sleep or are unable to sleep due to other environmental constraints). Under these circumstances, it would be inappropriate to diagnose an individual with insomnia disorder. Similarly, an insomnia disorder diagnosis should not be given if symptoms are better explained by another sleep disorder (Criterion F), are attributable to substance use/medication use (Criterion G), or are better explained by another mental/medical condition (Criterion H).[51]

The DSM-5 also includes important specifiers for a diagnosis of insomnia disorder, including: with other sleep disorder, with medical comorbidity, and with non-sleep-disorder mental health comorbidity.[51] There are also 4 specifiers for symptoms duration and episodes. *Acute* or *short-term insomnia* refers to insomnia symptoms with a duration of less than 3 months, but all other diagnostic criteria for insomnia disorder are met. In this situation a diagnosis of "other specified insomnia disorder" should be given. The episodic specifier refers to insomnia symptoms with a duration of more than 1 month, but less than 3 months. The persistent specifier refers to insomnia symptoms lasting 3 months of longer. The recurrent specifier refers to 2 or more episodes of insomnia symptoms within the previous year.[51]

Per the ICSD-3, insomnia is categorized into 3 separate diagnoses: chronic insomnia disorder, short-term insomnia disorder, and other insomnia disorder.[103] A diagnosis of chronic insomnia requires that a patient report difficulty with either sleep initiation or sleep maintenance and daytime consequences as the result of the insomnia symptoms despite adequate opportunity to sleep. Similar to the DSM-5, patients most report sleep disturbance at least 3 nights per week for at least 3 months, and symptoms should not be better explained by medication/substance use or another medical or mental condition.[103] Similar to the diagnostic specifiers in the DSM-5, a short-term insomnia disorder diagnosis is given when a patient meets all other criteria for chronic insomnia disorder, but symptoms have a duration of less than 3 months. A diagnosis of other insomnia disorder is given when a patient presents with insomnia symptoms, but does not meet the diagnostic criteria for either chronic insomnia disorder or short-term insomnia disorder.[103]

INSOMNIA DISORDER PRESENTATIONS

Insomnia presentations vary across patients. Some patients experiences difficulty falling asleep (i.e., sleep initiation), some patients experiences difficulty staying asleep (i.e., sleep maintenance), and some patients struggle with both sleep initiation and maintenance. Insomnia can also be characterized by non-restorative sleep. All these sleep-related challenges can contribute to daytime impairment for patients.

Sleep Initiation

A prototypical insomnia patient presents with a complaint related to sleep onset, meaning they get into bed and cannot fall sleep. Sleep onset latency refers to the amount of time it takes a patient to transition from wakefulness to sleep.[104] Sleep onset latency can be assessed with polysomnography (PSG); however, an objective sleep test is not required for a patient to be diagnosed with insomnia disorder, and often the perceived time to fall asleep is extended in insomnia patients. Insomnia disorder is diagnosed based on a patient's self-report of their sleep. Sleep onset insomnia is a frequently reported type of sleep disturbance, in which patients report difficulty falling asleep at night. Normal sleep onset latency ranges from 10 to 20 minutes, with longer latency being indicative of clinically significant sleep disturbance.[105]

Sleep Maintenance

In addition to difficulties falling asleep, patients with insomnia disorder frequently report difficulty maintaining sleep. This involves awakenings that occur following sleep onset, often in the middle of the night and often for extended periods of time.[104] This presentation may include multiple nighttime awakenings of short durations, or a single nighttime awakening of a longer duration. Some waketime following sleep onset is normal; however, total waketime after sleep onset that is longer than 30 minutes is considered excessive.[105] Difficulty maintaining sleep may also present as early morning awakenings, or when a patient consistently awakens earlier than desired and is not able to return to sleep.[104,106]

Factors Impeding Sleep

It is important to assess factors impacting the initiation and maintenance of sleep for patients presenting with insomnia symptoms, as this may inform future treatment. Hyperarousal at bedtime is a commonly reported experience, characterized by physical and cognitive anxiety symptoms.[107] Patients may report worry about current and/or future stressors.[108,109] It is not unusual for patients to experience anxiety about not being about to sleep and concerns about how lack of sleep will impact them. Additionally, some patients may report rumination of previous events.[108] In the context of comorbid nightmare disorder and/or PTSD, patients may report anticipatory anxiety regarding sleep onset due to the experience of nightmares.[110] Arousal symptoms can inform providers' understanding of patients' insomnia presentations and inform intervention strategies.

It should be noted that symptoms associated with comorbid sleep disorders and medical conditions may contribute to difficulties with initiating and maintaining sleep. Common examples include RLS symptoms hindering sleep onset and breathing difficulties associated with sleep apnea contributing to difficulty maintaining sleep,[52,55] although most commonly other sleep disturbances emerge over time. Medical conditions may also interact with the sleep environment to interfere with sleep. Chronic pain conditions and physical discomfort in the night are associated with sleep disturbance.[66] While it is important to determine whether sleep disturbance is fully attributable to other conditions, more often than not, insomnia symptoms and comorbidities are simultaneously contributing the presentation of the patient. As such, insomnia interventions often incorporate other behavioral medicine interventions to address medical comorbidities.

Non-Restorative Sleep and Daytime Impairment

In addition to difficulties initiating and maintaining sleep, patients with insomnia disorder may also report non-restorative sleep.[111] Non-restorative sleep refers to the experience of being "insufficiently rested or refreshed," which contributes to impairment. Non-restorative sleep can be reported despite the appearance of normal sleep parameters. It is estimated that 11%–25% of insomnia patients experience non-restorative sleep.[112,113] Experiences associated with non-restorative sleep include feeling unrested upon awakening and difficulty getting up in the morning. It remains unclear whether non-restorative sleep in the context of adequate sleep time represents a distinct form of insomnia disorder.

Sleep disturbance resulting from insomnia disorder results in clinically significant daytime impairment. Impairment may present across a single domain or across multiple domains, including: cognitive functioning, affect/mood, physical functioning, interpersonal functioning, and performance at work/school. Patients with insomnia report more frequent and more severe problems with attention and memory than patients without a diagnosis of insomnia disorder.[114] A meta-analysis found that, compared to individuals without insomnia, patients with insomnia demonstrated impairments in episodic memory, working memory, and aspects of executive functioning. As such, sleep disturbance is an important consideration when assessing neurodevelopmental and neurocognitive disorders.[115]

As previously noted in the psychiatric comorbidities section, insomnia and depression frequently co-occur. Insomnia symptoms are predictive of negative mood and increased emotion dysregulation.[116] Emotion dysregulation is an emotional experience and/or expression that interferes with goal-directed activity.[117] Evidence demonstrates that mood improves following insomnia interventions. Sleep disturbance and the severity of insomnia symptoms are associated with the overactivation of the hypothalamic-pituitary-adrenal (HPA) axis, which increases production of the stressor hormone cortisol.[118,119] Due to insomnia's relationship with HPA axis overactivation, it is not surprising that insomnia with short sleep duration (≤5 hours) is associated with higher risk of hypertension, diabetes, and mortality.[120–122]

Given the broad impact of insomnia on an individual patient's functioning, impairment may also impact a patient's relationships with others. Research has shown that poor sleep is predictive of greater relationship conflict in couples.[123] This is particularly important in sleep interventions, as providers consider the role of bed partners in the development and maintenance of insomnia symptoms. Outside of the home settings, insomnia can impair performance at work and school. In a study of children between 5 and 10 years of age, insomnia was associated with decreased performance in school. Similar findings were observed in adolescents between 11 and 17 years of age.[124] In adult subjects, research has shown that employees who report sleep problems are more likely to have decreased job performance than good sleepers.[125]

THE BROADER IMPACT OF INSOMNIA

Given the high prevalence of insomnia disorder and the consequences that individuals with insomnia disorder experience, there is a significant societal burden associated with insomnia. It is estimated that untreated insomnia costs the United States $100 billion each year. Costs can largely be attributed to hospitalizations and medical visits.[126] Data from the CMS Chronic Conditions Data Warehouse revealed that patients with insomnia had significantly higher rates of healthcare resource utilization than patients without insomnia. Additionally, compared to those without insomnia, patients with insomnia had $63 607 higher all-cause costs.[126] These findings were consistent with previous studies which have found that, compared to the general population, insomnia patients have 60% greater healthcare cost.[127] Individuals with insomnia also demonstrate a greater number of outpatient and emergency department visits and greater utilization of pharmacotherapy,[128] creating a significant burden on the healthcare system.

In terms of lost productivity, insomnia contributes to greater workplace absenteeism. In the United States, the annualized individual-level association of insomnia is approximately 11 days of missed days of work, resulting in a capital loss of $2280 at the individual level. At the population level, insomnia results in $63.2 billion of lost workplace productivity.[1] Insomnia also contributes to work-related accidents. The estimated average cost of insomnia-related accidents and errors at work is $32 062, which is higher than workplace accidents and errors that are not associated with insomnia ($21 914). There are approximately 274 000 workplace accidents and errors related to insomnia each year, resulting in an annual cost of $31.1 billion.[129]

Not only is insomnia linked to workplace accidents, it is also associated with increased risk of road traffic accidents.[130] Insomnia has been found to be a significant independent predictor of both motor vehicle accidents (OR: 1.82) and near-miss accidents (OR: 3.35).[130] One study found short sleep duration (<6 hours) the night preceding the accident to be the greatest predictor of fatal sleep-related motor vehicle accidents.[131] Individuals who experience insomnia are also significantly more likely than individuals without insomnia to experience road traffic injuries,[132] suggesting that insomnia is not only predictive of accidents, but also the severity accidents that occur.

Insomnia is also associated with self-inflicted injury and suicidal ideation.[133] Psychiatric comorbidities are common among patients with insomnia disorder, which is consistent with the negative impact of insomnia on cognition and mood. Short duration of sleep is associated with both suicidal ideation and suicide attempts.[134,135] Controlling for demographic variables and other comorbidities, insomnia is still found to be an independent predictor of suicide attempts, while sleep medicine visits are associated with reduced risk for suicide attempts.[136] A number of mechanisms have been proposed to mediate the relationships between insomnia and suicidal ideation, including depression symptoms, emotion dysregulation, and feelings of hopelessness.[133,137,138]

The relationship between insomnia and suicidal ideation is indicative of the overall reduction in quality of life experienced by patients with chronic insomnia.[139] Health-related quality of life can be understood as a quality of health, functioning, comfort, and happiness. Domains of quality of life include physical functioning, physical role limitation, bodily pain, vitality, mental health, emotional role limitation, social functioning, and health perception, all of which can be impacted by insomnia symptoms.[140] Quality-adjusted life-years (QALYs) is a measure of disease burden, which includes quality and quantity of life. In a recent epidemiological study of the United States, QALY population loss associated with insomnia was estimated to be 5.6 million, which was more than QALY losses for arthritis, hypertension depression, and anxiety.[141] In summary, the impact of insomnia symptoms is far reaching.

While insomnia is associated with multiple negative outcomes, the reverse is true for individuals who report good sleep. Healthy sleep is associated with enhanced cognitive functioning and improved mood and emotion regulation.[116,142] Following recommended sleep guidelines is associated with a 19% reduction in risk for premature all-cause mortality.[143] Fortunately, there are also effective treatments for insomnia disorder, including cognitive behavioral therapy for insomnia (CBT-I), which is also the first-line treatment for insomnia disorder.[144] CBT-I has been shown to improve sleep/wake patterns in individuals with a variety of medical and mental health comorbidities and has been studied across multiple subpopulations.[145]

SUMMARY AND CONCLUSION

Insomnia is a highly prevalent disorder in the United States and globally.[1,7] Women experience higher rates of insomnia than men, and these differences are observed from adolescence throughout the life span.[1,8] Insomnia disorder commonly occurs in the context of other sleep disorders, medical conditions, and psychiatric conditions.[144] Insomnia disorder may go undiagnosed in the presence of these comorbidities, which may result in delayed treatment for insomnia disorder when it occurs. Lower economic status and reduced resources are associated with increased rates of insomnia disorder,[47] which may be the result of increased stressors and exposure to multiple insomnia-precipitating events. The prevalence of insomnia disorder is understudied in certain subpopulations, including underserved groups who may be at an increased risk of experiencing insomnia (e.g., Hispanic/Latinx communities, immigrant populations, and transgender men and women).[22,45]

The main diagnostic systems for the assessment and diagnosis of insomnia disorder include the DSM-5 and ICSD-3, with significant overlap across these diagnostic systems.[51,103] The main features of insomnia include difficulty initiating sleep, difficulty maintaining sleep, and non-restorative sleep. Providers must assess duration of insomnia symptoms, frequency of insomnia symptoms, and the presence of comorbidities and substance and medication use to ensure that insomnia disorder is an appropriate diagnosis. It is equally important to understand the impairment that patients report as a result of their insomnia symptoms. This will vary across patients. Assessment should include physical, cognitive, psychological, and social consequences of sleep disturbance.[144] Impairment may more evident in certain settings (e.g., work or school). In some cases, patients may require education about healthy sleep to provide accurate information about their sleep experience and daytime functioning.

Insomnia is a risk factor for work-related accidents and motor vehicle accidents.[129,130] Providers should ask patients about their daytime sleepiness and assess risk for accidents and injury. Insomnia is also a predictor for suicidal ideation and suicide attempts.[135] Suicide risk assessment (and as appropriate, safety planning) should be a part of comprehensive assessment conducted with all patients presenting with insomnia symptoms. Insomnia is also associated with a wide range of long-term consequences for both individual patients and society at large.[127] Given the significant economic and health consequences, as well as overall loss of quality of life associated with this disorder, the identification and treatment of insomnia disorder should be a top healthcare priority.

REFERENCES

1. Kessler RC, Berglund PA, Coulouvrat C, et al. Insomnia and the performance of US workers: Results from the America insomnia survey. *Sleep*. 2011;34(9):1161–1171.
2. Ford ES, Cunningham TJ, Giles WH, Croft JB. Trends in insomnia and excessive daytime sleepiness among US adults from 2002 to 2012. *Sleep Med*. 2015;16(3):372–378.
3. Ford ES, Wheaton AG, Cunningham TJ, Giles WH, Chapman DP, Croft JB. Trends in outpatient visits for insomnia, sleep apnea, and prescriptions for sleep medications among US adults: Findings from the National Ambulatory Medical Care survey 1999–2010. *Sleep*. 2014;37(8):1283–1293.
4. Chaput J-P, Yau J, Rao DP, Morin CM. Prevalence of insomnia for Canadians aged 6 to 79. *Health Rep*. 2018;29(12):16.
5. Taylor DJ, Mallory LJ, Lichstein KL, Durrence HH, Riedel BW, Bush AJ. Comorbidity of chronic insomnia with medical problems. *Sleep*. 2007;30(2):213–218.
6. Buysse DJ, Angst J, Gamma A, Ajdacic V, Eich D, Rössler W. Prevalence, course, and comorbidity of insomnia and depression in young adults. *Sleep*. 2008;31(4):473–480.
7. Schutte-Rodin S, Broch L, Buysse D, Dorsey C, Sateia M. Clinical guideline for the evaluation and management of chronic insomnia in adults. *J Clin Sleep Med*. 2008;4(5):487–504.

8. Calhoun SL, Fernandez-Mendoza J, Vgontzas AN, Liao D, Bixler EO. Prevalence of insomnia symptoms in a general population sample of young children and preadolescents: Gender effects. *Sleep Med*. 2014;15(1):91–95.
9. Johnson EO, Roth T, Schultz L, Bresau N. Epidemiology of DSM-IV insomnia in adolescence: Lifetime prevalence, chronicity, and an emergent gender difference. *Pediatrics*. 2006;117(2):e247–e256.
10. Roberts RE, Roberts CR, Duong HT. Chronic insomnia and its negative consequences for health and functioning of adolescents: A 12-month prospective study. *J Adolesc Health*. 2008;42(3):294–302.
11. Hysing M, Pallesen S, Stormark KM, Lundervold AJ, Sivertsen B. Sleep patterns and insomnia among adolescents: A population-based study. *J Sleep Res*. 2013;22(5):549–556.
12. National Sleep Foundation. National Sleep Foundation: Sleep in America poll 2007 (Rep. No. 06-897). Washington, DC: Author; 2007. https://www.thensf.org/wp-content/uploads/2021/03/2007-SIA-Summary_Of_Findings.pdf
13. Zhang B, Wing Y-K. Sex differences in insomnia: A meta-analysis. *Sleep*. 2006;29(1):85–93.
14. Foley DJ, Monjan A, Simonsick EM, Wallace RB, Blazer DG. Incidence and remission of insomnia among elderly adults: An epidemiologic study of 6,800 persons over three years. *Sleep*. 1999.
15. Quan SF, Enright PL, Katz R, et al. Factors associated with incidence and persistence of symptoms of disturbed sleep in an elderly cohort: The Cardiovascular Health Study. *Am J. Med Sci*. 2005;329(4):163–172.
16. Galinsky AM, Ward BW, Joestl SS, Dahlhamer JM. Sleep duration, sleep quality, and sexual orientation: Findings from the 2013–2015 National Health Interview Survey. *Sleep Health*. 2018;4(1):56–62.
17. Fricke J, Sironi M. Dimensions of sexual orientation and sleep disturbance among young adults. *Prev Med Rep*. 2017;8:18–24.
18. Caceres BA, Hickey KT, Heitkemper EM, Hughes TL. An intersectional approach to examine sleep duration in sexual minority adults in the United States: Findings from the Behavioral Risk Factor Surveillance System. *Sleep Health*. 2019;5(6):621–629.
19. Blosnich JR, Farmer GW, Lee JG, Silenzio VM, Bowen DJ. Health inequalities among sexual minority adults: Evidence from ten US states, 2010. *Am J Prev Med*. 2014;46(4):337–349.
20. Caceres BA, Hickey KT. Examining sleep duration and sleep health among sexual minority and heterosexual adults: Findings from NHANES (2005–2014). *Behav Sleep Med*. 2020;18(3):345–357.
21. Harry-Hernandez S, Reisner SL, Schrimshaw EW, et al. Gender dysphoria, mental health, and poor sleep health among transgender and gender nonbinary individuals: A qualitative study in New York City. *Transgender Health*. 2020;5(1):59–68.
22. Auer MK, Liedl A, Fuss J, et al. High impact of sleeping problems on quality of life in transgender individuals: A cross-sectional multicenter study. *PLoS One*. 2017;12(2):e0171640.
23. Carpenter JS, Andrykowski MA. Psychometric evaluation of the Pittsburgh sleep quality index. *J Psychosom Res*. 1998;45(1):5–13.
24. Buysse DJ, Reynolds III CF, Monk TH, Berman SR, Kupfer DJ. The Pittsburgh Sleep Quality Index: A new instrument for psychiatric practice and research. *Psychiatry Res*. 1989;28(2):193–213.
25. Chaudhry SK, Susser LC. Considerations in treating insomnia during pregnancy: A literature review. *Psychosomatics*. 2018;59(4):341–348.
26. Sedov ID, Anderson NJ, Dhillon AK, Tomfohr-Madsen LM. Insomnia symptoms during pregnancy: A meta-analysis. *J Sleep Res*. 2021;30(1):e13207.
27. Sivertsen B, Hysing M, Dørheim SK, Eberhard-Gran M. Trajectories of maternal sleep problems before and after childbirth: A longitudinal population-based study. *BMC Pregnancy Childbirth*. 2015;15(1):1–8.
28. Patel D, Steinberg J, Patel P. Insomnia in the elderly: A review. *J Clin Sleep Med*. 2018;14(6):1017–1024.
29. Kamel NS, Gammack JK. Insomnia in the elderly: Cause, approach, and treatment. *Am J Med*. 2006;119(6):463–469.
30. Sarsour K, Morin CM, Foley K, Kalsekar A, Walsh JK. Association of insomnia severity and comorbid medical and psychiatric disorders in a health plan-based sample: Insomnia severity and comorbidities. *Sleep Med*. 2010;11(1):69–74.
31. Brewster GS, Riegel B, Gehrman PR. Insomnia in the older adult. *Sleep Med Clin*. 2018;13(1):13–19.
32. Kravitz HM, Ganz PA, Bromberger J, Powell LH, Sutton-Tyrrell K, Meyer PM. Sleep difficulty in women at midlife: A community survey of sleep and the menopausal transition. *Menopause*. 2003;10(1):19–28.
33. El Khoudary SR, Greendale G, Crawford SL, et al. The menopause transition and women's health at midlife: A progress report from the Study of Women's Health Across the Nation (SWAN). *Menopause (NY)*. 2019;26(10):1213.
34. Jaussent I, Dauvilliers Y, Ancelin M-L, et al. Insomnia symptoms in older adults: Associated factors and gender differences. *Am J Geriatr Psychiatry*. 2011;19(1):88–97.
35. Grandner MA, Martin JL, Patel NP, et al. Age and sleep disturbances among American men and women: Data from the US Behavioral Risk Factor Surveillance System. *Sleep*. 2012;35(3):395–406.
36. Martin JL, Schweizer CA, Hughes JM, et al. Estimated prevalence of insomnia among women veterans: Results of a postal survey. *Women's Health Issues*. 2017;27(3):366–373.
37. Williams NJ, Grandner MA, Snipes SA, et al. Racial/ethnic disparities in sleep health and health care: Importance of the sociocultural context. *Sleep Health*. 2015;1(1):28–35.
38. Nunes J, Jean-Louis G, Zizi F, et al. Sleep duration among black and white Americans: Results of the National Health Interview Survey. *J Natl Med Assoc*. 2008;100(3):317–322.
39. Pigeon WR, Heffner K, Duberstein P, Fiscella K, Moynihan J, Chapman BP. Elevated sleep disturbance among blacks in an urban family medicine practice. *J Am Board Fam Med*. 2011;24(2):161–168.
40. Kalmbach DA, Pillai V, Arnedt JT, Drake CL. DSM-5 insomnia and short sleep: Comorbidity landscape and racial disparities. *Sleep*. 2016;39(12):2101–2111.
41. Singareddy R, Vgontzas AN, Fernandez-Mendoza J, et al. Risk factors for incident chronic insomnia: A general population prospective study. *Sleep Med*. 2012;13(4):346–353.

42. Jackson CL, Kawachi I, Redline S, Juon H-S, Hu FB. Asian-White disparities in short sleep duration by industry of employment and occupation in the US: A cross-sectional study. *BMC Public Health*. 2014;14(1):1–11.
43. Taylor DJ, Pruiksma KE, Hale WJ, et al. Prevalence, correlates, and predictors of insomnia in the US Army prior to deployment. *Sleep*. 2016;39(10):1795–1806.
44. Grandner MA, Patel NP, Gehrman PR, et al. Who gets the best sleep? Ethnic and socioeconomic factors related to sleep complaints. *Sleep Med*. 2010;11(5):470–478.
45. Loredo JS, Soler X, Bardwell W, Ancoli-Israel S, Dimsdale JE, Palinkas LA. Sleep health in US Hispanic population. *Sleep*. 2010;33(7):962–967.
46. Gaston SA, Nguyen-Rodriguez S, Aiello AE, et al. Hispanic/Latino heritage group disparities in sleep and the sleep-cardiovascular health relationship by housing tenure status in the United States. *Sleep Health*. 2020;6(4):451–462.
47. Patel NP, Grandner MA, Xie D, Branas CC, Gooneratne N. "Sleep disparity" in the population: Poor sleep quality is strongly associated with poverty and ethnicity. *BMC Public Health*. 2010;10(1):1–11.
48. Mindell JA, Sadeh A, Kwon R, Goh DY. Cross-cultural comparison of maternal sleep. *Sleep*. 2013;36(11):1699–1706.
49. Léger D, Beck F, Richard JB. Sleep loss in the homeless—an additional factor of precariousness: Survey in a group of homeless people. *JAMA Intern Med*. 2017;177(2):278–279.
50. Roth T. Insomnia: definition, prevalence, etiology, and consequences. *J Clin Sleep Med*. 2007;3(5 suppl):S7–S10.
51. American Psychiatric Association. *Diagnostic and Statistical Manual of Mental Disorders*, 5th edition *(DSM-5®)*. American Psychiatric Association; 2013.
52. Luyster FS, Buysse DJ, Strollo Jr PJ. Comorbid insomnia and obstructive sleep apnea: Challenges for clinical practice and research. *J Clin Sleep Med*. 2010;6(2):196–204.
53. Pieh C, Bach M, Popp R, et al. Insomnia symptoms influence CPAP compliance. *Sleep Breath*. 2013;17(1):99–104.
54. Wickwire EM, Smith MT, Birnbaum S, Collop NA. Sleep maintenance insomnia complaints predict poor CPAP adherence: A clinical case series. *Sleep Med*. 2010;11(8):772–776.
55. Ferini-Strambi L, Marelli S. Pharmacotherapy for restless legs syndrome. *Expert Opin Pharmacother*. 2014;15(8):1127–1138.
56. Appleton SL, Gill TK, Lang CJ, et al. Prevalence and comorbidity of sleep conditions in Australian adults: 2016 Sleep Health Foundation national survey. *Sleep Health*. 2018;4(1):13–19.
57. Li SX, Zhang B, Li AM, Wing YK. Prevalence and correlates of frequent nightmares: A community-based 2-phase study. *Sleep*. 2010;33(6):774–780.
58. Schredl M. Nightmare frequency and nightmare topics in a representative German sample. *Eur Arch Psychiatry Clin Neurosci*. 2010;260(8):565–570.
59. Ohayon MM, Morselli P, Guilleminault C. Prevalence of nightmares and their relationship to psychopathology and daytime functioning in insomnia subjects. *Sleep*. 1997;20(5):340–348.
60. Katz DA, McHorney CA. Clinical correlates of insomnia in patients with chronic illness. *Arch Intern Med*. 1998;158(10):1099–1107.
61. LeBlanc ES, Smith NX, Nichols GA, Allison MJ, Clarke GN. Insomnia is associated with an increased risk of type 2 diabetes in the clinical setting. *BMJ Open Diabetes Res Care*. 2018;6(1).
62. Wu M-P, Lin H-J, Weng S-F, Ho C-H, Wang J-J, Hsu Y-W. Insomnia subtypes and the subsequent risks of stroke: Report from a nationally representative cohort. *Stroke*. 2014;45(5):1349–1354.
63. Lu JL, Freire AX, Molnar MZ, Kalantar-Zadeh K, Kovesdy CP. Association of chronic insomnia with mortality and adverse renal outcomes. In *Mayo Clinic Proceedings* (Vol. 93, no. 11, pp. 1563–1570). Elsevier; 2018.
64. Zheng B, Yu C, Lv J, et al. Insomnia symptoms and risk of cardiovascular diseases among 0.5 million adults: A 10-year cohort. *Neurology*. 2019;93(23):e2110–e2120.
65. Budhiraja R, Parthasarathy S, Budhiraja P, Habib MP, Wendel C, Quan SF. Insomnia in patients with COPD. *Sleep*. 2012;35(3):369–375.
66. Wei Y, Blanken TF, Van Someren EJ. Insomnia really hurts: Effect of a bad night's sleep on pain increases with insomnia severity. *Front Psychiatry*. 2018;9:377.
67. Morin CM, Gibson D, Wade J. Self-reported sleep and mood disturbance in chronic pain patients. *Clin J Pain*. 1998;14(4):311–314.
68. Louie GH, Tektonidou MG, Caban-Martinez AJ, Ward MM. Sleep disturbances in adults with arthritis: Prevalence, mediators, and subgroups at greatest risk. Data from the 2007 National Health Interview Survey. *Arthritis Care Res*. 2011;63(2):247–260.
69. Smith MT, Perlis ML, Park A, et al. Comparative meta-analysis of pharmacotherapy and behavior therapy for persistent insomnia. *Am J Psychiatry*. 2002;159(1):5–11.
70. Ford DE, Kamerow DB. Epidemiologic study of sleep disturbances and psychiatric disorders: An opportunity for prevention? *JAMA*. 1989;262(11):1479–1484.
71. McCall WV. A psychiatric perspective on insomnia. *J Clin Psychiatry*. 2001;62:27–32.
72. Breslau N, Roth T, Rosenthal L, Andreski P. Sleep disturbance and psychiatric disorders: A longitudinal epidemiological study of young adults. *Biol Psychiatry*. 1996;39(6):411–418.
73. Hertenstein E, Feige B, Gmeiner T, et al. Insomnia as a predictor of mental disorders: A systematic review and meta-analysis. *Sleep Med Rev*. 2019;43:96–105.
74. Harvey AG. Sleep and circadian rhythms in bipolar disorder: Seeking synchrony, harmony, and regulation. *Am J Psychiatry*. 2008;165(7):820–829.
75. Ogeil RP, Phillips JG. Commonly used stimulants: Sleep problems, dependence and psychological distress. *Drug Alcohol Depend*. 2015;153:145–151.
76. Clark I, Landolt HP. Coffee, caffeine, and sleep: A systematic review of epidemiological studies and randomized controlled trials. *Sleep Med Rev*. 2017;31:70–78.
77. Jaehne A, Loessl B, Bárkai Z, Riemann D, Hornyak M. Effects of nicotine on sleep during consumption, withdrawal and replacement therapy. *Sleep Med Rev*. 2009;13(5):363–377.

78. Chakravorty S, Chaudhary NS, Brower KJ. Alcohol dependence and its relationship with insomnia and other sleep disorders. *Alcohol Clin Exp Res*. 2016;40(11):2271–2282.
79. Hasin DS. US epidemiology of cannabis use and associated problems. *Neuropsychopharmacology*. 2018;43(1):195–212.
80. Conroy DA, Kurth ME, Strong DR, Brower KJ, Stein MD. Marijuana use patterns and sleep among community-based young adults. *J Addict Dis*. 2016;35(2):135–143.
81. Schweizer CA, Hoggatt KJ, Washington DL, et al. Use of alcohol as a sleep aid, unhealthy drinking behaviors, and sleeping pill use among women veterans. *Sleep Health*. 2019;5(5):495–500.
82. Jenkins MM, Colvonen PJ, Norman SB, Afari N, Allard CB, Drummond SP. Prevalence and mental health correlates of insomnia in first-encounter veterans with and without military sexual trauma. *Sleep*. 2015;38(10):1547–1554.
83. Plumb TR, Peachey JT, Zelman DC. Sleep disturbance is common among servicemembers and veterans of Operations Enduring Freedom and Iraqi Freedom. *Psychol Serv*. 2014;11(2):209.
84. Ohayon MM, Shapiro CM. Posttraumatic stress disorder in the general population. *Compr Psychiatry*. 2000;41(6):469–478.
85. Seelig AD, Jacobson IG, Smith B, et al. Sleep patterns before, during, and after deployment to Iraq and Afghanistan. *Sleep*. 2010;33(12):1615–1622.
86. Carlson G, Kelly, MR, Grinberg, AM, et al. Insomnia precipitating events among women veterans: The impact of traumatic and nontraumatic events on sleep and mental health symptoms. *Behav Sleep Med*. 2020:1–18.
87. Babson KA, Feldner MT. Temporal relations between sleep problems and both traumatic event exposure and PTSD: A critical review of the empirical literature. *J Anxiety Disord*. 2010;24(1):1–15.
88. Pruiksma KE, Taylor DJ, Wachen JS, et al. Residual sleep disturbances following PTSD treatment in active duty military personnel. *Psychol Trauma*. 2016;8(6):697.
89. Pigeon WR, Bishop TM, Krueger KM. Insomnia as a precipitating factor in new onset mental illness: A systematic review of recent findings. *Curr Psychiatry Rep*. 2017;19(8):1–11.
90. Corkum P, Tannock R, Moldofsky H. Sleep disturbances in children with attention-deficit/hyperactivity disorder. *J Am Acad Child Adolesc Psychiatry*. 1998;37(6):637–646.
91. Polimeni M, Richdale A, Francis A. A survey of sleep problems in autism, Asperger's disorder and typically developing children. *J Intellect Disabil Res*. 2005;49(4):260–268.
92. Phillips NL, Moore T, Teng A, Brookes N, Palermo TM, Lah S. Behavioral interventions for sleep disturbances in children with neurological and neurodevelopmental disorders: A systematic review and meta-analysis of randomized controlled trials. *Sleep*. 2020;43(9). doi:https://doi.org/10.1093/sleep/zsaa040
93. Mayer G, Jennum P, Riemann D, Dauvilliers Y. Insomnia in central neurologic diseases: Occurrence and management. *Sleep Med Rev*. 2011;15(6):369–378.
94. Bianchetti A, Scuratti A, Zanetti O, et al. Predictors of mortality and institutionalization in Alzheimer disease patients 1 year after discharge from an Alzheimer dementia unit. *Dement Geriatr Cogn Disord*. 1995;6(2):108–112.
95. Chen PY, Chiu HT, Chiu HY. Daytime sleepiness is independently associated with falls in older adults with dementia. *Geriatr Gerontol Int*. 2016;16(7):850–855.
96. Shamim SA, Warriach ZI, Tariq MA, Rana KF, Malik BH. Insomnia: Risk factor for neurodegenerative diseases. *Cureus*. 2019;11(10). doi:10.7759/cureus.6004.
97. O'Caoimh R, Mannion H, Sezgin D, O'Donovan MR, Liew A, Molloy DW. Non-pharmacological treatments for sleep disturbance in mild cognitive impairment and dementia: A systematic review and meta-analysis. *Maturitas*. 2019;127:82–94.
98. Mathias J, Alvaro P. Prevalence of sleep disturbances, disorders, and problems following traumatic brain injury: A meta-analysis. *Sleep Med*. 2012;13(7):898–905.
99. Taylor CA, Bell JM, Breiding MJ, Xu L. Traumatic brain injury–related emergency department visits, hospitalizations, and deaths—United States, 2007 and 2013. *MMWR Surveill Summ*. 2017;66(9):1.
100. Fichtenberg NL, Millis SR, Mann NR, Zafonte RD, Millard AE. Factors associated with insomnia among post-acute traumatic brain injury survivors. *Brain Injury*. 2000;14(7):659–667.
101. Mahmood O, Rapport LJ, Hanks RA, Fichtenberg NL. Neuropsychological performance and sleep disturbance following traumatic brain injury. *J Head Trauma Rehabil*. 2004;19(5):378–390.
102. Zeitzer JM, Friedman L, O'Hara R. Insomnia in the context of traumatic brain injury. *J Rehabil Res Dev*. 2009;46(6):827–836.
103. American Academy of Sleep Medicine. *International Classification of Sleep Disorders*: Diagnostic and Coding *Manual*. AASM; 2005:51–55.
104. Natale V, Léger D, Bayon V, et al. The consensus sleep diary: Quantitative criteria for primary insomnia diagnosis. *Psychosom Med*. 2015;77(4):413–418.
105. Littner MR, Kushida C, Wise M, et al., & Standards of Practice Committee of the American Academy of Sleep Medicine. Practice parameters for clinical use of the multiple sleep latency test and the maintenance of wakefulness test. *Sleep*. 2005;28(1):113–121. https://pubmed.ncbi.nlm.nih.gov/15700727/.
106. Carney CE, Buysse DJ, Ancoli-Israel S, et al. The consensus sleep diary: Standardizing prospective sleep self-monitoring. *Sleep*. 2012;35(2):287–302.
107. Riemann D, Spiegelhalder K, Feige B, et al. The hyperarousal model of insomnia: A review of the concept and its evidence. *Sleep Med Rev*. 2010;14(1):19–31.
108. Lancee J, Eisma MC, van Zanten KB, Topper M. When thinking impairs sleep: Trait, daytime and nighttime repetitive thinking in insomnia. *Behav Sleep Med*. 2017;15(1):53–69.
109. Tutek J, Gunn HE, Lichstein KL. Worry and rumination have distinct associations with nighttime versus daytime sleep symptomology. *Behav Sleep Med*. 2021;19(2):192–207.
110. Standards of Practice Committee, Aurora RN, Zak RS, Auerbach SH, et al. Best practice guide for the treatment of nightmare disorder in adults. *J Clin Sleep Med*. 2010;6(4):389–401.

111. Stone KC, Taylor DJ, McCrae CS, Kalsekar A, Lichstein KL. Nonrestorative sleep. *Sleep Med Rev*. 2008;12(4):275–288.
112. Ohayon MM. Prevalence and correlates of nonrestorative sleep complaints. *Arch Intern Med*. 2005;165(1):35–41.
113. Roth T, Jaeger S, Jin R, Kalsekar A, Stang PE, Kessler RC. Sleep problems, comorbid mental disorders, and role functioning in the national comorbidity survey replication. *Biol Psychiatry*. 2006;60(12):1364–1371.
114. Fortier-Brochu É, Morin CM. Cognitive impairment in individuals with insomnia: Clinical significance and correlates. *Sleep*. 2014;37(11):1787–1798.
115. Fortier-Brochu É, Beaulieu-Bonneau S, Ivers H, Morin CM. Insomnia and daytime cognitive performance: A meta-analysis. *Sleep Med Rev*. 2012;16(1):83–94.
116. Gruber R, Cassoff J. The interplay between sleep and emotion regulation: Conceptual framework empirical evidence and future directions. *Curr Psychiatry Rep*. 2014;16(11):500.
117. Gratz KL, Roemer L. Multidimensional assessment of emotion regulation and dysregulation: Development, factor structure, and initial validation of the difficulties in emotion regulation scale. *J Psychopathol Behav Assess*. 2004;26(1):41–54.
118. Vgontzas AN, Bixler EO, Lin H-M, et al. Chronic insomnia is associated with nyctohemeral activation of the hypothalamic-pituitary-adrenal axis: Clinical implications. *J Clin Endocrinol Metab*. 2001;86(8):3787–3794.
119. Vgontzas AN, Tsigos C, Bixler EO, et al. Chronic insomnia and activity of the stress system: A preliminary study. *J Psychosom Res*. 1998;45(1):21–31.
120. Vgontzas AN, Liao D, Bixler EO, Chrousos GP, Vela-Bueno A. Insomnia with objective short sleep duration is associated with a high risk for hypertension. *Sleep*. 2009;32(4):491–497.
121. Vgontzas AN, Liao D, Pejovic S, Calhoun S, Karataraki M, Bixler EO. Insomnia with objective short sleep duration is associated with type 2 diabetes: A population-based study. *Diabetes Care*. 2009;32(11):1980–1985.
122. Vgontzas AN, Liao D, Pejovic S, et al. Insomnia with short sleep duration and mortality: The Penn State cohort. *Sleep*. 2010;33(9):1159–1164.
123. Gordon AM, Chen S. The role of sleep in interpersonal conflict: Do sleepless nights mean worse fights? *Soc Psychol Personal Sci*. 2014;5(2):168–175.
124. Combs D, Goodwin JL, Quan SF, Morgan WJ, Shetty S, Parthasarathy S. Insomnia, health-related quality of life and health outcomes in children: A seven year longitudinal cohort. *Sci Rep*. 2016;6(1):1–10.
125. Kuppermann M, Lubeck DP, Mazonson PD, et al. Sleep problems and their correlates in a working population. *J Gen Intern Med*. 1995;10(1):25–32.
126. Wickwire EM, Shaya FT, Scharf SM. Health economics of insomnia treatments: The return on investment for a good night's sleep. *Sleep Med Rev*. 2016;30:72–82.
127. Ozminkowski RJ, Wang S, Walsh JK. The direct and indirect costs of untreated insomnia in adults in the United States. *Sleep*. 2007;30(3):263–273.
128. Hatoum HT, Kong SX, Kania CM, Wong JM, Mendelson WB. Insomnia, health-related quality of life and healthcare resource consumption. *Pharmacoeconomics*. 1998;14(6):629–637.
129. Shahly V, Berglund PA, Coulouvrat C, et al. The associations of insomnia with costly workplace accidents and errors: results from the America Insomnia Survey. *Arch Gen Psychiatry*. 2012;69(10):1054–1063.
130. Garbarino S, Magnavita N, Guglielmi O, et al. Insomnia is associated with road accidents: Further evidence from a study on truck drivers. *PLoS One*. 2017;12(10):e0187256.
131. Kalsi J, Tervo T, Bachour A, Partinen M. Sleep versus non-sleep-related fatal road accidents. *Sleep Med*. 2018;51:148–152.
132. Lin Y-C, Sun C-A, Lin H-T, et al. Increased risk of road traffic injuries in individuals with insomnia. *J Transport Health*. 2021;21:101030.
133. McCall WV, Blocker JN, D'Agostino R Jr, et al. Insomnia severity is an indicator of suicidal ideation during a depression clinical trial. *Sleep Med*. 2010;11(9):822–827.
134. Chakravorty S, Siu HK, Lalley-Chareczko L, et al. Sleep duration and insomnia symptoms as risk factors for suicidal ideation in a nationally representative sample. *Prim Care Companion CNS Disord*. 2015;17(6):402–422.
135. Lin H-T, Lai C-H, Perng H-J, et al. Insomnia as an independent predictor of suicide attempts: A nationwide population-based retrospective cohort study. *BMC Psychiatry*. 2018;18(1):1–11.
136. Bishop TM, Walsh PG, Ashrafioun L, Lavigne JE, Pigeon WR. Sleep, suicide behaviors, and the protective role of sleep medicine. *Sleep Med*. 2020;66:264–270.
137. Woosley JA, Lichstein KL, Taylor DJ, Riedel BW, Bush AJ. Hopelessness mediates the relation between insomnia and suicidal ideation. *J Clin Sleep Med*. 2014;10(11):1223–1230.
138. Hartwig E, Palmer C, Rufino K, Alfano C, Patriquin M. Sleep problems mediate the impact of emotion regulation on suicide ideation. *Sleep*. 2018;41:A357.
139. Scalo J, Desai P, Rascati K. Insomnia, hypnotic use, and health-related quality of life in a nationally representative sample. *Qual Life Res*. 2015;24(5):1223–1233.
140. Kyle SD, Morgan K, Espie CA. Insomnia and health-related quality of life. *Sleep Med Rev*. 2010;14(1):69–82.
141. Olfson M, Wall M, Liu S-M, Morin CM, Blanco C. Insomnia and impaired quality of life in the United States. *J Clin Psychiatry*. 2018;79(5). doi:10.4088/JCP.17m12020.
142. Barnes CM, Watson NF. Why healthy sleep is good for business. *Sleep Med Rev*. 2019;47:112–118.
143. Loprinzi PD, Joyner C. Meeting sleep guidelines is associated with better health-related quality of life and reduced premature all-cause mortality risk. *Am J Health Promot*. 2018;32(1):68–71.
144. Qaseem A, Kansagara D, Forciea MA, Cooke M, Denberg TD. Management of chronic insomnia disorder in adults: A clinical practice guideline from the American College of Physicians. *Ann Intern Med*. 2016;165(2):125–133.
145. Wu JQ, Appleman ER, Salazar RD, Ong JC. Cognitive behavioral therapy for insomnia comorbid with psychiatric and medical conditions: A meta-analysis. *JAMA Intern Med*. 2015;175(9):1461–1472.

Chapter 13

Pharmacotherapy for Insomnia

Abbey Dunn

INTRODUCTION

Insomnia is a common problem, with some estimates indicating that a third of the adult population experiences insomnia symptoms each year.[1] It is a frequent reason for which patients seek medical care, with the number of physician office visits for insomnia increasing 13% from 4.9 million visits in 1999 to 5.5 million visits in 2010.[2]

As defined by the International Classification of Sleep Disorders, insomnia is characterized primarily by difficulty initiating or maintaining sleep, including waking earlier than desired, with sleep latency or wake after sleep onset >30 minutes, or waking more than 30 minutes before the desired time, when given adequate opportunity and circumstances for sleep.[3] The diagnosis also requires at least 1 of the following associated daytime symptoms: fatigue/malaise; reduced motivation, energy, or initiative; daytime sleepiness; impairment of memory, attention, or concentration; impairment in social, family, occupational/vocational, or academic performance; proneness for errors/accidents; mood disturbance or irritability; behavioral problems; or patient-reported concerns or dissatisfaction with sleep. Insomnia is considered acute or short-term when symptoms are present for less than 3 months. Insomnia is considered chronic when it has occurred at least 3 times a week for at least 3 months. Chronic insomnia is a very common problem, which is thought to affect about 10% of the adult population.[4]

As with increasing office visits, the number of prescriptions for any sleep medication increased 293% from 5.3 million in 1999 to 20.8 million in 2010.[2] While medications are commonly prescribed for insomnia, medications are generally not recommended as the initial treatment for most patients. First-line treatment of acute, or short-term insomnia, should include identification and treatment of conditions and comorbidities interfering with sleep, as often in cases of acute insomnia, there is an identifiable precipitating event. Usually, symptoms remit with time as distress lessens or with resolution of the precipitant. However, for patients whose symptoms are severe, distressing, or interfering with daytime function, medications can be considered on an as-needed basis for a brief period.[28]

Cognitive behavioral therapy for insomnia (CBT-I) is considered first-line treatment for chronic insomnia and implements cognitive restructuring and behavioral modifications to improve sleep (the principles and implementation of CBT for insomnia are discussed elsewhere, outside of this chapter).[5–7] While CBT-I is the preferred first-line treatment of chronic insomnia, it is not effective in all cases. Additionally, not all patients will be willing or able to undergo this therapy, whether due to patient preference or lack of available providers. Ideally, initiating treatment with medications for sleep should be on a short-term basis and should be supplemented with behavioral and cognitive therapies when possible. Long-term use of medication may be indicated in conjunction with CBT-I techniques or alone, depending on individual circumstances, especially in severe or refractory cases or with chronic comorbid illnesses, with the goal to improve sleep quality, quantity, and improve daytime functioning.[7] A shared decision-making approach should be implemented, and the risks and benefits of treatment discussed with the patient. The use of medications for the treatment of insomnia must be considered in the context of the individual patient's treatment goals and preferences, costs, comorbidities, current medications, contraindications, side effects, and prior treatments.[7]

The following sections will discuss various pharmacologic treatments for insomnia, which encompass the following categories: medications with U.S. Food and Drug Administration (FDA) approved indications for insomnia; drugs used off-label for the treatment of insomnia; over the counter (OTC) sleep aids; and supplements.

The majority of the discussion will focus on the classes of medications with FDA indications for treatment of insomnia, which include:

- Benzodiazepine receptor agonists (BZRAs): including both non-benzodiazepine receptor agonists (nBZRAs) and traditional and benzodiazepine hypnotics (BZDs)
  - o nBZRAs: eszopiclone, zaleplon, and zolpidem
  - o BZDs: estazolam, flurazepam, temazepam, triazolam, and quazepam
- Dual orexin receptor antagonists (DORAs): lemborexant and suvorexant
- Melatonin receptor agonist: ramelteon
- Histamine receptor antagonist: doxepin

For most healthy adults, these medications, with the exclusion of some of the BZDs (due to higher risk-to-benefit ratio, discussed later in the chapter), are considered first-line treatment for insomnia.

While a wide range of medications including sedating anti-depressants, anti-psychotics, anti-epileptics, and antihistamines are prescribed off-label for treatment of insomnia, these medications are not recommended as a first-line treatment for insomnia. These classes of medications can be considered in cases where patients have comorbid conditions which may also respond to treatment, or in cases where particular classes of first-line medications must be avoided or were not effective.

CLINICAL ASSESSMENT

Patients presenting with insomnia complaints should be assessed for the presence of co-occurring conditions that can impact their treatment. This includes screening for mood and anxiety disorders. Insomnia has been identified as a prospective risk factor for psychiatric illness, especially the development of depression.[8] Clinical depression has been identified in 10%–25% of insomnia cases, and anxiety disorders in 20%–30%.[9] Insomnia has also been identified as a risk factor for suicide, and thus patients with depression or mood disorders should also be assessed for suicidal ideation prior to prescribing and during treatment.[10,11] There are shared warnings regarding the risk for worsening depression or suicidal ideation on all medications with FDA indications for treatment of insomnia.

It is also important to assess for current and remote substance abuse history. Of the FDA approved medications for insomnia, the BZDs, BZRAs, and DORAs are all schedule-IV controlled substances with risk for abuse or dependence and may need to be avoided. Doxepin for sleep maintenance or ramelteon for sleep-onset insomnia may be preferable with a prior history of substance abuse as they are not classified as controlled substances.

Patients should also be assessed for conditions causing compromised respiratory function which may be worsened with sedating medications, particularly BZDs, including chronic obstructive pulmonary disease and hypoventilation. There is a risk for respiratory depression with BZDs, which may translate to increased risk for complications such as acute respiratory failure or hypoventilation, especially in patients with underling lung disease.[12,13]

Screening for obstructive sleep apnea (OSA) is recommended, as insomnia and OSA are often comorbid conditions. A 2019 meta-analysis found worldwide pooled prevalence rates of OSA in insomnia patients at 35%.[14] Patients with comorbid insomnia and OSA may find it more difficult to adhere to positive airway pressure (PAP). While both OSA and insomnia are common, there are limited data on the use of hypnotic medications in untreated OSA, especially in cases of severe OSA, which tend to be excluded from clinical trials. Of the nBZRAs, limited data suggest that zolpidem and eszopiclone do not worsen the overall apnea hypopnea index (AHI) or oxygen desaturation index, but zolpidem at 20 mg (twice the recommended maximum dose) has been associated with a significant decrease in the minimum oxygen saturation.[15] Ramelteon, evaluated in a small double-blind, randomized, crossover study, has not been found to worsen mild or moderate OSA.[16] Of the DORAs, suvorexant at 40 mg, twice the recommended maximum dose, has not been found to worsen mild to moderate OSA in adults, and lemborexant has not been associated with worsening of OSA in elderly patients with mild OSA.[17,18] The data are extremely limited, and these drugs must be used with caution in patients with OSA, especially if severe.

PRESCRIBING PRACTICES

When initiating a medication for sleep, it should be prescribed at the lowest recommended dose and titrated based on individual response with frequent reassessment. Response to treatment should be reassessed at regular intervals. Sleep diaries can be helpful to show the overall trend, especially when patients may be more prone to only recall poor nights of sleep. Medication for sleep should be used for the shortest duration possible, although some patients with chronic insomnia may require long-term treatment.

Shared Warning and Precautions

Patients should be counseled on potential adverse effects of the selected medication. Concerns common to medications used to treat insomnia include the risk of severe allergic reactions, central nervous system depression, abnormal thinking including possible amnesia, behavioral and mood changes including risk for worsening depression or suicidal ideation, and the potential for residual next-day effects, including impaired mental alertness and the potential for impaired next-day driving (which can be present even if feeling awake). Patients should be counseled to avoid combining medication for sleep with alcohol, or other sedating medications, especially opioids, which may increase these risks. Patients should be advised to only use medication when they have ample time to devote to sleep to allow for drug clearance to minimize potential next-day effects, which is variable depending on the pharmacokinetic profile of individual drugs.

All medications with FDA-approved indications for insomnia also share a warning for the potential of complex sleep-related behaviors. These are abnormal behaviors occurring during sleep, which are typically associated with wakefulness, and of which the subject has little to no recall of the next day. Such behaviors can include somnambulism, sleep eating, sleep driving, and sexual activity. The nBZRAs have been associated with higher incidence of complex sleep-related behaviors, and there is a black box warning on zaleplon, eszopiclone, and zolpidem. The FDA issued this warning after a review of the medical literature and events submitted to the FDA Adverse Event Reporting System identified 66 cases of complex sleep behaviors resulting in severe injury, and including death, occurring over 26 years in patients using nBZRAs.[19] Twenty of these cases reported death, 46 reported serious injury, and 22 reported a previous known episode of complex sleep-related behavior. These behaviors can occur at any time in the course of treatment, whether on the first dose of medication or after a longer duration of use. Patients should be counseled to discontinue the medication should such behaviors occur, and further use of nBZRAs is contraindicated.

Elderly Patients

Insomnia is a very common condition in the elderly, and particular care should be taken when selecting a medication for insomnia in this population.[20] Benzodiazepine receptor agonists (both BZDs and nBZRAs) are listed on the Beers Criteria list of potentially inappropriate medications for elderly adults, citing increased sensitivity and decreased metabolism of long-acting agents in the elderly, as well as increased risk of cognitive impairment, delirium, falls, fractures, and motor vehicle crashes in this population.[21] A study looking at the adverse events of nBZRAs in older people (age 60 and older) found adverse cognitive events were 4.78 times more common, adverse psychomotor events were 2.61 times more common, and reports of daytime fatigue were 3.82 times more common with these drugs than with placebo.[22] Thus, these potential risks must be weighed against the potential benefits when considering these medications in an elderly patient. Use of lemborexant, suvorexant, doxepin (3–6 mg), or ramelteon is generally preferable in this population, as these medications have more favorable safety and adverse effect profile, they but are not without risks.

The medications discussed in the following sections are summarized in Table 13.1. Please note, these sections serve as an overview of classes of medications for insomnia but may be incomplete. Please refer to each drug's full prescribing information for additional considerations and complete drug interactions.

BENZODIAZEPINE RECEPTOR AGONISTS

The BZRAs include both nBZRAs and BZDs. The nBZRAs include eszopiclone, zaleplon, and zolpidem (with both immediate and controlled-release formulations). The BZDs with indications for insomnia include estazolam, flurazepam, temazepam, triazolam, and quazepam.

In terms of their mechanism of action, BZDs act as positive allosteric modulators on the gamma-aminobutyric acid (GABA)-A receptor, which is inhibitory, and reduces the excitability of neurons, producing amnestic, anticonvulsant, muscle relaxant, anxiolytic, and hypnotic effect.[23] Non-benzodiazepine receptor agonists are structurally unrelated to BZDs but also bind to the GABA-A subunit; they differ in their affinity for binding sites, binding more selectively to the alpha-1 subunit, which mediates sedation.[24] This selectivity in binding sites is felt to account for less physical dependence and lower abuse potential compared to BZDs, which have wider subunit binding affinity, including to the alpha-2 subunit, which mediates anxiolytic effects.[24] Notably, all of the BZRAs have been classified as schedule IV controlled substances by the U.S. Drug Enforcement Agency, carrying a relatively low risk for potential abuse and dependence compared to drugs in schedules I–III.

BENZODIAZEPINES

While estazolam, flurazepam, temazepam, triazolam, and quazepam have labeled indications for insomnia, many of these medications are not recommended as first-line agents for the treatment of insomnia due to significant risks and the availability of lower-risk alternative treatments. BZDs have been associated with significant adverse effects, including drowsiness, dizziness, lightheadedness, and cognitive impairment.[25] In addition to significant adverse effects, there is also the potential for abuse, misuse, addiction, as well as physical dependence and withdrawal reactions. If used habitually, benzodiazepines must be tapered off slowly to avoid abrupt discontinuation, which can lead to a withdrawal syndrome that can be severe or even fatal, especially with high-dose use. The risk of overdose or death is also increased with concomitant use of opioids as well as alcohol, and in 2020 the FDA updated the boxed warning on BZDs to include these potential risks.[26,27] Given these concerns, the American College of Physicians issued guidelines recommending against the use of any BZD for insomnia.[5] In 2017, the American Academy of Sleep Medicine (AASM) issued a Clinical Practice Guideline for the pharmacological treatment of insomnia in which, of the FDA-approved BZDs for insomnia, there was only sufficient evidence to recommend triazolam for sleep-onset insomnia and temazepam for

Table 13.1 **Prescription Drugs for Insomnia**

Drug: Generic (Brand name)	Indication*	Typical Dose for Adults+	Dose for Elderly (Age ≥65)+	Mean Half-Life in Hours (hrs)
Non-Benzodiazepine Receptor Agonists				
Eszopiclone (Lunesta)	Sleep onset and/or maintenance insomnia	1–3 mg	1–2 mg	6 hrs
Zaleplon (Sonata)	Sleep onset insomnia	5-20 mg	5–10 mg	1 hr
Zolpidem	Sleep onset insomnia	5–10 mg for males 5 mg for females	5 mg	2.6 hrs for 5 mg 2.5 hrs for 10 mg
Tablet (Ambien) Sublingual tablet (Edluar) Oral spray (Zolpimist)				
Zolpidem sublingual (Intermezzo)	Insomnia with middle of the night waking and difficulty returning to sleep	1.75–3.5 mg for males 1.75 mg for females	1.75 mg	2.5 hrs
Zolpidem extended release (Ambien CR)	Sleep onset and/or maintenance insomnia	6.25–12 mg for males 6.25 mg for females	6.25 mg	2.8 hrs
Benzodiazepines				
Estazolam (Prosom)	Sleep onset and/or maintenance insomnia	1–2 mg	0.5 mg	10–24 hrs
Flurazepam (Dalmane)	Sleep onset and/or maintenance insomnia	15–30 mg	15 mg	47–100 hrs
Temazepam (Restoril)	Sleep onset and/or maintenance insomnia	7.5–30 mg	7.5–15 mg	8.8 hrs
Triazolam (Halcion)	Sleep onset and/or maintenance insomnia	0.125–0.5 mg	0.125–0.25 mg	1.5–5.5 hrs
Quazepam (Doral)	Sleep onset and/or maintenance insomnia	7.5–15 mg	7.5 mg	39–73 hrs
Dual Orexin Receptor Antagonists				
Suvorexant (Belsomra)	Sleep onset and/or maintenance insomnia	10–20 mg	10–20 mg	15 hrs
Lemborexant (Dayvigo)	Sleep onset and/or maintenance insomnia	5–10 mg	5 mg–10 mg; exercise caution at doses >5 mg	17 hrs for 5 mg 19 hrs for 10 mg
Melatonin Receptor Agonist				
Ramelteon (Rozerem)	Sleep onset insomnia	8 mg	8 mg	1–2.6 hrs for drug 2–5 hrs for metabolite
Histamine (H1) Receptor Antagonist				
Doxepin (Silenor)	Sleep maintenance insomnia	3–6 mg	3–6 mg	15.3 hrs for drug 31 hrs for metabolite

* Appropriate clinical use may differ from FDA-approved indication.
+ Significant drug interactions exist which may require dosage adjustments or avoidance; consult full prescribing information guide for guidance. Downward dose adjustment may be necessary in patients on other central nervous system depressants because of potentially additive effects.

sleep-onset and maintenance insomnia versus no treatment.[28] In the analysis, triazolam 0.25 mg was found to reduce sleep latency by 9 minutes compared with placebo, and temazepam 15 mg was found to reduce sleep latency by 37 minutes and increase total sleep time by 99 minutes compared to placebo. There was inadequate data to provide clinical treatment recommendations regarding estazolam, quazepam, or flurazepam. Of the BZDs with indications for insomnia, these have the longest elimination half-lives and have been associated with adverse effects such as next day somnolence, cognitive impairment, and psychomotor impairment.[29–31]

NON-BENZODIAZEPINE RECEPTOR AGONISTS

Among the nBZRAs, one of the biggest pharmacologic and also clinically important differences in these medications is the onset and duration of action. Zaleplon has the shortest half-life, approximately 1 hour, and eszopiclone the longest, approximately 6 hours. Zolpidem has a half -life which is intermediate in comparison, 2.5–2.6 hours, though an extended-release version also exists. Thus clinically, the selection of appropriate nBZRA medication often depends on the pattern of the patient's insomnia. Patients with sleep-onset insomnia would typically benefit more from use of shorter-acting nBZRAs: zaleplon or zolpidem. Patients with sleep-maintenance insomnia would likely benefit most from those medications with longer half-lives such as eszopiclone, or the extended-release formulations of zolpidem. Although the immediate-release formulation of zolpidem has approved indication for sleep-onset insomnia, it can be effective for sleep maintenance in some patients. For those with middle of the night waking with at least 4 hours remaining before planned awakening, the lower dose sublingual version of zolpidem (Intermezzo) or zaleplon can be utilized, although off-label.

If an nBZRA is chosen for an elderly or debilitated patient with insomnia, lower dosages of nBRZRAs should be utilized to avoid increased side effects; nBZRAs should be avoided in those with severe hepatic impairment, and lower maximum doses are recommended for patients with mild to moderate hepatic impairment. These medications should not be taken with food or immediately after a meal as this can delay absorption and impair efficacy.

ESZOPICLONE

Eszopiclone has labeled indications for the treatment of sleep-onset and maintenance insomnia. The recommended starting dose is 1 mg taken immediately before bedtime with at least 7–8 hours remaining before planned awakening. The maximum dose is 3 mg. However, in the elderly, debilitated, those with severe hepatic impairment, or in patients taking concurrent potent CYP3A4 inhibitors, the recommended maximum dose is 2 mg. Notably, the 3 mg dose of eszopiclone has been associated with next-morning psychomotor and memory impairment and because of this, patients taking the 3 mg dose should be counseled against driving or engaging in other activities that could be hazardous or require complete mental alertness the day after use.[32]

In terms of efficacy, a 2018 meta-analysis of subjective patient-reported data demonstrated a 12-minute decrease in sleep onset latency (SOL), a 17-minute decrease in wake after sleep onset (WASO), and a 28-minute increase in total sleep time (TST) with eszopiclone compared to placebo.[33] Additionally, there was no evidence of tolerance or rebound insomnia on discontinuation. Likewise, the 2017 meta-analysis performed as part of the AASM Clinical Practice Guideline which showed a mean reduction in sleep latency of 14 minutes, a 10–14-minute reduction in WASO, and an increase in TST of 28–57 minutes with eszopiclone versus placebo.[28]

Eszopiclone also has demonstrated sustained long-term efficacy over a 12-month clinical trial which showed consistent improvement in patient-reported variables, including decreased sleep latency, wake time after sleep onset, and number of awakenings, and increased total sleep time.[34] There was also no evidence for tolerance developing over the course of the study with 12 months of daily treatment, with the most common adverse effect being unpleasant taste, reported by >5% of subjects.

Eszopiclone has also been studied in older adults (age 65–85) with primary insomnia. In this population, eszopiclone 2 mg a night for 12 weeks was associated with statistically significant decreases in mean subjective SOL and WASO, as well as a significant increase in mean subjective TST compared to placebo, without evidence of tolerance or rebound insomnia after discontinuation.[35]

ZALEPLON

Zaleplon has a labeled indication for sleep-onset insomnia. Because of its rapid onset, zaleplon should be taken immediately prior to bedtime or in bed, after being unable to initiate sleep. The recommended dose of zaleplon in non-elderly adults is 10 mg at bedtime, although 5 mg may be sufficient in some cases, with a maximum dose of 20 mg. In elderly adults the recommended initial dose is 5 mg, with a maximum of 10 mg. Coadministration of a potent CYP3A4 enzyme inducer is not recommended, as this could lead to ineffectiveness of zaleplon.

In terms of efficacy, in adults with primary insomnia, zaleplon 10 mg has been shown to reduce SOL by about 10 minutes compared with placebo, but does not have an effect on TST or WASO.[28] Zaleplon has also been shown to be effective in elderly patients (age >65) with insomnia, significantly reducing subjective sleep latency with both 5 and 10 mg doses.[36] In this study there was a weak indication of rebound insomnia after discontinuation of the 10 mg dose after 2 weeks of treatment, but this finding was not replicated in several other studies.[37,38]

ZOLPIDEM

Zolpidem is available in both immediate-release and long-acting formulations. The immediate release has labeled indications for the treatment of sleep-onset insomnia, and the extended release has indications for sleep-onset and/or maintenance insomnia. A lower dose version sublingual formulation of zolpidem (Intermezzo) has an indication for sleep maintenance insomnia, especially to be taken for middle of the night waking with difficulty returning to sleep, which is unique to the class.

The recommended dosage of immediate-release zolpidem in adults ranges from 5 to 10 mg at bedtime and 6.25 to 12.5 mg at bedtime for the extended-release formulation. Patients should be counseled to only take zolpidem if they have 7–8 hours to remain in bed before planned awakening. The recommended dosing for the sublingual middle of the night formulation is 1.75–3.5 mg and should only be taken with 4 or more hours remaining before planned awakening.

There are different maximum doses of zolpidem for men and women. The recommended maximum dose for women is 5 mg for immediate release, 6.25 mg for the extended-release formulation, and 1.75 mg of the immediate-release sublingual formulation taken for middle of the night insomnia. This change was made in 2013 based on data showing decreased clearance of zolpidem in women leading to higher drug levels the following morning, which may lead to significant impairment, especially with driving.[39] While next-day impairment can occur with both formulations, the risk is higher for the extended-release formulation. Thus, patients taking these medications should be counseled on the risks of next-day impairment during activities that require complete mental alertness (such as driving), which can occur even if feeling fully awake.

In terms of efficacy, a meta-analysis including 12 randomized controlled trials found that zolpidem 10 mg reduced mean sleep latency by 5–12 minutes, increased mean total sleep time by 29 minutes, and reduced mean WASO by 25 minutes compared to placebo.[28] It should be noted that at the time of the original approval for zolpidem, 10 mg a night was the recommended starting dose, which has since been reduced to 5 mg, and thus efficacy data for the 5 mg dose are not well established. Adverse effects include drowsiness, dizziness, and diarrhea.

There are no head-to-head trials comparing the extended-release and immediate-release formulations of zolpidem. When comparing extended-release and immediate-release forms of zolpidem, 12.5 mg of extended-release zolpidem produces higher plasma concentrations 3–6 hours after dosage than with 10 mg immediate-release zolpidem, but the differences in terms of residual plasma levels and pharmacodynamic effects are no longer significant by 8 hours after dosing.[40]

DUAL OREXIN RECEPTOR ANTAGONISTS: SUVOREXANT AND LEMBOREXANT

Suvorexant and lemborexant have labeled indications for the treatment of sleep-onset and maintenance insomnia. These medications are potent and selective orexin receptor antagonists which bind to orexin receptor 1 (OX1R) and orexin receptor 2 (OX2R), preventing the binding of the wake-promoting hormone orexin; this action suppresses the wake drive and promotes sleep.[41,42] When comparing the 2 drugs, lemborexant has a stronger inhibition effect on OX2R than OX1R compared to suvorexant and binds and dissociates more rapidly from orexin receptors.[43] Suvorexant was the first DORA with FDA approval, and lemborexant the most recent, gaining approval in 2019.

Both DORAs have indications for sleep-onset and/or maintenance insomnia and should be given within 30 minutes of bedtime and with at least 7 hours remaining before planned awakening. Taking suvorexant or lemborexant with food or soon after a meal may delay intended effects.

The recommended starting dose of suvorexant is 10 mg with a maximum dose of 20 mg. Concomitant use of strong inhibitors of CYP3A is not recommended with suvorexant. In patients using concomitant moderate CYP3A inhibitors, the recommended starting dose is 5 mg, which can be increased to 10 mg as needed if not effective.

The recommended starting dose of lemborexant is 5 mg with a maximum dose of 10 mg. Concomitant use of strong or moderate CYP3A inhibitors or inducers is not recommended. If used with weak CYP3A inhibitors, the maximum recommended dose is 5 mg.

Neither drug is recommended in cases of severe hepatic impairment. No dose adjustment is necessary in cases of mild to moderate hepatic impairment for suvorexant, but with lemborexant there are dose adjustments for moderate hepatic impairment, not to exceed 5 mg.

Somnolence is the most common adverse effect with both drugs, risk of which increases with dose. Patients taking 20 mg dose of suvorexant or the 10 mg dose of lemborexant should be advised against next-day driving and other activities requiring complete mental alertness; patients prescribed lower doses should also be informed of these potential risks.

Notably, orexin-1 deficiency is seen in narcolepsy with cataplexy, a sleep disorder characterized by excessive daytime sleepiness with instability of sleep-wake regulation with frequent lapses into rapid-eye movement (REM) sleep. Given the mechanism of action of these medications, as an orexin receptor antagonist, there is a theoretical risk for adverse effects similar to symptoms experienced in narcolepsy, such as hypnopompic or hypnogogic hallucinations, sleep paralysis, and cataplexy-like leg weakness. In clinical trials, such adverse effects appear to be rare, however.[44] Because of this, these medications are contraindicated in patients with narcolepsy.

In terms of efficacy, suvorexant, while approved for both sleep-onset and maintenance insomnia, appears to have more clinically significant impact on sleep maintenance than onset. A meta-analysis of 4 randomized clinical trials involving 3076 patients with primary insomnia treated with suvorexant found a reduction in subjective time to sleep onset (sTSO) by a weighted mean difference (WMD) of 9.20 minutes at 1 month and 9.45 minutes at 3 months, but no significant difference at 12 months, and increased subjective TST (sTST) by a WMD of 20.10 minutes at month 1, 18.54 minutes at 3 months, and 17.80 minutes at 12 months compared with placebo.[45] These findings were similar to and consistent with an earlier meta-analysis which found an improvement in sTST by a WMD of 20.16 minutes, and improvement in sTSO by a WMD 7.62 minutes.[43]

The long-term safety and tolerability of suvorexant have been evaluated in clinical trials lasting up to 12 months which did not demonstrate significant withdrawal symptoms or rebound insomnia with abrupt discontinuation compared with placebo.[44] It should be noted that the doses of suvorexant in this trial were higher than those currently approved for use in the United States.

Suvorexant has also been shown to be effective and safe in the elderly population (65 years and older), with significantly improved sleep maintenance and sleep onset compared to placebo over 3 months of nightly treatment.[46] Additionally, suvorexant has a unique indication for the treatment of insomnia in mild to moderate Alzheimer disease. In this population, suvorexant at doses of 10–20 mg was found to significantly decrease WASO and increase TST on polysomnography (PSG) by a mean difference of 28 minutes compared to placebo.[47]

Clinical trial data for lemborexant 5–10 mg per night have shown it to be effective over 6 months with significant improvement in sleep variables compared to placebo, with the median subjective sleep onset latency (sSOL) reduced by 21.81 and 28.21 minutes for the 5 mg and 10 mg doses respectively, subjective WASO reduced by 46.75 and 41.95 minutes respectively, and sTST increased by 69.95 and 74.08 minutes respectively compared to baseline values at month 6 of treatment.[48] Longer-term data showed that these improvements were maintained through month 12 without evidence of rebound insomnia or withdrawal upon discontinuation.[49]

RAMELTEON

Ramelteon is a melatonin receptor agonist and is the only drug of its class that is FDA approved for treatment of sleep-onset insomnia. The drug has high affinity for the M_1 and M_2 melatonin receptors, located primarily in the suprachiasmatic nucleus (the central pacemaker of circadian timing), which is considered to account for its sleep-promoting effects.[50] Ramelteon has higher binding affinity at these sites and longer half-life than melatonin. It is a rapidly acting medication with a short half-life, making it appropriate for the treatment of sleep-onset insomnia but not sleep maintenance. The recommended dose of ramelteon is 8 mg prior to bedtime. Ramelteon should not be used in conjunction with fluvoxamine, a strong CYP1A2 inhibitor, as this combination can significantly increase ramelteon levels, and should be used with caution in patients taking other CYP1A2-inhibiting drugs.

Notably unlike BZDs, nBZRAs, and DORAs, ramelteon is not classified as a controlled substance in the United States. It has no measurable affinity for other receptor sites, a characteristic which is felt to account for its lack of abuse potential.[50]

Ramelteon's effect on SOL is modest, with a reduction of around 9–9.5 minutes as demonstrated in meta-analysis.[28,51] The long-term efficacy of ramelteon was evaluated over 6 months in a randomized controlled trial of ramelteon 8 mg versus placebo in adults and demonstrated consistent reduction in PSG-measured latency to persistent sleep compared with baseline and placebo through month 6.[52] Additionally, over the 6 months of treatment, there were no significant next-day effects seen on measures of psychomotor function, immediate and delayed memory recall, level of alertness, or ability to concentrate. Ramelteon was well tolerated with an adverse-event profile similar to that of placebo and also was not associated with rebound insomnia or withdrawal symptoms upon discontinuation after 6 months of use. Ramelteon has also been studied in elderly patients, age 65 and older, and was found to be well tolerated and effective.[53]

DOXEPIN

Doxepin is a tricyclic antidepressant with sedative effects which, at low doses of 3–6 mg, has a labeled indication for sleep-maintenance insomnia. At these very low doses, doxepin is a highly selective antagonist of the histamine (H1) receptor, which is thought to account for its soporific effects.[54] At higher doses (75–150 mg), doxepin is thought to exert antidepressant effects by inhibiting norepinephrine and serotonin reuptake.[55]

The recommended dose is 6 mg in adults and 3 mg in the elderly, taken 30 minutes prior to bedtime. A dose of 3 mg is also recommended for patients with hepatic impairment and for individuals with a tendency for urinary retention. The medication should not be taken within 3 hours of a meal to reduce the potential for next-day side effects due to delayed onset of action.

Doxepin should not be administered with monoamine oxidase inhibitors (MAOIs) or within

2 weeks of stopping an MAOI due to the risk for hypertensive crisis and serotonin syndrome. Doxepin is also contraindicated in patients with untreated narrow angle glaucoma or severe urinary retention. There is a black box warning on anti-depressants about the risk of suicidal ideation in children, adolescents, and young adults; and while the dose for insomnia is about 10 to 100 times lower than the recommended doses for depression, this risk cannot be excluded.

In terms of efficacy, in meta-analysis, doxepin at 3–6 mg was associated with significant improvements in WASO and TST, with a mean reduction in WASO of 22–23 minutes and a mean increase in TST by 26–32 minutes compared to placebo.[28] In clinical trials, the most common adverse reactions with doxepin compared to placebo were somnolence/sedation, nausea, and upper respiratory tract infection.[28]

In the elderly, doxepin has been shown to be effective and well tolerated with a 12-week study of doxepin 1–3 mg showing significant improvement in measures of WASO, TST, overall SE, and SE in the last quarter of the night compared to placebo.[56] Additionally, during this study there was no rebound insomnia noted after discontinuation, as well as no significant next-day residual effects, including no reports of memory impairment, complex sleep behaviors, anticholinergic effects, weight gain, or increased appetite. These results are similar to that of a 4-week study of doxepin 6 mg versus placebo in elderly chronic insomnia patients which found sustained significant improvement in patient-reported TST and WASO compared to placebo without reported anticholinergic effects or memory impairment.[57]

OFF-LABEL MEDICATIONS

These medications are not recommended as a first-line treatment for primary insomnia but can be considered in cases where patients have comorbid conditions which may also respond to treatment, or in cases where first-line medications must be avoided or were not effective.

Antidepressants

Doxepin is the only antidepressant with FDA indication for insomnia; however, other sedating antidepressants are commonly prescribed in an off-label manner for the treatment of insomnia. In 2006, off-label antidepressants were prescribed significantly more frequently for insomnia than nBZRAs and BZDs.[58]

TRAZODONE

Trazodone is one of the most commonly prescribed off-label antidepressants for insomnia.[59] Trazodone has a hypnotic effect at low doses (~25–100 mg) due to blockade of serotonin receptors, histamine receptors, and $\alpha 1$ adrenergic receptors, and has antidepressant effects due to inhibition of the serotonin reuptake transporter at higher dosages (>150 mg).[60] While commonly prescribed, the data for trazodone for the treatment of primary insomnia are weak.

A 2018 meta-analysis including 7 randomized placebo-controlled trials of trazodone for insomnia did find that patients receiving trazodone perceived better sleep quality and had fewer awakenings than those receiving placebo; however, there was no significant improvement in objective measures of sleep efficiency, sleep latency, total sleep time, or wake after sleep onset.[61] It should be noted that only 2 of the 7 trials included in the meta-analysis were performed in subjects with primary insomnia; the other 5 trials included secondary causes of insomnia. A 2018 Cochrane review found equivocal data to support short-term use trazodone, given small improvement in sleep quality demonstrated in clinical trials, but with no evidence to support long-term use.[62]

The 2017 AASM Clinical Practice Guidelines for pharmacotherapy for chronic insomnia recommended against the use of trazodone for sleep-onset and maintenance insomnia, citing an absence of demonstrated efficacy and limited evidence regarding harms, which outweighed the benefits.[28] It should be noted that only a single study of trazodone 50 mg met the inclusion criteria, and while there was subjective improvement in sleep latency and duration, it did not meet the threshold for clinically significant improvement in this review.[63]

As with the evidence for efficacy, the evidence of trazodone's safety in primary insomnia is lacking. One small randomized, double-blind, placebo-controlled study of 16 patients with primary insomnia assessed the effects of

50 mg of trazodone on subsequent daytime impairments and found impaired next-day memory performance, equilibrium, and muscle endurance relative to placebo.[64] However, a larger meta-analysis found trazodone to be well tolerated with no serious adverse events reported in patients receiving trazodone compared to placebo.[61] The reported adverse effects were mild to moderate and included daytime sleepiness, gastrointestinal discomfort, dizziness, and dry mouth. Other potential additional adverse effects of trazodone include orthostatic hypotension, syncope, QT prolongation, priapism, blurred vision, activation of mania or hypomania, bleeding risk, and risk for serotonin syndrome.

MIRTAZAPINE

Mirtazapine is a tetra-cyclic antidepressant which enhances noradrenergic and serotonergic neurotransmission without inhibiting reuptake; however, its exact mechanism of action is not fully known.[65,66] Mirtazapine additionally has potent histamine blocking effects, which may account for its sedating effects. It has FDA indications for the treatment of major depressive disorder in adults with recommended doses of 15–45 mg per day, but doses used off-label for sleep are typically lower, 7.5–15 mg at bedtime.

There is a paucity of data in primary insomnia. There have been small studies evaluating the effects of mirtazapine on insomnia in patients with depression. In patients with major depressive disorder, mirtazapine 30 mg nightly for 9 weeks showed significant improvement in WASO and subjective insomnia severity ratings, in addition to a reduction in depressive symptoms. Similarly, a study randomizing patients with major depressive disorder to mirtazapine 15–45 mg/day or fluoxetine 20–40 mg/day found significant improvement in SOL, sleep efficiency (SE), and WASO, after only 2 weeks of mirtazapine treatment, while there were no significant changes with fluoxetine.[67] A case series of 28 male patients with depressive symptoms, insomnia, and suicidal ideation found improvement or resolution of insomnia symptoms and suicidal ideation over 8 weeks treatment with mirtazapine 7.5–30 mg at bedtime.[68] While there may be benefit in these populations, more research is needed prior to being able to recommend mirtazapine for the treatment of primary insomnia. It may be appropriate in patients with depression and comorbid insomnia.

TRICYCLIC ANTIDEPRESSANTS

There are no placebo-controlled studies of the tricyclic antidepressants, amitriptyline, and nortriptyline, for treatment of primary insomnia. In clinical practice, patients with comorbid conditions such as pain disorders, for which the drug is indicated, and which concomitantly impact sleep and contribute to insomnia, may benefit from the analgesic and sedating properties of these medications, but their use for primary insomnia is not typically recommended.

Antipsychotics

Quetiapine is a second-generation atypical antipsychotic medication with indications for schizophrenia, bipolar disorder, and as an adjunct treatment of major depressive disorder. Given its sedating properties, mediated by antagonism of histamine (H1) and serotonin (type 2A) receptors, it has been used off-label for insomnia but typically at doses much lower than those recommended for psychiatric disorders.

There is a paucity of data on quetiapine for insomnia. A small open-label pilot study of quetiapine at doses of 25–75 mg (which are below the typical antipsychotic dose of 150–800 mg) in 18 subjects with primary insomnia showed improvement in TST and SE over 6 weeks but no improvement in SOL.[69] A small (n = 13) randomized, double-blind, placebo-controlled study of quetiapine in patients with primary insomnia did not find any statistically significant improvement in TST or SOL.[70]

Based on the paucity of data and potential for possible adverse effects, including weight gain, hepatoxicity, restless legs syndrome, and akathisia, quetiapine is not recommended for treatment of primary insomnia.[28,71,72]

Anti-epilepticsThe alpha-2 detla ligand (gabapentinoid) drugs gabapentin and pregabalin are commonly used for the treatment of restless leg syndrome but have a limited role in the treatment of insomnia, primarily as an adjunct in patients with chronic pain conditions which interfere with sleep.

GABAPENTIN

There has been little investigation regarding the off-label use of the sedating anti-epileptic drug gabapentin for the treatment of insomnia. Gabapentin has FDA indications for post-herpetic neuralgia and as an adjunctive treatment for partial seizures. Gabapentin is structurally similar to the inhibitory neurotransmitter GABA, characterized by high-affinity binding to the α2δ protein, an auxiliary subunit of voltage-gated calcium channels in the central nervous system.[73] The complete mechanism of action of gabapentin remains unknown.

Randomized, double-blind, placebo-controlled studies utilizing gabapentin at doses of 250–500 mg in subjects who had reported experiencing "occasional disturbed sleep" showed benefit in terms of increasing total sleep time and decreasing wake after sleep onset with gabapentin compared to placebo.[74,75] Similarly, a study of gabapentin administered at doses of 200–900 mg in subjects with chronic insomnia showed improved sleep efficiency and decreased wake after sleep onset; however, this study was not placebo controlled.[76]

Outside of primary insomnia, there is some limited evidence that gabapentin subjectively improves insomnia symptoms related to alcohol dependence and withdrawal.[77–79]

PREGABALIN

Pregabalin is a novel compound, structurally related to gabapentin, which binds to the α2δ subunits of voltage-gated calcium channels and subtly reduces the synaptic release of several neurotransmitters[80] Pregabalin has FDA indications for the treatment of post-herpetic neuralgia, neuropathic pain associated with diabetic peripheral neuropathy and with spinal cord injury, fibromyalgia, and adjunctive treatment of partial onset seizures. While there have not been studies of pregabalin in primary insomnia, it has been studied in several conditions with associated insomnia or sleep disturbance. Treatment with pregabalin has been associated with improvement in insomnia in patients with generalized anxiety disorder presenting with high levels of insomnia.[81,82] Pregabalin has been shown to improve sleep continuity in patients with painful diabetic neuropathy, to improve subjective sleep quality in patients with fibromyalgia with moderate to severe pain, as well as improving sleep disturbances in those with post-herpetic neuralgia.[74,83,84]

Given the paucity of data, gabapentin and pregabalin are not recommended for treatment of primary insomnia but may be appropriate in patients with pain conditions that contribute to disrupted sleep.

Antihistamines

First generation anti-histamine drugs cross the blood brain barier and are well known to cause sedation, a side effect that has led to their use as off-label presciption and over counter sleep aids.

HYDROXYZINE

Hydroxyzine is a first-generation antihistamine and a potent histamine 1 (H1) antagonist which is used off-label for insomnia given its sedating properties.[85] Hydroxyzine has FDA-approved indications for treatment of anxiety, in allergic conditions such as pruritus or urticaria, and as adjunctive therapy for procedural or pre- or postoperative sedation. Despite off-label use for insomnia, there have not been any studies of hydroxyzine in subjects with primary insomnia. A small study investigated the effects of hydroxyzine 25–50 mg on sleep parameters measured by continuous electroencephalogram (EEG) in healthy volunteers and found significant reductions, about 50%, in SOL at both doses, compared to placebo, and significant increases in TST in female subjects only.[86] Given the lack of available data, hydroxyzine is not recommended for treatment of primary insomnia.

OVER-THE-COUNTER ANTIHISTAMINES

Diphenhydramine and doxylamine are two first-generation antihistamines sold over the counter, without prescriptions, as sleep aids. They are highly selective antagonists at the H1 receptor but also at the muscarinic receptor, which can lead to significant side effects such as dizziness, dry mouth, urinary retention, constipation, and confusion.[87]

Several literature reviews have found little evidence to support the use of diphenhydramine or doxylamine for insomnia, and given the lack of efficacy data and potential for adverse effects, these medications are not recommended for treatment of chronic insomnia but might be appropriate for short-term use of acute insomnia in otherwise healthy non-elderly adults.[87,88]

Supplements

Many dietary supplements are marketed for insomnia however, there is generally insufficient evidence supporting their use. In the US, the FDA does not regulate dietary supplements in the same manner as other presciption and ove the counter medications. Because of this, manufacturers are not required to demonstrate the effictiveness of their products before selling them to consumers.

MELATONIN

In the United States, melatonin is a commonly used supplement for insomnia. Melatonin is an endogenous hormone synthesized and released by the pineal gland, and its production and release are mediated by the suprachiasmatic nuclei of the hypothalamus, central circadian pacemaker, and thus melatonin secretion is an important physiologic sleep regulator in humans.[89]

Melatonin, in both controlled-release and immediate-release formulations, is widely available over the counter in many forms, including pills, patches, gummies, sprays, and liquids. As melatonin is classified as a dietary supplement, it does not require a prescription in the United States and is not subject to the same regulatory oversight by the FDA as prescription medications, and quality and purity can differ substantially, with one study showing melatonin content varying from −83% to + 478% of the labeled content.[90]

While generally regarded as safe, there is insufficient evidence to recommend melatonin for the treatment of insomnia, and methodologically there are inconsistencies in dosing and administration among available studies.[28,91] Of the available evidence, a 2013 meta-analysis found significant reduction in SOL with immediate-release melatonin (at varying doses) compared to placebo, with subjects randomly assigned to melatonin falling asleep 7 minutes earlier on average than those taking placebo; however, when looking at objective measures only, the reduction in SOL was 5.5 minutes.[92] The same analysis also found that melatonin also significantly increased TST compared to placebo by 8 minutes on average, but when stratified to objective measures, statistical significance was not reached.

There is limited evidence which suggests that prolonged-release melatonin given at a dose of 2 mg may be beneficial for elderly patients with insomnia, with demonstrated reduction in SOL by 9 to 19 minutes and improvement in self-reported sleep quality with use.[93–95] However, these studies have been criticized for publication bias, heterogeneity, and imprecision.[28] Further research in this area is needed.

OTHER SUPPLEMENTS

There is not sufficient evidence to recommend use of valerian root, kava kava, chamomile, tryptophan, or wuling for insomnia.[96,97] Significant adverse effects have been reported with kava kava, including case reports of fulminant liver failure and acute hepatitis.[98]

DISCONTINUING MEDICATION

The duration of treatment should be individualized for each patient. Given the limited and typically short duration of clinical trial data, the long-term effect of prolonged treatment is not well known. Several studies have shown an association between long-term use of BZDs (>1 year) and cognitive impairment, as well as an increased risk of Alzheimer disease.[99] However, a recent large-scale study did not find an association between use of BZDs or nBZRAs and subsequent dementia and found that patients with the highest use had the lowest odds of developing dementia.[100] Further research is needed on this topic.

If prescribing for extended periods of time, continued reassessment of risks, benefits, and potential adverse effects is necessary. When choosing to discontinue long-term treatment, slow tapering can be utilized, in conjunction with CBT-I, to lessen the effects of rebound insomnia and anxiety surrounding discontinuation, and to improve the likelihood of successful abstinence.[101,102]

CONCLUSION

Insomnia is a common condition for which patients seek medical care. In cases where medications are indicated, there are several classes of medications which can be utilized. Appropriate selection of medication should be individualized, taking into account the patient's pattern of sleep difficulty—whether sleep onset, sleep maintenance, or mixed insomnia—and the pharmacodynamic and pharmacokinetic properties of the available drugs, as well as potential adverse effects, risks, and benefits of treatment.

REFERENCES

1. Ohayon MM. Epidemiology of insomnia: What we know and what we still need to learn. *Sleep Med Rev*. 2002;6(2):97–111.
2. Ford ES, Wheaton AG, Cunningham TJ, Giles WH, Chapman DP, Croft JB. Trends in outpatient visits for insomnia, sleep apnea, and prescriptions for sleep medications among US adults: Findings from the National Ambulatory Medical Care survey 1999–2010. *Sleep*. 2014;37(8):1283–1293.
3. American Academy of Sleep Medicine. *International Classification of Sleep Disorders*. 3rd ed. American Academy of Sleep Medicine; 2014.
4. Roth T, Roehrs T. Insomnia: Epidemiology, characteristics, and consequences. *Clin Cornerstone*. 2003;5(3):5–15.
5. Qaseem A, Kansagara D, Forciea MA, Cooke M, Denberg TD, Clinical Guidelines Committee of the American College of Physicians. Management of chronic insomnia disorder in adults: A clinical practice guideline from the American College of Physicians. *Ann Intern Med*. 2016;165(2):125–133.
6. Riemann D, Baglioni C, Bassetti C, et al. European guideline for the diagnosis and treatment of insomnia. *J Sleep Res*. 2017;26(6):675–700.
7. Schutte-Rodin S, Broch L, Buysse D, Dorsey C, Sateia M. Clinical guideline for the evaluation and management of chronic insomnia in adults. *J Clin Sleep Med*. 2008;4(5):487–504.
8. Pigeon WR, Bishop TM, Krueger KM. Insomnia as a precipitating factor in new onset mental illness: A systematic review of recent findings. *Curr Psychiatry Rep*. 2017;19(8):44.
9. Ohayon MM. Observation of the natural evolution of insomnia in the American general population cohort. *Sleep Med Clin*. 2009;4(1):87–92.
10. Pigeon WR, Pinquart M, Conner K. Meta-analysis of sleep disturbance and suicidal thoughts and behaviors. *J Clin Psychiatry*. 2012;73(9):e1160–e1167.
11. Nadorff MR, Nazem S, Fiske A. Insomnia symptoms, nightmares, and suicide risk: Duration of sleep disturbance matters. *Suicide Life Threat Behav*. 2013;43(2):139–149.
12. Guilleminault C. Benzodiazepines, breathing, and sleep. *Am J Med*. 1990;88(3A):25S–S28.
13. Wang SH, Chen WS, Tang SE, et al. Benzodiazepines associated with acute respiratory failure in patients with obstructive sleep apnea. *Front Pharmacol*. 2018;9:1513.
14. Zhang Y, Ren R, Lei F, et al. Worldwide and regional prevalence rates of co-occurrence of insomnia and insomnia symptoms with obstructive sleep apnea: A systematic review and meta-analysis. *Sleep Med Rev*. 2019;45:1–17.
15. Mason M, Cates CJ, Smith I. Effects of opioid, hypnotic and sedating medications on sleep-disordered breathing in adults with obstructive sleep apnoea. *Cochrane Database Syst Rev*. 2015;7:CD011090.
16. Kryger M, Wang-Weigand S, Roth T. Safety of ramelteon in individuals with mild to moderate obstructive sleep apnea. *Sleep Breath*. 2007;11(3):159–164.
17. Sun H, Palcza J, Card D, et al. Effects of suvorexant, an orexin receptor antagonist, on respiration during sleep in patients with obstructive sleep apnea. *J Clin Sleep Med*. 2016;12(1):9–17.
18. Cheng JY, Filippov G, Moline M, Zammit GK, Bsharat M, Hall N. Respiratory safety of lemborexant in healthy adult and elderly subjects with mild obstructive sleep apnea: A randomized, double-blind, placebo-controlled, crossover study. *J Sleep Res*. 2020;29(4):e13021.
19. Harbourt K, Nevo ON, Zhang R, Chan V, Croteau D. Association of eszopiclone, zaleplon, or zolpidem with complex sleep behaviors resulting in serious injuries, including death. *Pharmacoepidemiol Drug Saf*. 2020;29(6):684–691.
20. Patel D, Steinberg J, Patel P. Insomnia in the elderly: A review. *J Clin Sleep Med*. 2018;14(6):1017–1024.
21. American Geriatrics Society Beers Criteria Update Expert Panel. American Geriatrics Society 2019 updated AGS Beers Criteria® for potentially inappropriate medication use in older adults. *J Am Geriatr Soc*. 2019;67(4):674–694.
22. Glass J, Lanctot KL, Herrmann N, Sproule BA, Busto UE. Sedative hypnotics in older people with insomnia: Meta-analysis of risks and benefits. *BMJ*. 2005;331(7526):1169.
23. Griffin CE III, Kaye AM, Bueno FR, Kaye AD. Benzodiazepine pharmacology and central nervous system-mediated effects. *Ochsner J*. 2013;13(2):214–223.
24. Sanger DJ. The pharmacology and mechanisms of action of new generation, non-benzodiazepine hypnotic agents. *CNS Drugs*. 2004;18(Suppl 1):9–15; discussion 41, 3–5.
25. Holbrook AM, Crowther R, Lotter A, Cheng C, King D. Meta-analysis of benzodiazepine use in the treatment of insomnia. *CMAJ*. 2000;162(2):225–233.
26. Hernandez I, He M, Brooks MM, Zhang Y. Exposure-response association between concurrent opioid and benzodiazepine use and risk of opioid-related overdose in Medicare Part D beneficiaries. *JAMA Netw Open*. 2018;1(2):e180919.

27. Gudin JA, Mogali S, Jones JD, Comer SD. Risks, management, and monitoring of combination opioid, benzodiazepines, and/or alcohol use. *Postgrad Med.* 2013;125(4):115–130.
28. Sateia MJ, Buysse DJ, Krystal AD, Neubauer DN, Heald JL. Clinical practice guideline for the pharmacologic treatment of chronic insomnia in adults: An American Academy of Sleep Medicine clinical practice guideline. *J Clin Sleep Med.* 2017;13(2):307–349.
29. Aden GC, Thatcher C. Quazepam in the short-term treatment of insomnia in outpatients. *J Clin Psychiatry.* 1983;44(12):454–456.
30. Bliwise D, Seidel W, Greenblatt DJ, Dement W. Nighttime and daytime efficacy of flurazepam and oxazepam in chronic insomnia. *Am J Psychiatry.* 1984;141(2):191–195.
31. Cohn JB, Wilcox CS, Bremner J, Ettinger M. Hypnotic efficacy of estazolam compared with flurazepam in outpatients with insomnia. *J Clin Pharmacol.* 1991;31(8):747–750.
32. Lunesta (eszopiclone). Package insert. Sunovion Pharmaceuticals; 2014.
33. Rosner S, Englbrecht C, Wehrle R, Hajak G, Soyka M. Eszopiclone for insomnia. *Cochrane Database Syst Rev.* 2018;10:CD010703.
34. Roth T, Walsh JK, Krystal A, Wessel T, Roehrs TA. An evaluation of the efficacy and safety of eszopiclone over 12 months in patients with chronic primary insomnia. *Sleep Med.* 2005;6(6):487–495.
35. Ancoli-Israel S, Krystal AD, McCall WV, et al. A 12-week, randomized, double-blind, placebo-controlled study evaluating the effect of eszopiclone 2 mg on sleep/wake function in older adults with primary and comorbid insomnia. *Sleep.* 2010;33(2):225–234.
36. Hedner J, Yaeche R, Emilien G, Farr I, Salinas E. Zaleplon shortens subjective sleep latency and improves subjective sleep quality in elderly patients with insomnia: The Zaleplon Clinical Investigator Study Group. *Int J Geriatr Psychiatry.* 2000;15(8):704–712.
37. Walsh JK, Vogel GW, Scharf M, et al. A five week, polysomnographic assessment of zaleplon 10 mg for the treatment of primary insomnia. *Sleep Med.* 2000;1(1):41–49.
38. Fry J, Scharf M, Mangano R, Fujimori M. Zaleplon improves sleep without producing rebound effects in outpatients with insomnia: Zaleplon Clinical Study Group. *Int Clin Psychopharmacol.* 2000;15(3):141–152.
39. Farkas RH, Unger EF, Temple R. Zolpidem and driving impairment: Identifying persons at risk. *N Engl J Med.* 2013;369(8):689–691.
40. Greenblatt DJ, Roth T. Zolpidem for insomnia. *Expert Opin Pharmacother.* 2012;13(6):879–893.
41. Beuckmann CT, Suzuki M, Ueno T, Nagaoka K, Arai T, Higashiyama H. In vitro and in silico characterization of lemborexant (E2006), a novel dual orexin receptor antagonist. *J Pharmacol Exp Ther.* 2017;362(2):287–295.
42. Winrow CJ, Gotter AL, Cox CD, et al. Promotion of sleep by suvorexant-a novel dual orexin receptor antagonist. *J Neurogenet.* 2011;25(1-2):52–61.
43. Kishi T, Nomura I, Matsuda Y, et al. Lemborexant vs suvorexant for insomnia: A systematic review and network meta-analysis. *J Psychiatr Res.* 2020;128:68–74.
44. Michelson D, Snyder E, Paradis E, et al. Safety and efficacy of suvorexant during 1-year treatment of insomnia with subsequent abrupt treatment discontinuation: A phase 3 randomised, double-blind, placebo-controlled trial. *Lancet Neurol.* 2014;13(5):461–471.
45. Kuriyama A, Tabata H. Suvorexant for the treatment of primary insomnia: A systematic review and meta-analysis. *Sleep Med Rev.* 2017;35:1–7.
46. Herring WJ, Connor KM, Snyder E, et al. Suvorexant in elderly patients with insomnia: Pooled analyses of data from phase III randomized controlled clinical trials. *Am J Geriatr Psychiatry.* 2017;25(7):791–802.
47. Herring WJ, Ceesay P, Snyder E, et al. Polysomnographic assessment of suvorexant in patients with probable Alzheimer's disease dementia and insomnia: A randomized trial. *Alzheimers Dement.* 2020;16(3):541–551.
48. Karppa M, Yardley J, Pinner K, et al. Long-term efficacy and tolerability of lemborexant compared with placebo in adults with insomnia disorder: Results from the phase 3 randomized clinical trial SUNRISE 2. *Sleep.* 2020;43(9):1–11.
49. Yardley J, Karppa M, Inoue Y, et al. Long-term effectiveness and safety of lemborexant in adults with insomnia disorder: Results from a phase 3 randomized clinical trial. *Sleep Med.* 2021;80:333–342.
50. Kato K, Hirai K, Nishiyama K, et al. Neurochemical properties of ramelteon (TAK-375), a selective MT1/MT2 receptor agonist. *Neuropharmacology.* 2005;48(2):301–310.
51. Kuriyama A, Honda M, Hayashino Y. Ramelteon for the treatment of insomnia in adults: A systematic review and meta-analysis. *Sleep Med.* 2014;15(4):385–392.
52. Mayer G, Wang-Weigand S, Roth-Schechter B, Lehmann R, Staner C, Partinen M. Efficacy and safety of 6-month nightly ramelteon administration in adults with chronic primary insomnia. *Sleep.* 2009;32(3):351–360.
53. Roth T, Seiden D, Sainati S, Wang-Weigand S, Zhang J, Zee P. Effects of ramelteon on patient-reported sleep latency in older adults with chronic insomnia. *Sleep Med.* 2006;7(4):312–318.
54. Goforth HW. Low-dose doxepin for the treatment of insomnia: Emerging data. *Expert Opin Pharmacother.* 2009;10(10):1649–1655.
55. Stahl SM. Selective histamine H1 antagonism: Novel hypnotic and pharmacologic actions challenge classical notions of antihistamines. *CNS Spectr.* 2008;13(12):1027–1038.
56. Krystal AD, Durrence HH, Scharf M, et al. Efficacy and safety of doxepin 1 mg and 3 mg in a 12-week sleep laboratory and outpatient trial of elderly subjects with chronic primary insomnia. *Sleep.* 2010;33(11):1553–1561.
57. Lankford A, Rogowski R, Essink B, Ludington E, Heith Durrence H, Roth T. Efficacy and safety of doxepin 6 mg in a four-week outpatient trial of elderly adults with chronic primary insomnia. *Sleep Med.* 2012;13(2):133–138.
58. Lai LL, Tan MH, Lai YC. Prevalence and factors associated with off-label antidepressant prescriptions for insomnia. *Drug Healthc Patient Saf.* 2011;3:27–36.
59. Vijay A, Becker JE, Ross JS. Patterns and predictors of off-label prescription of psychiatric drugs. *PLoS One.* 2018;13(7):e0198363.

60. Stahl SM. Mechanism of action of trazodone: A multifunctional drug. *CNS Spectr*. 2009;14(10):536–546.
61. Yi XY, Ni SF, Ghadami MR, et al. Trazodone for the treatment of insomnia: A meta-analysis of randomized placebo-controlled trials. *Sleep Med*. 2018;45:25–32.
62. Everitt H, Baldwin DS, Stuart B, et al. Antidepressants for insomnia in adults. *Cochrane Database Syst Rev*. 2018;5:CD010753.
63. Walsh JK, Erman M, Erwin CW, et al. Subjective hypnotic efficacy of trazodone and zolpidem in DSMIII-R primary insomnia. *Hum Psychopharm Clin*. 1998;13(3):191–198.
64. Roth AJ, McCall WV, Liguori A. Cognitive, psychomotor and polysomnographic effects of trazodone in primary insomniacs. J Sleep Res. 2011;20(4):552–558.
65. Davis R, Wilde MI. Mirtazapine. *CNS Drugs*. 1996;5(5):389–402.
66. Stimmel GL, Dopheide JA, Stahl SM. Mirtazapine: An antidepressant with noradrenergic and specific serotonergic effects. *Pharmacotherapy*. 1997;17(1):10–21.
67. Winokur A, DeMartinis NA III, McNally DP, Gary EM, Cormier JL, Gary KA. Comparative effects of mirtazapine and fluoxetine on sleep physiology measures in patients with major depression and insomnia. *J Clin Psychiatry*. 2003;64(10):1224–1229.
68. Gandotra K, Chen P, Jaskiw GE, Konicki PE, Strohl KP. Effective treatment of insomnia with mirtazapine attenuates concomitant suicidal ideation. *J Clin Sleep Med*. 2018;14(5):901–902.
69. Wiegand MH, Landry F, Bruckner T, Pohl C, Vesely Z, Jahn T. Quetiapine in primary insomnia: A pilot study. *Psychopharmacology (Berl)*. 2008;196(2):337–338.
70. Tassniyom K, Paholpak S, Tassniyom S, Kiewyoo J. Quetiapine for primary insomnia: A double blind, randomized controlled trial. *J Med Assoc Thai*. 2010;93(6):729–734.
71. Coe HV, Hong IS. Safety of low doses of quetiapine when used for insomnia. *Ann Pharmacother*. 2012;46(5):718–722.
72. Anderson SL, Vande Griend JP. Quetiapine for insomnia: A review of the literature. *Am J Health Syst Pharm*. 2014;71(5):394–402.
73. Sills GJ. The mechanisms of action of gabapentin and pregabalin. *Curr Opin Pharmacol*. 2006;6(1):108–113.
74. Rosenberg RP, Hull SG, Lankford DA, et al. A randomized, double-blind, single-dose, placebo-controlled, multicenter, polysomnographic study of gabapentin in transient insomnia induced by sleep phase advance. *J Clin Sleep Med*. 2014;10(10):1093–1100.
75. Furey SA, Hull SG, Leibowitz MT, Jayawardena S, Roth T. A randomized, double-blind, placebo-controlled, multicenter, 28-day, polysomnographic study of gabapentin in transient insomnia induced by sleep phase advance. *J Clin Sleep Med*. 2014;10(10):1101–1109.
76. Lo HS, Yang CM, Lo HG, Lee CY, Ting H, Tzang BS. Treatment effects of gabapentin for primary insomnia. *Clin Neuropharmacol*. 2010;33(2):84–90.
77. Karam-Hage M, Brower KJ. Gabapentin treatment for insomnia associated with alcohol dependence. *Am J Psychiatry*. 2000;157(1):151.
78. Mason BJ, Goodell V, Shadan F. Gabapentin treatment for alcohol dependence: Reply. *JAMA Intern Med*. 2014;174(7):1201–1202.
79. Malcolm R, Myrick LH, Veatch LM, Boyle E, Randall PK. Self-reported sleep, sleepiness, and repeated alcohol withdrawals: A randomized, double blind, controlled comparison of lorazepam vs gabapentin. *J Clin Sleep Med*. 2007;3(1):24–32.
80. Taylor CP, Angelotti T, Fauman E. Pharmacology and mechanism of action of pregabalin: The calcium channel alpha2-delta (alpha2-delta) subunit as a target for antiepileptic drug discovery. *Epilepsy Res*. 2007;73(2):137–150.
81. Holsboer-Trachsler E, Prieto R. Effects of pregabalin on sleep in generalized anxiety disorder. *Int J Neuropsychopharmacol*. 2013;16(4):925–936.
82. Montgomery SA, Herman BK, Schweizer E, Mandel FS. The efficacy of pregabalin and benzodiazepines in generalized anxiety disorder presenting with high levels of insomnia. *Int Clin Psychopharmacol*. 2009;24(4):214–222.
83. Boyle J, Eriksson ME, Gribble L, et al. Randomized, placebo-controlled comparison of amitriptyline, duloxetine, and pregabalin in patients with chronic diabetic peripheral neuropathic pain: Impact on pain, polysomnographic sleep, daytime functioning, and quality of life. *Diabetes Care*. 2012;35(12):2451–2458.
84. Sabatowski R, Galvez R, Cherry DA, et al. Pregabalin reduces pain and improves sleep and mood disturbances in patients with post-herpetic neuralgia: Results of a randomised, placebo-controlled clinical trial. *Pain*. 2004;109(1–2):26–35.
85. Monti JM, Monti D. Histamine H 1 receptor antagonists in the treatment of insomnia. *CNS Drugs*. 2000;13(2):87–96.
86. Alford C, Rombaut N, Jones J, Foley S, Idzikowski C, Hindmarch I. Acute effects of hydroxyzine on nocturnal sleep and sleep tendency the following day: AC-EEG study. *Human Psychopharmacol*. 1992;7(1):25–35.
87. Griend JPV, Anderson SL. Histamine-1 receptor antagonism for treatment of insomnia. *J Am Pharm Assoc*. 2012;52(6):e210–e219.
88. Culpepper L, Wingertzahn MA. Over-the-counter agents for the treatment of occasional disturbed sleep or transient insomnia: A systematic review of efficacy and safety. *Prim Care Companion CNS Disord*. 2015;17(6).
89. Claustrat B, Brun J, Chazot G. The basic physiology and pathophysiology of melatonin. *Sleep Med Rev*. 2005;9(1):11–24.
90. Erland LA, Saxena PK. Melatonin natural health products and supplements: Presence of serotonin and significant variability of melatonin content. *J Clin Sleep Med*. 2017;13(2):275–281.
91. Andersen LPH, Gögenur I, Rosenberg J, Reiter RJ. The safety of melatonin in humans. *Clin Drug Invest*. 2016;36(3):169–175.
92. Ferracioli-Oda E, Qawasmi A, Bloch MH. Meta-analysis: Melatonin for the treatment of primary sleep disorders. *PLoS One*. 2013;8(5):e63773.
93. Wade AG, Ford I, Crawford G, et al. Nightly treatment of primary insomnia with prolonged release melatonin for 6 months: A randomized placebo controlled trial on age and endogenous melatonin as predictors of efficacy and safety. *BMC Med*. 2010;8:51.

94. Lemoine P, Nir T, Laudon M, Zisapel N. Prolonged-release melatonin improves sleep quality and morning alertness in insomnia patients aged 55 years and older and has no withdrawal effects. *J Sleep Res*. 2007;16(4):372–380.
95. Luthringer R, Muzet M, Zisapel N, Staner L. The effect of prolonged-release melatonin on sleep measures and psychomotor performance in elderly patients with insomnia. *Int Clin Psychopharmacol*. 2009;24(5):239–249.
96. Leach MJ, Page AT. Herbal medicine for insomnia: A systematic review and meta-analysis. *Sleep Med Rev*. 2015;24:1–12.
97. Meolie AL, Rosen C, Kristo D, et al. Oral nonprescription treatment for insomnia: An evaluation of products with limited evidence. *J Clin Sleep Med*. 2005;1(2):173–187.
98. Clouatre DL. Kava kava: Examining new reports of toxicity. *Toxicol Lett*. 2004;150(1):85–96.
99. Barker MJ, Greenwood KM, Jackson M, Crowe SF. Cognitive effects of long-term benzodiazepine use: A meta-analysis. *CNS Drugs*. 2004;18(1):37–48.
100. Osler M, Jorgensen MB. Associations of benzodiazepines, z-drugs, and other anxiolytics with subsequent dementia in patients with affective disorders: A nationwide cohort and nested case-control study. *Am J Psychiatry*. 2020;177(6):497–505.
101. Morin CM, Bastien C, Guay B, Radouco-Thomas M, Leblanc J, Vallieres A. Randomized clinical trial of supervised tapering and cognitive behavior therapy to facilitate benzodiazepine discontinuation in older adults with chronic insomnia. *Am J Psychiatry*. 2004;161(2):332–342.
102. Takaesu Y, Utsumi T, Okajima I, et al. Psychosocial intervention for discontinuing benzodiazepine hypnotics in patients with chronic insomnia: A systematic review and meta-analysis. *Sleep Med Rev*. 2019;48:101214.

Chapter 14

Non-Pharmacological Treatments of Insomnia

Kyle Rexer, Libby Cardoni, and J. Todd Arnedt

Chronic insomnia is characterized by nocturnal complaints of difficulty falling asleep, staying asleep, and/or early morning awakenings that contribute to daytime impairment.[1] It is a highly prevalent disorder, impacting 5%–15% of adults in the United States,[1,2] with higher rates among women, older adults, and individuals from low socioeconomic status (SES) backgrounds. Chronic insomnia is associated with an increased risk for psychiatric disorders,[3,4] substance use disorders,[3,5] and medical problems,[6] and it worsens comorbid conditions[7] as well as quality of life.[8] Insomnia is one of the most burdensome disorders not only at the individual level, but at a societal level[9] as well, with estimated total costs as high as $108 billion annually.[10]

Despite the high prevalence and burden of insomnia, the availability of effective treatment options remains insufficient. While prescription medications and over-the-counter sleep aids are widely available and can provide rapid symptomatic relief, they are not a long-term solution for many. Medications can cause unpleasant side effects, increase fall risk, lead to tolerance, and many patients simply prefer non-pharmacological approaches.[11,12] For these reasons, several behavioral interventions have been developed, and evidence supports their use in many cases as first-line treatments for chronic insomnia.[13]

The purpose of this chapter is to describe current and emerging non-pharmacological approaches to treating insomnia. For each treatment, we will review the primary components, evidence regarding their efficacy, and offer some clinical considerations relevant to each non-pharmacological approach.

COGNITIVE BEHAVIORAL THERAPY FOR INSOMNIA (CBT-I)

Cognitive behavioral therapy for insomnia (CBT-I) is a relatively brief, empirically supported, multicomponent treatment targeting patients' maladaptive cognitions and behaviors that interfere with sleep. CBT-I is based on the most recognized conceptual model of chronic insomnia, commonly referred to as the 3-P model.[14] This model suggests that predisposing, precipitating, and perpetuating factors all contribute to the development and maintenance of insomnia over time. *Predisposing* factors refer to existing characteristics that make a person more sensitive to developing sleep issues, such as genetics. Acute insomnia may result when a predisposed individual encounters distressing circumstances, or *precipitating* events, such as the diagnosis of a medical condition or a major change in family structure. In many cases of acute insomnia, sleep will return to baseline once the stressor resolves. According to the 3-P model, chronic insomnia develops when individuals engage in maladaptive strategies to improve sleep or to mitigate the daytime consequences of insomnia. These strategies, referred to as *perpetuating* factors, may include spending excessive periods in bed, napping during the day, consuming excessive caffeine, and developing irregular sleep schedules. Individuals may additionally have unhelpful beliefs about sleep or develop worry and anxiety about their inability to sleep. In accordance with the 3-P model, CBT-I addresses the perpetuating factors that contribute to the maintenance of insomnia via (1) basic education about the sleep process, (2) altering maladaptive sleep behaviors, (3) altering maladaptive cognitions, and (4) addressing hyperarousal and/or anxiety about sleep.

The CBT-I protocol is often completed in 4–6 weekly or biweekly sessions, each lasting 30–60 minutes. Treatment can be delivered individually, in groups, by telephone or telemedicine, or via guided or unguided self-help strategies (e.g., bibliotherapy, internet-delivered). During treatment, patients are tasked with recording information about their sleep (in the form of a structured sleep diary) and practicing skills learned in-session. Each session is structured and involves a review of the sleep diary, adjustment of the prescribed sleep schedule, and introduction/review of sleep skills. Typically, CBT-I will include elements of sleep hygiene, stimulus control, sleep restriction, relaxation techniques, and cognitive therapy.

Empirical Evidence

Several meta-analyses have shown CBT-I to produce moderate to large treatment effects across numerous self-reported sleep parameters, including: (1) sleep latency, (2) wake after sleep onset, (3) number of awakenings, (4) total sleep time (TST), (5) sleep quality, as well as greater symptomatic improvement relative to placebo.[15–18] Another meta-analysis[19] examined 37 randomized clinical trials involving individuals with comorbid insomnia (i.e., insomnia co-occurring with another medical or mental health condition) found CBT-I to be effective, with larger effect sizes for insomnia comorbid with mental health disorders than for medical disorders. More recent analyses have demonstrated 33% higher remission rates for patients treated with CBT-I compared to control conditions.[20]

CBT-I is widely recognized as the gold standard treatment for insomnia. It has received a strong recommendation for treating insomnia by the American Academy of Sleep Medicine (AASM)[20] as well as other leading national and international medical organizations.[21,22] Research has generally shown CBT-I to be at least as effective as pharmacological interventions in the short term, with superior long-term results.[13,23–25] These findings have earned CBT-I its status as the recommended first-line intervention for chronic insomnia.

Components of CBT-I

The specific components of multicomponent CBT-I vary across treatment protocols but at a minimum include at least one behavioral strategy and one cognitive strategy. Most typically, CBT-I will include the behavioral strategies sleep restriction and stimulus control, a cognitive therapy strategy, and sleep hygiene education along with education about sleep/wake regulation Relaxation and counter-arousal strategies may or may not be added.[20] Each specific component of CBT-I is described below.

SLEEP HYGIENE EDUCATION

Educating patients on the nature of insomnia as well as the sleep process is an important component of CBT-I. Psychoeducation generally includes an overview of sleep hygiene, as an individual's lifestyle can contribute to their insomnia symptoms. Sleep hygiene refers to a set of behavioral and environmental guidelines to improve sleep. Common sleep hygiene practices targeted by CBT-I include refraining from taking daytime naps, avoiding sleep-interfering substances too close to bedtime, and ensuring a sleep-conducive sleeping environment (e.g., kept dark, cool, and quiet). While sleep hygiene is a common component of multicomponent CBT-I, the AASM recommends against using sleep hygiene as a standalone treatment.[20]

STIMULUS CONTROL THERAPY (SCT)

SCT, rooted in learning theory, proposes that insomnia patients come to associate the bed (or bedroom) with arousal.[26,27] It is not uncommon for insomnia patients to report feeling sleepy prior to entering their bedroom, but then feel wide awake as soon as they get into bed. As patients spend more time awake in bed trying to sleep, the bed becomes a cue for wakefulness and frustration as opposed to sleep and relaxation. In addition, when individuals engage in non-sleep activities while in bed (e.g., watching television, reading, eating, etc.), the bed-sleep association is weakened. SCT aims to strengthen the bed as a cue for sleep by eliminating any other behaviors in bed (with sex and recovering from illness being 2 exceptions).

Patients implementing SCT are encouraged to limit non-sleep-related behaviors in bed, which includes lying awake. To minimize the amount of time spent awake in bed, patients are encouraged to get into bed only when they are feeling sleepy. Once in bed, if they are unable to fall asleep within 20–30 minutes, then they are encouraged to get out of bed and to return when they feel sleepy. Although good sleep hygiene generally discourages napping, SCT principles suggest that any napping that does occur should take place in bed (to reinforce bed as a cue for sleep).

The use of SCT as a stand-alone treatment was given a conditional recommendation by the AASM.[20] SCT has been shown to improve sleep quality across numerous sleep parameters on its own,[28,29] but it is more commonly used as part of multicomponent CBT-I.

SLEEP RESTRICTION THERAPY (SRT)

As previously discussed, insomnia patients frequently respond to sleep disruption by engaging in maladaptive behaviors that perpetuate insomnia. For example, patients often extend sleep opportunity in an effort to obtain more sleep, which is typically counterproductive and can produce shallow and poor-quality sleep. SRT, introduced by Spielman and colleagues,[14] aims to improve sleep quality by restricting the amount of time spent in bed. The goal of sleep restriction is to initially increase a patient's need for sleep (sleep drive) to consolidate fragmented sleep. Once the patient is sleeping more efficiently (typically calculated with the aid of a daily sleep diary), time in bed opportunity is gradually extended until daytime functioning is optimized. SRT may also help patients fall asleep more quickly and establish a more consistent sleep-wake cycle.

Example of SRT

A patient is asked to track their sleep each day over a 1–2-week period, using a daily sleep diary (see Table 14.1). Average sleep time is calculated and used to determine the patient's sleep window. In the example in Table 14.1, the average sleep time was about 5.5 hours. If the patient needed to wake up for work each day at 5:00 AM, then their bedtime would be set at 11:30 PM (i.e., 5.5 hours sleep window). Note that sleep windows are never set below 5 hours to avoid excessive sleep deprivation. Sleep windows are extended when a patient (1) reports a need for more sleep and/or (2) demonstrates a sufficient level of sleep efficiency. Sleep efficiency is calculated by taking TST divided by total time in bed. Many CBT-I protocols call for a sleep efficiency of 85%–90% before increasing the time in bed opportunity. Once patients are sleeping efficiently and are no longer reporting high levels of sleep need, the time in bed opportunity is no longer extended. Patients should be advised that SRT may initially produce increased sleepiness, and appropriate safety precautions to mitigate sleepiness-related accidents should be discussed.

SRT is a critical component of CBT-I and can be used as a stand-alone treatment to treat insomnia effectively.[29,30] The treatment has received a conditional recommendation by the

Table 14.1 **Sample Sleep Diary**

	Day 1	Day 2	Day 3	Day 4	Day 5	Day 6	Day 7	Avg
Bedtime (hh:mm)	19:30	21:00	20:00	21:00	21:00	23:00	23:00	**21:12**
Lights out (hh:mm)	19:30	21:00	20:00	21:00	21:00	23:00	23:00	**21:12**
Sleep latency (min)	120.00	90.00	180.00	120.00	150.00	30.00	120.00	**115.71**
Awake in middle of night (min)	90.00	60.00	15.00	90.00	90.00	150.00	90.00	**83.57**
Wake time (hh:mm)	5:00	5:00	5:00	5:00	5:00	9:00	8:00	**6:00**
Rise Time (hh:mm)	5:00	5:00	5:00	5:00	5:00	10:00	9:00	**6:17**
Time in bed (hrs)	9.50	8.00	9.00	8.00	8.00	11.00	10.00	**9.07**
Total sleep time (hrs)	6.00	5.50	5.75	4.50	4.00	7.00	5.50	**5.46**
Sleep efficiency (%)	63.16	68.75	63.89	56.25	50.00	63.64	55.00	**60.10**

AASM,[20] and a recent meta-analysis[31] by Maurer and colleagues found SRT to produce large treatment effects comparable to CBT-I. The authors noted, however, that these results must be interpreted tentatively given the low quality and limited number of SRT trials included in their analysis. Additionally, the authors highlighted the need for long-term follow-up studies.

SLEEP COMPRESSION

Like SRT, sleep compression is designed to consolidate sleep and improve sleep efficiency.[32,33] However, sleep compression slowly reduces time in bed opportunity rather than acutely reducing time in bed as done in sleep restriction. For example, a patient who is getting 5 hours of sleep but spending 8 hours in bed each night may be asked to initially reduce time spent in bed to 7 hours and 40 minutes. Time spent in bed may be reduced by an additional 20 minutes every week until the patient's sleep efficiency sufficiently improves.

While not as extensively studied as SRT, sleep compression has demonstrated efficacy as a stand-alone treatment[32] and better outcomes at 1-year post-treatment compared to relaxation. [33]

Sleep compression can be incorporated into the CBT-I protocol and may be well suited for individuals more sensitive to abrupt changes in their sleep schedule.[34]

COUNTER AROUSAL OR RELAXATION THERAPY

Relaxation techniques are often included in CBT-I, as heightened physiological arousal is commonly seen in individuals experiencing chronic insomnia. This "hyperarousal" has been demonstrated in studies using various measurements of arousal, including: (1) higher frequency electroencephalogram (EEG) activity,[35,36] (2) increased cortisol levels,[37] (3) higher 24-hour metabolic rate,[38,39] (4) high-frequency heart rate variability,[40] and (5) increased brain metabolism.[41] One of the more commonly used relaxation techniques is progressive muscle relaxation (PMR). This technique involves tightening a particular muscle for about 10 seconds, then slowly releasing while focusing one's attention on the relaxing muscle. The exercise then continues with patients repeating this exercise with a different muscle. Another relaxation technique that is typically implemented in CBT-I is diaphragmatic breathing or deep breathing. Patients are taught to slowly inhale and exhale with an emphasis on belly movement (as opposed to chest movement). Many clinicians will encourage patients to first practice these skills during the daytime while in a relaxed state before implementing them at night. Finally, mindfulness is another technique that has been increasingly utilized in CBT-I protocols.

While PMR and diaphragmatic breathing may be particularly helpful for symptoms of physical arousal, scheduled worry time is designed to mitigate cognitive arousal. This technique involves having patients identify a specific time during the day to worry (typically not close to bedtime). During this period, patients may choose to write down their worries and how they might solve them, or they may choose to simply let their mind wander and sit with any worry that arises. Because it is very difficult to simply stop worrying on command, many individuals end up being "stuck in their minds" all day with worry. Implementing a scheduled worry time may help patients respond to worry differently. Instead of getting entangled with worrisome thoughts when they arise, patients remind themselves that they will have plenty of time to worry later, but for now should stay focused on the current task. PMR and deep breathing have been shown to reduce insomnia symptoms and improve sleep quality in elderly individuals with insomnia when compared to controls.[42] Another study by Nicassio and Bootzin[27] also provided evidence for the efficacy of PMR, as well as another form of relaxation (autogenic training), in treating insomnia. Rybarczyk and colleagues[43] found a home-based audio relaxation program to produce significant improvements in several self-reported sleep parameters, although outcomes were inferior to in-person group CBT. While the AASM has provided a conditional recommendation to utilize counter-arousal or relaxation therapy as a stand-alone treatment for insomnia,[20] most providers instead incorporate relaxation strategies into CBT-I.

COGNITIVE THERAPY (CT)

CT is a form of psychotherapy focused on how thoughts impact one's feelings and behaviors; it involves identifying and challenging maladaptive thought patterns. In the context of insomnia, common maladaptive thoughts relate to needing 8 hours of sleep a night as well as underestimating one's ability to function on little sleep the next day. To address these concerns, CT may involve psychoeducation regarding common sleep myths as well as challenging and changing maladaptive thoughts (cognitive restructuring; see Table 14.2). A patient who believes they will not be able to function the next day if they do not get 8 hours of sleep (black and white thinking) may be encouraged by a clinician to examine the evidence of the thought (e.g., have they ever made it through the day on less than 8 hours of sleep). They would then be asked to think of an alternative, more flexible thought that considers all the evidence (e.g., I may not be at my best if I do not sleep well tonight, but I often make it through the day on less than 8 hours of sleep).

CT is another core component of CBT-I that can be used as a stand-alone treatment for insomnia.[20,44] However, patients appear to benefit the most when cognitive techniques are combined with behavioral approaches as part of the CBT-I protocol. For example, Harvey and colleagues[45] compared behavior therapy alone (BT), CT alone, and CBT for the treatment of insomnia. The authors found both BT and CT to be effective stand-alone treatments, with BT demonstrating quicker improvements and CT producing greater gains at 6-month follow-up. However, full CBT was superior to BT and CT alone.

Table 14.2 **Common Cognitive Distortions in Insomnia**

Black-and-white thinking	"If I do not get 8 hours of sleep, I will not be able to function tomorrow."
"Should" statements	"I am too young to have sleep issues, I should be able to sleep easily."
Catastrophizing	"If I am not sleeping well, then my work will suffer. Then my boss will fire me, I will lose my house, and my spouse will leave me."
Disqualifying the positives	Recognizing poor nights of sleep and ignoring when one has a good night of sleep
Jumping to conclusions; fortune telling	Assuming after a poor night of sleep that one's insomnia has returned and will only worsen
Hypervigilance or night anxiety	"Staying alert at night keeps my family safe."

Delivery Modality

CBT-I is most often delivered via individual face-to-face format; however, high insomnia prevalence rates, coupled with limited providers, make this modality insufficient to meet demand. Group CBT-I offers the advantage of treating more individuals at once as well as allowing group members to learn from each other's experiences. Despite posing some logistical challenges, such as how to record and review participants' individual sleep diaries, research supports the efficacy of group CBT-I for treating chronic insomnia.[46] With advancing communication technology over the past decade, as well as the social distancing mandates brought on by the COVID-19 pandemic, providers have increasingly relied on telehealth. Telehealth-delivered CBT-I does not require major protocol changes, and a recent study found telehealth-delivered CBT-I to not be inferior to face-to-face delivery.[47]

Healthcare systems have also utilized self-guided internet-based programs, such as Sleepio™, to help meet the growing demand for insomnia treatment. Self-guided modalities have been shown to be effective in reducing insomnia symptoms while offering a more flexible and cost-effective treatment option.[48] One meta-analysis[49] found self-guided CBT-I to be efficacious and an appropriate first-step treatment, although some studies find that self-guided CBT-I outcomes may be enhanced with provider involvement.

Contraindications/Special Considerations

While CBT-I can be used across a diverse range of settings and populations, it is not indicated for patients with uncontrolled substance use or with sleep disturbances caused exclusively by other sleep disorders like sleep apnea or nightmares. CBT-I should not be used to treat circadian rhythm sleep-wake disorders or to address sleep disturbances stemming from night shift or rotating shift work schedules. Individuals with uncontrolled seizure disorder or bipolar disorder should refrain from engaging in SRT, as sleep deprivation can potentially induce seizures or manic episodes. Patients with comorbid medical and mental health conditions also benefit from CBT-I; however, clinicians need to consider the prominence of the comorbid condition, its role in perpetuating insomnia, and the probability that it would interfere with an individual's ability to engage successfully in CBT-I.

Modifications to the CBT-I protocol may be required for fall-risk patients; if it is unsafe for a patient to get out of bed during the night, they may instead choose to sit at the end of the bed or sit up in bed when unable to sleep. CBT-I principles have also been used to address disrupted sleep in inpatient settings. One way to introduce CBT-I principles on an inpatient floor would be to encourage patients to sit in a hospital chair during the day and return to their hospital bed at night (assuming it is safe for the patient to do so). For many patients on an inpatient service with insomnia, it may be more appropriate to implement the full protocol after they have recovered and have been discharged home.

BRIEF TREATMENTS FOR INSOMNIA (BTIS)

Brief treatments for insomnia (BTIs) are multicomponent treatments that provide a subset of the treatment elements typically contained in full-scale CBT-I. These abbreviated treatments were developed to address central barriers associated with the dissemination of CBT-I, such as the shortage of trained providers and the extensive patient resources required to participate in CBT-I. They were designed to be acceptable and more accessible to primary care patients, efficacious over a short period of time, and, in some cases, deliverable by healthcare providers without significant specialty training. The various BTIs all include behavioral strategies typical of CBT-I (SRT and SCT) as core treatment components. Some versions additionally include cognitive strategies[50–52] or other behavioral components commonly included in CBT-I (e.g., relaxation[53]). BTIs vary from 2–4 total sessions, conducted weekly or biweekly, with each session 15–60 minutes on average. Most are delivered to patients individually, although one version has been tested in a group delivery format, [50] and they could readily be translated to other delivery formats (e.g., telehealth, digital). Controlled studies of BTIs to date have used trained mental health providers to administer treatment, although one potential advantage of the strictly behavioral BTI protocols is that they could be delivered by providers with limited specialty training.

The most widely tested BTI, brief behavioral treatment for insomnia (BBT-I), is delivered in a 4-session manualized protocol, after patients complete an initial intake interview, standardized questionnaires, and 1–2 weeks of baseline sleep-wake diaries. Patients are provided with a workbook containing rationales, explanations of concepts, and written patient instructions (available from the authors upon request). Individual BBT-I sessions, like CBT-I, follow a predictable structure. A summary

Table 14.3 **Treatment Content Included in BBT-I**

Content	Approach
Session 1 (45–75 minutes, in-person)	
A. Healthy sleep practices	Education regarding good sleep hygiene practices
B. Two-process model of sleep regulation	Education regarding the homeostatic and circadian sleep regulatory systems
C. Four sleep rules	1. Reduce time in bed (TIB) 2. Consistent wake time 3. Go to bed when sleepy. 4. Get out of bed after 20 minutes if awake.
Session 2 (<20 minutes, via telephone)	
Check-in	Review self-reported sleep quality, daily sleep-wake diary results, daytime functioning, and recommendation adherence.
Session 3 (30 minutes, in-person)	
A. Check-in	Review self-reported progress, sleep-wake diary results, and address challenges with treatment implementation.
B. Sleep schedule titration	Adjust sleep schedule based on patient progress: • Increase TIB by 15 minutes if sleep onset latency (SOL) and wake after sleep onset (WASO) <30 minutes. • Decrease TIB by 15 minutes if SOL and WASO <30 minutes.
Session 4 (<20 minutes, via telephone)	
A. Check-in	1. Review self-reported progress, sleep-wake diary results, and address challenges with treatment implementation. 2. Titrate TIB further.
B. Relapse prevention	1. Anticipate triggers for insomnia recurrence and strategies for managing sleep. 2. Review TIB titration recommendations.

Adapted from Gunn and collegues[54]

of the 4-session BBT-I content is outlined in Table 14.3.[54]

The rationale for BBT-I is that insomnia is associated with sleep-related behaviors that interfere with the normal function of homeostatic and circadian systems and that modification of these disruptive sleep behaviors will restore them to optimal function. By focusing on behavioral techniques specifically and linking them to underlying physiological processes, the treatment avoids potential stigma associated with psychological treatments, broadening its appeal to more patients.

Empirical Evidence

Several randomized controlled trials have shown different BTIs to improve insomnia and self-reported sleep outcomes more than control conditions.[50–53,55–61] These studies have been conducted in veterans with insomnia[51,52,56,57,59] and in older adults with insomnia with and without comorbid mental health disorders.[53,55,58,60] In one of the first studies of BBT-I, Buysse and colleagues[55] found that, compared to an information control, BBTI-treated older adults with insomnia were more likely to experience treatment response (67% vs. 25%) and remission (55% vs. 13%) at post-treatment, with rates comparable to full CBT-I. BTI effects on daytime sequelae of insomnia, such as depression and anxiety, fatigue/sleepiness, and cognition, however, have been more variable and, when present, the effect sizes are considerably smaller. Sleep-related improvements produced by BTIs are maintained at 3- and 6-month follow-up, and nearly two-thirds of participants no longer met clinical criteria for insomnia at follow-up in one study.[55] Older adults with more severe baseline depression and anxiety symptoms, worse sleep quality, longer objective TST, and absence of nocturia may be more likely to respond to BBT-I, but more research is needed.[62,63] Based on these efficacy data, the AASM assigned BTIs a conditional recommendation for the treatment of chronic insomnia in adults, meaning that most patients should receive the treatment, but treatment may not be indicated in all cases.[20]

Contraindications/Special Considerations

Clinical considerations for the use of BTIs are similar to those for CBT-I. Given that SRT is a component of all BTIs, the treatment may be contraindicated in populations working in occupations where sleepiness would be dangerous (e.g., commercial drivers) or in patients with specific comorbid mental health or medical conditions where sleepiness could worsen the accompanying condition (e.g., bipolar disorder, seizure disorder). Like CBT-I, clinical judgment is indicated regarding the appropriate timing of BTIs in patients with insomnia and co-occurring disorders. While potential benefits of BTIs relative to CBT-I include increased access to care and delivery by providers without specialty training, future trials are needed that directly assess these issues. In addition, studies are needed that evaluate the efficacy and safety of BTIs in more diverse samples of patients with insomnia.

INTENSIVE SLEEP RETRAINING (ISR)

Intensive sleep retraining (ISR) is a brief laboratory-based behavioral treatment that was designed to leverage homeostatic and circadian sleep drive to improve sleep onset latency (SOL) and other symptoms of chronic insomnia. The treatment is carried out in a single session in a sleep laboratory across a period of 24–25 hours,[28] during which time patients are provided with multiple opportunities to fall asleep for brief periods. ISR is designed to decondition the arousal response associated with making an active attempt to fall asleep through the experience of several rapid sleep onsets, which help to reinforce cues for sleep in the bedroom environment.[64]

These sleep onsets happen with increasing frequency and shorter latencies throughout the intervention period as sleep pressure builds.[65] The experience of several successful sleep onsets, coupled with mild sleep deprivation, result in near immediate improvement in sleep onset as well as other insomnia symptoms.[28,65]

Intensive Sleep Retraining Protocol

ISR is conducted in a sleep lab over a period of 24–25 hours, during which time patients are monitored via EEG to allow for precise detection of sleep onset. The night before coming to the lab, patients are instructed to limit their time in bed to 5 hours to induce a state of mild sleep deprivation. Additionally, they are instructed to avoid naps and caffeine for the 24-hour period before participating in the intervention. Patients may be asked to keep a sleep diary starting 2 weeks before the intervention night and continuing for 6 weeks post-intervention to monitor their subjective sleep experience, including sleep onset latency and wake after sleep onset.[64] Once in the lab, the intervention period is divided into 30-minute intervals, each of which is an opportunity for the patient to fall asleep; there are approximately 48–50 sleep opportunities during the entire intervention period. If the patient is observed on EEG to have fallen asleep, they are awakened after 3 minutes and asked if they recognized that they had fallen asleep. This question serves as a form of sleep-wake discrimination training, which has been previously shown to improve sleep in individuals with insomnia.[28,64] The patient is then kept awake until the next 30-minute sleep opportunity starts. This cycle is repeated for the duration of the intervention. On the first night of recovery sleep following the intervention, patients are instructed to limit their TST to 8 hours to maintain homeostatic sleep pressure and to promote a regular sleep schedule.[64]

Empirical Evidence

Studies have demonstrated ISR to be efficacious, including 2 pilot studies and 1 randomized controlled trial.[66] In the randomized clinical trial, Harris and collegues[28] randomized participants with chronic sleep-onset insomnia, with or without sleep maintenance symptoms, to receive ISR alone, stimulus control therapy (SCT) alone, ISR plus SCT, or a sleep hygiene (SH) control intervention. ISR was delivered in a 25-hour protocol, while SCT and SH were delivered across 5 weekly sessions. Participants were assessed immediately after completion of treatment and then again 2- and 6-months post-intervention. Both the ISR and ISR plus SCT conditions resulted in immediate improvements in SOL and TST post-treatment, though the combined treatment group demonstrated a larger effect size for improvements in both measures. Overall, 61% of participants in the combined group reached "good sleeper" status on sleep diary measures; these gains were maintained over the 6-month follow-up period. [28] The ISR monotherapy group also demonstrated significant treatment benefits, but participants' subjective sleep parameters did not normalize over time. These findings suggest that durable sleep improvements are more likely achieved when ISR is paired with an existing behavioral intervention for insomnia. Given the limited available data, the most recent AASM Clinical Guidelines issued no recommendation regarding the efficacy and safety of ISR.[20] In addition, ISR has not been tested in other subtypes of chronic insomnia, including patients with a primary complaint of wake after sleep onset/early morning awakenings and those with comorbid insomnia.[64]

Contraindications/Special Considerations

A primary consideration for ISR is that of cost and resource utilization. In-lab studies require the staffing of a registered sleep technician during non-standard times, as well as use of the sleep lab resources for a period of 24–25 hours.[20] The resources and cost associated with ISR are therefore likely to be higher than for other sleep interventions.[20] To mitigate the costs associated with treatment, several at-home options are in development, including a mobile application and wearable devices.[65] In-home options may in fact lead to a superior treatment response because the conditioning is taking place in the environment where patients typically sleep and thus does not need to be transferred from the intervention setting to the home.[28] Another important consideration is that, because of the demanding nature of this intervention, some patients may elect another treatment option for their chronic insomnia.[20]

Contraindications for ISR include comorbid diagnoses of conditions that may be susceptible to sleep deprivation, including bipolar and seizure disorder.[64] Additionally, there are several acute side effects of treatment to be considered, including cognitive impairment, fatigue, and increased sleepiness following the intervention.[20] However, these risks are considered minimal and are outweighed by the potential benefits, including subjective reports of significant improvement in sleep latency and overall sleep quality.[20] In fact, the magnitude of the improvements in both sleep and daytime functioning are comparable to SCT alone, but are nearly immediate.[65]

ACCEPTANCE AND COMMITMENT THERAPY (ACT)

ACT is an empirically based third-wave CBT psychotherapy that aims to increase psychological flexibility. As opposed to changing the way patients think, ACT uses several techniques, such as acceptance and mindfulness, to help patients make contact with the present moment and change the way they relate to internal experiences to help them engage more effectively in value-congruent behaviors.[67] Take, for example, a patient who values good relationships but struggles with social anxiety. Traditional CBT may aim to reduce anxiety via relaxation or by modifying unhelpful cognitions. ACT shifts the focus of treatment away from avoiding illness and toward living a valued life; any effort to eliminate private events is referred to as experiential avoidance (the opposite of psychological flexibility), which is thought to be associated with mental illness. ACT utilizes techniques to help clients remain in the present moment and defuse from one's thoughts instead of becoming entangled in one's thoughts or "stuck in one's mind." Clients are then encouraged to allow thoughts and feelings to come and go as they engage in value congruent action.

Empirical Evidence

Although research examining the efficacy of ACT to treat insomnia is limited, existing literature suggests that ACT may be beneficial.

One systematic review[68] examined the impact of ACT on insomnia and sleep quality. The authors included 19 studies in their review, most of which reported that ACT improved insomnia symptoms and sleep quality. Fiorentino, Martin, and Alessi[69] have proposed an ACT-based protocol called Acceptance and Behavioral Changes to treat Insomnia (ABC-I). The protocol consists of 5 one-hour individual sessions and combines many CBT-I components (including psychoeducation, sleep hygiene, SCT, and SRT) with the 6 core processes of ACT (i.e., Hexaflex): (1) acceptance, (2) mindfulness, (3) values, (4) committed action, (5) cognitive defusion, and (6) self-as-context. The protocol was shown to be effective in 2 pilot studies treating older veterans with insomnia.[69] The authors posited that ACT techniques may help to increase adherence with CBT-I, which is critical to treatment success.[70] For example, patients struggling with increased distress during the sleep-restriction phase may choose to take a nap during the day. ACT would aim to change the way the client responds to these feelings, which might include increasing one's present moment awareness (mindfulness), learning to make room for discomfort (acceptance), and/or changing the way one relates to discomfort (cognitive defusion and self-as-context) to commit to value-congruent behavior (committed action and values). Although initial results look promising, future research is needed to evaluate the efficacy of this combined ABC-I treatment.

Contraindications/Special Considerations

Since an acceptance-based approach to treating insomnia would contain the same core elements of traditional CBT-I, the contraindications or special considerations discussed in the CBT-I section would also be applicable. Clinicians trained in both interventions are often confronted with the challenge of deciding whether a patient is better suited for ACT or traditional CBT. While further research is needed to evaluate who will respond better to ACT and traditional CBT, some guidelines to help in the decision process have been proposed.[71] In general, an acceptance-based approach is preferred for patients dealing with very intense emotions, engaging in attempts to avoid painful memories or emotions, or experiencing chronic stressors outside of their control. Alternatively, a change-based approach may be best for patients whose situation is more controllable, distressing thoughts are more distorted (e.g., "My career is over if I do not get this promotion" vs. "I have a chronic illness"), or when meta-cognitive beliefs about thoughts are present (e.g., believing worry is helpful because it keeps one on guard). Finally, it is important to consider client preference and comfort with each approach.

CONCLUSIONS

Among the non-pharmacological treatment options for chronic insomnia, CBT-I has been recognized as the gold standard. Several of the components that make up CBT-I, such as sleep restriction therapy (SRT) and stimulus control therapy (SCT), can also be used as stand-alone treatments. Providers should consider CBT-I as the first-line defense in the treatment of chronic insomnia when adequate resources are available.

While CBT-I is first-line, emerging non-pharmacological therapies offer alternative approaches. BBT-I is more efficient than CBT-I and appropriate for individuals for whom cognitions are minimally relevant to the insomnia. ACT is an evidence-based therapy for a variety of disorders and more recently has been implemented to treat insomnia. ABC-I is another emerging therapy that shares many of the same components as CBT-I and BBT-I (such as the critical component of sleep restriction). One possible advantage to the acceptance approach used in ABC-I is that it may be better suited to address negative thoughts more rooted in reality compared to the restructuring approach of CBT-I. Finally, although the costs and a lack of resources often make ISR prohibitive, initial results suggest the treatment may produce rapid improvements. In addition, protocols are ongoing to evaluate the efficacy and safety of ISR carried out in the home environment using a mobile application and wearable devices. There is an abundance of research supporting CBT-I as the first-line treatment for chronic insomnia, but future research is still needed to better establish the validity of these emerging therapies.

REFERENCES

1. American Academy of Sleep Medicine. *The International Classification of Sleep Disorders (ICSD-3)*. American Academy of Sleep Medicine; 2014.
2. American Psychiatric Association. *Diagnostic and Statistical Manual of Mental Disorders*. 5th edition. APA;2013. doi:10.1176/appi.books.9780890425596.893619.
3. Breslau N, Roth T, Rosenthal L, Andreski P. Sleep disturbance and psychiatric disorders: A longitudinal epidemiological study of young adults. *Biol Psychiatry*. 1996;39(6):411–418. doi:10.1016/0006-3223(95)00188-3.
4. Taylor DJ, Lichstein KL, Durrence HH, Reidel BW, Bush AJ. Epidemiology of insomnia, depression, and anxiety. *Sleep*. 2005;28(11):1457–1464. doi:10.1093/sleep/28.11.1457.
5. Pasman JA, Smit DJA, Kingma L, Vink JM, Treur JL, Verweij KJH. Causal relationships between substance use and insomnia. *Drug Alcohol Depend*. 2020;214:1–5. doi:10.1016/j.drugalcdep.2020.108151.
6. Taylor DJ, Laurel J. Mallory LJ, et al. Comorbidity of chronic insomnia with medical problems. *Sleep*. 2007;30(2):213–218.
7. Katz DA, Colleen MA. The relationship between insomnia and health-related quality of life in patients with chronic illness. *J Fam Pract*. 2002;51(3):229–234.
8. Ishak WW, Bagot K, Thomas S, et al. Quality of life in patients suffering from insomnia. *Innov Clin Neurosci*. 2012;9(10):13–26.
9. Gadermann AM, Alonso J, Vilagut G, Zaslavsky AM, Kessler RC. Comorbidity and disease burden in the national comorbidity survey replication (NCS-R). *Depress Anxiety*. 2012;29(9):797–806. doi:10.1002/da.21924
10. Stoller M. Economic effects of insomnia. *Clin Ther*. 1994;16(5):873–897.
11. Morin CM, Gaulier B, Barry T, Kowatch RA. Patients' acceptance of psychological and pharmacological therapies for insomnia. *Sleep*. 1992;15(4):302–305. https://academic.oup.com/sleep/article/15/4/302/2749271.
12. Vincent N, Lionberg C. Treatment preference and patient satisfaction in chronic insomnia. *Sleep*. 2001;24(4):411–417. https://academic.oup.com/sleep/article/24/4/411/2750018.
13. Rios P, Cardoso R, Morra D, et al. Comparative effectiveness and safety of pharmacological and non-pharmacological interventions for insomnia: An overview of reviews. *Syst Rev*. 2019;8(1):1–16. doi:10.1186/s13643-019-1163-9.
14. Spielman AJ, Caruso LS, Glovinsky PB. A behavioral perspective on insomnia treatment. *Psychiatr Clin North Am*. 1987;10:541–553.
15. Morin CM, Culbert JP, Schwartz SM. Nonpharmacological interventions for insomnia: A meta-analysis of treatment efficacy. *Am J Psychiatry*. 1994;151(8):1172–1180.
16. Murtagh DR, Greenwood KM. Identifying effective psychological treatments for insomnia: A meta-analysis. *J Consult Clin Psychol*. 1995;63(1):79–89.
17. Smith MT, Perlis ML, Park A, et al. Comparative meta-analysis of pharmacotherapy and behavior therapy for persistent insomnia. *Am J Psychiatry*. 2002;159(1):5–11.
18. Irwin MR, Cole JC, Nicassio PM. Comparative meta-analysis of behavioral interventions for insomnia and their efficacy in middle-aged adults and in older adults 55+ years of age. *Health Psychol*. 2006;25(1):3–14.
19. Wu JQ, Appleman ER, Salazar RD, Ong JC. Cognitive behavioral therapy for insomnia comorbid with psychiatric and medical conditions a meta-analysis. *JAMA Intern Med*. 2015;175(9):1461–1472. doi:10.1001/jamainternmed.2015.3006.
20. Edinger JD, Arnedt JT, Bertisch SM, et al. Behavioral and psychological treatments for chronic insomnia disorder in adults: An American Academy of Sleep Medicine systematic review, meta-analysis, and GRADE assessment. *J Clin Sleep Med*. 2021;17(2):263–298. doi:10.5664/JCSM.8988.
21. Qaseem A, Kansagara D, Forciea MA, Cooke M, Denberg TD. Management of chronic insomnia disorder in adults: A clinical practice guideline from the American College of Physicians Management of chronic insomnia disorder in adults. *Ann Intern Med*. 2016;165(2):123–133. doi:10.7326/M15-2175.
22. Wilson S, Anderson K, Baldwin D, et al. British Association for Psychopharmacology consensus statement on evidence-based treatment of insomnia, parasomnias and circadian rhythm disorders: An update. *J Psychopharmacol (Oxford, England)*. 2019;33(8):923–947.
23. Jacobs GD, Pace-Schott EF, Stickgold R, Otto MW. Cognitive behavior therapy and pharmacotherapy for insomnia: A randomized controlled trial and direct comparison. *Arch Intern Med*. 2004;164:1888–1896. https://jamanetwork.com/.
24. Mitchell MD, Gehrman P, Perlis M, Umscheid CA. Comparative effectiveness of cognitive behavioral therapy for insomnia: A systematic review. *BMC Fam Pract*. 2012;13(40):1–11. doi:10.1186/1471-2296-13-40.
25. Sivertsen B, Omvik S, Havik OE, et al. A comparison of actigraphy and polysomnography in older adults treated for chronic primary insomnia. *Sleep*. 2006;29(10):1353–1358. https://academic.oup.com/sleep/article/29/10/1353/2709223.
26. Bootzin RR. Stimulus control treatment for insomnia. *Proc Am Psychol*. 1972;7:395–396.
27. Nicassio P, Bootzin R. A comparison of progressive relaxation and autogenic training as treatments for insomnia. *J Abnormal Psychol*. 1974;83(3):253–260. doi:10.1037/h0036729.
28. Harris J, Lack L, Kemp K, Wright H, Bootzin R. A randomized controlled trial of intensive sleep retraining (ISR): A brief conditioning treatment for chronic insomnia. *Sleep*. 2012;35(1):49–60. doi:10.5665/sleep.1584.
29. Sidani S, Epstein DR, Fox M, Collins L. Comparing the effects of single-and multiple-component therapies for insomnia on sleep outcomes. *Worldviews Evid Based Nurs*. 2019;16(3):195–203. doi:10.1111/wvn.12367.
30. Drake CL, Kalmbach DA, Arnedt JT, et al. Treating chronic insomnia in postmenopausal women: A randomized clinical trial comparing cognitive-behavioral therapy for insomnia, sleep restriction therapy, and sleep hygiene education. *Sleep*. 2019;42(2):1–11. doi:10.1093/sleep/zsy217.
31. Maurer LF, Schneider J, Miller CB, Espie CA, Kyle SD. The clinical effects of sleep restriction therapy for insomnia:

A meta-analysis of randomised controlled trials. *Sleep Med Rev*. 2021;58:1–11. doi:10.1016/j.smrv.2021.101493.
32. Lichstein KL. Sleep compression treatment of an insomnoid. *Behav Ther*. 1988;19:625–632.
33. Lichstein KL, Riedel BW, Wilson NM, Lester KW, Aguillard RN. Relaxation and sleep compression for late-life insomnia: A placebo-controlled trial. *J Consult Clin Psychol*. 2001;69(2):227–239. doi:10.1037/0022-006X.69.2.227.
34. Lichstein KL, Thomas SJ, McCurry SM. Sleep compression. In: Perlis, Michael, Aloia, Mark, and Kuhn, Brett, eds. *Behavioral Treatments for Sleep Disorders*. Elsevier; 2011:55–59. doi:10.1016/B978-0-12-381522-4.00005-5.
35. Krystal AD, Edinger JD, Wohlgemuth William K, Marsh GR. NREM sleep EEG frequency spectral correlates of sleep complaints in primary insomnia subtypes. *Sleep*. 2002;25(6):630–640. https://academic.oup.com/sleep/article/25/6/626/2750129.
36. Perlis ML, Smith MT, Andrews PJ, Orff H, Giles DE. Beta/gamma EEG activity in patients with primary and secondary insomnia and good sleeper controls. *Sleep*. 2001;24(1):110–117. https://academic.oup.com/sleep/article/24/1/110/2749965.
37. Vgontzas AN, Bixler EO, Lin HM, et al. Chronic insomnia is associated with nyctohemeral activation of the hypothalamic-pituitary-adrenal axis: Clinical implications. *J Clin Endocrinol Metab*. 2001;86(8):3787–3794.
38. Bonnet MH, Arand DL. 24-hour metabolic rate in insomniacs and matched normal sleepers. *Sleep*. 1995;18(7):581–588. https://academic.oup.com/sleep/article/18/7/581/2749713.
39. Bonnet MH, Arand DL. Physiological activation in patients with sleep state misperception. *Psychosom Med*. 1997;59(5):533–540.
40. MacNeil S, Deschênes SS, Caldwell W, Brouillard M, Dang-Vu TT, Gouin JP. High-frequency heart rate variability reactivity and trait worry interact to predict the development of sleep disturbances in response to a naturalistic stressor. *Ann Behav Med*. 2017;51(6):912–924. doi:10.1007/s12160-017-9915-z.
41. Nofzinger EA, Buysse DJ, Germain A, Price JC, Miewald JM, Kupfer DJ. Functional neuroimaging evidence for hyperarousal in insomnia. *Am J Psychiatry*. 2004;161(11):2126–2128. http://ajp.psychiatryonline.org.
42. Jayarathne W, de Zoysa P. The impact of a progressive muscular relaxation exercise programme for reducing insomnia in an elderly population: Results from a preliminary study at two elderly homes in the Colombo District of Sri Lanka. *Sri Lanka J Soc Sci*. 2016;39(1):47–52. doi:10.4038/sljss.v39i1.7402.
43. Rybarczyk B, Lopez M, Benson R, Alsten C, Stepanski E. Efficacy of two behavioral treatment programs for comorbid geriatric insomnia. *Psychol Aging*. 2002;17(2):288–298. doi:10.1037/0882-7974.17.2.288.
44. Harvey AG, Sharpley AL, Ree MJ, Stinson K, Clark DM. An open trial of cognitive therapy for chronic insomnia. *Behav Res Ther*. 2007;45(10):2491–2501. doi:10.1016/j.brat.2007.04.007.
45. Harvey AG, Bélanger L, Talbot L, et al. Comparative efficacy of behavior therapy, cognitive therapy, and cognitive behavior therapy for chronic insomnia: A randomized controlled trial. *J Consult Clin Psychol*. 2014;82(4):670–683. doi:10.1037/a0036606.
46. Koffel EA, Koffel JB, Gehrman PR. A meta-analysis of group cognitive behavioral therapy for insomnia. *Sleep Med Rev*. 2015;19:6–16. doi:10.1016/j.smrv.2014.05.001.
47. Arnedt JT, Conroy DA, Mooney A, Furgal A, Sen A, Eisenberg D. Telemedicine versus face-to-face delivery of cognitive behavioral therapy for insomnia: A randomized controlled noninferiority trial. *Sleep*. 2021;44(1):1–11. doi:10.1093/sleep/zsaa136.
48. Grierson AB, Hobbs MJ, Mason EC. Self-guided online cognitive behavioural therapy for insomnia: A naturalistic evaluation in patients with potential psychiatric comorbidities. *J Affect Disord*. 2020;266:305–310. doi:10.1016/j.jad.2020.01.143.
49. Ho FYY, Chung KF, Yeung WF, et al. Self-help cognitive-behavioral therapy for insomnia: A meta-analysis of randomized controlled trials. *Sleep Med Rev*. 2015;19:17–28. doi:10.1016/j.smrv.2014.06.010.
50. Lovato N, Lack L, Wright H, Kennaway DJ. Evaluation of a brief treatment program of cognitive behavior therapy for insomnia in older adults. *Sleep*. 2014;37(1):117–126. doi:10.5665/sleep.3320.
51. Pigeon WR, Funderburk J, Bishop TM, Crean HF. Brief cognitive behavioral therapy for insomnia delivered to depressed veterans receiving primary care services: A pilot study. *J Affect Disord*. 2017;217:105–111. doi:10.1016/j.jad.2017.04.003.
52. Pigeon WR, Funderburk JS, Cross W, Bishop TM, Crean HF. Brief CBT for insomnia delivered in primary care to patients endorsing suicidal ideation: A proof-of-concept randomized clinical trial. *Transl Behav Med*. 2019;9(6):1169–1177. doi:10.1093/tbm/ibz108.
53. McCrae CS, Curtis AF, Williams JM, et al. Efficacy of brief behavioral treatment for insomnia in older adults: Examination of sleep, mood, and cognitive outcomes. *Sleep Med*. 2018;51:153–166. doi:10.1016/j.sleep.2018.05.018.
54. Gunn HE, Tutek J, Buysse DJ. Brief behavioral treatment of insomnia. *Sleep Med Clin*. 2019;14(2):235–243.
55. Buysse DJ, Germain A, Moul DE, et al. Efficacy of brief behavioral treatment for chronic insomnia in older adults. *Arch Intern Med*. 2011;171(10):887–895. doi:10.1001/archinternmed.2010.535.
56. Edinger JD, Sampson WS. A primary care "friendly" cognitive behavioral insomnia therapy. *Sleep*. 2003;26(2):177–182. doi:10.1093/sleep/26.2.177.
57. Gebara MA, DiNapoli EA, Lederer LG, et al. Brief behavioral treatment for insomnia in older adults with late-life treatment-resistant depression and insomnia: A pilot study. *Sleep Biol Rhythms*. 2019;17(3):287–295. doi:10.1007/s41105-019-00211-6.
58. Germain A, Moul DE, Franzen PL, et al. Effects of a brief behavioral treatment for late-life insomnia: Preliminary findings. *J Clin Sleep Med*. 2006;2(4):403–406. doi:10.5664/jcsm.26654.
59. Germain A, Richardson R, Stocker R, et al. Treatment for insomnia in combat-exposed OEF/OIF/OND military veterans: Preliminary randomized controlled trial. *Behav Res Ther*. 2014;61:78–88. doi:10.1016/j.brat.2014.07.016.

60. McCrae CS, McGovern R, Lukefahr R, Stripling AM. Research evaluating brief behavioral sleep treatments for rural elderly (RESTORE): A preliminary examination of effectiveness. *Am J Geriatr Psychiatry*. 2007;15(11):979–982. doi:10.1097/JGP.0b013e31813547e6.
61. Wang J, Wei Q, Wu X, Zhong Z, Li G. Brief behavioral treatment for patients with treatment-resistant insomnia. *Neuropsychiatr Dis Treat*. 2016;12:1967–1975. doi:10.2147/NDT.S110571.
62. Troxel WM, Conrad TS, Germain A, Buysse DJ. Predictors of treatment response to brief behavioral treatment of insomnia (BBTI) in older adults. *J Clin Sleep Med*. 2013;9(12):1281–1289. doi:10.5664/jcsm.3270
63. Tyagi S, Resnick NM, Perera S, Monk TH, Hall MH, Buysse DJ. Behavioral treatment of insomnia: Also effective for nocturia. *J Am Geriatr Soc*. 2014;62(1):54–60. doi:10.1111/jgs.12609.
64. Harris J, Lack L. Intensive sleep retraining: Conditioning treatment for primary insomnia. In: Perlis, Michael, Aloia, Mark, and Kuhn, Brett, eds. *Behavioral Treatments for Sleep Disorders*. Elsevier; 2011:127–131. doi:10.1016/B978-0-12-381522-4.00013-4.
65. Lack L, Scott H, Micic G, Lovato N. Intensive sleep re-training: From bench to bedside. *Brain Sci*. 2017;7(4):1–11. doi:10.3390/brainsci7040033.
66. Ong J. *Cognitive-Behavioral Therapies for Insomnia: An Issue of Sleep Medicine Clinics*. Elsevier; 2019.
67. Hayes SC, Strosahl KD, Wilson KG. *Acceptance and Commitment Therapy: The Process and Practice of Mindful Change*. 2nd ed. Guilford; 2012.
68. Salari N, Khazaie H, Hosseinian-Far A, et al. The effect of acceptance and commitment therapy on insomnia and sleep quality: A systematic review. *BMC Neurol*. 2020;20(1):1–18. doi:10.1186/s12883-020-01883-1.
69. Fiorentino L, Martin JL, Alessi CA. The ABCs of insomnia (ABC-I): An acceptance commitment therapy (ACT)-based insomnia treatment development study: Pilot results and future directions. In: Sedky K, Nazir R, Bennett D, eds. *Sleep Medicine and Mental Health: A Guide for Psychiatrists and Other Healthcare Professionals*. Springer; 2020:85–100.
70. Matthews EE, Arnedt JT, McCarthy MS, Cuddihy LJ, Aloia MS. Adherence to cognitive behavioral therapy for insomnia: A systematic review. *Sleep Med Rev*. 2013;17(6):1–26. doi:10.1016/j.smrv.2013.01.001.
71. Hallis L, Cameli L, Dionne F, Knäuper B. Combining cognitive therapy with acceptance and commitment therapy for depression: A manualized group therapy. *J Psychother Integr*. 2016;26(2):186–201. doi:10.1037/int0000028.

Chapter 15

Circadian Rhythm Sleep-Wake Disorders

Overview and Clinical Approach

Stephanie D. Ivins, Sabra M. Abbott, and Phyllis C. Zee

INTRODUCTION TO CIRCADIAN RHYTHMS

In this section we will provide an overview of circadian rhythms and circadian physiology.

Definition

Circadian rhythms are the approximately 24-hour, self-sustained oscillations that occur in nearly all biological processes and are present across the vast majority of living organisms. Because these rhythms are self-sustained, they persist and keep time in the absence of external signals from the social and physical environment. Because these rhythms are typically close to, but not exactly 24 hours, there is flexibility (within a range) to be able to adjust timing to align these rhythms in response to exposures to environmental stimuli—a process known as entrainment. The stimuli to which circadian rhythms can entrain (i.e., zeitgebers) include light (the strongest of the zeitgebers) and non-photic agents such as the hormone melatonin, physical activity, and social activity.[1] The ability of organisms to entrain in response to zeitgebers allows for adaptation to environmental changes in a way that confers survival benefit through optimization of the timing of physiological processes.

The sleep-wake cycle is undoubtedly the best-recognized of the human circadian rhythms. Through the use of rigorous protocols designed to study subjects under constant environmental, behavioral, and postural conditions (i.e., constant routine) or those that impose non-24-hour schedules on the sleep/wake cycle and other behavioral patterns (i.e., forced desynchrony), numerous other physiological processes—including core body temperature, blood pressure, mood and cognition, and the endocrine secretion of cortisol, melatonin, glucose, insulin, leptin, and the catecholamines—have also been shown to display circadian temporal patterns.[2]

Circadian Physiology

In the absence of time cues from the environmental light/dark cycle, or other zeitgebers, the endogenous human circadian period (i.e., tau) is described as "free-running." The average duration of the human circadian tau in constant dim light is approximately 24.2 hours.[3] This free-running period is genetically determined, largely by the expression of cell-autonomous transcription/translation feedback loops involving a core set of genes—circadian locomotor output cycles kaput (*CLOCK*), brain and muscle arnt-like protein 1 (*BMAL1*), period (*PER1*, *PER2*, *PER3*), and cryptochrome (*CRY1*, *CRY2*)—collectively referred to as the clock genes.[4,5] CREB (cAMP response element-binding protein) also plays a critical role in the initiation and maintenance of the circadian period via binding to the cAMP response element in the promoter regions of clock genes, *PER* and *CRY*.[6]

CREB, BMAL1, and CLOCK are transcription factors that together activate expression of the *PER* and *CRY* genes. Following translation of the *PER* and *CRY* mRNA, the resulting PER and CRY proteins accumulate in the cytoplasm. These are then translocated back to the nucleus, where they inhibit their own transcription in a negative feedback loop. The rate of build-up of PER/CRY dimers depends, in part, on the phosphorylation of PER. This process is mediated by the serine/threonine kinase, casein kinase 1 (CK1), and ultimately activates PER's proteasomal degradation, slowing the rate of dimerization and negative feedback.[7] As such, mutations that either increase or decrease the rate of phosphorylation of PER can respectively decrease or increase the overall rate of the transcription-translation feedback loop.

This oscillatory pattern of circadian gene expression occurs in nearly all tissues throughout the human body, allowing for the existence of independent and tissue-specific circadian rhythms—often referred to as peripheral clocks.[8] For optimal physiological function, the peripheral clocks in tissues are typically entrained by a central clock, the suprachiasmatic nucleus (SCN)—an anatomical structure composed of ~20,000 neurons, located in the anterior hypothalamus. Situated directly above the optic chiasm, the SCN receives light signals, allowing for entrainment to the light/dark cycle.

The path that light takes to reach the SCN begins in the retina, where light is initially perceived by specialized photoreceptor cells called intrinsically photosensitive retinal ganglion cells (ipRGCs). These cells contain the photopigment melanopsin, which has peak spectral absorption for blue wavelengths of light around 480 nm. Wavelengths of light on the green-yellow spectrum are also absorbed, but to a lesser extent.[9] When light reaches the melanopsin-containing ipRGCs, the photic input is converted to electrical impulses through a series of biochemical reactions.[10] These electrical impulses (i.e., action potentials) are directly transmitted to the SCN through the monosynaptic pathway of the retinohypothalamic tract. Following integration of these signals and subsequent modulation of the SCN's intrinsic rhythmic neural activity, rhythmic outputs are generated from the SCN. These outputs—conveyed via the autonomic nervous system, the hypothalamic-pituitary-adrenal axis, and by changes in core body temperature—adjust the rhythms of the peripheral clocks throughout the body, resulting in their synchronization.[11]

The SCN also sends signals through an indirect, multi-synaptic pathway to the pineal gland, to regulate the synthesis of melatonin—a hormone that also plays a key role in modulating timing of the sleep-wake cycle. The pathway starts with intrahypothalamic neuronal projections to the paraventricular nucleus (PVN). From the PVN, signals project to the intermediolateral cell column (IML) located in the upper thoracic spinal cord. Neurons of the IML project to the superior cervical ganglion (SCG). Postganglionic neurons of the SCG then release norepinephrine which, via binding of beta-1 adrenergic receptors in the pineal gland, ultimately stimulates increased melatonin production.[11,12] Notably, a direct physiological consequence of this is that common anti-hypertensives that block the beta-adrenergic system can also inadvertently suppress melatonin production.

The sensitivity of the ipRGCs to light, particularly of blue wavelengths, is associated with how easily an individual's circadian timing can be phase-shifted in response to light exposure. The greater the sensitivity, the more easily phase-shifting is expected to occur, as will be discussed in greater detail in the next section. This sensitivity can be estimated via post-illumination pupil response (PIPR). One might suspect that populations with greater tendencies to use electronic devices such as phones, tablets, or monitors late into the evening and who are more easily phase-shifted with blue light exposure are at greater risk of having a delayed sleep-wake phase relative to conventional norms. Indeed, such an association has been reported.[13]

Phase Response Curves (PRCs)

The plot in Figure 15.1 suggests that the phase response curves (PRCs) in each case are identical, just shifted (this is roughly true, though there are some technicalities beyond the scope of this chapter). Other noteworthy features are the core body temperature nadir and dim light melatonin onset (DLMO). The core body temperature nadir occurs ~3 hours before habitual wake-up time and marks the transition from light being phase-delaying to phase-advancing. The DLMO occurs ~2 hours before habitual sleep onset. Recall that measuring shifts in the DLMO in response to exogenously given melatonin is one way to construct PRCs.

The entraining effects of light and melatonin are sensitive to the timing of administration relative to an individual's circadian timing. Often, an individual's circadian timing is most easily determined through observation of habitual sleep-wake times (i.e., the sleep-wake cycle followed in the absence of alarm clocks). This is crucial for the clinician to keep in mind, as both light and melatonin can induce circadian phase advances or delays, depending

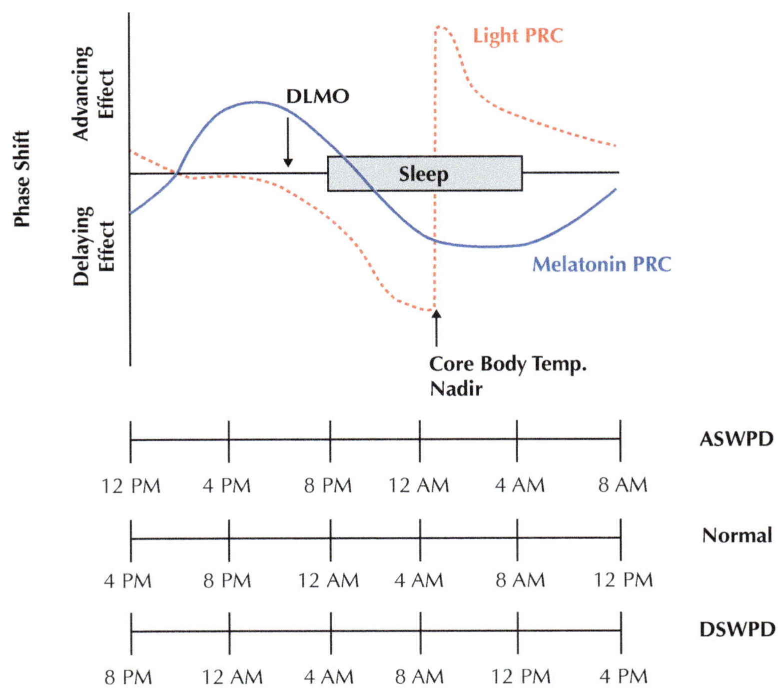

Figure 15.1. This plot depicts PRCs for light and melatonin. The PRC for light is in red (dotted line) while the exogenously administered melatonin PRC is in blue. The y-axis indicates the direction and magnitude of the phase shift induced by exposure to light/melatonin. Time-of-day is on the x-axis. We label the specific times on the x-axis using 3 schemes stylistically representative of 3 hypothetical patients: one with advanced sleep-wake phase disorder (ASWPD), one with a normal sleep schedule, and one with delayed sleep-wake phase disorder (DSWPD). ASWPD and DSWPD are discussed in detail in later sections, though the quick summary is that ASWPD (DSWPD) patients have advanced (delayed) sleep schedules relative to conventional norms. The gray box indicates when the patient is asleep.

upon the time of exposure. If treatment with either zeitgeber is mis-timed, it might have the opposite effect to what is intended. To help optimize the timing of such interventions, one can use PRCs. These plots indicate how circadian rhythms shift in response to a stimulus (e.g., how the sleep-wake cycle or other circadian markers change with exposure to light or melatonin; Figure 15.1). It should be noted that, in general, the magnitude of phase shifts produced from light are greater than those produced from melatonin, as can be seen from the PRCs in Figure 15.1 (i.e., the max [min] of the light PRC is greater [less] than the max [min] of the melatonin PRC).

Whether light is phase-delaying or phase-advancing depends on the timing of exposure relative to the timing of the endogenous circadian rhythm. Common circadian phase markers include timing of core body temperature nadir and timing of dim light melatonin onset (DLMO). The latter is measured more commonly in clinical practice, and generally occurs around 7 hours prior to core body temperature nadir (see Figure 15.1). Light has phase-advancing effects if an individual is exposed to light after the core body temperature nadir, while phase-delaying effects are observed before.

The effects of melatonin are roughly inverse to those of light. Melatonin administration has its peak phase-advancing effects prior to DLMO. Measuring shifts in the DLMO in response to light and exogenously administered melatonin is one way to construct PRCs.[14] Melatonin's maximal phase-delaying effects occur around an individual's habitual wake-up time.

Note that PRCs reflect results from an average of healthy control individuals. How any specific individual responds to light and melatonin can depart from these guidelines. Furthermore, when extrapolating information from PRCs, one should keep in mind that these curves are based on subjects without evidence of circadian misalignment, so those with circadian rhythm sleep-wake disorders (CRSWDs) may respond differently.

CIRCADIAN RHYTHM SLEEP WAKE DISORDERS (CRSWDS)

The goals of the next section are to define the main circadian rhythm sleep-wake disorders CRSWDs and discuss their diagnosis, pathophysiology, and treatment.

General Diagnostic Criteria

Circadian rhythm sleep-wake disorders (CRSWDs) can arise from disturbance of the circadian system, and/or misalignment between the timing of endogenous circadian rhythms and the social/physical environments and behavior. *According to the International Classification of Sleep Disorders* (ICSD-3),[15] for diagnosis, the following 3 criteria must be satisfied:

A. A chronic or recurrent pattern of sleep-wake rhythm disruption primarily due to alteration of the endogenous circadian timing system or misalignment between the endogenous circadian rhythm and the sleep-wake schedule desired or required by an individual's physical environment or social/work schedules;
B. The circadian rhythm disruption leads to insomnia, excessive sleepiness, or both;
C. The sleep and wake disturbances cause clinically significant distress or impairment in mental, physical, social, occupational, educational, or other important areas of functioning.

Symptoms of insomnia and excessive daytime sleepiness can be prominent features of multiple sleep disorders and comorbid medical or psychiatric conditions, making it difficult to differentiate CRSWDs from other sleep disorders. Therefore, while not required for diagnosis of CRSWDs, the use of biomarkers to confirm circadian phase is recommended. The ICSD-3 defines 6 CRSWDs: advanced sleep-wake phase disorder (ASWPD); delayed sleep-wake phase disorder (DSWPD); non-24 hour sleep-wake rhythm disorder (N24SWD); irregular sleep-wake rhythm disorder (ISWRD); shift work disorder (SWD); and jet lag disorder (JLD). While there are underlying biological differences that can make individuals susceptible to the impacts of shift work or jet lag, the latter 2 disorders are often viewed in a separate category, as they only develop as a result of extrinsic changes to environmental schedules. For that reason, we will focus on the first 4 disorders, ASWPD, DSWPD, N24SWD and

ISWRD, for this chapter. The clinical approach to diagnosis of those CRSWDs, and their management, is discussed in the following sections.

Advanced Sleep-Wake Phase Disorder

Advanced sleep-wake phase disorder (ASWPD) is characterized by sleep-wake times that typically occur 2 or more hours earlier than societal norms. When patients are allowed to sleep during their natural sleep period, sleep quality and duration will be normal.

Having an advanced circadian phase is not sufficient for diagnosis; functional impairment is also required. Because there are many contexts in which patients with an advanced circadian phase are not bothered by or may even benefit from having an advanced phenotype, the prevalence of this disorder is generally thought to be less than DSWPD. For example, 1 study reported that, in a sleep clinic, one might expect 1 out of every 300 patients to have an advanced phase, while only 1 out of every 2500 patients will have ASWPD.[16] When encountered in a clinical setting, ASWPD tends to be seen in older patients, given that some degree of advancement of the circadian phase may be age-associated.

DIAGNOSIS

The key step in diagnosing ASWPD is characterizing the patient's habitual sleep-wake timing. In a clinical setting, sleep logs, actigraphy, and questionnaires are commonly used for this purpose. Diagnosis requires documenting that there is a stable advance of sleep-wake timing over at least 7 days when allowed to sleep on their preferred schedule. The use of circadian phase markers, such as collecting salivary melatonin to determine DLMO, can be considered, but is not required. Other medical or psychiatric conditions should also be considered, such as depression, which could present with similar sleep patterns.

PATHOPHYSIOLOGY

The exact cause of ASWPD is not fully understood. However, at least in some cases, it appears to be an inherited trait associated with mutations in several circadian genes, including *PER2*, *CK1*, *PER3*, *CRY2*, and *TIMELESS*.[10]

Theoretically altered light sensitivity may also play a role if there is either increased sensitivity to the phase-advancing effect of morning light conditions or decreased sensitivity to the phase-delaying effect of evening light conditions. However, this has not yet been documented clinically.

TREATMENT

Evidence from large-scale clinical trials on the efficacy of treatment options for ASWPD is limited (see Table 15.1 later in the chapter for a summary of recommendations).

Based on what is known, evening bright light exposure for 1–2 hours is typically recommended.[17] Recall from the PRC to light that light has a phase-delaying effect during the time window starting before natural sleep onset and ending around the time of the nadir of core body temperature.

From the PRC to melatonin, one might also hypothesize that morning melatonin administration might be helpful in the treatment of ASWPD as well, since the maximal phase-delaying effects of melatonin occur near natural sleep offset time. Unfortunately, there is currently no robust clinical evidence to support this; however, it is an alternative approach sometimes employed in practice.[18]

Delayed Sleep-Wake Phase Disorder

Delayed sleep-wake phase disorder (DSWPD) is characterized by sleep-wake times that are delayed by 2 hours or more relative to conventional norms. Because of this delay, patients will experience insomnia when trying to fall asleep, and excessive daytime sleepiness (EDS) when trying to stay awake at typical socially accepted times. Symptoms must have persisted for 3 or more months. The presence of functional impairment (e.g., difficulty in making it to work or school on time) is also a requirement for diagnosis.

DSWPD is often diagnosed as chronic insomnia. To help distinguish between these 2 overlapping disorders, it is important to inquire, when allowed to sleep on their desired schedule, whether insomnia and symptoms of excessive sleepiness improve or even mostly abate, as would be expected in the case of DSWPD.[19]

Table 15.1 **Summary of Current Treatment Recommendations for Circadian Rhythm Sleep-Wake Disorders**

Disorder	Light	Melatonin/Melatonin Agonist	Other
Advanced sleep-wake phase disorder	*1–2 hours of bright light in the evening, prior to natural sleep onset	(Theoretical) 0.5 mg of melatonin on awakening in the middle of the night	Limit bright light exposure immediately after awakening.
Delayed sleep-wake phase disorder	1–2 hours of bright light, within the first 2 hours of natural wake time	* 0.5 mg of melatonin 1 hour prior to desired bedtime, and get into bed at desired bedtime. If shifts >1–2 hours are desired, can take 0.5 mg of melatonin 5 hours prior to natural bedtime, and gradually move bedtime earlier.	Avoid bright light starting at least 2–3 hours prior to bedtime. Wear blue blocking glasses in the morning if required to wake before natural wake time.
Non-24 hour-sleep-wake rhythm disorder	(Sighted) Bright light for 1–2 hours when waking at desired time	* (Blind) 0.5 mg of melatonin or 20 mg of tasimelteon 1 hour prior to desired bedtime (Sighted) In addition to above, can also take 0.5 mg of melatonin 5 hours prior to desired bedtime.	(Sighted) Avoid bright light starting at least 2–3 hours prior to bedtime.
Irregular sleep-wake rhythm disorder	* Increase daytime light exposure	* (Children/adolescents only) 2–10 mg of melatonin within 1 hour of desired bedtime	Limit bright light and noise at night. Increase daytime activity.

* Indicates recommendation included in the current American Academy of Sleep Medicine guidelines.[17] Additional recommendations based on current clinical practice have also been included for reference.

It is especially important to keep DSWPD in mind when adolescents present with reports of insomnia in conjunction with difficulty waking up for school, as the prevalence of this disorder is greater in this population.

DIAGNOSIS

In addition to the clinical history described in the preceding, to diagnose DSWPD, a stable delay in sleep patterns for at least 7 days must be demonstrated via techniques including either a sleep log or actigraphy monitoring. It may also be helpful to have the patient fill out a questionnaire such as the Horne-Östberg Morningness-Eveningness Questionnaire or the Munich Chronotype Questionnaire. Though less practical in a clinical setting, melatonin sampling to determine DLMO or establishment of the nadir of core body temperature measurement can aid in diagnosis. Comorbid disorders, such as depression, anxiety, and other factors, including poor sleep hygiene, late evening light exposure, and side effect of medications, should be considered in patients with suspected DSWPD. Furthermore, even in the absence of such factors, there appears to be a subset of patients with clinical features of DSWPD, in which sleep-wake behaviors are delayed, however the DLMO is not delayed.[20] This phenotype of DSWPD is further described in Figure 15.2.

PATHOPHYSIOLOGY

Although the exact cause of this disorder is not known, there is evidence that the cause is multi-factorial, with contributing elements including genetics, light sensitivity, and behavioral/psychological factors.

In some cases, there appears to be an inherited susceptibility. For example, mutations in the *CRY1* and *PER2* genes have been found in familial cohorts of DSWPD.[21,22]

Environmental and behavioral influences are thought to play a role in this disorder in some individuals, including tendencies to either sleep in or stay up late, which influences the timing of light exposure, and consumption of stimulants like caffeine or nicotine which can impact the ability to sleep.[19] Increased bright light exposure during the phase delay portion

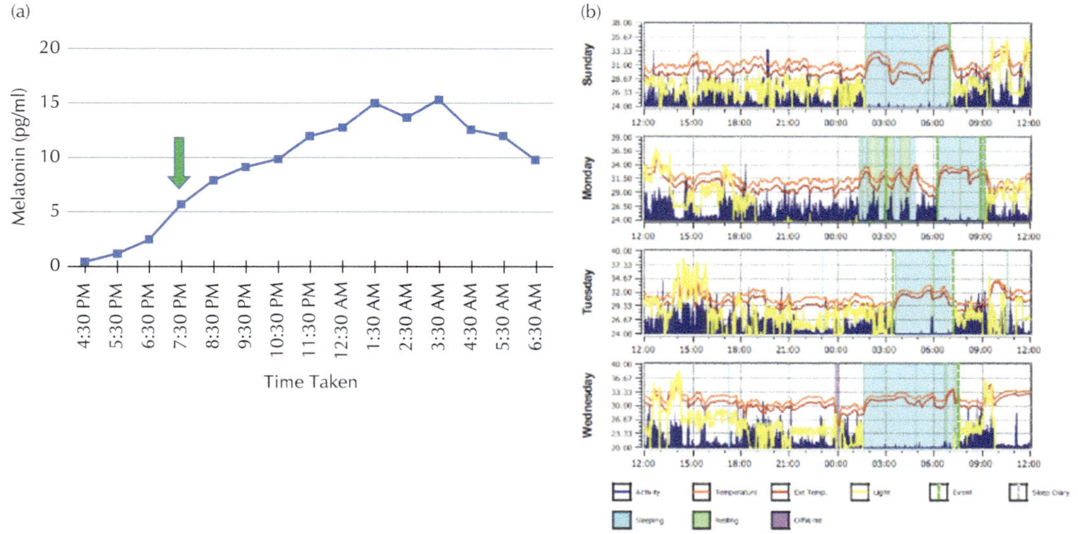

Figure 15.2. Timing of DLMO is not always delayed relative to sleep-wake timing in individuals with DSWPD. Part A shows salivary melatonin levels collected from a person with a stably delayed sleep-wake timing. The *x*-axis shows the time of sample collection in hours. The *y*-axis shows salivary melatonin levels in pg/ml. The green arrow indicates the person's DLMO (defined here as the point at which the salivary melatonin level is ≥4 pg/ml). Part B shows a sample of the corresponding actigraphy for this person's sleep-wake pattern. Given this person's onset of sleep is ~2 AM, the expected DLMO would be 11 PM–midnight. However, as shown in part A, this person's DLMO does not exhibit the expected delay, instead occurring at ~7:30 PM.

of the light PRC (such as from blue-light emitting smartphones, laptops, or energy-efficient lightbulbs) may occur in those with habitually late bedtimes, and is thought to play a role in the development/maintenance of DSWPD in some individuals. An alternative, or additional contributing factor in some cases, may be decreased bright light exposure during the phase advance portion of the light PRC—most notably during the latter third of the phase advance region.[23]

Altered light sensitivity, including reduced sensitivity to morning light and/or increased sensitivity to evening light, can also make the ability to appropriately entrain to the environmental light-dark timing more challenging. Recently, pupillometry has been used as a tool to distinguish individuals with DSWPD and either high or low light sensitivity.[24,25]

TREATMENT

Based on our understanding of circadian physiology and limited clinical evidence, appropriately timed bright light therapy and melatonin administration are recommended to treat DSWPD,[17] as described below and summarized in Table 15.1.

The appropriate timing of these treatments depends on estimating circadian phase, in order to target treatments during the time at which light and melatonin would be expected to produce maximal phase advances, based on the known PRCs for light and melatonin (see introduction to this chapter).

Maximal phase-advancing effects of bright light therapy occur slightly after the minimum core body temperature is reached. Typically, this point is roughly 2–3 hours prior to the natural sleep offset.[26] Therefore, administering light therapy at the time it would have a maximal effect is typically impractical as it would require waking the patient up before their natural wake-up time. However, pilot studies have demonstrated some improvement in sleep-wake timing using a combination of light flashes administered while asleep, in conjunction with cognitive behavioral therapy.[27] Alternatively, clinical recommendations typically suggest 1–2 hours of bright light therapy within the first 2 hours after waking up.

Unfortunately, maximal phase-delaying effects of bright light therapy occur slightly before the minimum core body temperature is reached. If the estimation of this point is inaccurate, or the patient's wake-up time is significantly earlier than their natural wake time, morning light exposure can inadvertently lead to further phase delay.

Some studies offer evidence that light avoidance during the phase-delay portion of the light PRC may potentially aid in the treatment of DSWPD. This phase-delay portion begins around 5–6 hours before minimum core body temperature is reached, which is often the time window right before bedtime, emphasizing the importance of dimming lights and minimizing electronic screen time in the hours before bed.[17]

Low-dose melatonin administration, particularly in conjunction with behavioral sleep-wake scheduling, has been effectively leveraged in the treatment of DSWPD. For instance, 1 study concluded that adults treated with 0.5 mg of fast-release melatonin an hour before desired bedtime showed improved outcomes in terms of objective and subjective measurements of sleep quality when compared to a control group.[28]

Accurately timed melatonin treatment has been shown to improve sleep-related metrics like total sleep duration, number of night-time awakenings, and sleep onset latency in other populations, including children and adolescents with neurodevelopmental disorders such as autism spectrum disorder.[29]

It is important to note that the bioavailability of melatonin is affected by food. To maximize the therapeutic effects of melatonin—whether one is aiming to advance or delay phase—it is advised to take it roughly 60 minutes before or after a meal. Additionally, taking melatonin apart from food makes sense given the modulation of insulin secretion by melatonin, and potential subsequent impact on glucose levels.[30]

Non-24-Hour Sleep-Wake Rhythm Disorder

In non-24 hour sleep-wake rhythm disorder (N24SWD), the timing of the sleep-wake schedule does not align with a 24-hour light-dark cycle. Often, the schedule is longer, though shorter schedules are possible. Patients with N24SWD present with a progressive shifting of their sleep-wake phase (advances for patients with less than 24-hour schedules, delays for patients with longer schedules). Due to the constant shifting of this schedule, sometimes patients will sleep in synchrony with their environment. However, as days pass and their natural schedule becomes misaligned with their environment, they will present with several days of insomnia or EDS. They will soon drift into having a synchronized schedule again, only to have this shifting process repeated.

N24SWD is more prevalent in blind populations. Estimates vary, but the rates are relatively high, perhaps 18%–50% in those who are legally blind.[31] That some individuals lacking conscious light perception maintain normal circadian rhythms can be explained by the observation that photoreception by the ipRGCs may remain intact in the setting of loss or impairment of rod/cone mediated photoreception,[32] or that these individuals may entrain with nonphotic sources like social or physical activity.

It is also possible for sighted individuals to be diagnosed with N24SWRD. The exact prevalence is unknown, though it is considered rarer (albeit under-recognized) compared to blind populations, and in sighted individuals is frequently described in individuals who initially present with extreme DSWPD and may alternate between being very delayed and following a non-24-hour pattern.

DIAGNOSIS

In addition to confirming that a patient's clinical history is consistent with the description of N24SWD, sleep logs or actigraphy must also be performed to make the diagnosis. Results, in this case, must be obtained over longer periods than the 7 days required for diagnosing DSWPD, ASWPD, and ISWRD: usually 14 days or longer are recommended. This distinction is made because, for N24SWD, we are trying to demonstrate the gradual evolution of a sleep-wake schedule, rather than characterize a fixed sleep-wake schedule.

Performing supplemental testing on other circadian markers like DLMO or urinary 6-sulfatoxy-melatonin can help confirm the diagnosis.[15] Because we expect these rhythms to shift, taking measurements on multiple days is crucial. Observations should be separated by enough time for a shift in the sleep-wake schedule to occur (but obviously not limited to amounts of time over which we'd expect the schedule to go through a complete 24-hour shift—e.g., do not test every 24 days for a patient with a suspected 25-hour sleep-wake schedule).

PATHOPHYSIOLOGY

N24SWD has been reported in association with polymorphisms in *PER3*.[10]

In blind populations, lack of light entrainment is postulated in N24SWD pathogenesis. Many individuals in these populations simply do not possess this means of entrainment, either due to loss or destruction of the retinal ganglion cells, which prevents light from reaching the endogenous circadian pacemaker. As most humans have an endogenous period of slightly longer than 24 hours, they require daily light signals to maintain entrainment to the 24-hour light-dark cycle.[15] Recall that non-photic sources for entrainment are often less effective.

Less is known about the pathogenesis of N24SWD in sighted populations. N24SWD can develop following traumatic brain injury or chemotherapy.[10] Psychiatric disorders such as depression may also contribute to the extent that they induce behaviors in patients that reduce exposure to important means of entrainment, like light or social activity.

It is well documented that in sighted populations with N24SWD that DWSPD commonly precedes it. This is because their endogenous circadian pacemaker periods tend to be significantly longer than 24 hours. In addition, it has been documented that these individuals have impaired melanopsin function, which may decrease their ability to respond to the phase-advancing inputs of light.[24]

TREATMENT

In blind populations, the first line treatment of N24SWD is the administration of either melatonin or the FDA-approved melatonin receptor agonist tasimelteon (see Table 15.1). In the former case, the timing of the melatonin dose should be consistent on a nightly basis (often roughly 1–2 hours before desired sleep onset). The dosage is typically between .1 and .5 mg.[33] Tasimelteon is recommended to be given 1 hour before desired sleep onset. In clinical trials, 20% (3%) of patients taking tasimelteon (controls) achieved entrainment after 1 month, and moreover, 90% (20%) were able to maintain it with continued administration.[34]

Other management strategies for N24SWD in blind populations include further strengthening non-photic entrainment cues via scheduling meals, physical activity, and socialization.

Evidence is limited on the efficacy of N24SWD treatments (see Table 15.1) in sighted populations. No large-scale clinical trials have been performed to date. However, some support for treatment approaches based on combining photic and non-photic means of entrainment has been reported.[35] Melatonin administration can also be attempted, as in the case of blind populations.

Irregular Sleep-Wake Rhythm Disorder

The defining characteristic of irregular sleep-wake rhythm disorder (ISWRD) is the absence of a primary consolidated sleep period. Instead, a patient with ISWRD will sleep during 3 or more randomly distributed blocks over the course of a day. Typically, these blocks will be at most 4 hours in length. Despite this fragmentation, total sleep duration over a 24-hour period will often be normal for age.

Patients usually present with insomnia or EDS, and symptoms must have persisted for 3 or more months. In addition, the patient's dispersed sleep schedule must be involuntary (i.e., not dictated by external schedule demands) and not better explained by sleep hygiene or another disorder.

ISWRD commonly arises in association with neurodevelopmental or neurodegenerative disorders. The frequency in male and female populations is similar.

DIAGNOSIS

Clinical history must be consistent with the preceding in order to diagnose ISWRD. In addition, documenting the lack of discernible patterns in a patient's sleep schedule over at least 7 days is also required. Either sleep logs or actigraphy can be used in principle, though actigraphy may be far more practical when ISWRD is associated with neurodevelopmental or neurodegenerative disorders and the patient is unable to track their own sleep-wake patterns, though caregivers can also be asked to assist with sleep logs.

Unlike the diagnostic approach for DSWPD, melatonin sampling to determine DLMO is not usually helpful in diagnosing ISWRD. If this is done, however, one may find that the patient with ISWRD exhibits a melatonin profile with a dampened amplitude.

Although we observed earlier that ISWRD commonly arises in association with neurodevelopmental or neurodegenerative disorders (e.g., Alzheimer disease, Lewy body dementia), whether ISWRD should be diagnosed in this case is debatable: the ICSD3 states that the random dispersal of sleep does not have a better explanation. However, there is likely a connection between many of these disorders and the pathophysiology of ISWRD (see the following).

PATHOPHYSIOLOGY

One potential cause of the diminished circadian entrainment in patients with ISWRD is impaired light input to the suprachiasmatic nucleus.[10] In some cases, pathology in the optic nerve or retina might be responsible. Input can also be impaired if individuals are living in an environment where daytime light exposure is insufficient.

Diminished circadian rhythm amplitude could be due to impaired output from the SCN as well. This might occur as part of either a neurodegenerative or neurodevelopmental disorder. These populations have been reported to exhibit unusual melatonin rhythms and lowered melatonin secretion amplitude.[15,36]

TREATMENT

Behavioral interventions are often utilized in the treatment of ISWRD. In general, the goal is to implement a structured schedule which promotes activity during the daytime and sleep and rest during the nighttime. For instance, schedules which facilitate engagement in regular daytime social activities and physical movement/exercise, and which provide nighttime environments conducive to sleep (e.g., dark, quiet, cool), may be beneficial.[37]

Data is conflicting as to the effectiveness of bright light therapy for the treatment of ISWRD, including in patients with neurodegenerative disorders. Interestingly, the combined use of morning bright light exposure and evening melatonin was shown to be beneficial in patients with dementia, as evidenced by higher rest-activity rhythms and decreased daytime sleep.[38] However, the AASM advises against the use of melatonin in elderly patients with dementia, given concern that it may negatively impact mood.[39]

In children and adolescents, including those with neurodevelopmental disorders, melatonin has been shown to be safe and effective for management of ISWRD, and is supported by AASM guidelines (see Table 15.1).

OUTLOOK

During the past decade, we have seen major advances in our understanding of the mechanisms regulating circadian rhythms and of the ubiquitous effects of circadian rhythms in metabolism, inflammation, cardiovascular, and neurological disorders.[40,41] Furthermore, there is increased recognition that the circadian system and circadian misalignment have broader impacts on health beyond sleep and wake timing. For example, simply having a delayed phenotype has previously been associated with an increase in allcause mortality.[42]

Circadian disruption in the form of exposure to shift work has long been recognized as a probable carcinogen. In addition, circadian disruption has an apparent role in the progression of cancer. One study reported that patients with metastatic colorectal cancer had a 5-fold higher risk of dying within 2 years if they experienced poor circadian rhythmicity.[43] The promotion of tumor growth has been associated with circadian disruption in additional cancers, including breast and prostate cancers.[40]

Circadian misalignment is highly correlated with mood disorders. Whether the former causes the latter or vice versa is still unknown, but it is known that circadian systems and neurological systems associated with mood disorders, including the reward and serotonergic systems, are strongly linked. Medicines aimed at treating mood disorders such as lithium, ketamine, and selective serotonin reuptake inhibitors (SSRIs) have been shown to affect circadian rhythms too.[44]

Neurodegenerative diseases, including Alzheimer disease, Parkinson disease, and Huntington disease, are associated with circadian rhythm disruption. It is thought that multiple pathways might link such disruption with these conditions, and in this context, the former can be a risk factor, an early symptom, and/or a direct contributor to progression of the latter. Both sleep fragmentation and deprivation are known risk factors for Alzheimer disease.[45]

Given these wide-ranging associations, recognizing the role of circadian disruption in disease may lead to better optimization of already existing therapies for many illnesses. In addition, there is the potential to develop new circadian-based treatment strategies.

Some strategies—namely, chrono-pharmacology and chronotherapy—aim to both improve treatment efficacy and reduce adverse side effects by optimizing the timing of either treatment administration or release once administered. Giving bright light and melatonin-based therapies in accordance with a patient's individual PRCs when treating CRSWDs are simple examples. However, research has also shown potential for improved treatment outcomes when circadian rhythms inform the timing of administration or release of medications in a broad range of conditions.[46] Certain medications for the treatment of hypertension, for instance, have been shown to be significantly more effective if administered at night. Further benefits of nighttime administration over morning administration can include reduction of cardiovascular disease risk and side effects including edema.[47]

Dosage time also has an impact on the efficacy of glucocorticoids and disease-modifying antirheumatic drugs in the context of rheumatoid arthritis treatment. This may seem sensible, as key symptoms of rheumatoid arthritis like morning stiffness themselves exhibit a circadian rhythm. In one study, patients given a modified-release formulation of prednisone at night experienced diminished morning joint stiffness compared to patients given an immediate-release formulation of prednisone in the morning.[48]

Future studies are needed to address these gaps, along with the development of clinically scalable diagnostic tools and biomarkers of sleep, cardiometabolic, and immune dysfunction to assess the effectiveness of circadian-based treatments.

The field of circadian medicine is an expanding field and an active area of research. Findings will have significance for CRSWDs, the primary focus of this chapter, but as highlighted previously, will likely impact numerous other conditions.

REFERENCES

1. Abbott S, Reid KJ, Zee PC. Circadian Disorders of the Sleep-Wake Cycle. In: Kryger M, Roth T, Goldstein C, Dement W, eds. *Principles and Practice of Sleep Medicine Seventh Edition* (pp.). Elsevier; 2022: 441–450.
2. Klerman EB, Brager A, Carskadon MA, et al. Keeping an eye on circadian time in clinical research and medicine. *Clinic Transl Med*. 2022 Dec;12(12):e1131.
3. Middleton B, Arendt J, Stone MB. Human circadian rhythms in constant dim light (8 lux) with knowledge of clock time. *J Sleep Res*.1996 Jun;5(2);69–76.
4. Gallego M, Virshup DM. Post-translational modifications regulate the ticking of the circadian clock. *Nat Rev Mo Cell Biol*. 2007 Feb;8(2):139–148.
5. Ko CH, Takahashi JS. Molecular components of the mammalian circadian clock. *Hum Mol Genet*. 2006 Oct 15;15:R271–R277.
6. Lee Y, Lee J, Kwon I, et al. Coactivation of the CLOCK–BMAL1 complex by CBP mediates resetting of the circadian clock. *J Cell Sci*. 2010 Oct 15;123(20):3547–3557.
7. Hirota T, Lee JW, Lewis WG, et al. High-throughput chemical screen identifies a novel potent modulator of cellular circadian rhythms and reveals CKIα as a Clock regulatory kinase. *PLoS Biol*. 2010 Dec 14;8(12):e1000559.
8. Vitaterna MH, Shimomura K, Jiang P. Genetics of circadian rhythms. *Neurol Clin*. 2019 Aug;37(3):487–504.
9. Wahl S, Engelhardt M, Schaupp P, Lappe C, Ivanov IV. The inner clock: Blue light sets the human rhythm. *J Biophotonics*. 2019 Dec;12(12):e201900102.
10. Meyer N, Harvey AG, Lockley SW, Dijk D-J. Circadian rhytms and disorders of the timing of sleep. *Lancet*. 2022 Sep 14;400:1061–1078.

11. Colwell CS, Witkovsky P, Silver R. The Suprachiasmatic Nucleus (SCN): Critical Points. In Colwell CS, ed. *Circadian Medicine*. Wiley; 2015.
12. Benarroch EE. Suprachiasmatic nucleus and melatonin: Reciprocal interactions and clinical correlations. *Neurology*. 2008 Aug;71(8):594–598.
13. van der Meijden P, Someren JL, Te Lindert BH, et al. Individual differences in sleep timing relate to melanopsin-based phototransduction in healthy adolescents and young adults. *Sleep*. 2016 Jun;39(6):1305–1310.
14. Emens JS, Burgess HJ. Effect of light and melatonin and other melatonin receptor agonists on human circadian physiology. *Sleep Med Clin*. 2015 Dec;10(4):435–453.
15. American Academy of Sleep Medicine. *International Classification of Sleep Disorders*. 3rd ed. American Academy of Sleep Medicine; 2014.
16. Curtis BJ, Ashbrook LH, Young T, et al. Extreme morning chronotypes are often familial and not exceedingly rare: The estimated prevalence of advanced sleep phase, familial advanced sleep phase, and advanced sleep–wake phase disorder in a sleep clinic population. *Sleep*. 2019 Oct;42(10):zsz148.
17. Auger RR, Burgess HJ, Emens JS, Derly LV, Thomas SM, Sharkey KM. Clinical practice guideline for the treatment of intrinsic circadian rhythm sleep-wake disorders: Advanced sleep-wake phase disorder (ASWPD), delayed sleep-wake phase disorder (DSWPD), non-24-hour sleep-wake rhythm disorder (N24SWD), and irregular sleep-wake rhythm disorder (ISWRD). An update for 2015: An American Academy of Sleep Medicine Clinical Practice Guideline. *J Clin Sleep Med*. 2015;11(10):1199–1236.
18. Zee PC. Melantonin for the treatment of advanced sleep phase disorder. *Sleep*. 2008 Jul;31(7):923.
19. Bjorvatn B, Pallesen S. A practical approach to circadian rhythm sleep disorders. *Sleep Med Rev*. 2009;13(1):47–60.
20. Murray JM, Sletten TL, Magee M, et al. Prevalence of circadian misalignment and its association with depressive symptoms in delayed sleep phase disorder. *Sleep*. 2017 Jan 1;40(1):zsw002.
21. Patke A, Murphy PJ, Onat OE, et al. Mutation of the human circadian clock gene CRY1 in familial delayed sleep phase disorder. *Cell*. 2017 Apr 6;169(2):203–215.
22. Miyagawa T, Hida A, Shimada M, et al. A missense variant in PER2 is associated with delayed sleep-wake phase disorder in a Japanese population. *J Hum Genet*. 2019 Dec;64(12):1219–1225.
23. Wilson J IV, Reid KJ, Braun RI, Abbott SM, Zee PC. Habitual light exposure relative to circadian timing in delayed sleep-wake phase disorder. *Sleep*. 2018 Nov 1;41(11):zsy166.
24. Abbott SM, Choi J, Wilson J, Zee PC. Melanopsin-dependent phototransduction is impaired in delayed sleep–wake phase disorder and sighted non–24-hour sleep–wake rhythm disorder. *Sleep*. 2021 Feb;44(2):zsaa184.
25. Watson LA, Phillips AJ, Hosken IT, et al. Increased sensitivity of the circadian system to light in delayed sleep–wake phase disorder. *J Physiol*. 2018 Dec 15;596(24):6249–6261.
26. Czeisler CA, Buxton OM. Human Circadian Timing System and Sleep-Wake Regulation. In: Kryger M, Roth T, Goldstein C, Dement W, eds. *Principles and Practice of Sleep Medicine*. 7th ed. Elsevier; 2017:375–389.
27. Kaplan KA, Mashash M, Williams R, Batchelder H, Starr-Glass L, Zeitzer JM. Effect of light flashes vs sham therapy during sleep with adjunct cognitive behavioral therapy on sleep quality among adolescents: A randomized clinical trial. *JAMA Network Open*. 2019 Sep 25;2(9):e1911944.
28. Sletten TL, Magee M, Murray JM, et al. Efficacy of melatonin with behavioural sleep-wake scheduling for delayed sleep-wake phase disorder: A double-blind, randomised clinical trial. *PLoS Med*. 2018 Jun 18;15(6):e1002587.
29. Rossignol DA, Frye RE. Melatonin in autism spectrum disorders: A systematic review and meta-analysis. *Dev Med Child Neurol*. 2011 Sep;53(9):783–792.
30. Espino J, Pariente JA, Rodríguez AB. Role of melatonin on diabetes-related metabolic disorders. *World J Diabetes*. 2011 Jun 15;2(6):82–91.
31. Flynn-Evans EE, Tabandeh H, Skene DJ, Lockley SW. Circadian rhythm disorders and melatonin production in 127 blind women with and without light perception. *J Biol Rhythms*. 2014 Jun;29(3):215–224.
32. Lockley SW, Arendt J, Skene DJ. Visual impairment and circadiam rhythm disorders. *Dial Clin Neurosci*. 2007 Sep;9(7):301–314.
33. Lewy AJ, Emens JS, Lefler BJ, Yuhas K, Jackman AR. Melatonin entrains free-running blind people according to a physiological dose-response curve. *Chronobiol Int*. 2005;22(6):1093–1106.
34. Lockley SW, Dressman MA, Licamele L, et al. Tasimelteon for non-24-hour sleep-wake disorder in totally blind people (SET and RESET): Two multicentre, randomised, double-masked, placebo-controlled phase 3 trials. *Lancet*. 2015 Oct 31;386(10005):1754–1764.
35. Malkani RG, Abbott SM, Reid KJ, Zee PC. Diagnostic and treatment challenges of sighted non-24-hour sleep-wake disorder. *J Clin Sleep Med*. 2018 Apr 15;14(4):603–613.
36. Abbott SM, Zee PC. Irregular sleep-wake rhythm disorder. *Sleep Med Clin*. 2015 Dec;10(4):517–522.
37. Roth HL. Dementia and sleep. *Neurologic Clin*. 2012 Nov;30(4):1213–1248.
38. Dowling GA, Burr RL, Van Someren EJ, et al. Melatonin and bright-light treatment for rest-activity disruption in institutionalized patients with Alzheimer's disease. *J Am Geriatr Soc*. 2008 Feb;56(2):239–246.
39. Riemersma-van der Lek RF, Swaab DF, Twisk J, Hol EM, Hoogendijk WJ, Van Someren EJ. Effect of bright light and melatonin on cognitive and noncognitive function in elderly residents of group care facilities: A randomized controlled trial. *JAMA*. 2008 Jun 11;299(22):2642–2655.
40. Hou Y, Liu L, Chen X, Li Q, Li J. Association between circadian disruption and diseases: A narrative review. *Life Sciences*. 2020 Dec 1;262:118512–118519.
41. Bishehsari F, Levi F, Turek FW, Keshavarzian A. Circadian rhythms in gastrointestinal health and diseases. *Gastroenterology*. 2016;151(3):e1–e5.

42. Knutson KL, von Schantz M. Associations between chronotype, morbidity and mortality in the UK Biobank cohort. *Chronobiol Int*. 2018 Aug;35(8):1045–1053.
43. Mormont M-C, Waterhouse J, Bleuzen P, et al. Marked 24-h rest/activity rhythms are associated with better quality of life, better response, and longer survival in patients with metastatic colorectal cancer and good performance status. *Clin Cancer Res*. 2000 Aug 1;6(8):3038–3045.
44. Agnorelli C, Fagiolini A. Circadian neuromarkers of mood disorders. *J Affect Dis Rep*. 2022 Dec;10:100384.
45. Musiek ES, Holtzman DM. Mechanisms linking circadian clocks, sleep, and neurodegeneration. *Science*. 2016 Nov 25;354(6315):1004–1008.
46. Odho S, Koyanagi S, Matsunaga N. Chronopharmacological strategies focused on chrono-drug discovery. *Pharmacol Ther*. 2019 Oct;202:72–90.
47. Hermida RC, Ayala DE, Mojon A, Fernandez JR. Influence of circadian time of hypertension treatment on cardiovascular risk: Results of the MAPEC study. *Chronobiol Int*. 2010 Sep;27(8):1629–1651.
48. To H. Chronotherapy for rheumatoid arthritis: Current perspectives. *Chronophysiol Ther*. 2016 Aug;6:47–53.

Chapter 16

Narcolepsy and the Hypersomnias

Sandhya Kumar, Gnanaraj Joseph, Sheila Maurer, and Rupendra Ghatak

INTRODUCTION

Central disorders of hypersomnolence, also referred to as hypersomnias, are particularly distinct from other sleep disorders, such as sleep apnea, restless legs syndrome, or circadian rhythm disorders, in that they have excessive daytime sleepiness (EDS) as a key clinical symptom. Hypersomnias include: (1) narcolepsy type 1 and 2; (2) idiopathic hypersomnia; (3) Kleine Levin syndrome; (4) hypersomnia due to medical or neurological disorder; (5) hypersomnia due to medication or substance abuse; (6) hypersomnia associated with psychiatric disorders; and (7) insufficient sleep syndrome. Herein we will focus on narcolepsy, a chronic and debilitating instability of the sleep-wake states due to destruction of orexin (also known as hypocretin)–containing neurons at the lateral hypothalamus.

The *International Classification of Sleep Disorders* (ICSD), 3rd edition, classifies narcolepsy into narcolepsy type 1 (NT1) and narcolepsy type 2 (NT2); these were previously classified as narcolepsy with and without cataplexy, respectively. We will provide an overview of the epidemiology, pathophysiology, clinical features, diagnosis, and management of narcolepsy.

EPIDEMIOLOGY

Narcolepsy is the most common type of hypersomnias. It is a rare sleep disorder, which usually starts in the initial decades of life. Prevalence of narcolepsy in children age 5–19 years is estimated to be 20–50 cases per 100,000 people, and the diagnosis is often missed.[1–2]

The prevalence of narcolepsy is highest in the Japanese population, with160 per 100,000 in school-aged children, and 590 per 100,000 among adults in Japan. The lowest frequency, 0.2 per 100,000, has been found among Israeli Jews.[3–7] Prevalence studies reported 50–67 per 100,000 individuals in the United States[8] and 47 individuals per 100,000 individuals in a European population.[9]

PATHOPHYSIOLOGY

The pathophysiology of narcolepsy is still not completely understood, but appears to involve a combination of genetic susceptibility, destruction of orexin-containing neurons in the lateral hypothalamus, autoimmune microglial activation, and dysregulation of sleep-wake and rapid eye movement (REM) sleep mechanisms.

Narcolepsy has a strong genetic association with the human leukocyte antigen (HLA) class II alleles in the major histocompatibility region, particularly the HLA-DQB1*06:02 allele.[10,11,12] HLA-DQB1*06:02 is found in over 90% of narcoleptic patients with cataplexy and approximately 50% of patients without cataplexy, but only in 12%–30% of the general population in the United States, Europe, and Japan.[13] While HLA-DQB1*06:02 significantly increases the risk of developing narcolepsy, it alone is not sufficient to cause it, indicating that other factors play a crucial role in the disorder's development. Narcolepsy is sporadic; the risk that an affected parent will have an affected child is only 1%. If one monozygotic twin has narcolepsy, there is a roughly 30% chance of the other twin developing narcolepsy.[13]

The discovery of orexin also known as hypocretin has been a pivotal breakthrough in understanding narcolepsy. Orexin is produced by neurons in the lateral hypothalamus, which play a critical role in regulating wakefulness and sleep-wake transitions (Figure 16.1). In the late 1990s, researchers asserted that type

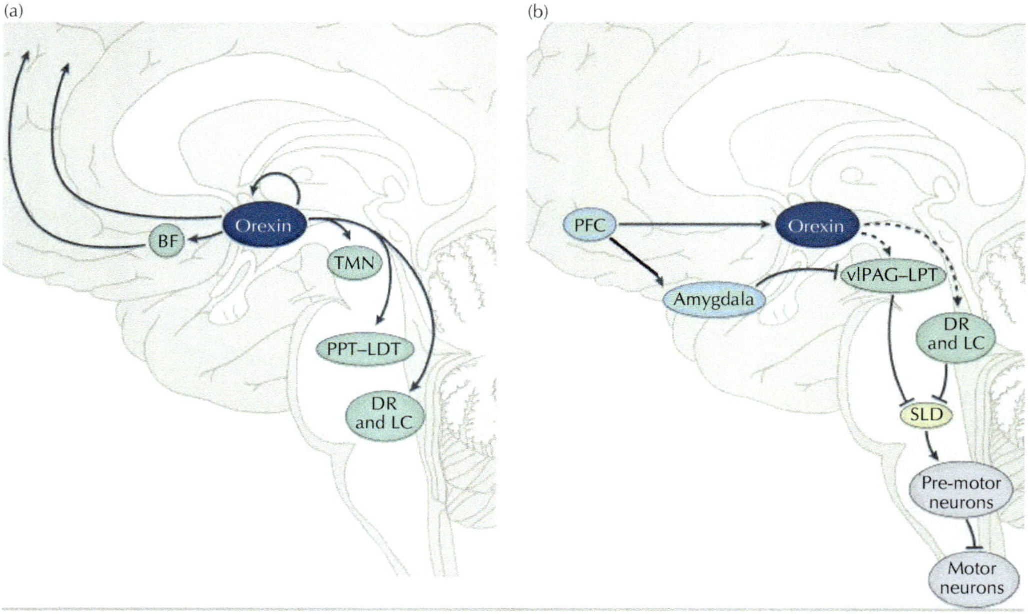

Figure 16.1. Wake-promoting and cataplexy-suppressing orexin pathways.

a: Orexin neurons (dark blue) maintain wake by exciting various wake promoting neurons (green), including those in the cortex, basal forebrain (BF), tuberomammillary nucleus (TMN), pedunculopontine and laterodorsal tegmental nuclei (PPT–LDT), dorsal raphe (DR), and locus coeruleus (LC). Orexin neurons may also undergo auto-excitation, helping drive sustained activity in the orexin neurons and their targets. **b**: Normally, orexin neurons (dark blue) block the occurrence of muscle paralysis during wake by activating rapid eye movement (REM) sleep-suppressing regions (green), such as neurons in the ventral lateral periaqueductal gray and lateral pontine tegmentum (vlPAG-LPT), DR and LC. All these nuclei inhibit the sublaterodorsal nucleus (SLD), a region which during REM sleep drives muscle paralysis by activating GABAergic pre-motor neurons that inhibit motor neurons (purple). With strong emotional stimuli, signals from the medial prefrontal cortex (mPFC) probably activate orexin neurons and neurons in the central nucleus of the amygdala, which have opposing effects on the vlPAG-LPT, DR, and LC. However, in narcolepsy, the excitatory drive from the orexin neurons is absent, and signals from the amygdala can inhibit these REM sleep-suppressing regions, enabling activity in the SLD and resulting in cataplexy.

Mahoney CE, Cogswell A, Koralink IJ, Scammell TE. The neurobiological basis of narcolepsy. *Nat Rev Neurosci*. 2019 Feb;20(2):83–93. Figure reproduced with permission.

1 narcolepsy is caused by a selective loss of orexin-containing neurons[14–16] by an autoimmune process. Why this autoimmune attack targets orexin-producing neurons remains unclear, but it is thought to involve a combination of genetic susceptibility, young age, and environmental triggers. In individuals with a genetic predisposition (HLA-DQB1*06:02 positive), an environmental trigger such as an infection (e.g., streptococcus or influenza) might abnormally activate the immune system (T-cell response) where it mistakenly attacks and destroys the orexin-producing neurons, perhaps through molecular mimicry,[17,18] leading to an autoimmune response. Microglial activation in the hypothalamus, with suggested inflammation and immune response involvement (as indicated by cytokines, e.g., IL-4, IL-6, IL-8, and TNF-alpha, detected in sera or plasma of patients with narcolepsy),[19] likely contributes to the destruction of orexin-producing neurons, further exacerbating narcolepsy.[20]

Orexin (hypocretin) promotes wakefulness by stimulating other wake-promoting systems in the brain, such as the noradrenergic, serotonergic, and histaminergic systems. Loss of orexin producing neurons leads to orexin (hypocretin) deficiency, decreased activity of wake-promoting systems, sleep-wake cycle disruption, and EDS.

Narcolepsy is also associated with abnormalities in REM sleep regulation. Normally, there is an orderly progression of sleep stages, with REM sleep occurring after a period of non-rapid eye movement (NREM) sleep; however, in narcolepsy, REM sleep can occur quite early after sleep onset or can intrude into wakefulness, resulting in phenomena like sleep paralysis and hypnagogic hallucinations.

CLINICAL PRESENTATION OF NARCOLEPSY

Narcolepsy has 5 cardinal features:

1. *Excessive daytime sleepiness (for at least 3 months)*: required for a diagnosis of narcolepsy and occurs even after adequate hours of sleep at night. This can range from being excessively sleepy during the daytime while inactive, to falling asleep under circumstances requiring attention, to sleep attacks (described as uncontrollable sleepiness lasting from a few seconds to a few minutes that can occur even while engaging in active tasks like eating or talking).
2. *Cataplexy*: loss of muscle tone in response to an emotional trigger. Loss of deep tendon reflex occurs with complete cataplexy. Cataplexy episodes usually last a few seconds to minutes and vary in frequency from less than once a year to several times during the day. There is no loss of consciousness during cataplexy. Status cataplecticus, characterized by repeated attacks occurring for hours to days, is a very rare presentation.[21] Symptom severity can fluctuate across the life span, as well as with hormonal changes (e.g., puberty, pregnancy, and menopause), schedule changes, and life stressors. Early symptoms that may be overlooked or mistaken for other disorders and noted retrospectively include: abnormal napping; clumsiness; facial hypotonia with ptosis, jaw drop, tongue thrust, head roll, and/or shoulder drop.
3. *Hallucinations*: Vivid hallucinations occur upon wakefulness (hypnopompic) or at the onset of sleep (hypnogogic) as a REM-mediated phenomenon. Narcolepsy is characterized by the loss of the orderly progression of varying stages of sleep, with REM sleep intruding into wakeful states, causing hallucinations.
4. *Sleep paralysis*: a brief phenomenon that usually occurs upon awakening where patients feel that they are paralyzed; they are aware of their surroundings, but just do not have the ability to move. This is thought to be associated with a delay of the spinal cord control mediated by REM sleep neurons remaining active upon awakening while the brain's neurotransmitters controlling REM sleep are inactive.
5. *Disturbed nocturnal sleep*: Ironically, though excessive daytime sleepiness is a cardinal feature of narcolepsy, narcoleptics are unable to maintain a good, consolidated sleep at night. They usually do not have difficulties with sleep initiation but have significant sleep fragmentation through the night.

PROCEDURES AND TESTING REQUIREMENTS

Apart from clinical features, sleep studies are an integral part in the diagnosis of narcolepsy. This entails an overnight baseline polysomnogram to be followed by a multiple sleep latency testing (MSLT) the next day. Details of the testing are summarized in Box 16.1. The American Academy of Sleep Medicine (AASM) has published recommendations for MSLT testing, and full details of these recommendations can be found on the AASM website.[22]

DIAGNOSIS

Apart from the clinical features mentioned above, the diagnosis of narcolepsy is made if patients present with a mean sleep latency of 8 minutes or less along with 2 or more sleep onset REM periods (SOREM) in a mean sleep latency testing. A SOREM within 15 minutes of sleep onset on the previous night polysomnogram could replace one of the SOREMs on the MSLT.

Differentiating between narcolepsy type I (NT1) and type II (NT2) is the presence of

Box 16.1 Sleep Study Setup

Preparing for the Sleep Test

- Before the test, set sleep goals, especially the nightly sleep time duration, with the doctor.
- Have patients keep a sleep diary; it is helpful to use a sleep tracker like an actigraphy for 2 weeks before the study.
- If the patient is already on positive airway pressure (PAP) therapy or other modalities of treatment for sleep-disordered breathing, ensure adequate control of the underlying sleep-disordered breathing prior to the MSLT. Review of compliance data and ensuring adequate compliance with therapy is needed. Patient should be on PAP at their home settings during the night of the study. A titration using PAP should be avoided

Medication and Therapy Plan

- Decide on using medications and therapies.
- Taper and stop certain medications 2 weeks before the MSLT due to their effects on suppressing REM sleep or causing excessive sleepiness or inability to fall asleep. This list includes antidepressants, anti-anxiety medications, antipsychotics, antihistamines, sedatives, stimulants, wake-promoting agents, prednisone. This should always be done in collaboration with the prescribing provider. For medications with a longer half-life, a longer wash-out period up to 6 weeks might be required.
- Make patient aware of informing the physician if any new medications are prescribed by any providers
- Discuss caffeine limits to avoid affecting the test
- Aim for no caffeine, or reduce gradually to prevent withdrawal symptoms on the test day

(*Continued*)

Box 16.1 Sleep Study Setup (cont.)

During Study

- MSLT follows a previous overnight baseline polysomnogram (PSG) with a minimum of 7 hours of recording time and 6 hours of total sleep time.
- Patients should wear comfortable clothes.
- Patients need to avoid alcohol, caffeine, or marijuana/drugs on test day.
- If using nicotine and unable to avoid its use, then this must be stopped 30 minutes before a nap trial.
- Use prescribed breathing therapies (PAP or dental device for treatment of sleep disordered breathing) during PSG and MSLT. Keep settings and mask consistent with home use

Recording Setup

- Use a minimum of 7-channel recordings for MSLT (3 channels of EEG, right and left EOG, EMG, and EKG).
- Remove unnecessary devices for comfort.

Monitoring

- Record audiovisual data during nap trials; continuous monitoring throughout the day also is needed.

Nap Trials Structure

- MSLT has 5 nap trials.
- First trial starts 1.5–3 hours after the end of polysomnogram recording.
- Subsequent trials start 2 hours after the prior trial.
- Offer restroom use and check comfort before each nap trial.
- Avoid stimulating or vigorous activities, including use of electronic devices, at least 30 minutes before each nap trial.
- Avoid prolonged bright light exposure the day of the study.
- Patient should be off the bed once each nap trial is concluded and stays off bed between nap trials.

During Nap Trials

- Ensure a dark, quiet, and comfortable room.
- Patient lies in bed for all nap trials.

Trial Instructions

- Instruct patient to lie quietly with eyes closed and allow sleep.
- Testing starts immediately, once lights are turned off.

(Continued)

Box 16.1 Sleep Study Setup (cont.)

Trial Duration and Sleep Onset

- End each trial if no sleep in 20 minutes.
- If sleep onset is achieved, which is the first epoch of any stage of sleep, continue for 15 more minutes, so a nap could last anywhere from 20 to 35 minutes.

Preparation Before Trials

- Conduct bio-calibrations before each nap trial.

Meals

- Have a light breakfast 1 hour before the first trial.
- Eat a light lunch after the second nap trial.

Drug Screening

- Use urine drug screening when needed for accurate results.

cataplexy and/or cerebrospinal fluid (CSF) hypocretin level less than or equal to 110 pg/ml in NT1, and absence of cataplexy and CSF levels of hypocretin not measured or greater than 110 pg/ml in NT2.

MANAGEMENT OF NARCOLEPSY AND HYPERSOMNIA

Management of narcolepsy includes symptomatic treatment of EDS, disruptive nighttime sleep, and cataplexy. Hypersomnia interferes with work, school, relationships, and social life. Driving safety must be discussed and encouraged since in studies with narcoleptics about 66% had reported falling asleep at the wheel and a statistically significant increase in driving accidents of 36.8% due to sleepiness.[23] Management requires combined nonpharmacological/behavioral and pharmacological treatment strategies (Box 16.2). Behavioral strategies can be effective in managing early and mild narcolepsy symptoms.

Pharmacotherapy should aim to achieve normal alertness during waking hours or maximum alertness during important activities such as work, school, and driving. Despite optimal therapy, some residual sleepiness is expected. There are only a few comparative randomized controlled studies available regarding therapy choice. Hence, medication management is primarily based on clinical experience and expert opinion. Initial selection should be individualized based on primary symptoms, severity, efficacy, comorbidities, side effects, and cost.

Hypnogogic hallucinations and sleep paralysis improve with treatment of cataplexy. Ideally, monotherapy with first-line medications should be optimized based on side effects and efficacy. Depending on symptoms, the first agent may be titrated down or discontinued and a second-line agent may be considered. Many patients may need combination therapy for wake promotion and cataplexy control.[27]

The inability to adhere to safety requirements of alerting agents, comorbidities, or concurrent use of medications such as narcotics, sedatives which increase the risk of central nervous system (CNS) suppression, would disallow prescribing. Substance abuse will be a limiting factor.

Table 16.1 summarizes pharmacological therapies used for narcolepsy.

Box 16.2 Narcolepsy Management

Non-Pharmacological/Behavioral

- Maintain good sleep hygiene with a regular sleep-wake schedule and sufficient sleep time for age.
- Schedule one or two 15–30-minute naps in a day to reduce the risk of severe sleepiness and improve alertness.
- Schedule naps prior to events requiring attention. Some patients may need at least 1 hour of nap.
- Avoid:
  - sleep deprivation;
  - sedating drugs and substances that can worsen sleepiness, worsen sleep quality, or have drug interactions;
  - medications that can worsen cataplexy (e.g., alpha-1 antagonists);
  - large meals, sugar, caffeine, nicotine, and other alerting agents and activities at least 3–4 hours before bedtime.
- Ensure adequate treatment of:
  - coexistent sleep disorders: OSA, RLS, and REM behavior disorder;
  - coexistent psychiatric comorbidities: depression, anxiety, bipolar disorder;
  - other medical problems, including chronic pain.
- Perform regular exercise during the day to promote alertness.
- Work with school/employer for adaptive modifications.
- Weight management is encouraged.
- Psychosocial support: local mental health support groups; online resources; individual and family psychological counseling; CBT–I with narcolepsy adaptations[24];
- Driving safety: proper sleep, break after long drives; take turns driving; should not drive if daytime sleepiness is not controlled.

Pharmacological Approaches

Standard of Care

- Alerting agents: modafinil, armodafinil, pitolisant, solriamfetol, methyl phenidate, and amphetamines.[25–27]
- Oxybates and pitolisant can treat both sleepiness and cataplexy.[25–27]
- Oxybates act primarily through consolidating nighttime sleep and offer the best symptom control with monotherapy.
- Disadvantages of oxybates include: inability to adhere to safety requirements; comorbidities; concurrent use of medications such as narcotics, sedatives would disallow prescribing as the combination increases the risk of CNS suppression; and potential for substance abuse.

(*Continued*)

Box 16.2 Narcolepsy Management (cont.)

Mild to Moderate Sleepiness

- Mild to moderate sleepiness with or without cataplexy: use first-line wake-promoting agents (see Table 16.1).
- Modafinil or armodafinil is usually started as a first drug due to large experience and drug safety profile.
- Persistent sleepiness after monotherapy dose optimization: pitolisant or solriamfetol can be added. Also adding or switching to oxybates could be considered.
- Alternatives: second-line wake-promoting agents such as methylphenidate and amphetamines (reminder: these have high sympathomimetic side effects).

Severe Disabling Sleepiness

- Adding or switching to oxybates may be indicated when (1) monotherapy with modafinil/other first-line agents is insufficient to control sleepiness severity; and/or (2) patients report severe nighttime disruption;
- Limiting factors: side effects, cost, adherence to safety, concurrent medications, and comorbidities;
- Alternatives: solriamfetol, high dose of amphetamine or methylphenidate, and/or combination therapy.

Residual Cataplexy

- Patients with mild to moderate sleepiness whose symptoms are controlled on wake-promoting agents but still have residual cataplexy can be treated with venlafaxine, selective serotonin reuptake inhibitors (SSRIs), and tricyclic antidepressants in addition to alerting agents.
- Pitolisant can be added or be switched to if the above treatment is ineffective.
- Oxybates will be a good choice if there is severe cataplexy or severe excessive daytime sleepiness and no contraindications for its use.

Disrupted Sleep

- Insomnia with frequent arousals and fragmented sleep is commonly reported in patients with narcolepsy.
- In patients with mild insomnia, zolpidem can be considered.
- Oxybates will be a good choice if no contraindication for their use; should not be combined with any benzodiazepines, other sleep aids.
- Dual orexin receptor antagonists: contraindicated for treatment of insomnia.

Follow-up

- Symptoms of sleepiness and cataplexy need to be reassessed during follow-up visits.
- Persistent sleepiness: caution patients as to avoid potentially dangerous activities (e.g., driving, operating heavy machinery).

(Continued)

Box 16.2 Narcolepsy Management (cont.)

- Maintenance of wakefulness test: to assess any residual sleepiness if required (e.g., for some commercial drivers).
- Monitor blood pressure and heart rate closely on patients taking wake-promoting agents.
- Caution young women taking modafinil or armodafinil about loss of efficacy of contraceptive pills; suggest adding a second contraceptive method.

Considerations for Special Populations

Pregnancy and Lactation

- Compare risks associated with medication intake vs. uncontrolled sleepiness due to discontinuation.
- Most medications are contraindicated during first trimester with high rate of medication discontinuation.[28]
- Non-pharmacological options of symptom control are preferred during pregnancy.
- Medication alternatives: extended sleep time, frequent naps, discontinued working, and discontinued driving.
- Congenital risks of infants to mothers exposed to methylphenidate or amphetamines have been noted and FDA recommends against its use during pregnancy though it states that methylphenidate may be used with caution.[29]
- Amphetamines can lead to lasting effects on a child's behavior. Illicit use can increase the risk of prematurity and intrauterine growth restriction.

Elderly

- Dosing of wake-promoting agents may need to be reduced due to cardiovascular side effects.

Pediatric

- Oxybates have been approved for treatment of narcolepsy in the pediatric population 7 years or older. Stimulants (amphetamine salts and methylphenidates) are approved for pediatric ADHD and are considered safe first-line treatment for pediatric hypersomnia and narcolepsy. There are many formulations, including liquids, dissolvable, and transdermal, that allow for ease of administration and titration (see Table 16.1 for details). Other medications in Table 16.1 have limited clinical trials. Recommendations are based on case reports, case series in children, and adult efficacy.[30–33]

Perioperative and Inpatient Care

- Usually, medications for narcolepsy are discontinued during the hospital stay. The risk of using the medication needs to be weighed against the benefits of continuing the wake-promoting agents. They may also impact recovery from anesthesia.

Notes: OSA: obstructive sleep apnea; RLS: restless legs syndrome; REM: rapid eye movement.

Table 16.1 **Medications Used for Narcolepsy**

Drug	Dosage	Indications	Mechanism	Adverse Effects
Modafinil (Provigil)	100–200 mg every morning Can be titrated up to 400 mg in divided doses Pediatric: 50 mg every morning; titration to 200 mg in 1–2 divided doses.	EDS; first line of therapy	Dopamine reuptake inhibitor CSA-IV	Headache, nervousness, nausea, insomnia, severe rash (Steven Johnson syndrome) Reduced effectiveness of oral contraceptives; need additional contraceptive method
Armodafinil (Nuvigil)	150–250 mg every morning Pediatric: 50 mg every morning; titration up to 250 mg.			
Solriamfetol (Sunosi)	75–150mg daily Initially 75 mg daily, can be titrated up to 150 mg daily	EDS; first line of therapy	Unclear; probably dopamine and norepinephrine reuptake inhibitor; CSA-IV	Headache, nausea, reduced appetite, increased blood pressure and heart rate Note: Ensure blood pressure is adequately controlled prior to initiating treatment.
Pitolisant (Wakix)	8.9–35.6 mg once/day Initially 8.9 mg (two 4.45 mg tabs) can titrate to 35.6 mg once daily Pediatric: (Europe >6 years; USA >18 years): Dose by weight: <40 kg: 4.45 mg starting dose and titrate to 8.9–17.8 mg every morning >40 kg: 4.45–8.9 starting dose and titrate to 17.8–35.6 mg	EDS with cataplexy; first line of therapy	Histamine H3 receptor inverse agonist; CSA-N	Headache, insomnia, nausea, anxiety, severe rash, QT prolongation
Methylphenidate (Ritalin)	10–30 mg twice/day or 20 mg extended release every morning with 10–20 mg immediate release every afternoon Extended release: 10–60 mg every morning.			Reduced appetite, nausea, headache, insomnia, addiction, abuse, psychosis, mania, seizures, tachycardia, hypertension, priapism, myocardial infarction.

	Pediatric (>6 years): Immediate release: Start at 5 mg before breakfast and lunch, can titrate in increments of 5 mg/day every week to <25 kg: 35 mg maximum dose >25 kg: 60 mg maximum dose			In pediatrics: poor growth, weight loss, tics, mood lability, aggression, jitters, sleep disturbance: insomnia, arousals Check UDS to ensure use and no drug diversion. UN
Dextroamphetamine (Dexedrine, Procentra)	5–30 mg twice per day **or** 10 mg extended release every morning with 10–20 mg immediate or extended release every afternoon Pediatric (>6 years): 5 mg every morning. Titration to 5–40 mg in 1–2 divided doses.	EDS; second line of therapy	Dopamine and norepinephrine, and serotonin reuptake inhibitor CSA-II	Reduced appetite, nausea, headache, insomnia, addiction, abuse, psychosis, mania, seizures, tachycardia, hypertension, priapism, myocardial infarction, arrhythmias .
Amphetamine–dextroamphetamine (Adderall)	10–30 mg twice/day **or** 20 mg extended release twice/day Pediatric (>6 years): 5 mg every morning; titration to 10–40 mg in 1–2 divided doses			In pediatrics: poor growth, weight loss, tics, mood lability, aggression, jitters, sleep disturbance: insomnia, arousals Check UDS to ensure use and no drug diversion
Lisdexamphetamine (Vyvanse)	30 mg–70 mg/day Pediatric dose >6 years: 20 mg every morning; titration to 30–70 mg every morning			
Amphetamine sulfate (Evekeo)	10–60 mg per day in 2 or 3 divided doses			
Atomoxetine (Strattera)	40 mg/day, can titrate to maximum of 100 mg/day Pediatric (>6 years): Initially 0.5 mg/kg/day every morning; titration to 1.2 mg/kg/day in 1–2 divided doses Max dose:Lesser of 1.4 mg/kg or 100 mg/day	EDS; second line, when can't tolerate stimulants	Selective norepinephrine reuptake inhibitor	Headache, abdominal pain, nausea, loss of appetite, weight loss, changes in sleep patterns, suicidal ideation, psychosis, mania, cardiovascular events, priapism, hepatotoxicity

Continued

Table 16.1 *Continued*

Drug	Dosage	Indications	Mechanism	Adverse Effects
	2.25–4.5 g (grams) at bedtime and repeated 3–4 hours later (2 doses at night)			
Oxybates (gamma hydroxybutyrate) Oral suspension: Xyrem: Sodium Oxybate	Pediatric (>7 years with type 1 narcolepsy): by weight: 20–<30 kg: ≤2 g per night in 2 divided doses; max dose 6 g divided 30–<45 kg: ≤3 g per night in 2 divided doses; max dose 7.5 g divided >45 kg: ≤4.5 g per night in 2 divided doses; max dose 9 g divided	EDS, cataplexy and disrupted night sleep; Usually second line agent except in severe disabling EDS or cataplexy, when it can be used as first-line therapy	GHB, a metabolite of gamma aminobutyric acid (GABA) acts at GABA-B receptors	Morning sedation, nausea, dizziness, urinary incontinence, weight loss, sleepwalking, enuresis, tremors, confusion, severe sedation, central apnea, worsening OSA, coma. Slow escalation of dose recommended May take around 3 months to see the full effects Can be combined with wake-promoting agents
Extended suspension (Lumryz)	4.5 g as a single dose at bedtime. May increase nightly dose by 1.5 g at weekly intervals based on efficacy and tolerability; recommended: 6–9 g once daily at night. Maximum dose: 9 g/night		CSA-III.	Contraindicated with concurrent use of alcohol, sedatives, and hypnotics. Avoid use of any CNS suppressive medications.
Oxybate salts: calcium, potassium, magnesium and sodium (Xywav)	2.25–4.5 g at bedtime; repeated 4 hours later (2 doses at night)			Avoid driving at least for 6 hrs after taking the medication. Abuse potential: beware of misuse and/or diversion.
Reduced sodium load				
Venlafaxine (Effexor)	37.5–75 mg twice/day or 37.5–150 mg extended release every morning Pediatric (>6 years): 25 mg every morning; titration to 37.5–75 mg every morning≤	Cataplexy, sleep paralysis, hypnogogic hallucinations	Norepinephrine, serotonin reuptake inhibitor (SNRI)	Transient nausea, headache, dizziness, weight loss, constipation, sedation, insomnia, tremor,increase in BP, suicidal ideation, QT prolongation, serotonin syndrome

Fluoxetine (Prozac)	20–80 mg every morning Pediatric (>6 years): 5–10 mg every morning; titration to 10–30 mg every morning	Cataplexy, sleep paralysisa, hypnogogic hallucinations	Selective serotonin reuptake inhibitor (SSRI)	Nausea, dry mouth, insomnia, tremor, suicidal ideation, sexual dysfunction, QT prolongation; serotonin syndrome
Clomipramine	25–200 mg every morning, in single or divided doses Pediatric (>10 years): 25 mg at bedtime; titration to 25–100 mg at bedtime	Cataplexy	Nonspecific monoamine reuptake inhibitor (TCA)	Dry mouth, constipation, sweating; dizziness; blurred vision, somnolence. weight gain, orthostatic hypotension, cardiac arrhythmia, seizures, suicidal ideation, bone marrow suppression, serotonin syndrome
Protriptyline	5–60 mg every morning, in single or divided doses Pediatric (>10 years): 5 mg once daily; titration to 5–10 mg/day in 1–2 divided doses			
Investigational Drugs: Orexin agonists - Danavorexton ((TAK-925)[34,36] - Firazorexton (TAK-994): Under investigation in clinical trial	Single dose injectable	EDS; cataplexy	Orexin (OXR2) agonist	Study stopped prematurely due to increased hepatotoxicity
Monoaminergics: Flecanide/modafinil[35]	200 mg/day modafinil + 2 mg/day flecainide[31]	EDS associated with Parkinson disease	Antiarrhythmic and dopamine reuptake inhibitor	Headache, nausea, nasopharyngitis, dry mouth, fatigue, insomnia, chest pain, confusional state, nightmare, muscle spasm

Notes: GABA: gamma-aminobutyric acid; GHB: gamma hydroxybutyrate; SSRI: Sselective serotonin reuptake inhibitor; CSA: controlled substance act; SNRI: serotonin and norepinephrine reuptake inhibitor; EDS: excessive daytime sleepiness; OXR: orexin receptor; TCA: tricyclic antidepressant; UDS: Urine drug screen[29–32]

OTHER HYPERSOMNIAS

There are very few controlled trials available to guide the treatment decisions for management of hypersomnolence other than narcolepsy.

IDIOPATHIC HYPERSOMNIA

Management is predominantly the treatment of excessive daytime sleepiness. Oxybates has been approved by the U.S. Food and Drug Administration (FDA) in the treatment of idiopathic hypersomnia. Other wake-promoting agents that are used for narcolepsy can be used as off-label medications.

HYPERSOMNIA DUE TO MEDICAL NEUROLOGICAL DISEASE

Excessive sleep time and EDS can be related to several neurodegenerative diseases, including Parkinson's disease, dementia with Lewy bodies, genetic, Prader-Willi syndrome, muscular dystrophy, tumor, vascular or inflammatory insults to the CNS. Around 10% of patients with severe obstructive sleep apnea may suffer from residual EDS in spite of using adequate positive airway pressure treatment. Traumatic brain injury may lead to post-traumatic hypersomnia or insomnia. Post-viral hypersomnia may occur shortly after infections like Epstein-Barr virus. Unfortunately, there is a paucity of randomized control trial data available to guide management for hypersomnia due to medical neurological disorders. For residual hypersomnia after optimal treatment of obstructive sleep apnea, modafinil, armodafinil, and Solriamfetol have been approved by the FDA, but for remaining medical disorders a wake-promoting agent can be used as an off-label drug. Modafinil has been used in Parkinson disease, traumatic brain injury, and myotonic dystrophy.

HYPERSOMNOLENCE DUE TO MEDICATION/SUBSTANCE

Multiple medications are well known to cause hypersomnia including narcotics, sedatives. Evaluation of patient, review of medication list and discontinuation of the offending drug if possible is the recommended treatment.

HYPERSOMNOLENCE DUE TO PSYCHIATRIC DISORDERS

Excessive daytime sleepiness (EDS) and excessive sleepiness at night can be associated with psychiatric disorders such as atypical depression, bipolar disorder, and anxiety. Adequate treatment of these underlying disorders is essential for symptom control.

INSUFFICIENT SLEEP SYNDROME

Though National Sleep Foundation guidelines recommend 7–9 hours of sleep for adults, about one third of the adult population fail to adhere to these guidelines. Behavioral modification and sleep duration extension are recommended.

KLEINE LEVIN SYNDROME

Kleine Levin syndrome is a rare disorder characterized by recurrent episodes of excessive sleepiness along with other cognitive, psychiatric, or behavioral difficulties that could include voracious eating, hypersexuality, a sense of derealization, apathy, and disinhibition. Symptom onset is usually in the second decade, with males more commonly affected. An infection or use of alcohol can be a trigger for the onset of these symptoms. Episodes can last from 3 to 15 days, with recurrence usually 1–2 per year; the syndrome usually resolves after a median of about 14 years. Treatment is mostly supportive; lithium and a few anti-epileptic medications have been explored. Lithium may be beneficial in patients who have frequent episodes and has been shown to have low-quality evidence based on AASM Medical Practice Guidelines.[29]

REFERENCES

1. Scheer D, Schwartz SW, Parr M, Zgibor J, Sanchez-Anguiano A, Rajaram L. Prevalence and incidence of narcolepsy in a US health care claims database, 2008–2010. *Sleep*. 2019 Jul 8;42(7):zsz091. doi:10.1093/sleep/zsz091. PMID: 31004158.

2. Challamel MJ, Mazzola ME, Nevsimalova S, Cannard C, Louis J, Revol M. Narcolepsy in children. *Sleep*. 1994 Dec;17(Suppl 8):S17–S20. doi:10.1093/sleep/17.suppl_8.s17. PMID: 7701194.
3. Honda Y. Census of narcolepsy, cataplexy and sleep life among teenagers in Fujisawa city. *Sleep Res*. 1979;8:191.
4. Tashiro T, Kanbayashi T, Iijima S, Hishikawa Y. An epidemiological study on prevalence of narcolepsy in Japanese. *J Sleep Res*. 1992;1(Suppl):228.
5. Lavie P, Peled, R. Letter to the editor: Narcolepsy is a rare disease in Israel. *Sleep*. 1987;10:608–609.
6. Pollack S, Gideoni 0, Peled R, Lavie P. HLA-DR2 in Israeli Jews with narcolepsy-cataplexy. *Isr J Med Sci*. 1988;24:123–125.
7. Wilner A, Steinman L, Lavie P, Peled R, Friedmann A, Brautbar C. Narcolepsy-cataplexy in Israeli Jews is associated exclusively with the HLA DR2 haplotype: A study at the serological and genomic level. *Hum Immunol*. 1988 Jan;21(1):15–22. doi:10.1016/0198-8859(88)90077-8. PMID: 2896649.
8. Dement W, Zarcone W, Varner V, et al. The prevalence of narcolepsy. *Sleep Res*. 1972;1:148.
9. Ohayon MM, Priest RG, Zulley J, Smirne S, Paiva T. Prevalence of narcolepsy symptomatology and diagnosis in the European general population. *Neurology*. 2002 Jun 25;58(12):1826–1833. doi:10.1212/wnl.58.12.1826. PMID: 12084885.
10. Langdon N, Welsh KI, Van Dam M, Vaughn RV, Parkes D. Genetic markers in narcolepsy. *Lancet*. 1984; 2(8413):1178–1180.
11. Mignot E, Lin X, Arrigoni J, et al. DQB1*0602 and DQA1*0102 (DQ1) are better markers than DR2 for narcolepsy in Caucasian and black Americans. *Sleep*. 1994.
12. Tafti M. Genetic aspects of normal and disturbed sleep. *Sleep Med*. 2009 Sep;10(Suppl 1):S17–S21. doi:10.1016/j.sleep.2009.07.002. PMID: 19660984.
13. Scammell TE. Overview of sleep: The neurologic processes of the sleep-wake cycle. *J Clin Psychiatry*. 2015 May;76(5):e13. doi:10.4088/JCP.14046tx1c. PMID: 26035194.
14. Peyron C, Faraco J, Rogers W, et al. A mutation in a case of early onset narcolepsy and a generalized absence of hypocretin peptides in human narcoleptic brains. *Nat Med*. 2000 Sep;6(9):991–997. doi:10.1038/79690. PMID: 10973318.
15. Thannickal TC, Moore RY, Nienhuis R, et al. Reduced number of hypocretin neurons in human narcolepsy. *Neuron*. 2000 Sep;27(3):469–474. doi:10.1016/s0896-6273(00)00058-1. PMID: 11055430; PMCID: PMC8760623.
16. Crocker A, España RA, Papadopoulou M, et al. Concomitant loss of dynorphin, NARP, and orexin in narcolepsy. *Neurology*. 2005 Oct 25;65(8):1184–1188. doi:10.1212/01.wnl.0000168173.71940.ab. PMID: 16247044; PMCID: PMC2254145.
17. Aran A, Lin L, Nevsimalova S, et al. Elevated anti-streptococcal antibodies in patients with recent narcolepsy onset. *Sleep*. 2009 Aug;32(8):979–983. doi:10.1093/sleep/32.8.979. PMID: 19725248; PMCID: PMC2717204.
18. Mahlios J, De la Herrán-Arita AK, Mignot E. The autoimmune basis of narcolepsy. *Curr Opin Neurobiol*. 2013 Oct;23(5):767–773. doi:10.1016/j.conb.2013.04.013. PMID: 23725858; PMCID: PMC3848424.
19. Tafti M, Nishino S, Aldrich MS, Liao W, Dement WC, Mignot E. Major histocompatibility class II molecules in the CNS: Increased microglial expression at the onset of narcolepsy in canine model. *J Neurosci*. 1996 Aug 1;16(15):4588–4595. doi:10.1523/JNEUROSCI.16-15-04588.1996. PMID: 8764647; PMCID: PMC6579009.
20. Gerashchenko D, Shiromani PJ. Different neuronal phenotypes in the lateral hypothalamus and their role in sleep and wakefulness. *Mol Neurobiol*. 2004 Feb;29(1):41–59. doi:10.1385/MN:29:1:41. PMID: 15034222.
21. Panda S. Status cataplecticus as initial presentation of late onset narcolepsy. *J Clin Sleep Med*. 2014 Feb 15;10(2):207–209. doi:10.5664/jcsm.3456. PMID: 24533005; PMCID: PMC3899324.
22. Krahn LE, Arand DL, Avidan AY, et al. Recommended protocols for the Multiple Sleep Latency Test and the Maintenance of Wakefulness Test in adults: Guidance from the American Academy of Sleep Medicine. *J Clin Sleep Med*. 2021;17(12):2489–2498.
23. Broughton R, Ghanem Q, Hishikawa Y. Life effects of narcolepsy in 180 patients from North America, Asia and Europe compared to matched controls *Can J Neurol Sci*. 1981 Nov;8(4):299–304. doi:10.1017/s0317167100043419.
24. Nowakowski S, Garland S, Grandner MA, Cuddihy L, eds. *Adapting Cognitive Behavioral Therapy for Insomnia*. Elsevier; 2021.
25. Maski K, Trotti LM, Kotagal S, et al. Treatment of central disorders of hypersomnolence: An American Academy of Sleep Medicine clinical practice guideline. *J Clin Sleep Med*. 2021 Sep 1;17(9):1881–1893. doi:10.5664/jcsm.9328. PMID: 34743789; PMCID: PMC8636351.
26. Maski K, Trotti LM, Kotagal S, et al. Treatment of central disorders of hypersomnolence: An American Academy of Sleep Medicine systematic review, meta-analysis, and GRADE assessment. *J Clin Sleep Med*. 2021 Sep 1;17(9):1895–1945. doi:10.5664/jcsm.9326. PMID: 34743790; PMCID: PMC8636345.
27. Bassetti CLA, Kallweit U, Vignatelli L, et al. European guidelines and expert statements on the management of narcolepsy in adults and children. *J Sleep Res*. 2021 Dec;30(6):e13387. doi:10.1111/jsr.13387. PMID: 34173288.
28. Thorpy M, Zhao CG, Dauvilliers Y. Management of narcolepsy during pregnancy. *Sleep Med*. 2013 Apr;14(4):367–376. doi:10.1016/j.sleep.2012.11.021.
29. Trotti LM, Arnulf I. Idiopathic hypersomnia and other hypersomnia syndromes. *Neurotherapeutics*. 2021 Jan;18(1):20–31. doi:10.1007/s13311-020-00919-1. PMID: 32901432; PMCID: PMC8116415.
30. Babiker MO, Prasad M. Narcolepsy in children: A diagnostic and management approach. *Pediatr Neurol*. 2015;52:557.
31. Lecendreux M. Pharmacological management of narcolepsy and cataplexy in pediatric patients. *Paediatr Drugs*. 2014;16:363.
32. Hodgkins P, Shaw M, Coghill D, Hechtman L. Amfetamine and methylphenidate medications for attention-deficit/hyperactivity disorder: Complementary treatment options. *Eur Child Adolesc Psychiatry*. 2012;21:477.

33. Lecendreux M, Plazzi G, Dauvilliers Y, et al. Long-term safety and maintenance of efficacy of sodium oxybate in the treatment of narcolepsy with cataplexy in pediatric patients. *J Clin Sleep Med*. 2022; 18:2217.
34. Evans R, Kimura H, Alexander R, et al. Orexin 2 receptor-selective agonist danavorexton improves narcolepsy phenotype in a mouse model and in human patients. *Proc Natl Acad Sci U S A*. 2022 Aug 30;119(35):e2207531119. doi:10.1073/pnas.2207531119. PMID: 35994639; PMCID: PMC9436334.
35. Corvol JC, Azulay JP, Bosse B, et al.; THN102-202 Study Investigators. THN 102 for Excessive Daytime Sleepiness Associated with Parkinson's Disease: A Phase 2a Trial. *Mov Disord*. 2022 Feb;37(2):410–415. doi:10.1002/mds.28840. PMID: 34709684.
36. Mignot E, Bogan RK, Emsellem H, et al. Safety and pharmacodynamics of a single infusion of danavorexton in adults with idiopathic hypersomnia. *Sleep*. 2023 Sep 8;46(9):zsad049. doi:10.1093/sleep/zsad049. PMID: 36883238; PMCID: PMC10485568.

SECTION IV

Abnormal Sleep Behaviors

Chapter 17

Restless Legs Syndrome

Charles Davies

INTRODUCTION

Restless legs syndrome (RLS), also known as Willis-Ekbom Disease, is a condition first described by Ekbom.[1] Key features include uncomfortable urges to move the legs which are worse at night, worse at rest, and improved with repetitive movement of the legs. Approximately 80% of persons with RLS also have periodic leg movements of sleep.[2] In the past 2 decades, recognition of RLS mimics including peripheral neuropathy, positional discomfort, habitual leg movement, and akathisia have improved prevalence estimates. The Cambridge-Hopkins diagnostic questionnaire[3] provides a validated instrument to accurately diagnose RLS. RLS prevalence is estimated to be 5%–14.3% in the general population.[4] Severity can be determined using the International Restless Legs Scale (IRLS).[5] The role of low dopaminergic tone and low normal iron stores have long been understood as drivers of RLS symptoms. Serotonergic tone is also known to influence restless legs symptoms. Dopamine agonists have traditionally been a mainstay of treatment. However, compulsive behaviors and augmentation have tempered enthusiasm for these medications as first line agents for the treatment of RLS. Alpha-2-delta ligands provide an alternative treatment without risk for these side effects. The role of supplemental iron in the oral and IV form has increased over the past 20 years to ameliorate symptoms for persons with low normal iron stores.[6] Opioids are reserved for severe RLS symptoms which are refractory to standard treatments.[7] Future work will explore the potential association between RLS and hypertension found in some reports, as well as the hypothesis that RLS and associated PLMS can increase sympathetic activity in a manner similar to obstructive sleep apnea.

EPIDEMIOLOGY/RISK FACTORS

Restless legs syndrome is a common disorder which occurs in 3.9%–14.3% of North American adults[4] using criteria developed by the International Restless Legs Syndrome Study Group.[8,9] There is an approximate 2:1 ratio for RLS in women compared to men.[10,11]

When a differential diagnosis is applied to exclude mimics such as peripheral neuropathy, nocturnal leg cramps, habitual foot tapping, and akathisia, the prevalence is 1.9%–4.6% in European adults.[4] The prevalence is generally below 2% in Asian populations.[12-15] In African populations the prevalence is <1%–11%.[24–18]

In populations with selected comorbidities, RLS prevalence may be much higher. Iron deficiency anemia has the highest reported association, with 41% of such patients exhibiting RLS symptoms.[19] For patients with end-stage renal disease undergoing hemodialysis, the prevalence may be up to 20%.[20] The risk of RLS is notably higher in persons with peripheral neuropathy. One report found an RLS prevalence of 26.5% in persons with hereditary neuropathy.[21]

During pregnancy, a recent meta-analysis has indicated overall RLS prevalence at 21%. Prevalence in the first, second, and third trimesters is 8%, 16%, and 22%, respectively.[22] This may be related to generally lower iron stores in women during pregnancy (see Figure 17.1).

INHERITANCE

A positive family history has been reported in up to 60% of RLS patients.[23–26] A younger age of symptom onset is typically seen for patients with hereditary RLS. Genetic anticipation has been suggested by several studies of extended families with RLS. Trenkwalder et al. described a family with RLS symptoms appearing at a progressively earlier age over four generations.[27] Although the majority of familial RLS follow an autosomal dominant pattern, recessive patterns appear in the literature as well.[28,29] Twin studies have provided further evidence for a genetic form of RLS. Ondo and coworkers showed an 83.3% concordance rate for RLS among 12 monozygotic sets of twins.[30]

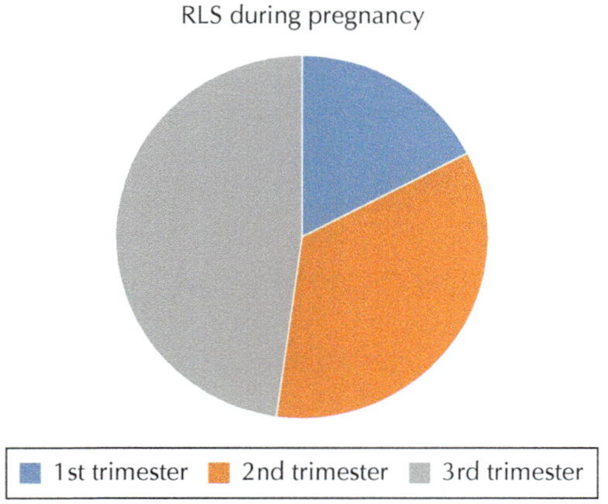

Figure 17.1. Distribution of RLS during pregnancy by trimester.

Genome wide association studies (GWAS) have been valuable in identifying multiple variants associated with RLS.[31] Single-nucleotide polymorphisms (SNP) on genes *PTPRD* and *BTBD9* were significantly associated with RLS with an odds ratio (OR) of 2.05 in a Korean population.[32] A GWAS performed by Winkelmann et al. found a significant association between RLS and SNP on the *MEIS1* gene (OR = 1.74.[33] Notably, *MEIS1* has been linked to iron metabolism.[34] Multiple SNPs on the *MAP2K5/SKOR1* gene have been associated with RLS with an OR up to 1.53.[33]

At least 2 genetic variants have been significantly associated with a decreased risk for RLS. An SNP on the *vitamin D3 receptor* gene had an OR = 0.61.[35] A repeat within the *alpha-synuclein (SNCA)* gene promoter (conferring risk for Parkinson disease) was inversely associated with RLS with an OR = 0.58.[36]

PATHOPHYSIOLOGY

A large body of evidence and clinical experience have supported the concept of reduced iron stores as central to the pathophysiology of RLS. Early clinical studies showed an association between RLS and low iron stores.[37,38] In fact, 2 of the most common risk factors, as listed earlier, end-stage renal disease and pregnancy, can be explained by the fact that both disorders are associated with low iron stores. Resolution of RLS symptoms after renal transplantation or delivery further supports the notion that iron deficiency is central to the pathophysiology of RLS.[39,40] This led Allen and Earley to propose that "[a]ll conditions that compromise iron availability will increase the risk of RLS leading to a higher than expected prevalence of RLS in these conditions."[41pS440] In some instances, RLS is noted without peripheral iron deficiency.

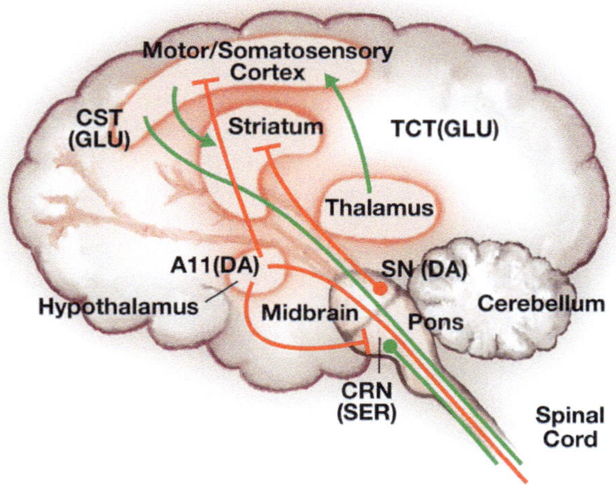

Figure 17.2. Proposed neural pathways for RLS brain.
Nuclei/regions: CRN: caudal raphe nucleus; SN: substantia nigra. Neurotransmitters: DA: dopamine; SER: serotonin; GLU: glutamine; GLY: glycine; GABA: gabapentin. Tracts: A11: dopaminergic; CST: corticospinal; TCT: thalamocortical; RST: rubrospinal; RaST: raphespinal.

A more robust association has been demonstrated between RLS and brain iron status. MRI studies have shown reduced iron in the substantia nigra and a negative correlation between iron concentration and RLS symptoms.[42,43] Analysis of iron stores in cerebrospinal fluid has also yielded an inverse correlation with RLS.[44,45] Autopsy studies provide further confirmation of the connection between decreased brain iron in the substantia nigra and RLS.[46] The role of iron as a co-factor for the synthesis of tyrosine hydroxylase, the rate-limiting step in dopamine synthesis, helps to explain how dopaminergic tone can affect RLS symptoms.

Anatomically, dopaminergic nuclei originating in the dorsal-posterior hypothalamus (Figure 17.2), project down the spine via A11 neurons to synapse in the spinal cord (Figure 17.3). The therapeutic effects of exogenous levodopa (converted to dopamine) and dopamine receptor agonists are related to uptake via D3 receptors which are inhibitory and can ameliorate sensory RLS symptoms when targeting the dorsal horn.[47] The predominance of D1 type receptors in the ventral horn of the spinal gray matter mediate input from A11 neurons to modulate leg movements.[47] It has been postulated that the high dopamine affinity D3 receptors allow relief of sensory symptoms with low dopamine concentrations.[48] However, high dopamine concentrations may target excitatory D1 type receptors, leading to motor manifestations of RLS including periodic limb movements (PLMs). This may also explain one of the adverse effects of prolonged dopamine therapy, augmentation, given the increased expression of D1 receptors with aging.[49] In addition, animal data support the idea that long-term treatment with D3 receptor agonists leads to up-regulation of excitatory D1 receptors with resultant augmentation.[50]

Whereas dopamine can improve RLS symptoms in appropriate concentrations, this is balanced by serotonergic tone, which can worsen symptoms. Serotonin produced in the Dorsal Raphe nucleus (Figure 17.2) is carried via autonomic circuits down the spine and also targets the dorsal horn of the spinal gray matter. Clemens proposed that increased serotonin levels would increase spinal sympathetic tone and lead to worsening of RLS symptoms.[51] In fact, reports have shown the positive association between SSRI medications and RLS symptoms.[52,53]

Glutamate has also been implicated in the pathophysiology of RLS. Allen et al. completed MR spectroscopy on RLS patients and controls to evaluate thalamic glutamate/glutamine (Glu/Gln) signal.[54] They found a significantly higher Glu/Gln level for RLS patients compared to controls. In addition, this signal was significantly correlated with wake time during the sleep period. The implication of thalamo-cortical activation provides some rationale for the associated sleep disruption that often accompanies other RLS symptoms. Furthermore, this may help explain the clinical finding that RLS patients often do not have excessive daytime sleepiness, despite significantly disrupted sleep. It has been proposed that dopaminergic systems mediate the sensory and motor symptoms (PLMs) of RLS, whereas glutamatergic systems mediate the hyper-arousal and sleep disturbance aspects of RLS.[55] The ability of α2δ ligands such as gabapentin and pregabalin to improve RLS symptoms is therefore explained by involvement of glutamatergic systems in the pathophysiology of RLS. These compounds lead to a reduction of calcium channel expression at nerve terminals and therefore diminish release of excitatory neurotransmitters including glutamate.[56] Figures 17.2 and 17.3 illustrate proposed neural pathways for RLS.

A third neurotransmitter thought to underlie RLS symptoms is adenosine.[55] Upregulation of adenosine A_{2A} receptors with iron deficiency[57] likely promotes RLS symptoms as a result of heteromer formation with dopamine type 2 receptors (D2R). This corresponds to a hypoadenosinergic state that translates to the sensorimotor and hyperarousal symptoms seen with RLS.[58] Indirect evidence supporting this concept was provided by the effective treatment of akathisia using an A2AR antagonist.[59] A small case series using the A2AR antagonist, Istradefylline, resulted in amelioration of RLS symptoms.[60]

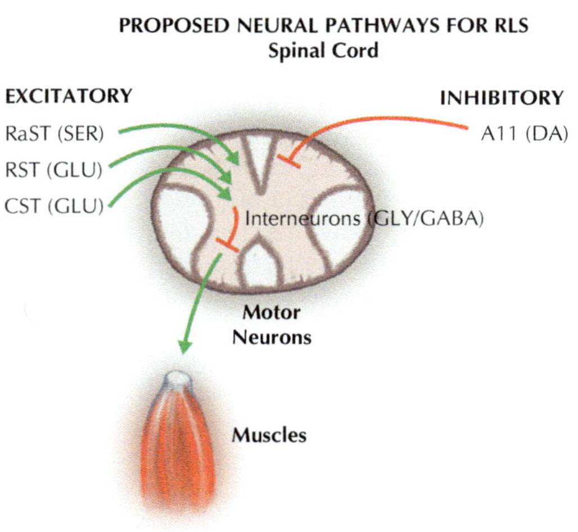

Figure 17.3. Proposed neural pathways for RLS spinal cord. Neurotransmitters: DA: dopamine; SER: serotonin; GLU: glutamine; GLY: Glycine; GABA: gabapentin. Tracts: A11: dopaminergic; CST: corticospinal; RST: rubrospinal; RaST: raphespinal. Adapted from: References 59, 62.

Vitamins and other molecules may also play a role in the pathophysiology of RLS. Vitamin D is indirectly linked to RLS due to its protective effect on dopaminergic neurons.[61] Furthermore, cerebrospinal fluid (CSF) vitamin D binding protein levels correlate with RLS.[62] Wali et al. demonstrated a significant association between vitamin D deficiency and RLS with an OR = 3.4.[63] Nitric oxide synthase, thiol, and other markers of oxidative stress have been associated with RLS.[64]

DIAGNOSIS

Diagnosis of RLS is made by clinical history using updated criteria developed by the International Restless Legs Syndrome Study Group (IRLSSG). Key features include: (1) uncomfortable urges to move the legs; (2) worsening of symptoms at night; (3) worsening of symptoms at rest; (4) Improvement with *repetitive* leg movement (see Table 17.1).

The updated criteria also include evaluation for possible RLS mimics, such as peripheral neuropathy, nocturnal leg cramps, akathisia, positional discomfort, and habitual foot tapping.[9] For persons with circadian rhythm disturbances due to either shift-work sleep-wake phase disorder or delayed sleep-wake phase disorder, symptoms may be prominent in the morning just prior to habitual bedtime. Common terms used by patients with RLS include: "crawling sensations," "jimmy legs,"

Table 17.1 **Symptoms of RLS**

U	Uncomfortable **urges** to move the legs
R	Worse at **rest**
G	**Gets** better with repetitive movement
E	Most prominent in the **evening**

and "restlessness." Often patients have a hard time putting their symptoms into words and simply report leg discomfort.

The presence of frank pain and or numbness with pins and needles sensations, aching, throbbing, or temperature intolerance should point the examiner toward peripheral neuropathy. Neuropathy patients may indicate improvement while walking on a cold floor but worsening when walking on a rug or textured surface due to dysesthesias. A description of leg muscle tensing, hardening, or "charlie horse" with improvement after massage suggests leg cramps. If the patient has been on long-term neuroleptic medication and reports a "whole-body" inner restlessness, akathisia is likely. Improvement with one position change without repetitive leg movement while sitting or walking is consistent with positional discomfort. Repetitive leg movement which is not bothersome most likely represents a normal variant. In some cases, the report of a spouse or family member describing their own irritation while the patient unconsciously taps their feet confirms this.

Formal instruments may be used and have been refined to include the latest criteria. The Cambridge-Hopkins diagnostic questionnaire has a sensitivity of 87.5%, specificity of 94.4% and positive predictive value of 87.2%.[3] Although an attended polysomnogram may provide enumeration of periodic limb movements during sleep as supportive data, no sleep study is required for the diagnosis of RLS. Laboratory evaluation of iron status is helpful in guiding therapy but is not required for the initial diagnosis. Electro-physiologic (such as nerve conduction studies) and imaging studies are typically unrevealing, and neither is required to make a diagnosis of RLS.

EVALUATION

Due to the strong association between RLS and iron deficiency, laboratory evaluation of iron stores is recommended. Ferritin is considered the best single measure of iron stores.[41] Recent guidelines[6] indicate a ferritin level ≤75 ng/ml as clinically significant for RLS sufferers. Treatment with supplemental iron (see the following) may improve symptoms. It is important to note that ferritin is an acute phase reactant and may be falsely elevated with acute or chronic inflammation. Ferritin should be performed as a fasting test delayed roughly 4 weeks after any acute illness. For cases of chronic inflammation due to chronic illness or even significant obesity, percent iron transferrin saturation and total iron binding capacity (TIBC) can serve as more accurate measures of true iron status. Iron transferrin saturation <20% and or TIBC <400 ug/dl indicate iron deficiency.[41] While erythrocyte sedimentation rate or other indices may be used to assess for inflammatory state, a simpler approach is to routinely check ferritin, percent iron transferrin saturation, and TIBC.

Assessment for exacerbating factors, including insomnia, poor sleep hygiene, antihistamines, caffeine, and sedentary lifestyle, may yield additional opportunities for improvement through behavioral modification without the risk of side effects for treatment with prescription medications. In cases of subclinical, episodic restless legs symptoms, sporadic increases in leg activity during the day may provide an explanation for symptoms at night. Medications should be reviewed for potential side effects of exacerbating RLS. For patients taking SSRI or SNRI medications, RLS symptoms may improve after switching to an alternative anti-depressant such as buproprion. Dopamine blocking agents such as antipsychotics may also worsen RLS.

The IRLSSG rating scale is a validated instrument for semi-quantitative assessment of RLS severity over the past week.[5] Although primarily used in a research setting, this questionnaire can be used to determine response to treatment in a clinical setting.

Evaluation for impaired sensation in the lower extremities during the physical exam is a valuable means of identifying peripheral neuropathy rather than RLS as an explanation for symptoms.

ASSOCIATED CONDITIONS

Over the past 2 decades, a growing body of literature has explored the possibility of RLS as a risk factor for hypertension. A recent meta-analysis showed an increased risk of hypertension for persons with RLS with an OR = 1.13.[65] However, after controlling for cardiovascular risk factors, there was not a significant increase. For patients with a combination of frequent RLS (≥2 episodes/week) and PLMS index ≥26/hour, there was a significantly increased risk for resistant hypertension (OR = 2.2) even after adjusting for common confounders.[66] PLMS as a mechanism for hypertension via sympathetic activation is supported by studies showing elevated blood pressure associated with PLMS.[67,68] This may in turn explain the association between RLS and cardiovascular disease.[69–71] Other conditions associated with RLS include multiple sclerosis, spinal cord pathology, and Parkinson disease. These forms are considered secondary RLS, in contrast to primary or idiopathic RLS for persons without such comorbidities.

TREATMENT

In all cases, behavioral strategies, including minimizing caffeine intake, obtaining adequate sleep each night, and regular exercise, can be helpful in minimizing RLS symptoms.

Iron

When low normal iron levels are established (ferritin ≤75 ng/ml, or iron transferrin saturation <20%), treatment with oral iron has been shown to improve RLS symptoms. A randomized, placebo-controlled study showed significant improvement in the IRLS scale (10.3) with oral iron compared to placebo (1.1) after 12 weeks.[72] Another study showed similar improvement in IRLS scores for oral iron and pramipexole after 12 weeks.[73] Recommended treatment includes ferrous sulfate 325 mg (65 mg elemental) twice a day with 100–200 mg of vitamin C with each dose. Calcium supplements and dairy products should be avoided when taking iron. Dark, hard stools and constipation may be associated with oral iron supplementation. Miralax or other stool softeners can be used to aid in constipation symptoms. Ferritin and iron studies should be checked every 3 months while taking supplemental iron to evaluate for iron overload.[6] If patients cannot tolerate oral iron, IV iron infusion with ferric carboxymaltose 1000 mg is effective in treating RLS for ferritin <300 ng/ml and transferrin saturation <45%.[74,75] In some patients, repletion of iron stores over a brief period may result in sustained symptom improvement with subsequent normal iron levels. For others, especially women of child-bearing age, or those with impaired iron absorption due to bariatric surgery or other cause, long-term iron supplementation (oral or IV) may be required.

Dopaminergic Medications

Long considered first-line treatment for RLS, dopaminergic medications offer the benefit of relatively rapid relief of symptoms.[76] Initially, carbidopa-levodopa was used extensively.[77] By the mid-1990s, however, augmentation was recognized as a significant side effect. Onset of RLS symptoms earlier in the day was noted in 82% of RLS patients taking carbidopa-levodopa by Allen and Earley.[78] Augmentation has since been defined to include spread of symptoms to the upper limbs and the need for medication dose escalation. Dopamine agonists with a longer half-life (10–12 hours) than carbidopa-levodopa (2 hours) were later introduced as an alternative treatment to avoid augmentation.[79] Over time, ropinirole and pramipexole emerged as the medications of choice for the treatment of RLS. In a meta-analysis, pramipexole improved the IRLS rating scale by 6.7 points compared with placebo. This was clinically significant. In a separate meta-analysis, ropinirole resulted in a 4-point improvement in the IRLS rating scale compared with placebo.[80] Over the past decade and a half, compulsive behaviors have been rarely reported with use of dopaminergic medications, including compulsive shopping, gambling, eating, and hyper-sexuality.[81–83] Dopamine agonists continue to be used to treat RLS with close monitoring for adverse effects such as compulsive behaviors and augmentation. Total dosing should not exceed 4 mg/day for ropinirole, 0.75 mg/day for pramipexole, and 3 mg/day for the transdermal dopamine agonist rotigotine, to minimize adverse effects.[84] Intermittent use of medications is ideal if tolerable; daily treatment should be initiated only when RLS symptoms are routinely affecting quality of life.[84] When augmentation or compulsive behaviors occur, the dose of dopamine agonists should be gradually tapered with initiation of an alternative treatment as clinically indicated.[84]

α2δ Ligands

This class of medication, including gabapentin, gabapentin enacarbil, and pregabalin, may now be considered as first-line therapy for RLS to avoid adverse effects associated with dopaminergic medications.[90] There is strong evidence that gabapentin enacarbil and some evidence that gabapentin and pregabalin are effective in treating RLS.[80] Gabapentin was shown to decrease the IRLS rating scale by 8.4 points compared with placebo. Pregabalin decreased the IRLS rating scale by 8 points compared with placebo.[85] Recommended initial and maintenance doses can be found in the accompanying medication Table 17.2.

Opioids

The treatment of RLS began with opioids[86] and now returns to opioids for persons with severe, refractory symptoms.[7] As recommended by Silber et al.,[7] tramadol, codeine, oxycodone, hydrocodone, or methadone all may be reasonable choices. Short-acting opioids may be more useful in cases of intermittent need for use, whereas longer-action opioids may be more helpful if treatment is needed daily or multiple times per day. It is important to avoid opioid treatment for any person with a history or concern for substance abuse. Common side effects of opioids include sedation, constipation, and itching. Miralax or diphenhydramine may be

Table 17.2 **Medications and Dosages for the Treatment of Restless Legs Syndrome (Willis-Ekbom Disease)***

Medication	Starting Dose	Maximum Dose	Common Side Effects	Comments
Dopaminergic				
Pramipexole	0.25–0.5 mg/day	0.75 mg/day	Compulsive behaviors, augmentation	May be divided to reduce side effects
Ropinirole	0.5–2mg/day	4mg/day	Compulsive behaviors, augmentation	May be divided to reduce side effects
Carbidopa-levodopa	25 mg/100 mg, 1–2 tablets as needed	Should not be taken daily	Oversedation, hypotension	May chew tablet for quick onset
Rotigotine	1 mg/day	3 mg/day	Compulsive behaviors, augmentation, skin irritation	Transdermal patch
α2δ ligands				
Gabapentin	300 mg/day	2400 mg/day	Weight gain, tremors, lower extremity edema	
Pregabalin	75 mg/day	450 mg/day	Weight gain, tremors, lower extremity edema	
Gabapentin Enacarbil	600 mg/day	1200 mg/day	Weight gain, tremors, lower extremity edema	Taken once a day
Opioids				
Hydrocodone	10 mg/day	45 mg/day	Oversedation, respiratory suppression, constipation, pruritus	Avoid with other sedatives
Oxycodone	5 mg/day	30 mg/day		
Methadone	2.5 mg/day	20 mg/day		
Tramadol	50 mg/day	200 mg/day		

* Based on references 15, 90, 91.

used for the latter two side effects, respectively. Recommended initial and maintenance doses of opioids may be found in Table 17.2.

CONCLUSIONS

Restless legs syndrome (RLS), also known as Willis-Ekbom disease is a common neurological disorder which can impact sleep and daytime function. Multiple polymorphisms have been found to be associated with RLS, including those on the *MEIS1*, *BTBDP*, *MAP2K5/LBOXCOR1*, *PRPRD*, and *TOX3* genes,[87–93] supporting an inherited as well as sporadic form. These findings complement epidemiologic reports that a majority of persons with RLS have a positive family history. Substantial evidence has accumulated implicating the neuro-transmitter dopamine as central to the pathophysiology. Recently, animal models have expanded understanding of the pathophysiology of RLS. Glutamate has been incorporated into the model of RLS to explain the absence of excessive sleepiness despite the sleep disruption and deprivation that are often noted in persons with RLS. Adenosine has also been hypothesized to contribute to RLS symptoms.[58] RLS is strongly associated with decreased iron stores, the evaluation of which can provide an opportunity to improve symptoms. Current first-line treatment for persistent symptoms includes α2δ ligands.[94] When using dopamine agonists, it is important to monitor regularly for augmentation and compulsive behaviors. Future work will focus on further elucidation of the pathophysiology to provide insights into novel treatments.

REFERENCES

1. Ekbom KA. Restless legs. *Acta Med Scand.* 1945;158(Suppl.):1–123.
2. Montplaisir J, Boucher S, Poirier G, et al. Clinical polysmnographic, and genetic characteristics of restless legs syndrome: A study of 133 patients diagnosed with new standard criteria. *Mov Disord.* 1997;12:61.
3. Allen RP, Burchell BJ, MacDonald B, Hening WA, Earley CJ. Validation of the self-completed Cambridge-Hopkins questionnaire (CH-RLSq) for ascertainment of restless legs syndrome (RLS) in a population survey. *Sleep Med.* 2009;10:1097–1100.
4. Ohayon MM, O'Hara R, Vitiello MV. Epidemiology of restless legs syndrome: A synthesis of the literature. *Sleep Med Rev.* 2012;16(4):283–295.
5. Walters AS, LeBrocq C, Dhar A, et al. Validation of the international restless legs syndrome study group rating scale for restless legs syndrome. *Sleep Med.* 2003;4(2):121–132.
6. Allen RP, Picchietti DL, Auerbach M, et al. Evidence-based and consensus clinical practice guidelines for the iron treatment of restless legs syndrome/Willis-Ekbom disease in adults and children: An IRLSSG task force report. *Sleep Med.* 2018;41:27–44.
7. Silber MH, Becker PM, Buchfuhrer MJ, et al. The appropriate use of opioids in the treatment of refractory restless legs syndrome. *Mayo Clin Proc.* 2018;93:59–67.
8. Allen RP, Picchietti D, Hening WA, Trenkwalder C, Walters AS, Montplaisir J. Restless legs syndrome: Diagnostic criteria, special considerations, and epidemiology. A report from the restless legs syndrome diagnosis and epidemiology workshop at the National Institutes of Health. *Sleep Med.* 2003;4:101–119.
9. Allen RP, Picchietti DL, Garcia-Borreguero D, et al. Restless legs syndrome/Willis-Ekbom disease diagnostic criteria: Updated International Restless Legs Syndrome Study Group (IRLSSG) consensus criteria—history, rationale, description, and significance. *Sleep Med.* 2014;15:860–873.
10. Tison F, Crochard A, Leger D, Bouee S, Lainey E, El Hasnaoui A. Epidemiology of restless legs syndrome in French adults: A nationwide survey: The instant study. *Neurology.* 20054;65:239–246.
11. Wesstrom J, Nilsson S, Sundstrom-Poromaa I, Ulfberg J. Restless legs syndrome among women: Prevalence, co-morbidity, and possible relationship to menopause. *Climacteric.* 2008;11:422–428.
12. Chen NH, Chuang LP, Yang CT, et al. The prevalence of restless legs syndrome in Taiwanese adults. *Psych Clin Neurosci.* 2010;64:170–178.
13. Mizuno S, Miyaoka T, Inagaki T, Horiguchi J. Prevalence of restless legs syndrome in non-institutionalized Japanese elderly. *Psych Clin Neurosci.* 2005;59:461–465.
14. Shi Y, Yu H, Ding D, Yu P, Wu D, Hong Z. Prevalence and risk factors of restless legs syndrome among Chinese adults in a rural community. *PLoS One.* 2015;10:e0121215.
15. Kim T-J, Yoon JE, Park JA, et al. Prevalence and characteristics of restless legs syndrome in Korean adults: A study in two independent samples of the general population. *Neuro-epidem.* 2019;52:193–204.
16. Burtscher C, Baxmann A, Kassubek J, et al. Prevalence of restless legs syndrome in an urban population of eastern Africa (Tanzania). *J Neurol Sci.* 2014;346:121–127.
17. Shalash AS, Elrassas HH, Monzem MM, Salem HH, Moneim AA, Moustafa RR. Restless legs syndrome in Egyptian medical students using a validated Arabic version of the restless legs syndrome rating scale. *Sleep Med.* 2015;16:1528–1531.
18. Fawale MB, Ismaila IA, Mustapha AF, Komolafe MA, Adedeji TA. Restless legs syndrome in a Nigerian elderly population. *J Clin Sleep Med.* 2016;12(7):965–972.
19. Akyol A, Kiylioglu N, Kadikoylu G, Bolaman AZ, Ozgel N. Iron deficiency anemia and restless legs syndrome: Is there an electrophysiological abnormality? *Clin Neurol Neurosurg.* 2003;106:23–27.
20. Lin X-W, Zhang J-F, Qiu M-Y, et al. Restless legs syndrome in end stage renal disease patients undergoing hemodialysis. *BMC Neurol.* 2019;19:47.

21. Hattan E, Chalk C, Postuma RB. Is there a higher risk of restless legs syndrome in peripheral neuropathy. *Neurology*. 2009;72:955–960.
22. Chen S-J, Shi L, Bao Y-P, Sun Y-K, et al. Prevalence of restless legs syndrome during pregnancy: A systematic review and meta-analysis. *Sleep Med Rev*. 2018;40:43–54.
23. Ondo W, Jankovic J, Restless legs syndrome: Clinicoetiologic correlates. *Neurology*. 1996;47:1435–1441.
24. Walters AS, Hickey K, Maltzman J, et al. A questionnaire study of 138 patients with restless legs syndrome: The "Night-Walkers" survey. *Neurology*. 1996;46:92–95.
25. Montplaisir J, Boucher S, Poirier G, Lavigne G, Lapierre O, Lesperance P. Clinical, polysomnographic, and genetic characteristics of restless legs syndrome: A study of 133 patients diagnosed with new standard criteria. *Mov Disord*. 1997;12:61–65.
26. Winkelmann J, Wetter TC, Collado-Seidel V, et al. Clinical characteristics and frequency of the hereditary restless legs syndrome in a population of 300 patients. *Sleep*. 2000;23:597–602.
27. Trenkwalder C, Seidel VC, Gasser T, Oertel WH. Clinical symptoms and possible anticipation in a large kindred of familial restless legs syndrome. *Mov Disord*. 1996;11:389–394.
28. Lazzarini A, Walters AS, Hickey K, et al. Studies of penetrance and anticipation in five autosomal-dominant restless legs syndrome pedigrees. *Mov Disord*. 1999;14:111–116.
29. Esteves AM, Pedrazzoli M, Bagnato M, Moreira F, Mello MT, Tufik S. Two pedigrees with restless legs syndrome in Brazil. *Braz J Med Biol Res*. 2008;41:106–109.
30. Ondo WG, Vuong KD, Wang Q. Restless legs syndrome in monozygotic twins: Clinical correlates. *Neurology*. 2000;55:1404–1406.
31. Jimenez-Jimenez FJ, Alonso-Navarro HA, Garcia-Martin E, Agundez JAG. Genetics of restless legs syndrome: An update. *Sleep Med Rev*. 2018;39:106–121.
32. Kim MK, Cho YW, Shin WC, et al. Association of restless legs syndrome variants in Korean patients with restless legs syndrome. *Sleep*. 2013;36:1787–1791.
33. Winkelmann J, Schormair B, Lichtner P, et al. Genome-wide association study of restless legs syndrome identifies common variants in three genomic regions. *Nat Genet*. 2007;39:1000–1006.
34. Catoire H, Dion PA, Xiong L, et al. Restless legs syndrome-associated *MEIS1* risk variant influences iron homeostasis. *Ann Neurol*. 2011;70:170–175.
35. Jimenez-Jimenez FJ, Garcia-Martin E, Alonso-Navarro H, et al. Association between vitamin D receptor rs731236(Taq1) polymorphism and risk for restless legs syndrome in the Spanish Caucasian population. *Medicine (Baltimore)*. 2015;94:E2125.
36. Lahut S, Vadasz D, Depboylu C, et al. The PD-associated alpha-synuclein promotor Rep1 allele 2 shows diminished frequency in restless legs syndrome. *Neurogenetics*. 2014;15:189–192.
37. Nordlander NB. Therapy in restless legs. *Acta Med Scand*. 1953;145:453–457.
38. Okeeffe ST, Noel J, Lavan JN. Restless legs syndrome in the elderly. *Postgrad Med J*. 1993;69:701–703.
39. Winkelmann J, Stautner A, Samtleben W, Trenkwalder C. Long-term course of restless legs syndrome in dialysis patients after kidney transplantation. *Mov Disord*. 2002;17:1072–1076.
40. Manconi M, Govoni V, De Vito A, et al. Pregnancy as a risk factor for restless legs syndrome. *Sleep Med*. 2004;5:305–308.
41. Allen RP, Earley CJ. The role of iron in restless legs syndrome. *Mov Disord*. 2007;22:S440–S448.
42. Earley CJ, Barker PB, Horska A, Allen RP. MRI-determined regional brain iron concentration in early- and late onset restless legs syndrome. *Sleep Med*. 2006;7:459–461.
43. Allen RP, Barker PB, Wehrl F, Song HK, Earley CJ. MRI measurement of brain iron in patients with restless legs syndrome. *Neurology*. 2001;56:2163–265.
44. Mizuno S, Mihara T, Miyaoka T, Inagaki T, Horiguchi J. CSF iron, ferritin, and transferrin levels in restless legs syndrome. *J Sleep Res*. 2005;14:43–47.
45. Earley CJ, Connor JR, Beard JL, Malecki EA, Epstein DK, Allen RP. Abnormalities in CSF concentrations of ferritin and transferrin in restless legs syndrome. *Neurology*. 2000;54:1698–1700.
46. Connor JR, Boyer PJ, Menzies SL, Dellinger B, Allen RP, Earley CJ. Neuropathological examination suggests impaired brain iron acquisition in restless legs syndrome. Neurology. 2003;61:304–309.
47. Trenkwalder C, Allen R, Hogl B, et al. Comorbidities, treatment, and pathophysiology in restless legs syndrome. *Lancet Neurol*. 2018;17:994–1005.
48. Keeler BE, Baran CA, Brewer KL, Clemens S. Increased excitability of spinal pain reflexes and altered frequency-dependent modulation in the D3-receptor knockout mouse. *Exp Neurol*. 2012;238:273–283.
49. Samir S, Yllanes AP, Lallemand P, Brewer KL, Clemens S. Aging-related morphine tolerance in dopamine D3 receptor knockout mice reversed by block of D1 receptor function. *Neurosci*. 2017;349:87–97.
50. Dinkins M-L, Lallemand P, Clemens S. Long-term treatment with dopamine D3 receptor agonists induces a behavioral switch that can be rescued by blocking the dopamine D1 receptor. *Sleep Med*. 2017;40:47–52.
51. Clemens S, Rye D, Hochman S. Restless legs syndrome revisiting the dopamine hypothesis from the spinal cord perspective. *Neurology*. 2006;67:125–130.
52. Picchietti D, Winkelman JW. Restless legs syndrome, periodic limb movements in sleep, and depression. *Sleep*. 2005;28:891–898.
53. Nofzinger EA, Fasiczka A, Berman S, Thase ME. Buproprion SR reduces periodic limb movements associated with arousals from sleep in depressed patients with periodic limb movement disorder. *J Clin Psychiatry*. 2000;61:858–862.
54. Allen RP, Barker PB, Horska A, et al. Thalamic glutamate/glutamine in restless legs syndrome: increased and related to disturbed sleep. *Neurology*. 2013;80:2028–2034.
55. Ferre S, Earley C, Gulyani S, Garcia-Borreguero D. In search of alternatives to dopaminergic ligands for the treatment of restless legs syndrome: Iron, glutamate, and adenosine. *Sleep Med*. 2017;31:86–92.
56. Bauer CS, Nieto-Rostro M, Rahman W, et al. The increased trafficking of the calcium channel subunit alpha2delta-1 to presynaptic terminals in neuropathic pain is inhibited by the alpha2delta ligand pregabalin. *J Neurosci*. 2009;29:4076–4088.

57. Quiroz C, Pearson V, Gulyani S, Allen R, Earley C, Ferre S. Up-regulation of striatal adenosine A_{2a} receptors with iron deficiency in rats: Effects on locomotion and cortico-striatal neurotransmission. *Exp Neurol.* 2010;224:292–298.
58. Ferré S, Quiroz C, Rea W, Guitart X, Garcia-Borreguero D. Adenosine mechanisms and hypersensitive corticostriatal terminals in restless legs syndrome: Rationale for the use of inhibitors of adenosine transport. In: Clemens S, Ghorayeb I, eds, *Advances in Pharmacology*. Elsevier; 2019:84:3.
59. Bleickardt CJ, Kazdoba TM, Jones NT, et al. Antagonism of the adenosine A2A receptor attenuates akathisia-like behavior induced with MP-10 or aripiprazole in a novel non-human primate model. *Pharmacol Biochem Behav.* 2014;118:36–45.
60. Nuermaimaiti M, Oyama G, Kasemsuk C, Hattori N. Istradefylline for restless legs syndrome associated with Parkinson's Disease. *Tremor Other Hyperkinet Mov.* 2018;8:521.
61. Ibi M, Sawada H, Nakanishi M, et al. Protective effects of 1 alpha,25-(OH)(2) D(3) against the neurotoxicity of glutamate and reactive oxygen species in mesencephalic culture. *Neuropharm.* 2001;40(6):761–771.
62. Patton SM, Cho YW, Clardy TW, Allen RP, Earley CJ, Connor JR. Proteomic analysis of the cerebrospinal fluid of patients with restless legs syndrome/Willis-Ekbom disease. *Fluid Barriers CNS.* 2013;10:20.
63. Wali S, Alsafadi S, Abaalkhail B, et al. The association between vitamin D level and restless legs syndrome: A population-based case-control study. *J Clin Sleep Med.* 2018;14(4):557–564.
64. Baskol G, Korkmaz S, Erdem F, et al. Assessment of nitric oxide, advanced oxidation protein products, malondialdehyde, and thiol levels in patients with restless legs syndrome. *Sleep Med.* 2012;13:414–418.
65. Hwang IC, Na K-S, Yu JL, Kang S-G. Higher prevalence of hypertension among individuals with restless legs syndrome: A meta-analysis. *Psychiatry Invest.* 2018;15(7):701–709.
66. Hein M, Lanquart J-P, Hubain P, Loas G. Risk of resistant hypertension associated with restless legs syndrome and periodic limb movements during sleep: A study on 673 treated hypertensive individuals. *Sleep Med.* 2019;63:46–56.
67. Pennestri MH, Montplaisir J, Colombo R, Lavigne G, Lanfranchi PA. Nocturnal blood pressure changes in patients with restless legs syndrome. *Neurology.* 2007;68:1213–1218.
68. Siddiqui F, Strus J, Ming X, Lee IA, Chokroverty S, Walters AS. Rise of blood pressure with periodic limb movements in sleep and wakefulness. *Clin Neurophysiol.* 2007;118:1923–1930.
69. Winkelman JW, Finn L, Young T. Prevalence and correlates of restless legs syndrome symptoms in the Wisconsin sleep cohort. *Sleep Med.* 2006;7:545–552.
70. Winkelman JW, Shahar E, Sharief I, Gottlieb DJ. Association of restless legs syndrome and cardiovascular disease in the Sleep Heart Health Study. *Neurology.* 2008;70:35–42.
71. Ferini-Strambi L, Walters AS, Sica D. The relationship among restless legs syndrome (Willis-Ekbom Disease), hypertension, cardiovascular disease, and cerebrovascular disease. *J Neurol.* 2014;261:1051–1068.
72. Wang J, O'Reilly B, Venkataraman R, Mysliwiec V, Mysliwiec A. Efficacy of oral iron in patients with restless legs syndrome and low normal ferritin: A randomized, double-blind, placebo-controlled study. *Sleep Med.* 2009;10:973–975.
73. Lee CS, Lee SD, Kang S-H, Park HY, Yoon I-Y. Comparison of the efficacies of oral iron and pramipexole for the treatment of restless legs syndrome patients with low serum ferritin. *European J Neurol.* 2014;21:260–266.
74. Allen RP, Adler CH, Du W, et al. Clinical efficacy and safety of IV ferric carboxymaltose (FCM) treatment of RLS: A multi-centred, placebo-controlled preliminary clinical trial. *Sleep Med.* 2011;12:906–913.
75. Cho YW, Allen RP, Earley CJ. Clinical efficacy of ferric carboxymaltose treatment in patients with restless legs syndrome. *Sleep Med.* 2016;25:16–23.
76. Akpinar S. Restless legs syndrome treatment with dopaminergic drugs. *Clin Neuropharmacol.* 1987;10:69–79.
77. Montplaisir J, Godbout R, Poirier G, Bedard MA. Restless legs syndrome and periodic movements in sleep: Physiopathology and treatment with L-dopa. *Clin Neuropharmacol.* 1986;9:456–463.
78. Allen RP, Earley CJ. Augmentation of the restless legs syndrome with carbidopa/levodopa. *Sleep.* 1996;19(3):205–213.
79. Earley CJ, Allen RP. Pergolide and carbidopa/levodopa treatment of the restless legs syndrome and periodic leg movements in sleep in a consecutive series of patients. *Sleep.* 1996;19(10):801–810.
80. Aurora RN, Kristo DA, Bista SR, et al. The treatment of restless legs syndrome and periodic limb movement disorder in adults-an update for 2012: Practice parameters with an evidenced-based systematic review and meta-analysis. *Sleep.* 2012;35:1039–1062.
81. Driver-Dunckley ED, Noble BN, Hentz JG, et al. Gambling and increased sexual desire with dopaminergic medications in restless legs syndrome. Clin Neuropharmacol. 2007;30(5):249–255.
82. Quickfall J, Suchowersky O. Pathological gambling associated with dopamine agonist use in restless legs syndrome. *Parkinsonism Relat Disord.* 2007;13(8):535–536.
83. Pourcher E, Remillard S, Cohen H. Compulsive habits in restless legs syndrome patients under dopaminergic treatment. *J Neurol Sci.* 2010;290:52–56.
84. Garcia-Borreguero D, Silber MH, Winkelman JW, et al. Guidelines for the first-line treatment of restless legs syndrome/Willis-Ekbom disease, prevention and treatment of dopaminergic augmentation: A combined task force of the IRLSSG, EURLSSG, and the RLS-foundation. *Sleep Med.* 2016;21:1–11.
85. Allen R, Chen C, Soaita A, et al. A randomized, double-blind, 6-week, dose-ranging study of pregabalin in patients with restless legs syndrome. *Sleep Med.* 2010;11:512–519.
86. Ekbom KA. Restless legs syndrome. *Neurology.* 1960;10:868–873.
87. Stefansson H, Rye DB, Hicks A, et al. A genetic risk factor for periodic limb movements in sleep. *N Engl J Med.* 2007;357:639–647.
88. Kim MK, Cho YW, Shin WC et al. Association of restless legs syndrome variants in Korean patients with restless legs syndrome. *Sleep.* 2013;36:1787.

89. Schormair B, Kemlink D, Roeske D, et al. PTPRD (protein tyrosine phosphatase receptor type delta) is associated with restless legs syndrome. *Nat Genet*. 2008;40:946.
90. Winkelmann J, Schormair B, Lichtner P, et al. Genome-wide association study of restless legs syndrome identifies common variants in three genomic regions. *Nat Genet*. 2007;39:1000.
91. Yang Q, Li L, Chen Q, et al. Association of variants in MEIS1, BTBD9, and MAP2K5/SKOR1 with restless legs syndrome in a US population. *Sleep Med*. 2011;12:800.
92. Yang Q, Li L, Yang, R, et al. Family-based and population-based association studies validate PTPRD as a risk factor for restless legs syndrome. *Mov Disord*. 2011;26:516.
93. Schormair B, Zhao C, Bell S, et al. Identification of novel risk loci for restless legs syndrome in genome-wide association studies in individuals of European ancestry: A meta-analysis. *Lancet Neurol*. 2017;16:898.
94. Winkelman JW, Berkowski JA, DelRosso LM, et al. Treatment of restless legs syndrome and periodic limb movement disorder: an American Academy of Sleep Medicine clinical practice guideline. *J Clin Sleep Med*. 2025;21:137–152.

Chapter 18

Periodic Limb Movements of Sleep

Qurratul (Afifa) Shamim-Uzzaman, Syed Kamal Nasser, and Ejaz A. Shamim

INTRODUCTION

"Periodic leg movements of sleep" were first described by Sir Thomas Willis as a key feature of restless legs syndrome (RLS).[1] However, it was not until 1953 that they were reported as a distinct clinical entity. Termed *nocturnal myoclonus*, they were originally described as "involuntary clonic movements at night which are greatly in excess of those which may occur in normal persons"[2p] and were first recorded on polysomnography (PSG) in 1965.[3]

Today, we understand periodic limb movements of sleep (PLMS) to be repetitive contractions of large muscle groups that occur at regular intervals during sleep. Typically, they are seen in the lower extremities, but they may affect the upper extremities and (rarely) the torso. In the extremities, they may affect one or both limbs simultaneously.

It is important to understand that not all leg movements that occur during sleep are PLMS. Movements during sleep must meet specific electromyographic (EMG) morphology and periodicity criteria to be classified as PLMS.

DIAGNOSTIC CRITERIA

Like other movements during sleep, periodic limb movements of sleep (PLMS) are defined by polysomnographic (PSG), not clinical, criteria. Recordings of EMG tone in large muscle groups of the lower extremities are used to identify PLMS. The muscles most commonly monitored for PLMS are the tibialis anterior muscles, as these are the muscles most frequently involved in *periodic* movement activity during sleep.[4,5]

Both lower extremities are monitored simultaneously, with the limb movements captured via 2 separate EMG channels. Two surface electrodes are placed longitudinally in the middle of each tibialis anterior muscle, such that the electrodes are either 2–3 cm apart or span a third of the length of the muscle, whichever is shorter[6] (see Figure 18.1 for a picture of electrode placement).

Diagnosis of PLMS is made when at least 4 sets of muscle activations, measured by elevations in EMG tone, are recorded in a periodic series meeting the specific criteria outlined in the following.

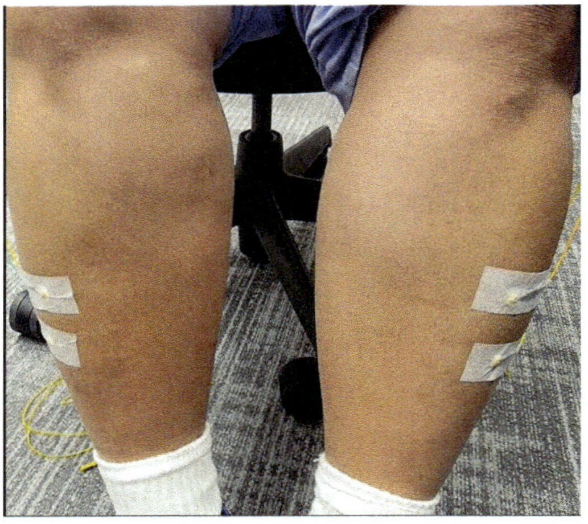

Figure 18.1. Assessing PLMS on PSG. This image shows the placement of EMG leads on bilateral anterior tibialis muscles for measurement of periodic limb movements during polysomnography.

PLMS: periodic limb movements of sleep; PSG: polysomnogram; EMG: electromyography.

Terminology

To score PLMS on PSG, we must first understand the nomenclature used in scoring these movements. Figures 18.2 and 18.3 show the EMG features of PLMS.[7]

Leg movement activity (LMA): LMA refers to any activity in the tibialis anterior muscle of one leg that is at least 8 μV higher than the baseline EMG tone in that muscle and ends when the tone decreases to within 2 μV of the baseline.

Leg movement (LM): An LMA that lasts at least 0.5 seconds, with the median amplitude being ≥ 8 μV higher than the baseline, is called a leg movement (LM). There is no maximum duration of an LM per se.

Candidate leg movements (CLM): LM that are <10 seconds in duration (i.e., LMA lasting 0.5–10 seconds in duration) are called candidate leg movements (CLM)—movements that are "candidates" for occurring in a periodic limb movement series. LM/CLM may occur in both legs simultaneously, or start in the second leg within 0.5–5 seconds of the first leg; in such cases, they are scored as a single bilateral LM (or a single CLM if the duration of the combined leg movements is less than 15 seconds, per WASM) (see Figure 18.2).

Inter-movement interval (IMI): The distance between the start of one CLM and the start of the next is called the inter-movement interval (IMI). This is also sometimes referred to as the period length.

Periodicity index: The proportion of all IMI that are periodic (i.e., the proportion of all IMI that have at least 3 consecutive IMI occurring between 4 consecutive PLM, with each index lasting 10–90 seconds in duration).

Periodic limb movements (PLM): A series of at least 4 CLM separated by an

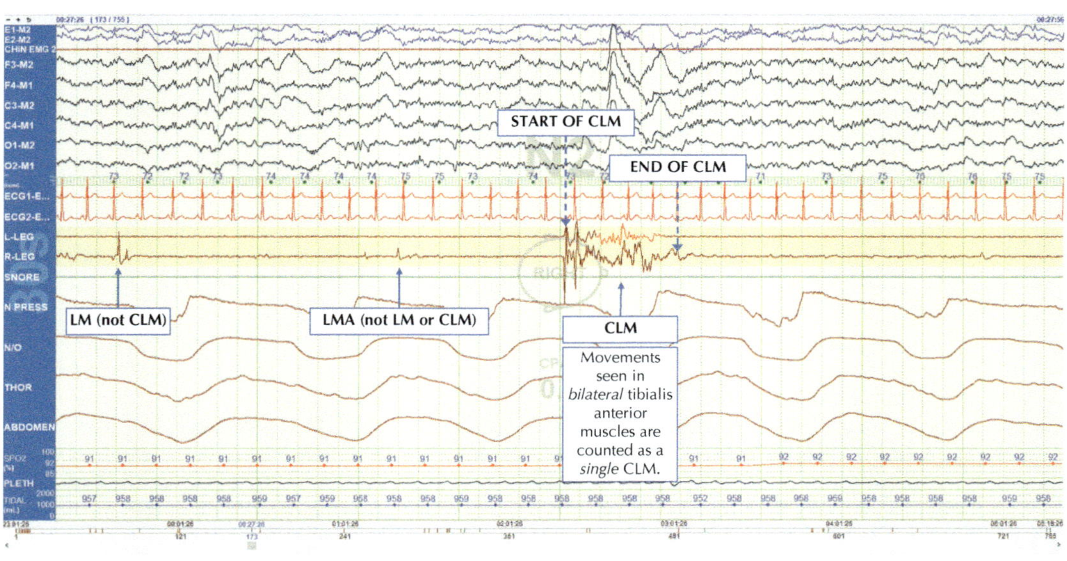

Figure 18.2. The anatomy of EMG activations. This is a 30-second epoch from a PSG showing the different types of activity recorded on limb EMG.

LM: leg movement; LMA: leg movement activity, CLM: candidate leg movement.

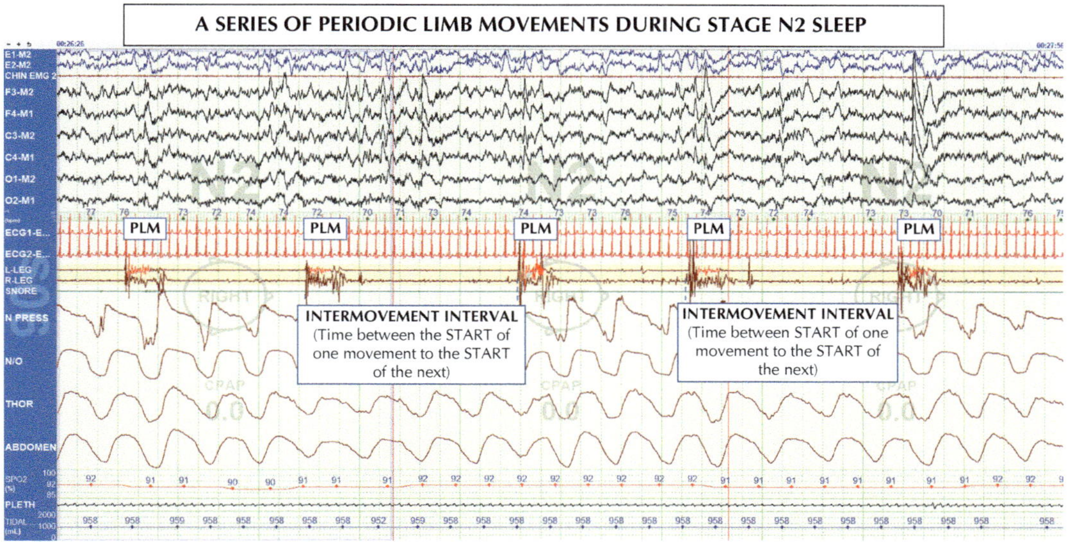

Figure 18.3. A periodic limb movement series. Ninety seconds from a PSG showing a series of periodic limb movements during stage N2 sleep.

inter-movement interval of 10–90 seconds (if WASM standards are used) or 5–90 seconds (if AASM criteria are used). PLM that occur during epochs of sleep are called **periodic limb movements of sleep (PLMS)** and those that occur during wake are known as **periodic limb movements of wakefulness (PLMW)** (see Figure 18.3).

Periodic limb movements of sleep index (PLMS index): The number of PLM that occur per hour of sleep, representing the frequency of PLMS during the night. This term is often represented on PSG as PLMI sleep or PLMSI.

Periodic limb movement disorder: A condition in which elevated PLMS index (≥15 in adults or ≥5 in children) impairs sleep or daytime functioning.

PSG Scoring Criteria

There are 2 primary sets of criteria for scoring periodic limb movements during sleep:

- Combined recommendations set forth by the World Association of Sleep Medicine (WASM) and International Restless Legs Syndrome Study Group (IRLSSG)
- Criteria recommended by the American Academy of Sleep Medicine (AASM).

Use of one set of rules over another does not appear to significantly affect the PLMS indices in any clinically meaningful way,[8] although PLMS indices may be lower in pediatric cases using the WASM rules than with the AASM rules (see later discussion).

Both the WASM/IRLSSG and the AASM agree that a periodic limb movement (PLM) is an 8 µV increase above the resting EMG tone in one or both anterior tibialis channels, lasting 0.5–10 seconds in duration, with return to no higher than 2 µV above the baseline EMG by the end of the movement, and occurring as a series of at least 4 such repeated motor movements[6,9] (see Figures 18.2 and 18.3). However, the AASM specifies that an LM should NOT be scored if it occurs in association with a respiratory event [(i.e., within 0.5s preceding and 0.5 seconds following an apnea, hypopnea, or respiratory effort related arousal (RERA)].

The 2 classification systems differ most prominently on the bilaterality of leg movements and the duration of the inter-movement interval (IMI). Whereas the AASM recommends that the IMI should be 5–90 seconds,[6] as was originally proposed by the WASM/IRLSSG in 2006,[5] the WASM updated their recommendations in 2016 to require at least 10 seconds (i.e., IMI of 10–90 seconds) between CLM,[9] based on automated algorithms and mathematical parameters utilized since their original proposal in 2006. The AASM has not adopted this at the time of writing this chapter.

It is notable that the WASM rules for scoring PLMS may result in lower PLMS counts in children than the AASM rules. Children tend to have shorter IMIs than adults, with younger children having shorter intervals than older children.[10] CLM occurring in series with short intervals, which may be <10s in younger children, may not be scored as PLM with the WASM rules. Because of this consideration, the WASM strongly recommends including both LMS and PLMS counts and indices in pediatric reports.[9] When CLM occur in both legs simultaneously, or within seconds of each other, they are scored as a single bilateral CLM. The AASM rules indicate that the CLM in the 2 legs must start within 5 seconds of each other to be scored as a single bilateral CLM. However, the WASM classification requires that either the CLM in both legs overlap or the CLM in the second leg start within 0.5 seconds of the first leg, as long as the duration of the combined leg movements is less than 15 seconds. Table 18.1 highlights the AASM and WASM criteria for scoring PLM.

CLINICAL FEATURES

In addition to the EMG scoring criteria for periodic limb movements, there are key characteristic clinical features associated with periodic limb movements.

Description of Movements

Periodic limb movements of sleep are repetitive contractions of *large* muscle groups that occur at regular intervals during sleep. These movements may be unilateral or bilateral and involve the lower extremity most frequently; but they may also occur in the upper extremities and trunk.[11]

Most commonly, PLMS originate in the tibialis anterior muscle (53%). PLMS may also originate in other muscles of the lower extremity, albeit much less frequently, including the gastrocnemius (18%), biceps femoris (13%), and rectus femoris (7%) muscles. Although significantly less common, PLMS may originate in upper extremity muscles such as the triceps brachii (5%) and biceps brachii (3%). Axial muscles such as the thoracolumbar paraspinales (0.8%) and rectus abdominis (0.3%) muscles may rarely be the originator of PLMS.[4]

Table 18.1 **PSG Scoring Criteria for PLMS**

Criteria		WASM/IRLSSG (2016 Standards)*	AASM (2020 Criteria)**
EMG Morphology	Amplitude	***Sustained*** increase in anterior tibialis EMG tone Onset: ≥8 μV increase above baseline Offset: ≤2 μV above baseline	***Absolute*** 8 μV increase in anterior tibialis EMG tone Onset: ≥8 μV increase above baseline Offset: ≤2 μV above baseline
	Duration	0.5–10 seconds	0.5–10 seconds
Periodicity	Frequency	Minimum of 4 in a series	Minimum of 4 in a series
	Inter-movement interval	10–90 seconds	5–90 seconds
Bilaterality	CLM in 2 legs considered a single bilateral CLM if:	• CLM in both legs overlap • If not overlapping, the ***offset*** of the CLM in one leg occurs ***<0.5 s*** before the onset of the subsequent CLM in the contralateral leg AND the combined duration of the CLM in both legs is <15 s	• ***Onset*** of the CLM in the first leg is ***<5 s*** before the onset of the subsequent CLM in the contralateral leg

* WASM = World Association of Sleep Medicine; CLM = candidate leg movement; * IRLSSG = International Restless Legs Syndrome Study Groups; EMG = electromyogram; **AASM = American Academy of Sleep Medicine.

Regardless of originating site, the electromyographic (EMG) activity spreads from its point of origin, but no consistent pattern of muscle recruitment has been identified (i.e., no specific rostral nor caudal propagation of the EMG activity has been shown).[4] However, the resultant contractions have a characteristic triple flexion pattern—dorsiflexion of the toe and ankle with flexion of the knee, and sometimes hip.[11] Similar triple-flexion patterns are seen with PLMS occurring in the upper extremities. A single limb may be affected, or contralateral extremities affected together.

Though not required for scoring PLMS, cortical arousals or autonomic arousals may be seen before, during, or immediately following the movement. The affected individuals may even awaken from the movement. However, the movements themselves are not typically reported by the patient as being bothersome; usually, it is the bedpartners that complain of the patients' leg movements, not the patients themselves.

The frequency of PLMS is not consistent throughout the night; in fact, they may vary during different parts of the night, as well as between nights.

Temporal Distribution of PLMS

The distribution of PLMS may vary throughout the night and may show variability between nights.

Two types of time-of-night patterns (i.e., distribution of PLMS within a single night) have been demonstrated.[12] The first (type I) tends to cluster around the late evening or early part of the night. In this pattern of distribution, the majority (60%) of PLMS activity occurs in the first 3 hours of sleep onset, then decreases over the remainder of the night, even when adjusted for increased REM sleep time later in the night. The second pattern (type II) shows PLMS activity to be more evenly distributed throughout the night, increasing across the first half of the night, then decreasing across the second half to a level similar to the beginning of the night. In the type II pattern, 50% of the PLMS activity occurs in the last 4 hours of the sleep period. Of note, in Culpepper's study, patients with the type I pattern had more PLMS overall than those with the type II pattern.

Early studies showed relatively good correlation in PLMS activity between nights, though with the type I pattern showing more stability (less variability between nights) than the type II pattern in patients with idiopathic PLMS.[12] However, later studies have shown significant night-to-night variability in PLMS activity,[13–15] especially when PLMS are seen in association with other disorders such as restless legs syndrome (RLS), insomnia secondary to psychiatric disorders, primary insomnia, sleep apnea, and organic hypersomnias (narcolepsy or idiopathic hypersomnia). In one study, this variance was seen across 2 nights in 27% of 115 patients studied, with the greatest night-to-night variability occurring in patients with RLS.[16] The clinical impact of the temporal distribution of PLMS activity is yet to be elucidated. Patients with the type II pattern tend to be younger, male, and sleepier during the day.[12] There is controversy as to the validity of single-night indices of PLMS on a routine sleep study; as PLMS indices may vary between nights in patients with different sleep comorbidities, these factors should be taken into account when using the PLMS index for diagnostic purposes. Furthermore, although the frequency of movements (PLMS index) may vary between nights, the inter-movement interval (IMI) and periodicity index tend to be consistently stable across nights within the same individual,[17,18] suggesting an underlying biological factor regulating the IMI.

PLMS Index

The PLMS index is commonly used to denote the frequency of PLMS throughout the night, per hour of sleep. A PLMS index <15 in adults and <5 in children is within normal limits.[19] Recent reports suggest that the clinical relevance of PLMS should not be based on the PLMS index alone, especially given the significant intrasubject night-to-night variability related to comorbidities. Therefore, the PLMS index should be interpreted in context with the periodicity index (a more stable measure in PLMS) and time of night distribution of PLMS.

PREVALENCE

The exact prevalence of PLMS in the general population is not well known. However, it is now well established that the presence of PLMS increases with age, occurring less frequently in children and more frequently in adults, with the greatest prevalence in older age groups.[20,21]

One large epidemiological study in Europe found a general population prevalence of 3.9% using the International Classification of Sleep Disorders (ICSD) criteria of PLMD in 18980 non-institutionalized individuals ages 15+ years from the United Kingdom, Spain, Germany, Italy, and Portugal; however, PSGs were not performed, and diagnosis was made solely through phone interviews.[22] Using PSG to identify PLMS, Scofield et al. found a prevalence of 7.6% in 592 individuals from Detroit, Michigan,[23] with a mean age of 41 years. In comparison, Ancoli-Israel found a prevalence of 45% in 427 randomly selected community-dwelling individuals over the age of 65 years living in San Diego, California.[24]

In 2006, Pennestri et al. demonstrated that PLMS index >5 was rarely seen below the age of 40 years, but above the age of 40, PLMS prevalence and frequency increased with each decade.[20] Longitudinal evaluations performed on 525 individuals of the Wisconsin Sleep Cohort having at least 3 PSGs showed that prevalence of PLMI ≥15 was 25.3% at a mean age of 56.7 ± 7.4 (SD), 30.1% at mean age 60.6 ± 7.2 (SD), and 43.4% at mean age 65.0 ± 7.1 (SD); prevalence of PLMI ≥15 increased significantly over the 8 years of observation, with an odds ratio of 2.26 (95% CI: 1.74–2.94).[25]

Recently, using an observational cohort study design, Ferri et al. assessed the age-related changes of PLMS in 165 patients with RLS using the IRLSSG diagnostic criteria of 2014. Leg movement and periodicity indices were analyzed in the following age groups: 16 preschoolers (≤5 years of age), 24 school-age children (age 6–12 years), 19 adolescents (age 13–17 years), 17 young adults (age 19–40 years), 47 adults (age 41–60 years), and 37 seniors (age >60 years). They found that PLMSI showed a decrease before age 10 years, steadily increased to age 30 years, then remained relatively stable until age 60 years, after which they increased to age 80 years. This pattern was due almost entirely to the frequency of PLM.[21]

Neither ethnic/racial disparities nor sex differences in PLMS are fully delineated yet. PLMS do appear to be more frequent in men than women,[23,26,27] and less prevalent in African American than Caucasian adults (4.3% versus 9.3%, respectively).[23] PLMS index >15/hour was found in 28.6% (31.3% in men, 26% in women) of 2162 general community-dwelling adults of the HypnoLaus Cohort (from Lausanne, Switzerland, an almost exclusively Caucasian population),[26] and 33% of 1090 participants of the Wisconsin Sleep Cohort.[27]

The exact prevalence of PLMS is not entirely clear in the pediatric population. In healthy children, studies suggest >5 events/hr are seen in 1.2%[28]–7%[29] of the general pediatric population, but may be higher in subsets of children. As in adults, African American children have a lower prevalence of PLMS compared to Caucasian children (7% versus 16.5%, respectively).[30]

Predisposing and Precipitating Factors

PLMS are dependent on stage of sleep, being most frequent in N1, then N2, and finally N3 sleep. They are least often seen in REM sleep.[19]

A positive family history of RLS also confers increased risk for PLMS as well as PLMD, and the genetic variants noted in the following may be mediators of this risk. PLMS have been precipitated with use of several medications, most commonly tricyclic antidepressants (TCAs), selective serotonin reuptake inhibitors (SSRIs), dopamine receptor antagonists (DAs), and lithium. Low brain iron, reflected by serum ferritin level, may worsen PLMS via the role of iron-dopamine pathways. And small studies suggest that, in individuals who sleep at night, both circadian influences and homeostatic sleep-dependent factors independently predispose to PLMS, especially in a type I pattern.[31]

Multivariate analyses of the HypnoLaus Sleep Cohort found age, male gender, antidepressant intake, presence of RLS, and SNP alleles of rs3923809, rs3104788 and rs2300478 to be independently associated with PLMSI >15.[26]

A German study[32] invited participants of 2 cohorts (1107 subjects from the SHIP-TREND Cohort of the Study of Health in Pomerania[33] and 247 subjects from the BiDirect Study[34]) for in-lab PSGs and confirmed the previous finding that being male and being older increases the likelihood of increased PLMS. Having

RLS and being on an antidepressant is strongly associated with higher prevalence of PLMS. Physical inactivity, smoking, obesity, diabetes, antidepressant use, and lower magnesium levels also correlated with higher PLMS activity.

Children with PLMS index >5/hour have higher prevalence of RLS, snoring, insomnia, mood disorders, chronic kidney disease, epilepsy, and chronic heart diseases. Children with PLMS indices >5 also report more morning headaches and have more behavioral problems. Use of antidepressants, antipsychotics, and antiseizure medications are more prevalent in children with PLMS index >5 than those with PLMS index <5. No difference in age, sex, or ferritin levels have been noted in children with PLMS index >5 versus those without elevated PLMS indices.[35] Children with a history of prematurity have higher prevalence of RLS (8.4%) and PLMD (7.8%), with 50% of patients having a PLMS index >5.[36] Iron deficiency is thought to play a role in this population.

FAMILIAL PATTERNS AND GENETICS

Familial patterns of PLMS have not yet been clearly defined. Recent literature has begun to uncover genetic associations of PLMS with the *BTBD9* gene (strongest association) as well as the *TOX3* and *MEIS1* genes.

A single nucleotide polymorphism (SNP) marker, rs3923809, in an intron of the *BTBD9* gene on chromosome 6p21.2 showed a strong association with PLMS and RLS in patients from Iceland and the United States (odds ratio: 1.7; $p = 3 \times 10^{-14}$).[37] Though all patients had RLS symptoms, this association was not present in patients who did not have PLMS (odds ratio: 1.0; $p = 0.81$), but persisted in patients with PLMS who did not meet full diagnostic criteria for RLS (odds ratio: 2.3; $p = 2 \times 10^{-6}$).

Of the Icelandic subjects, 943 were further genotyped for SNP marker rs3923809, as AA homozygotes, AG heterozygotes (carriers), and GG homozygotes (noncarriers). The at-risk allele is allele A. The odds of having allele A of marker rs3923809 increased as the PLMI increased, and the frequency of movements was greater in AA homozygotes than AG heterozygotes ($p = 0.003$), and greater in AG heterozygotes than GG homozygotes ($p < 0.001$), with AA homozygotes having twice as many PLMS than GG homozygotes ($p < 0.001$).

Haba-Rubio also found significant associations between PLMSI >15/hour and rs3923809(A) on BTBD9, with AA homozygotes having 3-fold higher frequency of PLMS compared to AG heterozygotes.[26] Significant but weaker associations were also seen with rs3104788 (gene *TOX3*), and rs2300478 (*MEIS1* gene) in this same European study.

ETIOLOGY/PATHOPHYSIOLOGY

Though much still needs to be learned about the possible etiology and pathogenesis of PLMS, current knowledge hints to genetic risk factors (described previously), the nervous system, and systemic as well as psychiatric conditions underlying the generation of PLMS.

In the central nervous system, both cortical and subcortical structures appear to play a role in the pathogenesis of PLMS. A small study of 6 patients with periodic limb movements of sleep underwent prolonged electroencephalogram (EEG) monitoring and found increased cortical activations before and after the PLMS.[38] Spectral analysis of heart rate variability and EEG show autonomic activation starting several seconds before EEG changes and movement onset, suggesting an independent sympathetic nervous system etiology.[39,40] Increased frequency of PLMS in Parkinsonian patients[41] and reduction in PLMS indices with dopaminergic therapy in patients with dopamine hypoactivity states suggest a central dopaminergic etiology;[41–44] and iron stores may play a role in PLMS, similar to RLS.[45] Disinhibition of muscles innervated at the lumbosacral L4 to S1 levels, and possibly cervical segments C6 to C7, has been suggested.[4] A common spinal mechanism in PLMS and RLS may intensify spinal cord activity[46] and may explain the typical triple-flexion pattern of the PLM.

CLINICAL IMPLICATIONS

The clinical impact of PLMS per se are not clearly known. However, PLMS may be associated with sleep disruption, daytime sleepiness, and cardiovascular outcomes secondary to autonomic hyperactivity; and PLMS are known to occur in greater frequency with other conditions. PSG studies in individuals with higher PLM rates (PLMI ≥15) show a shorter total sleep time and higher wake after sleep onset.[27]

The PLMS coexist with other sleep- and non-sleep-related conditions. When PLMS are increased (PLMSI ≥15 in adults or ≥5 in children) and result in significant sleep or daytime impairment (be it mental, social, behavioral, or physical) that is not better explained by another disorder, they result in a condition called periodic limb movement disorder (PLMD).[11]

Increased PLMS show strong associations with dopamine deficiency/hypoactivity states. Parkinsonian patients (such as those with idiopathic Parkinson's disease, multisystem atrophy, post-encephalitic Parkinsonism, drug-induced Parkinsonism, etc.) not on dopaminergic therapy have significantly greater rates of PLMS than patients with other non-hypodopaminergic neurodegenerative conditions such as Alzheimer disease.[41] Up to 80% of patients with RLS have PLMS.[47] PLMS are more commonly seen in people with idiopathic REM sleep behavior disorder (RBD),[48] in narcoleptics,[49] and in those with attention deficit hyperactivity disorder (ADHD).[50] In fact, PLMS are seen in up to 75% of patients with narcolepsy.[51] Individuals taking SSRIs[52] and TCAs[53] tend to have more PLMS.

Elevated PLMS indices have also been found in other conditions. Patients with obstructive sleep apnea have higher frequency of PLMS and consequently decreased quality of sleep.[54] Elevated PLMS are seen after traumatic brain injury (TBI)[55] and in patients with PTSD.[56] PLMS are also seen in spinal cord injury, end-stage renal disease, and congestive heart failure.[57]

It is possible that PLMS may be a risk factor for stroke and heart attack, though a direct association has never been made. Sieminski showed increases in systolic blood pressure and heart rate following PLMS in patients with RLS. Indirectly, PLMS are thought to be associated with nocturnal hypertension, increased heart rate, and arrhythmias,[58] postulated to occur through sympathetic hyperactivity. However, the data are not clear cut. PLMS were associated with arterial hypertension in one study,[59] but multivariate regression modeling did not reveal any significant association;[60] nor was there an association in 2793 community-dwelling older men unless they had structural heart disease and were not on inotropic agents (calcium channel blockers or beta-blockers).[61] While it is not clear if PLMS are an independent risk factor for heart attacks and strokes, presence of PLMS has been associated with increased mortality risk in patients with end-stage renal disease (ESRD)[62] and systolic heart failure;[63] in patients with ESRD, total number of arousals during sleep was a good prognosticator of mortality.[62] Those individuals sleeping more than 9 hours per day have a higher frequency of stroke-related mortality.[64] Left ventricular hypertrophy has been associated with PLMS,[65] which may aggravate underlying cardiovascular disease.

Children with increased PLMS are at higher risk for nocturnal hypertension, and their blood pressures may also be higher during the daytime.[66] A small control-matched study found that children with nocturnal enuresis had higher PLMS and sleep fragmentation.[67] Elevated PLMS have also been seen in sickle cell disease,[68] Asperger syndrome,[69] and Williams syndrome.[70]

DIFFERENTIAL DIAGNOSES

Periodic limb movements of sleep (PLMS) must be distinguished from a variety of other movements during sleep. The more common ones are described in the following and displayed in Figure 18.4.

Interestingly, many patients confuse PLMS with restless legs syndrome (RLS), often reporting that their sleep study showed RLS. It is important to note that although they are frequently seen in patients with RLS, PLMS are EMG activations (a series of 4 or more occurring with periodicity, as defined previously) during sleep; if they occur with increased frequency and result in clinical consequences, they are known as a clinical entity called periodic limb movement disorder (PLMD). In contrast, RLS is a disorder of wake defined by clinical criteria (urge to move that increases with immobility, improves with movement, and displays a circadian preference for the evening/night). Therefore, the differential diagnoses listed in this section, and summarized in Table 18.2, include only those conditions that may resemble PLMS via EMG criteria.

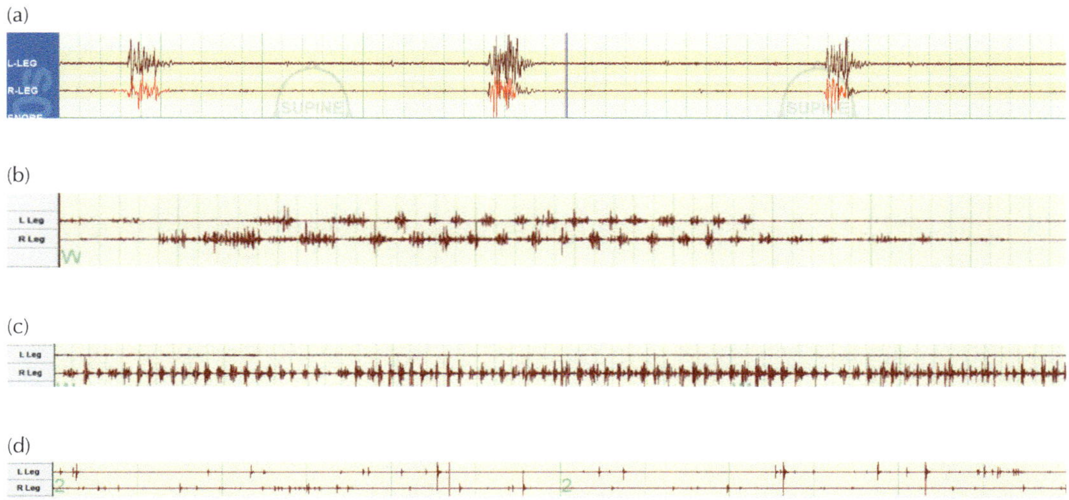

Figure 18.4. Various types of movements during sleep. Limb EMG leads comparing PLM (a), with alternating leg muscle activations (b), hypnagogic foot tremor (c), and excessive fragmentary myoclonus (d).

Table 18.2 Characteristic Features of Common Sleep-Related Movements

	PLMS	ALMA	EFM	HFT	HJ	SRRMD	RSWA
Amplitude of EMG burst (above baseline EMG)	Onset: 8μV Offset: 2μV	Onset: 8μV Offset: 2μV	>50 μV	50–200 μv	—	2 × background EMG	4 × background EMG
Duration	0.5–10 s	100–500 ms	≤150 ms	250–1000 ms	<1 s	1–59 min long runs	variable
Frequency	Occur every 5-90s	0.5–3.0 Hz	≥ 5/min (not at fixed intervals)	0.3–4.0 Hz	Not periodic—usually a single movement	0.5–2.0 Hz	Bursts in >50% of 10 consecutive 3 s mini-epochs
Minimum # of movements required in series	4	4	—	4	—	4	— (no fixed periodicity)
Description of movements	Triple-flexion, unilateral or bilateral	Movements alternate between legs	Small twitches	Rhythmic, oscillating movement of the whole foot or toes during pre-sleep wakefulness and N1, N2[52]	Myoclonic body jerk at sleep onset	Head rocking/ rolling Body rocking/ rolling Leg rocking/ rolling	Complex movements, may appear goal-directed
Body parts affects	Large muscle groups of LE, UE, and torso	Lower extremities	Small muscles and joints of hands/ feet and face	Lower extremities	Head, trunk and limbs	Any large muscle groups of the body	Any body part may be involved
Clinical consequences?	YES	Possible?	NO	NO	if excessive	NO	YES

PLMS = periodic limb movements of sleep; HFT = hypnagogic foot tremor; RSWA = REM sleep without atonia; ALMA = alternating leg muscle activation; HJ = hypnic jerk; EFM = excessive fragmentary myoclonus; SRRMD = sleep related rhythmic movement disorder.

Alternating Leg Muscle Activation

As the name suggests, ALMA is a high frequency leg movement consisting of alternating leg muscle activations (ALMA) of the tibialis anterior muscles that resemble normal bipedal locomotion.[71] Like PLMS, a minimum of 4 muscle activations are needed in an ALMA series.[72,73] However, unlike PLMS, the movements of ALMA are much shorter, lasting 100–500 ms; faster, occurring at a frequency of 0.5–3 Hz (typically 1–2 Hz); and usually alternate between the legs. The trains of ALMA usually last less than 20 seconds. They most often occur at wake-to-sleep or sleep-to-wake transitions but rarely persist into consolidated sleep; when they do, they have been seen in all stages of sleep.[11,73]

Excessive Fragmentary Myoclonus

Excessive fragmentary myoclonus (EFM) is characterized by very small movements of the corners of the mouth, fingers, or toes, often not visible to the naked eye, usually observed during non-rapid eye movement (NREM) sleep. Morphologically, EMG bursts of EFM occur for at least 20 minutes during NREM sleep with at least 5 bursts per minute, each with a duration of approximately 150 milliseconds.[74,75] EFM may be a benign movement phenomenon and there have been no reported clinical consequence.

Hypnagogic Foot Tremor

Hypnagogic foot tremor (HFT), first described as grouped phasic tremor potentials by Broughton in 1998,[76] is a common and benign PSG finding seen during pre-sleep wake as well as stage N1 and N2 sleep.[72] These are visible as rhythmic movements of the foot and toes occurring at a frequency of 0.3–4 Hz.[6] There are no known clinical consequences; treatment typically consists of reassuring and educating the patient on the benign nature of the movements.

Hypnic Jerks (aka Sleep Starts)

Hypnic jerks are brief (<1 second in duration), myoclonic jerks of one or more body segments occurring at sleep onset. They usually involve flexion of the head, trunk, and limbs and are often seen as a single contraction affecting the body asymmetrically. If the movements are severe or excessive in frequency, they can delay sleep onset or disrupt sleep maintenance. EMG shows brief high-amplitude potentials, typically 75–250 milliseconds in duration, during wake-to-sleep transitions or stage N1 sleep.[77]

REM Sleep Without Atonia

Loss of muscle tone is a characteristic feature of REM sleep and is commonly referred to as atonia during REM sleep. REM sleep *without* atonia (RWA) occurs when excessive sustained (tonic) elevations are seen in the chin EMG (>50% of the epoch having chin EMG tone that is at least 2 times greater than the baseline atonia of REM), or excessive transient (phasic) elevations are seen in the chin or limb EMG. Excessive phasic activity is defined as transient EMG elevations seen in ≥50% of 3-second mini-epochs during an epoch of REM sleep (when each epoch of REM is divided into ten 3-second mini epochs) with each EMG burst being at least 2 times greater in amplitude than the baseline REM atonia and lasting 0.1–5 seconds in duration.[6]

Though seen in other disorders such as narcolepsy[78] and trauma-related sleep disorder,[79] RWA is a cardinal feature of REM sleep behavior disorder (RBD), a parasomnia in which the normal atonia of REM sleep is lost, and patients appear to "act out" their dreams. The dreams of RBD are usually vivid and oftentimes have frightening or violent content with themes of being chased, attacked, or fighting back; less frequently, nonviolent dreams have also been reported. Witnessed behaviors are usually complex, appear to be goal-directed, and are often violent; they may range from benign hand gestures or foot movements to violent thrashing, punching, or kicking movements and may result in injury to the individual or their bed partner.[11]

Sleep-Related Rhythmic Movements

Sleep-related rhythmic movements are involuntary, non-epileptiform, stereotypical, large-amplitude movements occurring rhythmically before sleep onset; occasionally they may persist into consolidated sleep. Often manifested as body rocking, head banging, or head rolling, these movements occur repetitively and rhythmically at a frequency of 0.5–2 Hz.[11,80] Rhythmic or inarticulate vocalizations, even humming, have been reported with the movements.[11]

Typically, these movements are prevalent in children, most commonly in infancy, and decrease as the child ages. Rarely, they may persist into adulthood. Though non-volitional, both adults and children use these rhythmic movements as a method of self-soothing to help initiate sleep, and many children do not even remember performing the movements.[81] Thus, they are generally considered a benign phenomenon. However, injuries have been reported, especially with head banging; and sometimes the affected individuals sleep wearing helmets to prevent injury. If the rhythmic movements disrupt sleep, cause injury, or lead to daytime impairment, they meet criteria for sleep-related rhythmic movement disorder.[11]

ONGOING CONSIDERATIONS/ FUTURE DIRECTIONS:

There is much that still needs to be learned about PLMS. Scoring guidelines exist to quantify periodic limb movements, but better qualitative examination of PLMS is needed. Movements meeting criteria for PLMS during REM sleep should be further evaluated to ensure they are truly PLMS and not a form of parasomnia. Currently, we do not score PLMS that occur during respiratory events, even if they occur with regular periodicity. How does this potential under-reporting of PLMS indices affect clinical outcomes? And what of the periodicity intervals; more research is needed to understand their clinical import. Scoring criteria for PLMS are not consistent. Can computer algorithms be developed or artificial intelligence (AI) used to assist in standardizing PSG scoring of PLMS? Could AI-assisted scoring also separate PLMS occurring in REM sleep from RWA?

Much research is needed on the clinical implications of PLMS. Some PLMS are associated with arousals while others are not; do these disruptions in sleep continuity resulting from PLMS impact clinical outcomes or affect chronic health conditions? We have just started to identify associations between PLMS and cardiovascular disease—is this a causal relationship or are other mediators involved? If a causal relationship does exist, can treatment of PLMS/PLMD improve cardiovascular outcomes? Randomized controlled trials, currently lacking, can help elucidate these relationships. In the future, identification of genetic and environmental factors affecting PLMS may help in the treatment of associated comorbidities. To facilitate further research, a unified definition and accurate identification of PLMS are needed, in addition to the collection of longitudinal data regarding comorbidities and significant health-related events. A centralized database/registry may be helpful in this regard.

KEY POINTS

- PLMS should be differentiated from other movements during sleep.
- PLMS have a typical triple flexion movement; these have been described in the lower extremities as a characteristic toe extension with (dorsi-)flexion of the ankle, knee, and sometimes hip.
- PLMS may occur in normal sleep, but a PLMS index ≥15 in adults or ≥5 in children is usually considered excessive.
- Some night-to-night variability exists in the PLMS index; however, the IMI and PI tend to be more stable between nights than the PLMSI.
- There is still much to be learned about the pathophysiology of PLMS, but current knowledge points to CNS, autonomic, and/or genetic factors.
- PLMS have been associated with other conditions, especially dopamine-deficient states such as Parkinson's disease and RLS, OSA, and use of antidepressants.
- More research is needed to understand the health consequences of PLMS.

REFERENCES

1. Wilis T. De anima brutorum uae hominis viatlis ac sentivia est: exercitationes duae. In: *Oxon Londay: Typis E.F. impensis* R. Davis; 1672.
2. Symonds CP. Nocturnal myoclonus. *J Neurol Neurosurg Psychiatry*. 1953;16:166–171.

3. Lugaresi E, Coccogna G, Tassinari CA, et al. Rilievi poligrafici sui fenomeni motori nella syndrome delle gambe senza riposo [Polygraphic data on motor phenomena in the restless legs syndrome]. *Riv Neurol.* 1965;35:550–561.
4. Provini F, Vetrugno R, Meletti S, et al. Motor pattern of periodic limb movements during sleep. *Neurology.* 2001;57:300–304.
5. Zucconi M, Ferri R Allen RP, et al. World Association of Sleep Medicine (WASM) standards for recording and scoring periodic leg movements in sleep (PLMS) and wakefulness (PLMW) developed in collaboration with a task force from International Restless Legs Syndrome Study Groups (IRLSSG). *Sleep Med.* 2006;7:175–183.
6. Berry RB, Quan SF, Abreu AR, et al.; for the American Academy of Sleep Medicine. *The AASM Manual for the Scoring of Sleep and Associated Events: Rules, Terminology and Technical Specifications.* Version 2.6. American Academy of Sleep Medicine; 2020.
7. Ferri R. Time structure of leg movements activity during sleep: The theory behind the practice. *Sleep Med.* 2012;13:433–441.
8. Ferri R, Manconi M, Rundo F, et al. A data-driven analysis of the rules defining bilateral leg movements during sleep. *Sleep.* 2016;39(2):413–421.
9. Ferri R, Fulda S, Allen RP, et al. World Association of Sleep Medicine (WASM) 2016 standards for recording and scoring leg movements in polysomnograms developed by a joint task force from the International and the European Restless Legs Syndrome Study Groups (IRLSSG and EURLSSG). *Sleep Med.* 2016;26:86–95.
10. Ferri R, Manconi M, Lanuzza B, et al. Age-related changes in periodic leg movements during sleep in patients with restless legs syndrome. *Sleep Med.* 2008;9:790–798.
11. American Academy of Sleep Medicine. *International Classification of Sleep Disorders.* 34th ed. American Academy of Sleep Medicine; 2014.
12. Culpepper W, Badia P, Shaffer J. Time-of-night patterns in PLMS activity. *Sleep.* 1992;15(4):306–311.
13. Sforza E, Haba-Rubio J. Night-to-night variability in periodic leg movements in patients with restless legs syndrome. *Sleep Med.* 2005;6:259–267.
14. Trotti LM, Bliwise DL, Greer SA, et al. Correlates of PLMs variability over multiple nights and impact upon RLS diagnosis. *Sleep Med.* 2009;10:668–671.
15. Picchietti M, Picchietti D, England S, et al. Children show individual night-to-night variability of periodic limb movements in sleep, *Sleep.* 2009;32(4):530–535. https://doi.org/10.1093/sleep/32.4.530.
16. Hornyak M, Kopasz M, Feige B, Riemann D, Voderholzer U. Variability of periodic leg movements in various sleep disorders: implications for clinical and pathophysiologic studies, *Sleep.* 2005 Mar;28(3):331–335. https://doi.org/10.1093/sleep/28.3.331.
17. Ferri R, Fulda S, Manconi M, et al. Night-to-night variability of the periodic leg movements during sleep in restless legs syndrome and periodic limb movement disorder: Comparison between the periodicity index and the PLMS Index. *Sleep Med.* 2013;14:293–296. http://dx.doi.org/10.1016/j.sleep.2012.08.014.
18. Skeba P, Hiranniramol K, Earley C, Allen R. Intermovement interval as a primary stable measure of periodic limb movements of sleep. *Sleep Med.* 2016 Jan;17:138–143. doi:10.1016/j.sleep.2015.10.004.
19. Frauscher B, Gabelia D, Mitterling T, et al. Motor events during healthy sleep: A quantitative polysomnographic study. *Sleep.* 2014;37(4):763–773.
20 Pennestri MH, Whittom S, Adam B, Petit D, Carrier J, Montplaisir J. PLMS and PLMW in healthy subjects as a function of age: prevalence and interval distribution. *Sleep.* 2006 Sep;29(9):1183–1187. doi:10.1093/sleep/29.9.1183. PMID: 17040005.
21. Ferri R, DelRosso LM, Silvani A, et al. Peculiar lifespan changes of periodic leg movements during sleep in restless legs syndrome. *J Sleep Res.* 2020 Jun;29(3):e12896. doi:10.1111/jsr.12896. PMID: 31313413.
22. Ohanyon MM, Roth T. Prevalence of RLS and PLMD in general population. *J Psychosom Res.* 2002;53:547–554.
23. Scofield H, Roth T, Drake C. PLM during sleep: Population, prevalence, clinical correlates and racial differences. *Sleep.* 2008 Sep;31(9):1221–1227.
24. Ancoli-Israel S, Kripke DF, Klauber MR, et al. Periodic limb movements in sleep in community-dwelling elderly. *Sleep.* 1991;14: 496–500.
25. Leary EB, Moore HE IV, Schneider LD, Finn LA, Peppard PE, Mignot E. Periodic limb movements in sleep: Prevalence and associated sleepiness in the Wisconsin Sleep Cohort. *Clin Neurophysiol.* 2018;129(11):2306–2314. doi:10.1016/j.clinph.2018.08.022.
26. Haba-Rubio J, Marti-Soler H, Marques-Vidal P, et al. Prevalence and determinants of periodic limb movements in the general population. *Ann Neurol.* 2016 Mar;79(3):464–474. doi:10.1002/ana.24593. PMID: 26703954.
27. Moore H, Winkelmann J, Lin L, Finn L, Peppard P, Mignot E. Periodic leg movements during sleep are associated with polymorphisms in BTBD9, TOX3/BC034767, MEIS1, MAP2K5/SKOR1, and PTPRD. *Sleep.* 2014;37(9):1535–1542. doi:10.5665/sleep.4006.
28. Kirk VG, Bohn S. Periodic limb movements in children: Prevalence in a referred population. *Sleep.* 2004;27(2):313–315.
29. Marcus CL, Traylor J, Gallagher PR, et al. Prevalence of periodic limb movements during sleep in normal children. *Sleep.* 2014;37(8):1349–1352.
30. O'Brien LM, Holbrook CR, Jones F, Gozal D. Ethnic difference in PLM in children. *Sleep Med.* 2007 Apr;8(3):240–246. doi:10.1016/j.sleep.2006.08.009.
31. Duffy J, Lowe A, Silva E, Winkelman J. Periodic limb movements in sleep exhibit a circadian rhythm that is maximal in the late evening/early night. *Sleep Med.* 2011 Jan;12(1):83–88. doi:10.1016/j.sleep.2010.06.007.
32. Szentkirályi A, Stefani A, Hackner H, et al. Prevalence and associated risk factors of periodic limb movement in sleep in two German population-based studies. *Sleep.* 2019;42(3):zsy237. doi:10.1093/sleep/zsy237.
33. Völzke H, Alte D, Schmidt CO, et al. Cohort profile: The study of health in Pomerania. *Int J Epidemiol.* 2011;40(2):294–307.
34. Teismann H, Wersching H, Nagel M, et al. Establishing the bidirectional relationship between depression and subclinical arteriosclerosis: Rationale, design, and characteristics of the BiDirect Study. *BMC Psychiatry.* 2014;14:174.

35. Delrosso LM, Lockhart C, Wrede JE, et al. Comorbidities in children with elevated periodic limb movement index during sleep. *Sleep*. 2020 Feb 13;43(2):zsz221. doi:10.1093/sleep/zsz221. PMID: 31555831.
36. Cielo CM, DelRosso LM, Tapia IE, et al.; Caffeine for Apnea of Prematurity–Sleep Study Group. Periodic limb movements and restless legs syndrome in children with a history of prematurity. *Sleep Med*. 2017 Feb;30:77–81. doi:10.1016/j.sleep.2016.02.009. PMID: 28215268; PMCID: PMC5321628.
37. Stefansson H, Rye DB, Hicks A, et al. A genetic risk factor for periodic limb movements in sleep. N Engl J Med. 2007 Aug 16;357(7):639–647. doi:10.1056/NEJMoa072743. PMID: 17634447.
38. Iriarte J, Urrestarazu E, Alegre M, Valencia M, Artieda J. Oscillatory cortical changes during periodic limb movements. *Sleep*. 2004 Dec 15;27(8):1493–1498.
39. Guggisberg A, Hess C, Mathis J. The significance of the sympathetic nervous system in the pathophysiology of periodic leg movements in sleep. *Sleep*. 2007;30(6):755–766.
40. Sasai T, Matsuura M, Inoue Y. Change in heart rate variability precedes the occurrence of periodic leg movements during sleep: an observational study. *BMC Neurol*. 2013 Oct 6;13:139. doi:10.1186/1471-2377-13-139. PMID: 24093585; PMCID: PMC3852097.
41. Bliwise D, Trott L, Yesavage J, Rye D. Periodic leg movements in sleep in elderly patients with Parkinsonism and Alzheimer's disease. *Eur J Neurol*. 2012 Jun;19(6):918–923. doi:10.1111/j.1468-1331.2012.03673.x.
42. Benes H, Kurella B, Kummer J, Kazenwadel J, Selzer R, Kohnen R. Rapid onset of action of levodopa in restless legs syndrome: A double-blind, randomized, multicenter, crossover trial. *Sleep*. 1999; 22:1073–1081.
43. Allen R, Becker PM, Bogan R, et al. Ropinirole decreases periodic leg movements and improves sleep parameters in patients with restless legs syndrome. *Sleep*. 2004;27:907–914.
44 Partinen M, Hirvonen K, Jama L, et al. Efficacy and safety of pramipexole in idiopathic restless legs syndrome: A polysomnographic dose-finding study—the PRELUDE study. *Sleep Med*. 2006; 7:407–417.
45. Li J, Moore H IV, Lin L, et al. Association of low ferritin with PLM in the Wisconsin Sleep Cohort. *Sleep Med*. 2015 Nov;16(11):1413–1418. doi:10.1016/j.sleep.2015.05.015. PMID: 26498245; PMCID: PMC7987065.
46. Bara-Jimenez W, Aksu M, Graham B, Sato S, Hallett M. Periodic limb movements in sleep: state-dependent excitability of the spinal flexor reflex. *Neurology*. 2000 Apr 25;54(8):1609–1616.
47. Montplaisir J, Boucher S, Poirier G, Lavigne G, Lapierre O, Lespérance P. Clinical, polysomnographic, and genetic characteristics of restless legs syndrome: a study of 133 patients diagnosed with new standard criteria. *Mov Disord*. 1997 Jan;12(1):61–65.
48. Fantini ML, Michaud M, Gosselin N, Lavigne G, Montplaisir J. Periodic leg movements in REM sleep behavior disorder and related autonomic and EEG activation. *Neurology*. 2002 Dec 24;59(12):1889–1894.
49. Dauvilliers Y, Pennestri MH, Petit D, Dang-Vu T, Lavigne G, Montplaisir J. Periodic leg movements during sleep and wakefulness in narcolepsy. *J Sleep Res*. 2007 Sep;16(3):333–339.
50. Pockett C, Kirk V. Periodic limb movements in sleep and attention deficit hyperactivity disorder: Are they related? *Paediatr Child Health*. 2006 Jul;11(6):355–358.
51. Frauscher B, Ehrmann L, Mittelring T, et al. Delayed diagnosis, range of severity, and multiple sleep comorbidities: A clinical and polysomnographic analysis of 100 patients of the Innsbruck narcolepsy cohort. *J Clin Sleep Med*. 2013; 9:805–812.
52. Goerke M, Rodenbeck A, Cohrs S, Kunz D. The influence of the tricyclic antidepressant amitriptyline on periodic limb movements during sleep. *Pharmacopsychiatry*. 2013 May;46(3):108–113.
53. Cohrs S, Rodenbeck A, Hornyak M, Kunz D. [Restless legs syndrome, periodic limb movements, and psychopharmacology]. *Nervenarzt*. 2008 Nov;79(11):1263–1264, 1266–1272.
54. Budhiraja R, Javaheri S, Pavlova MK, Epstein LJ, Omobomi O, Quan SF. Prevalence and correlates of periodic limb movements in OSA and the effect of CPAP therapy. *Neurology*. 2020 Apr 28;94(17):e1820–e1827.
55. Castriota R et al. Treatment of sleep disorders after traumatic brain injury. *JCSM*. 2009; 5(2): 137–144.
56. Ross RJ, Ball WA, Dinges DA, et al. Motor dysfunction during sleep in posttraumatic stress disorder. *Sleep*. 1994; 17(8):723–732.
57. Koo BB, Blackwell T, Ancoli-Israel S, Stone KL, Stefanick ML, Redline S; Osteoporotic Fractures in Men (MrOS) Study Group. Association of incident cardiovascular disease with periodic limb movements during sleep in older men: Outcomes of sleep disorders in older men (MrOS) study. *Circulation*. 2011 Sep 13;124(11):1223–1231. doi:10.1161/CIRCULATIONAHA.111.038968. PMID: 21859975; PMCID: PMC3265562.
58. Sieminski M, Pyrzowski J, Partinen M. Periodic limb movements in sleep are followed by increases in EEG activity, blood pressure, and heart rate during sleep. *Sleep Breath*. 2017;21:497–503.
59. Shin D-S, Yang K-I, Kim D-E, Hwangbo Y, Koo BB, Cho YW. Periodic limb movements during sleep is not associated with hypertension in a clinical cohort of Korean adults. *Am J Hypertens*. 2018; 31(11):1228–1233. https://doi.org/10.1093/ajh/hpy114.
60. Sieminski M. Periodic limb movements in sleep and blood pressure. *Am J Hypertens*. 2018;31(11): 1178–1179. https://doi.org/10.1093/ajh/hpy132.
61. Koo BB, Mehra R, Blackwell T, Ancoli-Israel S, Stone KL, Redline S; Osteoporotic Fractures in Men (MrOS) Study Group. Periodic limb movements during sleep and cardiac arrhythmia in older men (MrOS sleep). *J Clin Sleep Med*. 2014;10(1):7–11. doi:10.5664/jcsm.3346.
62. Benz RL, Pressman MR, Hovick ET, Peterson DD. Potential novel predictors of mortality in end-stage renal disease patients with sleep disorders. *Am J Kidney Dis*. 2000;35:1052–6010.1016/S0272-6386(00)70039-4
63. Yumino D, Wang H, Floras JS, et al. Relation of periodic leg movements during sleep and mortality in patients with systolic heart failure. *Am J Cardiol*. 2011 Feb 1;107(3):447–451. doi:10.1016/j.amjcard.2010.09.037. PMID: 21257013.
64. McDermott M, Brown DL Chervin RD. Sleep disorders and the risk of stroke. *Expert Rev*

Neurother. 2018 July;18(7):523–531. doi:10.1080/14737175.2018.1489239.
65. Mirza M, Shen WK, Sofi A, Jahangir A, Mori N, Tajik AJ. Frequent periodic leg movement during sleep is associated with left ventricular hypertrophy and adverse cardiovascular outcomes. *J Am Soc Echocardiogr*. 2013;26:783–790. doi:10.1016/j.echo.2013.03.018.
66. Wing YK, Zhang J, Ho CKW, Au CT, Li AM. Periodic limb movement during sleep is associated with nocturnal hypertension in children. *Sleep*. 2010;33(6):759–765.
67. Dhondt K, Baert E, van Herzeele C, Raes A, Groen LA, van de Walle J. Sleep fragmentation and increased periodic limb movements are more common in children with nocturnal enuresis. *Acta Paediatr*. 2014;103(6):e268–e272. doi:10.1111/apa.12610.
68 Rogers V, Marcus C, Jawad A, et al. Periodic limb movements and disrupted sleep in children with sickle cell disease. *Sleep*. 2011;34(7):899–908. https://doi.org/10.5665/SLEEP.1124.
69. Tuisku K, Tani P, Nieminen-von Wendt T, et al. Lower limb motor restlessness in Asperger's disorder, measured using actometry. *Psychiatry Res*. 2004;128(1):63–70. doi:10.1016/j.psychres.2002.06.001.
70. Arens R, Wright B, Elliott J, et al. Periodic limb movement in sleep in children with Williams syndrome. *J Pediatr*. 1998 Nov;133(5):670–674. doi:10.1016/s0022-3476(98)70110-6. PMID: 9821427.
71. Chervin RD, Consens FB, Kutluay E. Alternating leg muscle activation during sleep and arousals: A new sleep-related motor phenomenon? *Mov Disord*. 2003 May;18(5):551–559. doi:10.1002/mds.10397. PMID: 12722169.
72. Bergmann M, Stefani A, Brandauer E, Holzknecht E, Hackner H, Högl B. Hypnagogic foot tremor, alternating leg muscle activation or high frequency leg movements: Clinical and phenomenological considerations in two cousins. *Sleep Med*. 2019 Feb;54:177–180. doi:10.1016/j.sleep.2018.10.024. PMID: 30580191.
73. Yang C, Winkelman JW. Clinical and polysomnographic characteristics of high frequency leg movements. *J Clin Sleep Med*. 2010 Oct 15;6(5):431–438. PMID: 20957842; PMCID: PMC2952745.
74. Broughton R, Tolentino MA, Krelina M. Excessive fragmentary myoclonus in NREM sleep: a report of 38 cases. *Electroencephalogr Clin Neurophysiol*. 1985; 61:123–133. doi:10.1016/0013-4694(85)91050-8.
75. Frauscher B, Kunz A, Brandauer E, Ulmer H, Poewe W, Högl B. Fragmentary myoclonus in sleep revisited: A polysomnographic study in 62 patients. *Sleep Med*. 2011 Apr;12(4):410–415. doi:10.1016/j.sleep.2010.08.016. PMID: 21316297.
76. Broughton R. Pathological fragmentary myoclonus, intensified hypnic jerks, and hypnagogic foot tremor: Three unusual sleep related movement disorders. In: Koella WP, Obal F, Shulz H, Visser P, eds. *Sleep '86*. G. Fischer Verlag; 1988:240e3.
77. Calandra-Buonaura G, Alessandria M, Liguori R, Lugaresi E, Provini F. Hypnic jerks: Neurophysiological characterization of a new motor pattern. *Sleep Med*. 2014 Jun;15(6):725–727. doi:10.1016/j.sleep.2014.01.024. PMID: 24815789.
78. Khalil A, Wright M-A, Walker M, Ericksson S. Loss of rapid eye movement sleep atonia in patients with REM sleep behavior disorder, narcolepsy, and isolated loss of REM atonia. *J Clin Sleep Med*. 2013;9(10):1039–1048. http://dx.doi.org/10.5664/jcsm.3078.
79. Mysliwiec V, Brock MS, Creamer JL, O'Reilly BM, Germain A, Roth BJ. Trauma associated sleep disorder: A parasomnia induced by trauma. *Sleep Med Rev*. 2018 Feb;37:94–104. doi:10.1016/j.smrv.2017.01.004. PMID: 28363448.
80. Trotti LM. Restless legs syndrome and sleep-related movement disorders. *Continuum (Minneap Minn)*. 2017 Aug;23(4, Sleep Neurology):1005–1016. doi:10.1212/CON.0000000000000488. PMID: 28777173.
81. DelRosso LM, Cano-Pumarega I, E SSA. Sleep-related rhythmic movement disorder. *Sleep Med Clin*. 2021 Jun;16(2):315–321. doi:10.1016/j.jsmc.2021.02.007. PMID: 33985656.
82. Stefani A, Högl B. Diagnostic criteria, differential diagnosis, and treatment of minor motor activity and less well-known movement disorders of sleep. *Curr Treat Options Neurol*. 2019 Jan 19;21(1):1. doi:10.1007/s11940-019-0543-8. PMID: 30661130; PMCID: PMC6339673.

Chapter 19

Non-Rapid Eye Movement Parasomnias

Alon Y. Avidan

INTRODUCTION

The *International Classification of Sleep Disorders*, 3rd edition (ICSD-3) defines 4 district non-rapid eye movement (NREM) parasomnias, or disorders of arousal (DOA)[1]: confusional arousals, sleep terrors, sleepwalking, and sleep-related eating disorder (SRED).[2–4] Sexsomnia is classified under confusional arousals. NREM parasomnias consist of abnormal subjective and emotional experiences or motor behaviors that manifest during the incomplete transition in and out of NREM sleep.[5–9] These events may manifest in response to external stimuli such as noise and internal factors, including CNS-suppressing medications or substances, fever, and apneas. NREM parasomnias are associated with universal amnesia as a rule and manifest as partial arousals from slow-wave, stage N3 sleep. The episodes are brief and commonly emerge during the first half of the night when slow wave sleep (SWS) is most prominent. Universal behavioral manifestations of NREM parasomnias are summarized in Figure 19.1.

Classification of the NREM Parasomnias

NREM parasomnias are universally classified based on common characteristics which share the underlying pathophysiology of increased venerability due to sleep fragmentation, impaired arousal from N3 sleep with impaired cognitive functioning during the event, followed by complete/partial amnesia for the event, and predisposition conferred through familial patterns of genetic inheritance.[4,7,10–13]

The ICSD-3 described key diagnostic criteria for the NREM parasomnias (NREM parasomnias Dx Criteria), which include[1]:

1. Recurrent nocturnal episodes of partial arousal from NREM sleep. The events emanate as partial arousals during the first third of the night during stage N3 sleep and rarely last beyond 30 minutes.
2. Abnormal response by patient to efforts of the observers to intervene during the episode

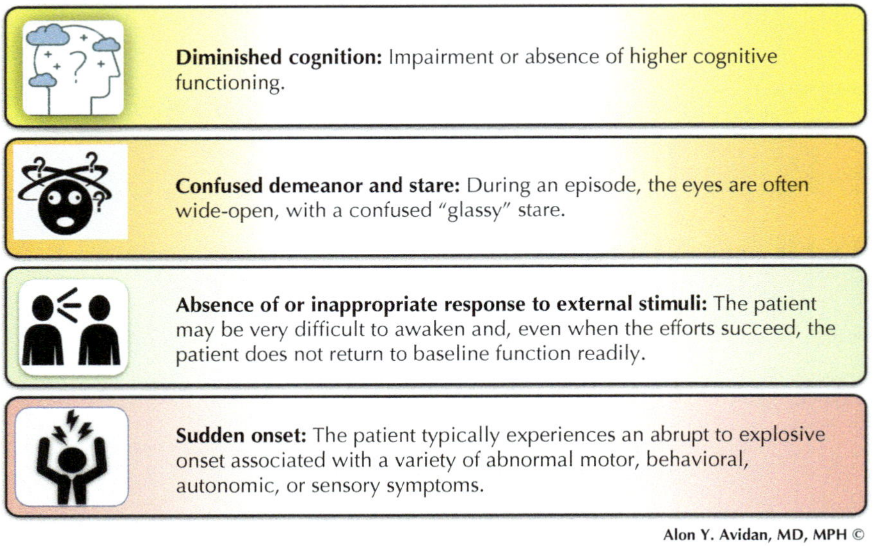

Figure 19.1. Universal behavioral manifestations of NREM parasomnias.

3. Partial or absent cognition or dream imagery following the event
4. Complete or partial amnesia for the episode. This is a universal feature of NREM parasomnias. While most patients with NREM parasomnias are amnestic to these events, some may report dream-like mentation.[14] Specific factors that might trigger NREM parasomnias might include anxiety and emotional stress, febrile illness, acute sleep deprivation, and central nervous system (CNS)-acting medications.[15–19]
5. Absence of other primary sleep disorders, mental disorders, medical conditions, medication, or substance use to help explain the disturbance. NREM parasomnias are universal in children where they might be viewed as age-related sleep manifestations, generally not requiring specific interventions.[12,15] In both adults and children, primary sleep disorders such sleep apnea and disruptive periodic limb movements also may provoke disorders of arousal.[20]

Table 19.1 highlights how unique behavioral manifestations may help differentiate between the various subtypes of NREM parasomnias.

Clinical Attributes of Disorders of Arousal

NREM parasomnias are phenomenologically distinguished and differentiated by their unique semiology—"a fingerprint" of unique clinical presentations and behaviors.

Confusional arousals (CA, also referred to as sleep drunkenness or excessive sleep inertia) present with abrupt awakening associated with confusion, disorientation, and, at times, utterances of unintelligible speech.[7,12,21] If displacement occurs out of bed, the event is reclassified as sleepwalking. CA consist of abnormal arousal behaviors, with abnormal duration rarely manifesting in explosive distress or motor behavior.[21–23]

Sleepwalking (SW, aka *somnambulism* or *noctambulism*) consists of amnestic displacement from the bed and non-goal-oriented ambulation associated with a range of behaviors from simple automatic locomotion, which is most common, to complex, violent, inappropriate, agitated behavior, which tends to be less common.[3,7] SW consists of normal arousal behaviors at onset, proceeding to non-agitated motor behavior, including walking with lack of distress.[24,25]

Sleep terrors (ST, aka *pavor nocturnus* or night terrors) initiate with an abrupt, sudden,

Table 19.1 **Key Similarities and Differentiating Features Among the NREM Parasomnias**[126]

General criteria	1. Recurrent episodes of incomplete awakening from NREM sleep 2. Absent or inappropriate responsiveness to efforts of bystanders to intervene or redirect the person during the event 3. Limited sleep-related mentation 4. Fragmented or no recollection for the episode 5. Absence of another primary sleep disorder, mental disorder, medical condition, medication, or substance use to help explain the disturbance		
	Confusional arousal (CA)	**Sleepwalking (SW)**	**Sleep terror (ST)**
Distinctive features	• Arousals characterized by mental confusion in the absence of displacement from bed • Absence of terror or ambulation outside the bed • Mild autonomic arousal during the event	• Arousals associated with ambulation or other complex behaviors out of bed	• Arousals characterized by an abrupt awakening accompanied by a scream • Intense fear and signs of autonomic arousal (mydriasis, tachycardia, tachypnea, diaphoresis) during the episode

Modified from: American Academy of Sleep Medicine. *The International Classification of Sleep Disorders, Revised: Diagnostic and Coding Manual.* 3rd edition. American Academy of Sleep Medicine; 2014.

and explosive sympathetic activity, uniquely differentiating these episodes from confusional arousals and sleepwalking. To an observer, the patient appears to be in a state of distress. ST events are typically accompanied by a piercing scream signaling abnormal arousal, associated with increased sympathetic activity, expression of fear, and aggression, which diminish over time.[23]

The unique clinical attributes of the disorders of NREM parasomnias are summarized in Figure 19.2 and in the following:

Complex behavioral semiology: Semiology refers to the clinically observed behavioral and motor events. In the case of NREM parasomnias, these are complex with variable clinical features. While the patient's eyes are open, there is a universal lack of interaction between the patient and their environment and the observers.

Age at onset during early life: Onset is common in childhood or the teens, generally after puberty, but may persist into young adulthood.

Infrequent occurrence: Events usually occur only a few times per month or week but rarely with more than 1 event per night. One should consider potential priming factors such as underdiagnosed sleep apnea and sleep deprivation contributing to the events.

Timing of events in the first half of the night: Arousals usually occur in the first half of the night.

Brief duration of episodes: NREM parasomnias typically lasts less than a minute, but episodes may be protracted when sleep inertia is prolonged.[23]

Figure 19.3 extrapolates in a graphic format the spectrum of behavioral manifestations of the arousal disorders against time, depicting characteristic attributes for each: the magnitude of displacement/ambulation and the degree and intensity of distress as a function of time.[13] Occasionally, an admixture of multiple behavior types may wax and wane simultaneously.[13] All events usually emerge out of stage N3 NREM sleep and terminate either in wakefulness or during lighter NREM sleep. The episodes are typically short-lived, but if an attempt is made by an observer to interrupt the behavior, there is a risk of prolonging their duration.[13]

Pathophysiology of the Disorders of Arousal

The passage between wakefulness and NREM sleep represents a period of increased vulnerability to incomplete and impaired arousal.

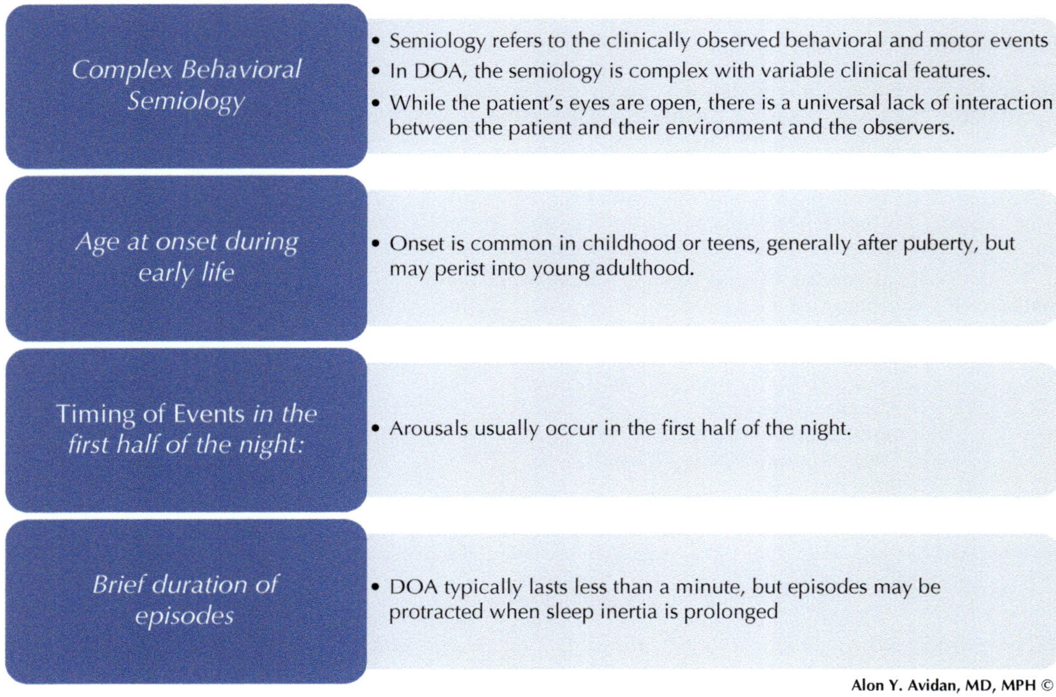

Figure 19.2. The unique clinical attributes of NREM parasomnias.

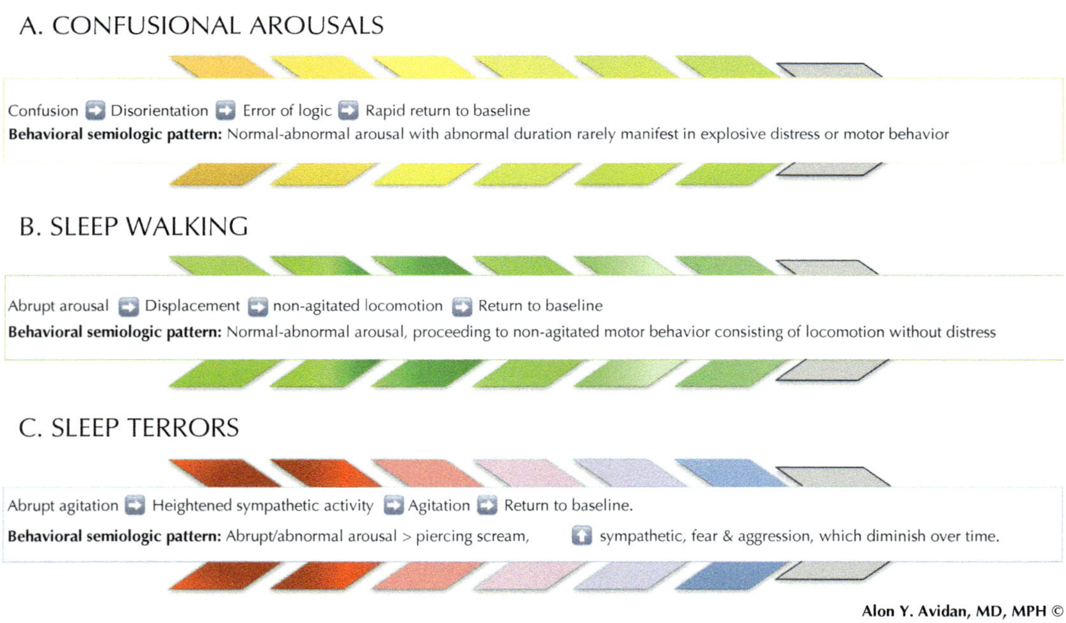

Figure 19.3. Clinical properties of the disorders of arousal. The figure illustrates the specific clinical attributes of arousal disorders during their evolution. *Confusional arousals* are characterized by normal to abnormal arousal with an expression of abnormal error of logic and prolongation of the period of observed confusion. *Sleepwalking* starts with an arousal proceeding to non-agitated motor behavior and displacement from the bed. Unlike confusional arousals and sleepwalking, which lack distress and agitation, patients with *sleep terror* experience abrupt and dramatic arousal, accompanied by a scream and heightened sympathetic activity (tachycardia, tachypnea). Aggression and abnormal prolongation of the episodes may occur if one attempts to intervene. The episode subsides with the patient returning to baseline and amnesia for the episode.

Abnormal intrusion of wakefulness into sleep during this process could result in complex behaviors characterized by disorientation, confusion, and amnesia.[5,10,17] NREM parasomnias result from the activation of discrete central pattern generators (CPG) in the CNS, independently leading to the expression of involuntary complex motor behaviors such as speech, eating, sexual behaviors, and locomotion, but also defensive, predatory, and emotional behaviors.[26]

Confusional Arousals

CASE ILLUSTRATION

James is a 32-year-old emergency room nurse presenting for evaluation of unusual nocturnal spells observed by his wife. These consist of experiencing awakening where he makes unintelligent requests or statements such as "the bridge is too far," or "turn off the radio," between 1 to 2 in the morning. The episodes emerged about 3 months ago when he changed his work schedule and began to work during the 6 PM to 6 AM shift, which he is struggling with. A recent example included an awakening where he appeared to have his eyes open but appeared confused and disoriented, asking for a "banana bag"; a few minutes later, he said, "sorry—never mind." The episodes rarely last for longer than 20 seconds, and he returns to sleep immediately afterward without recollecting the events the next day. James was never observed to experience displacement or agitation during the events, and he never appeared aggressive to his wife. He denies having any dreams where he is confronted, and his wife confirms that he never seems to act out what he says.

ICSD-3 Criteria for Confusional Arousals

To establish the diagnosis of confusional arousals (CA), the following criteria must be met[1]:

A. The patient needs to meet NREM parasomnias Dx Criteria.
B. While the patient is physically in bed, he/she/they experience spells, which are distinguished by confused mentation, or confused behavior demeanor.
C. Terror is absent and there is absence of ambulation outside of the bed.
D. During the duration of the episode, the patient should not demonstrate any evidence of autonomic hyperarousal such as tachycardia, tachypnea, diaphoresis, or mydriasis.

CA is also known as morning sleep inertia, sleep drunkenness, or Elpenor syndrome. These represent the least dramatic NREM parasomnias and consist of arousals from N3 sleep followed by a brief period of disorientation and confusion.[27,28] The episodes manifest in the early part of the night when N3 sleep is most prominently expressed.[29] To an observer, patients appear disoriented, confused, and displaying inappropriate and unintelligent speech and behaviors with characteristic slow or poor mentation, hence the term "sleep drunkenness." CA are brief, typically lasting less than a minute, and remit when the patient falls asleep. Patients are unable to recall the events after the arousal (retrograde amnesia) and are unable to form new memories following the arousal (anterograde amnesia). CA are not uncommon among children younger than 3 years of age and less common in older childhood. The prevalence in the adult population is approximately 4%.[30] In the setting of sleep apnea, one notes an important observation indicating that 13.2% of patients with confusional arousals had obstructive sleep apnea, compared with 2% of those without such arousals.[22] This observation suggests a potential mechanism attributed to breathing cessation precipitating abnormal arousals during sleep, which has semiologic similarities to confusional arousals.[22]

The proposed mechanism responsible for confusional arousals relates to the characteristic prolongation of the normal period of sleep inertia. An incomplete awakening from N3 leads to intensification and prolongation of the normal period of sleep inertia. The case of James serves as a reminder that predisposing factors, such as sleep deprivation and recovery from sleep deprivation, are critical in adult patients with confusional arousals, as in any patient with insufficient sleep for their age group.[21] Other factors include shift work disorder, fever, untreated sleep apnea, and exposure to CNS depressants such as sedative-hypnotics and antihistamines.[29,31]

Objectively Verifiable Indicators

Polysomnographic (PSG) features of confusional arousals include an abnormal intrusion of wakefulness into NREM sleep (Figure 19.4).[29] On closer observation of the PSG, arousals from N3 sleep are accompanied by stage N1 theta patterns with diffuse and poorly reactive alpha rhythm with delta-to-theta range activity.[29,32] New data support the belief that NREM parasomnias in the form of CA represent the expression of peculiar brain states, consistent with a partial and incomplete re-emergence of consciousness.[33]

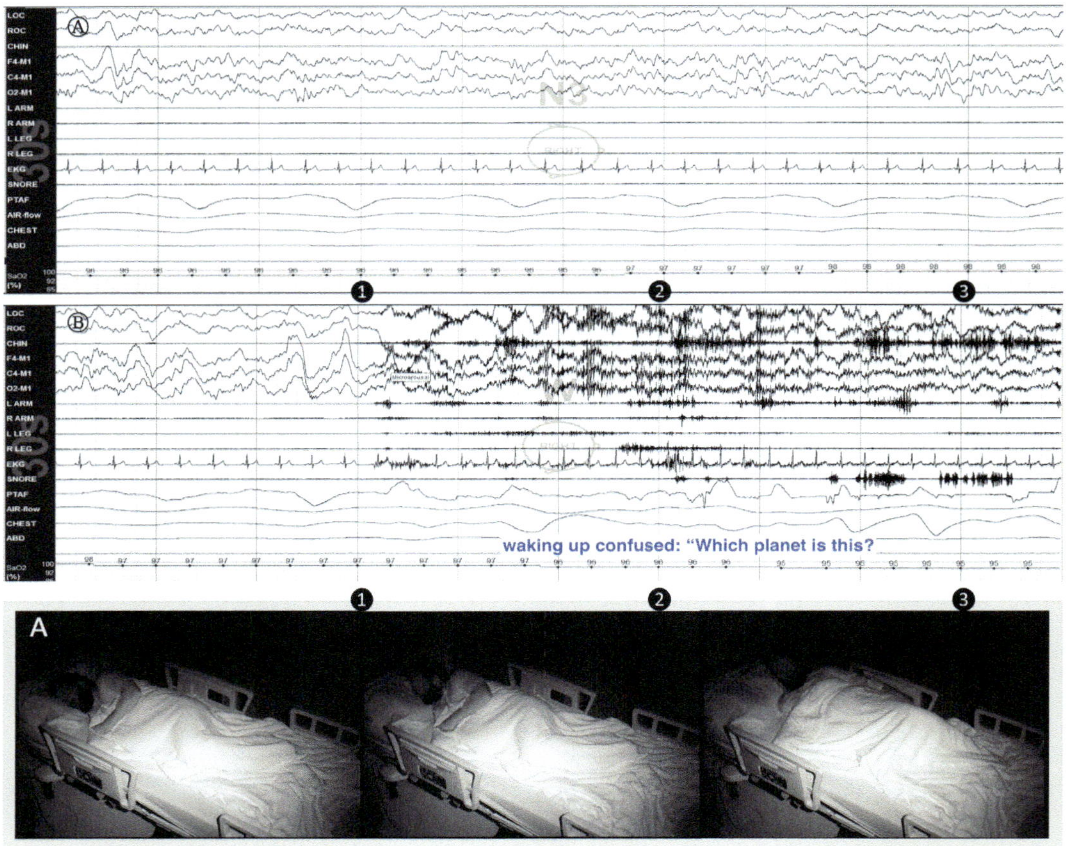

Alon Y. Avidan, MD, MPH ©

Figure 19.4. The evolution of a confusional arousal out of stage N3 sleep. The PSG recording is from a patient with recurrent nocturnal confusion. The episode is highly representative of the patient's abnormal arousal out of N3 sleep. The spell was remarkable for abrupt arousal accompanied by the eye-opening facial expression of confusion and perplexed vocalization (asking, "Where am I?" and "Which planet is this?"). The event was not preceded by a respiratory event, and the EEG showed no epileptiform abnormalities (Panel A and Panel B). Panel C illustrates the demeanor of his behavior during the spell, from the abrupt arousal (1) to the expression of confusion (2) and return to baseline (3). The patient reported no recall of the event upon awakening in the morning. Panel A: 30-second epoch just before an episode of confusion arousal experienced by the patient, highlighting normal stage N3 sleep. Panel B: 30-second epoch illustrating hypersynchronous delta activity preceding episode of confusional arousal experienced by the patient, who woke up asking, "Which planet is this?" Electrooculogram LOC and ROC left and respectively right outer cantus electrooculography (EOG) electrodes; CHIN: chin electromyogram (EMG).

Electroencephalogram (EEG) = M1: Left mastoid electrode location.

F3, C4, O2, right frontal, central, and respectively, occipital electroencephalography electrodes. Limb EMG (L = left LEG/ARM, R = right LEG/ARM). LEG limb placement: tibialis anterior, ARM limb placement: biceps. EKG = electrocardiogram; SNORE = snore sensor sound. PTAF = pressure transducer airflow; AIR-flow = nasal-oral airflow.

CHEST and ABD, chest and abdominal wall motion effort. SpO_2 = percent oxygen saturation by pulse oximetry by finger probe. Copyright remains with author, Alon Y. Avidan, MD, MPH ©.

Sexsomnia, Sleep Sex

CASE ILLUSTRATION

Benjamin is presenting to the clinic with his fiancé, Gina, as she is concerned about his disturbing abnormal behaviors at night. At first, Benjamin seemed somewhat reluctant to present for this evaluation as he felt extremely uncomfortable and embarrassed to discuss these behaviors. Gina opens the conversation and appears teary-eyed as she describes Benjamin's aggressive and uncharacteristic sexual acts toward her over the past 2 years. She perceives these behaviors to represent subconscious attitudes toward her. The episodes occur in the early part of the night, typically an hour after falling asleep, and are highly uncharacteristic of his usual sexual behavior, as well as lacking affection and appearing aggressive and "animalistic." Gina is more concerned, as Benjamin denies the aggressive episodes but remembers "having sex with her." More recent behaviors included forced nonconsensual anal sex, which was extremely uncomfortable and painful for Gina. Gina suspects that Benjamin may have subconscious aggression toward her, and she is frightened of his aggressive personality that pierces out of the night. Benjamin discloses a 30-pound weight gain over the past 2 years associated with the pandemic of Coronavirus disease 2019 (COVID-19) and has begun to experience snoring episodes and choking spells.

CLINICAL FEATURES AND TYPICAL CHARACTERISTICS

Sleepsex, aka "atypical sexual behavior during sleep," "somnambulistic sexual behavior," and "sexsomnia," represents a form of confusional arousal characterized by inappropriate amnestic sexual behaviors.[34–37] Sexsomnias are characterized by abrupt nocturnal episodes during N3 sleep of inappropriate and aggressive sexual behaviors manifesting with very limited awareness and amnesia during the sexual act and relative unresponsiveness to the external environment.[37] As with other complex nocturnal behaviors, complex sexual behaviors at night can occur in a variety of disorders, including as part of disorders of arousal, REM sleep behavior disorder (RBD), epileptic seizures, and psychiatric events.[38]

Patients with sexsomnia engage in often inappropriate amnestic sexual behavior ranging from masturbation to sexual activity that is not customary for the patient and his/her/their partners. The behavioral semiology of sexsomnia ranges from gentle and affectionate with the bed partners to violent explosive sexual acts, typically out of character for the affected person.[38] Attempting sexual activity with a non-partner co-sleeping in the same bed or an airline seatmate may have forensic and legal repercussions.[39] The consequences of sexsomnia can be serious, leading to relationship distress, as in the case of Benjamin and Gina, and even forensic repercussions in aggressive, inappropriate cases or those involving minor children and bystanders.[39] Although the underlying cause of sexsomnia is unknown, factors such as untreated sleep apnea, fatigue, stress, and substance abuse can precipitate the episodes.[38] The prevalence of sexsomnia is unknown, and the disorder probably is under-reported. A recent case series provides new data about hand dominance shift during sleep in sexsomnia, which provides new clues about the pathophysiology of NREM parasomnias in general, and sexsomnia in particular. The report highlights a lateral distribution of motor activity during sleep that is opposite to what would be expected based on wakeful hand dominance.[40] The prominent left-hand dominance during sleep reflects possible sleep-related cerebral reorganization. Alternatively, sleep may promote disinhibited, unorganized movements originating in the brainstem or spinal central pattern generators. Furthermore, the apparent shift in laterality of sexsomnias d may be an important verifiable indicator in forensic cases with suspected sexsomnias.[40]

Differential Diagnosis of Confusional Arousals and Sexsomnias

Confusional arousals (CA) are differentiated from somnambulism based on the lack of locomotion in the latter. CA are differentiated from sleep terrors based on the lack of intense screaming, sympathetic hyperarousal, and agitation in CA. The absence of complex dream enactment behaviors helps differentiate CA from REM sleep behavior disorder (RBD), a condition more likely to occur later in life and later during the night.[41] Unlike in RBD, episodes of CA tend to manifest in children during stage N3 sleep and in the first half of the night. Amnesia for the event preceding the arousal is typical in CA. Complex partial nocturnal seizures of the frontal lobe or inferomesial temporal origin may manifest with confusional amnestic semiology, which is also seen in CA. However, SRED with ictal confusion episodes begin with more stereotypical behavior, have a variable frequency, and may be associated with an ictal electroencephalogram (EEG) waveform which helps in differentiating these events from CA.[42,43]

Kleine-Levin syndrome (KLS) is a rare disorder of periodic and recurring hypersomnolence hyperphagia and megaphagia, abnormal behavior, and cognitive dysfunction associated with sleep inertia/drunkenness.[44] The latter may lead to diagnostic challenges, as it may be difficult to differentiate from confusional arousals, owing to the prolonged sleep inertia common in CA and KLS. During their symptomatic phase, patients with KLS present with other behavioral features which improve differentiation from CA, including hypersomnia, impaired cognition, amnesia, derealization, apathy, anxiety, depressed mood, hallucinations, delusions, mental confusion, and incoherent speech and abnormal behaviors of irritability, more protracted cognitive impairment, and hypersexuality during the active phase of the disease.[44–46] KLS also may be associated with episodes of sleep eating and sleep sexual activity, which further blurs the clinical distinction, but the other sleep features help distinguish this disorder from NREM parasomnias.[47]

Sleep Walking, Somnambulism

CASE ILLUSTRATION

Tarik is a 17-year-old high school student presenting with his parents due to concerns about abnormal nocturnal behaviors related to sleepwalking. He has had previous sleepwalking spells between the ages of 5 and 7, but they disappeared and returned more recently, coinciding with his preparation for the Scholastic Aptitude Test (SAT). Tarik is also enrolled in advanced placement classes and spends long hours after school preparing for class. He is currently getting about 5 hours of sleep and trying to "push through" by consuming energy drinks and Mountain Dew to give him a "kick" when he feels drowsy in the early evening. His father recently installed a bed alarm that allows his parents to redirect Tarik to his bedroom during sleepwalking episodes. The patient and his parents are worried as he plans to move to a new dorm in 2 months. His parents raise concerns about his safety as Tarik was recently found to be swimming at their family pool in the middle of the night and had no recollection of this event.

ICSD-3 Criteria for Somnambulism (SW)

To establish the diagnosis of SW, the following criteria must be met[1]:

A. The patient needs to meet NREM parasomnias Dx Criteria.
B. The arousals are associated with ambulation but could also include other complex behaviors out of bed.

Somnambulism, or sleepwalking (SW), emerges as complex behaviors during SWS and culminate within amnestic ambulation lasting for a few minutes. Episodes consist of various behaviors with a spectrum of complexities ranging from simple and calmly sitting up in bed to non-goal-oriented walking to agitated walking. In extremely rare cases, patients may engage in panic-laden efforts to flee a perceived threatening situation. During these escape behaviors, patients may pursue inappropriate behavior, such as displacing objects, urinating in a wastebasket, and sometimes even violence, such as attempts to suffocate a bed partner.[48,49] Seventeenth-century reports described a phenomenon in people known as the *noctambuli* who were observed to awaken and perform their chores but also attempted high-risk behaviors such as attempts to climb rooftops.[50] Typical SW frequency ranges from several times a week to episodes that manifest when specific precipitating factors (i.e., acute sleep deprivation, use of sedative-hypnotic) are present.[8,51] SW has been reported to result in falls and injuries to self and others during failed attempts to "escape," or while walking into sharp objects or during exposure to the elements (e.g., when walking outdoors in extreme weather). Rare reports of falling off balconies and even self-strangulation (i.e., parasomnia pseudosuicide) have been reported to have considerable forensic, social, religious, and insurance implications for surviving friends and family members.[52,53]

Although most sleepwalking events are benign and self-limiting, events may be associated with violent behaviors, injury to the sleepwalker or the bed partner, sleep disruption and deprivation, forced arousals, hypersomnia, anxiety, psychological distress, and altered quality of life.[54–56] Precipitating factors include sedatives, hypnotics, untreated sleep apnea, acute sleep deprivation, and extrinsic stimuli (such as noise).[55] Medications implicated in SW include selective serotonin reuptake (SSRIs),[57,58] bupropion,[59] mirtazapine,[60] paroxetine,[61] norepinephrine reuptake inhibitor,[62] and atypical antipsychotic agents.[63] In the case of zolpidem-induced somnambulism, it is hypothesized that desensitization of gamma-aminobutyric acid (GABA) receptors located on serotonergic neurons might facilitate SW, promoting a delay between desensitization of GABAergic receptors and a compensatory decrease in serotonin release.[64]

Other medical conditions, such as fever, untreated sleep apnea, and factors related to stress, and distended bladder may exacerbate the frequency of sleepwalking episodes. Attributes that promote sleep fragmentation and deprivation increase sleepwalking episodes and support the pathophysiologic hypothesis that impairment of either the sleep homeostatic mechanism or the arousal mechanism precipitates these events.[50,51]

DEMOGRAPHIC FEATURES AND EPIDEMIOLOGY

The prevalence of sleepwalking in the general pediatric population is between 1% and 17% and approaches 4% in adults.[65,66] A large study involving more than 1000 children from Los Angeles reported a prevalence of 2.5% of sleepwalking,[67] and 38% among Pakistani children[68] and 7% among Swedish schoolchildren,[69] peaking between the ages of 4 and 8 years.[70,71] Males and females are effected equally and familial patterns are common.[6] Recently, a specific human leukocyte antigen gene (DQB1) was found to increase susceptibility to sleepwalking.[72]

OBJECTIVE VERIFIABLE INDICATORS

Polysomnographic Features

A formal PSG is not required in the typical course of SW evaluation. However, PSG might help shed light when differentiating SW from potential mimics such as sleep-related epilepsy (SRE) and RBD. It may also help evaluate when patients are at risk for other primary sleep disorders that may potentially contribute to fragmentation of NREM sleep (i.e., OSA) and improve when the primary sleep disorder is treated (with positive airway pressure therapy).[73] However, 2 fundamental difficulties may impede the ability to accurately describe SW episodes: (1) somnambulistic behaviors may be missed as they do not occur nightly, and (2) when the episodes do occur, they are often less dramatic or complex than previously described by the patient or family members. While some literature suggests a method of acute sleep deprivation of up to 25 hours to precipitate SW events during the PSG,[74] the practical application of this technique in clinical practice is limited.

Consistent polysomnographic findings in patients with SW depict frequent arousals from N3 and emergence of hypersynchronous slow wave EEG just before and during the SW event. These findings may represent instability of slow wave sleep in the early portion of the sleep period.[14,75,76] However, these frequent polysomnographic variables are neither diagnostic nor confirmatory for sleepwalking. The lack of specificity and sensitivity for these biomarkers degrades their usefulness as tools in the clinical or forensic confirmation of parasomnias.[76,77]

Imaging and Electroencephalogram (EEG)

EEG spectral analyses and imaging studies confirmed that the motor manifestations during sleepwalking events are preceded by arousal-related activation of the cingulate motor area.[18] Patients with SW experience diminished delta EEG functional connectivity in the parietooccipital regions while experiencing enhanced alpha connectivity over a frontoparietal network and augmented beta connectivity involving symmetric inter-hemispheric networks, implicating the role of blunting of the arousal-related disinhibition of cortical geographies in playing a role in somnambulism.[74]

DIFFERENTIAL DIAGNOSIS

Sleepwalking should be differentiated from other NREM parasomnias, such as ST and CA, and REM parasomnias, such as RBD. Whereas in RBD, patients experience dream enactment during REM sleep, with some preserved recall of the dream mentation, patients with NREM parasomnias experience abrupt arousal with a typical association of hypersynchronous and high-amplitude delta activity on polysomnography.[78,79] It is worth noting that in the setting of RBD, the presence of sleepwalking, as a dream-enactment behavior, is associated with higher odds of phenoconversion to Parkinsonism-related neurodegeneration.[80]

Early reports of sleep-related partial complex seizures with ambulatory automatisms were originally described by Pedley and Guilleminault, who termed these events "episodic nocturnal wanderings," sleep phenomena characterized by paroxysmal ambulation and bizarre behavioral manifestations during sleep.[50,68] Episodic nocturnal wandering episodes may represent complex partial seizures but also can be seen as a postictal state, in alcohol intoxication (differentiated by drunken behavior while awake), dementia, and CNS drug-related effects.[81] Episodic nocturnal wanderings involving unintelligible speech, screaming, ambulation, and complex, violent behavior may also be encountered in the setting of nocturnal partial epilepsy with good therapeutic responses to anticonvulsants.[82]

Sleep-Related Eating Disorder (SRED)

Sleep-related eating disorder is a parasomnia associated with impaired consciousness and abnormal eating behavior and which may be associated with use of certain medications.

ICSD-3 CRITERIA FOR SRED

To establish the diagnosis of SRED, the following criteria must be met[1]:

A. Recurrent events of dysfunctional eating that occur after arousal during the patient's main sleep period
B. The presence of at least one of the following is associated with recurrent episodes of involuntary eating:
   a) Consumption of unusual/bizarre forms or combinations of edible or inedible, or toxic substances
   b) Sleep-related injurious or potentially injurious behaviors encountered while foraging for food or while preparing/cooking food
   c) Adverse health consequences from recurrent nocturnal eating (i.e., injury, weight gain, poorly controlled blood glucose in the setting of diabetes)
C. There is a partial or complete loss of conscious awareness during the eating episode, with subsequent lack of or impaired recall.
D. The disturbance is not better explained by another current sleep disorder, medical disorder, mental disorder, or medication/substance use.

SRED consists of episodes of amnestic nocturnal sleepwalking associated with compulsive eating behavior, occurring with fluctuating levels of impaired consciousness, and sometimes associated exposure to psychotropic agents (e.g., zolpidem, olanzapine).[19,83,84] These events of eating occur after partial arousal from sleep (Figure 19.5), and the patient may consume unusual food items, such as inedible substances (e.g., bar of soap) or unusual/odd food choices/combination (e.g., eating mayonnaise out of a jar, consuming a frozen pizza, or preparing a cat food–dish soap sandwich). The main concerns with SRED are related to the safety and welfare of the patient during the preparation of food (i.e., cutting and cooking) and the potential metabolic consequences (obesity, poor glucose control).

Differential Diagnosis of Somnambulism and SRED

SRED must be differentiated from nocturnal eating syndrome (NED). The latter is characterized by the conscious overindulgent consumption of food with a particularly high carbohydrate content before bedtime and is often associated with psychiatric comorbidities such as depression, eating disorders, and obesity, and is associated with psychosocial stressors.[85] NED and SRED share smoking, sleepwalking, and use of hypnotic medication

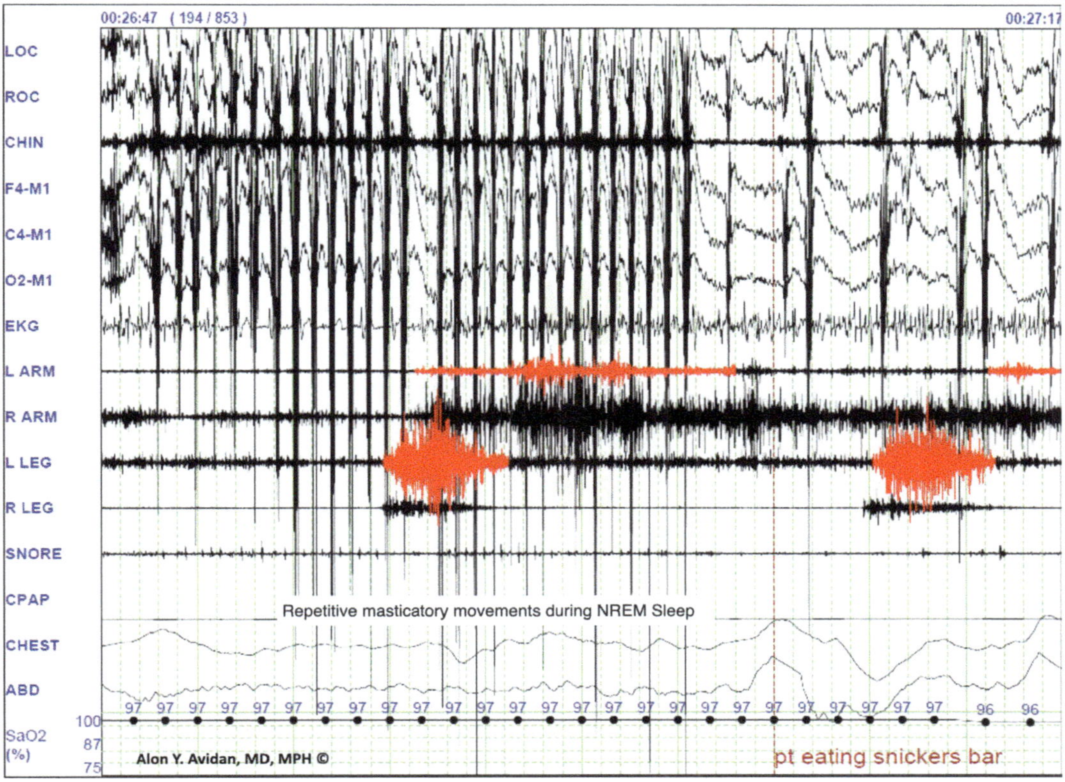

Figure 19.5. A 30-second epoch depicting sleep-related eating disorder. Related muscle activity was identified by repetitive masticatory movements during NREM sleep as the patient was eating a candy bar. There was no recollection of eating in the morning.

Electrooculogram LOC and ROC left and respectively right outer cantus electrooculography (EOG) electrodes; CHIN: chin electromyogram (EMG); electroencephalogram (EEG) = M1: left mastoid electrode location. F3, C4, O2, right frontal, central, and respectively, occipital electroencephalography electrodes. Limb EMG (L= left LEG/ARM, R= right LEG/ARM). LEG limb placement: tibialis anterior, ARM limb placement: biceps. EKG = electrocardiogram; SNORE = snore sensor sound; PTAF = pressure transducer airflow; AIR-flow = nasal-oral airflow.

CHEST and ABD, chest and abdominal wall motion effort. SpO_2 = percent oxygen saturation by pulse oximetry by finger probe. Copyright remains with author, Alon Y. Avidan, MD, MPH ©.

as risk factors, but NED is more likely to be associated with a sleep-awake phase delay, supporting the observation that it may represent an underlying pathophysiology of NED.[86]

Sleep Terrors

CASE ILLUSTRATION

Kurt is a 33-year-old attorney who has been experiencing nocturnal episodes consistent of violent outbursts witnessed by his wife. The episodes occur about 2 to 3 times a week, particularly when he is "burning the midnight oil" working on cases. His wife, Lilly, became concerned as the episodes became extremely distressing when Kurt was aggressive toward her when she was trying to interrupt his episodes. She is perplexed at the way he is responding to her when she's trying to come to his assistance and interrupt the behaviors. She describes the episodes as abrupt, occurring in the first one hour of his falling asleep. Typical spells consist of a scream followed by Kurt appearing agitated, disoriented, anxiety stricken, diaphoretic, hyperventilating, and appearing confused. The episodes end within a minute and are followed by reinitiation of sleep. Surprisingly, Kurt says he has very little recollection of the events or his acting aggressively towards Lilly immediately after the episodes or when waking up in the morning, although he notes that he was a bit short of breath.

ICSD-3 Criteria for Sleep Terrors (ST)

To establish the diagnosis of ST, the following criteria must be met[1]:

A. The patient needs to meet NREM parasomnias Dx Criteria.
B. Episodes are characterized by the presence of an abrupt terror, usually beginning with a startling vocalization such as a frightening scream.
C. The patient exhibits intense fear and signs of autonomic arousal, including mydriasis, tachycardia, tachypnea, and diaphoresis during an episode.

Essential Features and Associated Characteristics

Sleep terrors (ST), also known as night terrors (*pavor nocturnus*), consist of abrupt agitated arousal from NREM sleep, characterized by a piercing scream. The patient appears distressed, and the episodes are characteristically accompanied by heightened autonomic hyperarousal and manifestations of extreme fear, where the patient appears panic-stricken. ST represents the most dramatic NREM parasomnias and is characterized further by extreme agitation, panic, and confusion associated with heightened sympathetic activity. The latter is manifested by tachycardia, tachypnea, reduced galvanic skin resistance reflecting diaphoresis, flushing of the skin, and mydriasis (dilated pupils). Affected patients are in a state of cerebral hyperresponsiveness manifested by extreme agitation, disorientation, escape behavior, and marked confusion.[3,91] Patients may experience prominent motor activity and displacement resulting in bodily injury.[8,87–89] Sleep terror episodes may become violent, potentially resulting in injury to the patient and bed partner. Spells of ST are terminated by amnesia or very fragmented recall of the episode. The duration of the event usually is between 30 seconds to a few minutes. A universal feature of ST is inconsolability, while any attempt by the observer to interrupt the episode has a paradoxical outcome of intensifying, exacerbating, and prolonging the severity and duration of the sleep terror episode. A patient experiencing ST may appear to be awake, with eyes open, and may sometimes misperceive the nature of the environment or engages in automatic activity such as running for a door or window.[90] The medical literature has previously reported on cases of sleep terror episodes with unfortunate forensic implications.[91,92]

Demographic Features and Epidemiology

The estimated prevalence of ST is approximately 1%–6.5% among children 1–12 years of age, and ST affects up to 1% of adults.[93] Males are more frequently affected than females, with a peak incidence between 5 and 7 years of age.[94,95] The natural history of ST reveals significant diminution during early adolescence when the event frequency diminishes or ceases. While psychopathology, as a predisposition to ST, is uncommon in affected children, it may have a more significant role in adult sufferers.[92] As with sleepwalking, sleep terrors are perhaps more prevalent in adults than generally acknowledged.[90] The natural history of sleep terrors indicates that most children will outgrow the disorder by late adolescence.[93]

Objectively Verifiable Indicators

POLYSOMNOGRAPHIC FEATURES

The diagnosis of sleep terrors is based on ICSD-3 clinical criteria alone.[1] However, in selected patients, in the setting of episodes with atypical features (i.e., repetitive, frequent, or stereotyped episodes) or patients with possible underlying primary sleep disorders or neurologic or psychiatric disorders, the use of video PSG utilizing expanded electromyographic (EEG) and/or EEG montage may be essential to improve the diagnostic precision.[29,76,96]

Polysomnographic features in ST typically demonstrate high-voltage, symmetric, hypersynchronous slow wave activity. This is typically followed by an abrupt and incomplete arousal from N3, accompanied by a marked increase in EMG tone, tachypnea, tachycardia, a piercing scream, inconsolable crying (in a child), and sympathetic hyperactivation.[93–95] Although changes to these PSG attributes may be difficult to pick up or appreciate consistently, the brisk arousal from N3 sleep, as noted by the star (✪) in Figure 19.6, is strongly supportive of this parasomnia on PSG.

In the pediatric setting, sleep-disordered breathing and disruptive periodic limb movements in sleep may precipitate sleepwalking or sleep terrors. When patients with NREM parasomnias undergo formal PSG, the interpreting clinician should carefully interrogate the nasal cannula/pressure transducer and esophageal manometry signals (if available). These attributes would promote greater precision to the possibility of sleep-disordered breathing in general, but upper airway resistance, in particular, could facilitate the parasomnia.[16]

Differential Diagnosis

The differential diagnosis of ST is extensive and includes REM parasomnias such as REM nightmares and RBD, NREM parasomnias, sleep-related epilepsy, medical comorbidities such as gastroesophageal reflux disease (GERD), and uncommon psychiatric conditions as dissociative phenomena.[93] Nightmares are distinguishable from ST by the patient's recollection of vivid dream imagery, temperate clinical semiology, and the relative absence of autonomic hyperarousal, an attribute uniquely

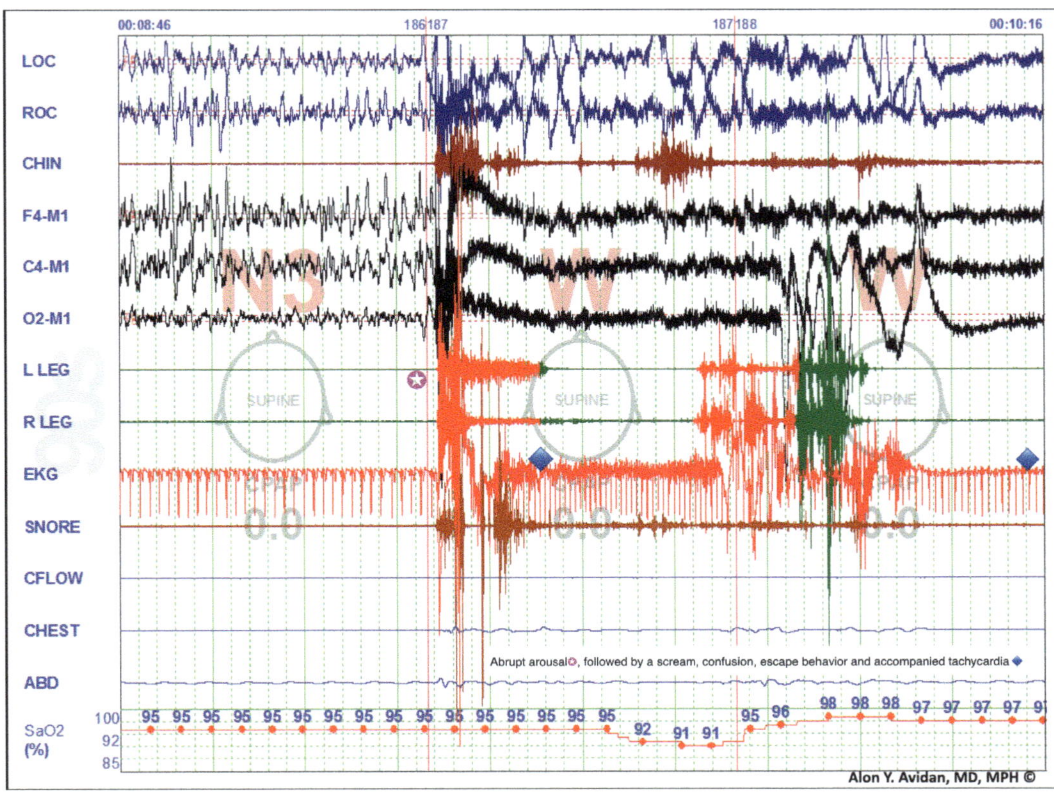

Figure 19.6. A 90-second epoch depicting sleep terror. The recording captured the patient's representative spells: an abrupt arousal out of slow-wave sleep demarcated by the star, accompanied by screaming, tachycardia, and amnesia for the event in the morning. The abrupt arousal is demarcated by ✪, followed by, a scream, confusion, escape behavior, and accompanied tachycardia ◈. Channels are as follows: electrooculogram (left: E1-M2, right: E2-M1), chin EMG (Chin1-chin2), EEG (right: frontal-F4, central-C4, occipital-O2, right mastoid-M2), 2 ECG, 2-limb EMG (LAT, RAT), snore, nasal-oral airflow-N/O, nasal pressure signal-NPRE, respiratory effort (thoracic, abdominal), and oxygen saturation (SaO_2). ECG = electrocardiogram; EEG = electroencephalogram; EMG = electromyogram; LAT = left anterior tibialis; RAT = right anterior tibialis.

characteristic of ST.[93] ST preferentially occurs during deep slow wave stage N3 sleep, while nightmares are stage REM sleep specific.[95] The presence of amnesia is a universal characteristic of ST, although fragmentary and vaguely described indistinct recollections of threatening images of reptile, insect, and monsters, from which patients have to defend themselves, have previously been reported.[16] Nocturnal events such as nocturnal anxiety attacks related in the setting of untreated obstructive sleep apnea, nocturnal cardiac ischemia, GERD, and sleep-related epilepsy (SRE) should also be entertained in the differential.[93] Differentiation from nightmares is most important, however. Differentiating between sleep terrors and SRE is sometimes challenging and requires electroencephalography when events are atypical by virtue of increased frequency or lacking response to traditional management.[97,98] Nocturnal seizures, especially complex partial seizures of temporal and frontal origin, may have a major fear component and manifest with many of the characteristics found in sleep terrors, including screaming, panic, fear, tachycardia, and vague frightening perceptions (Figure 19.6).[97] Polysomnography with expanded EEG montage is helpful when the history and clinical semiology alone are insufficient to differentiate ST from SRE conclusively. PSG-EEG is essential when the spells are frequent, repetitive, assume a stereotyped semiology, or when episodes are refractory to conventional therapy or have atypical features.[98–104] Videopolysomnographic recordings capturing multiple events may help demonstrate stereotypic behaviors suggestive of an epileptic origin.[102]

Clinical Evaluation of NREM Parasomnias

The clinical evaluation of patients suspected to have NREM parasomnias should be validated collaterally by an observer, such as a family member/bed partner, with specific attention to predisposing, priming, and precipitating factors, as delineated in Figure 19.7.[10,12,75,105]

Patients with NREM parasomnias generally do not require in-laboratory investigation. The exceptions include scenarios such as untreated sleep apnea, central disorders of hypersomnolence, periodic limb movement disorders, and comorbid sleep or medical disorders that lead to insomnia, hypersomnia, or impaired daytime

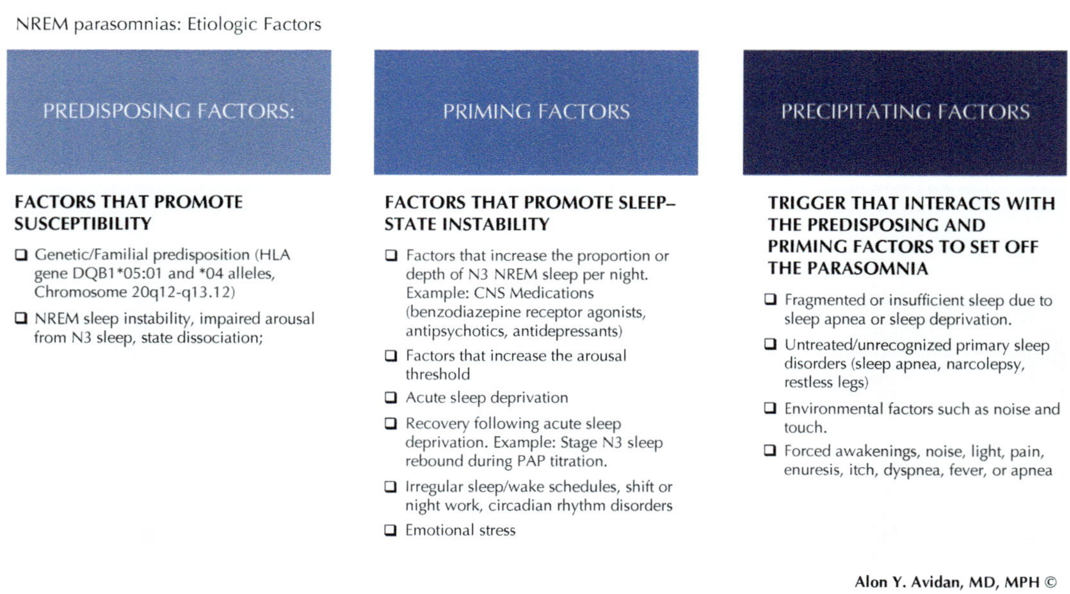

Figure 19.7. NREM parasomnias: etiologic factors. Predisposition to NREM parasomnias is conferred by genetic susceptibility. Priming factors promote slow-wave sleep or deepen N3 sleep. Precipitating factors promote NREM parasomnias by or trigger the episodes in those with the predisposition and priming conditions.[74]

functioning. The clinical history in patients suspected of having NREM parasomnia should focus on the key elements of the clinical semiology, the age at onset, timing during the night, frequency, severity, complexity, and duration.[5,23,26] A clear and detailed description of the events, from both the patient's and the witness's perspective, is essential to uncover the etiology. Patients may provide video recordings captured by eyewitnesses, usually demonstrating the later portions of an event. Although these recordings may be helpful, important details regarding the start of the events may be missed as the witnesses may be asleep. In addition to a detailed history, it is helpful for patients to undergo a general physical exam and a detailed upper airway and neurological exam to evaluate for clues of other sleep or neurological disorders. Most of these patients have normal findings, but the presence of physical or neurological findings may suggest the need for further evaluation. Furthermore, signs of injury should be questioned and considered as to the potential for the patient's injurious behaviors during events. These findings reinforce the need for polysomnography and help support safety interventions or pharmacotherapy.[29,105]

NREM parasomnias behaviors may also include a variety of utterances and random dialogue; however, talking in sleep in isolation with no other behavior or movement is considered a normal variant.[10] The clinician should also include consideration of REM-related parasomnias, sleep-related epilepsies (SREP), and other causes of paroxysmal encephalopathies.[13,99,106] The most common 2 etiologies that need specific differentiation from NREM parasomnias are REM parasomnias and SRE[107]:

a. REM sleep behavior disorder (RBD) is a disorder of loss of skeletal muscle tone demarcated by REM sleep without atonia (RSWA) and with dream enactment behavior (DEB).[108,109] DEB is more common in the later third of the night and may occur as multiple events throughout the night. Patients typically have their eyes closed, and the behaviors vary with the dream. RBD is typically more common in older individuals and associated with abnormal dream mentation and reasonable recollection.[110] Patients with RBD rarely get more than a few feet from the bed, usually instantly waking and realizing their dream enactment.[110] However, the appearance of somnambulism in the setting of RBD is associated with higher odds of having Parkinson disease (PD).[80] RBD can present in patients younger than 50, where it is related to the use of serotonergic antidepressants, with narcolepsy, other NREM parasomnias, attention deficit hyperactivity disorder (ADHD) spectrum, and epilepsy.[111–113]
b. SRE is stereotypic in behavior. Patients may be confused following events. Memory for the events is highly variable as the seizure must involve both medial temporal lobe structures to cause amnesia.[42] SRE typically emerges between the ages of 10 and 20 years but can manifest later in life.[114,115] In comparison with SRE, NREM parasomnias are typically less frequent and more complex and polymorphic, as opposed to the stereotypical semiology, and manifest at a higher frequency of events in a given night.[97] Recently developed tools such as the *Arousal Disorders Questionnaire (ADQ)* enhance diagnostic accuracy when confronting NREM parasomnias at sleep and epilepsy centers.

MANAGEMENT OF DISORDERS OF AROUSAL

Universal Treatment

The universal treatment of all NREM parasomnias is to promote the patient's safety. Patients, bed partners, and parents of pediatric patients should conduct a careful environmental survey of the sleep environment for possible safety issues. To minimize risk, the following interventions are suggested: removing sharp objects/furniture, placing the mattress on the floor, covering windows, locking balconies and main entrance doors, hiding car keys, and removing knobs from ovens.

Scheduled (Anticipatory) Awakenings (SA)

Scheduled or anticipatory awakenings may be utilized in the setting of NREM parasomnias and are ideal for children who have frequent and predictable parasomnia events occurring several times per week and manifesting at consistent times each night.[116] It is performed about 30 minutes before the patient typically expresses the experience of their typical event and has efficacy in confusional arousal, sleepwalking, and sleep terror episodes.[93,117,118] The technique of anticipatory or scheduled awakening consists of 3 distinct phases[119]:

A. The *baseline phase* enlists the parents/observers to keep a diary of the timing of the parasomnia events. This period typically lasts about 1–2 weeks until sufficient data are available to calculate the optimal time for awakenings.
B. The *intervention phase* follows next; it requires the parents/observers to awaken the child lightly 15–30 minutes before the usual occurrence of episodes. This period usually occurs 90–180 minutes after sleep onset. The parents/observers are instructed to ensure that when the child/patient awakens that he/she responds with their eyes open. Once the child/patient responds, parents/observers are instructed to allow the child to fall back asleep.
C. The SA protocol concludes with the *treatment fading and termination phase*, where one would expect to note an improvement and reduction in the frequency of awakenings while the sleep diary continues to be monitored. Parents are instructed to maintain the SA protocol for up to a month and to log the frequency of the episodes during this period.[120]

The interventions follow in the original sequence of A → B → C in the event that the events recur in the future. The mechanism is hypothesized to be related to an alteration of the sleep state and subsequent diminution of their frequencies. The advantage is comparable efficacy of the technique to medications but without the side effects of sedation or daytime somnolence. Potential complications include the impact on the parents' sleep and risk of sleep fragmentation or deprivation.[119] The theory behind the SA technique suggests that altering the patient's sleep patterns decreases the disruption in N3 sleep.[117] An alternative hypothesis is that the technique may condition the patient for self-arousal just before the NREM parasomnia event, thereby extinguishing it altogether. Ultimately, the SA technique may normalize the patient's total sleep time and improve sleep efficiency.[120]

SPECIFIC MANAGEMENT OF NREM PARASOMNIAS

Confusional Arousals and Sexsomnias

In most cases, the disorder remits with age, and episodes can be prevented or limited by avoidance of the facilitating factors (e.g., sleep deprivation, psychostimulants, and CNS agents with temporal association with the observed parasomnia). CA may be managed conservatively by avoiding sleep deprivation, preventing irregular sleep-wake schedule patterns, limiting exposure to CNS depressants, and managing coexisting sleep disorders. If present, other primary sleep disorders, such as insomnia, RLS, and sleep apnea, should be treated.

Pharmacologic management often is not necessary because the arousal episodes are self-limiting. In refractory cases, tricyclic antidepressants such as clomipramine (see Table 19.2) may be needed.

Anecdotal evidence suggests that successful amelioration of sexsomnia events entails the following approach: providing patient and bed partner education about the episodes and the lack of intent, optimizing safety, promoting sleep hygiene measures, ensuring optimal sleep duration, and, especially in patients with anxiety, psychotherapy and stress management techniques.[34,36,121] Benzodiazepines, particularly clonazepam, may be considered for first-line pharmacotherapy for refractory cases, with a recommended dosage ranging from 0.25 mg to 2 mg at bedtime (Table 19.2).[122]

SOMNAMBULISM

Maximizing safety interventions is the best-practice approach in the management of sleepwalking. This may be achieved by avoiding the precipitating factors and ensuring a safe living environment by removal of sharp furniture, covering windows, eliminating obstacles that may lead to injury during a sleepwalking episode, locking doors, using door alarms, and

Table 19.2 **Treatment Options for Disorders of Arousal: Prevention, Behavioral Approach, and Pharmacotherapy**[125,128]

	Confusional Arousal	Sexsomnias	Somnambulism	SRED	Sleep Terrors
Environmental Safety	X	X	X	X	X
Scheduled, Anticipatory awakening	X		X		X
Behavioral Management	Reassurance of benign nature, Avoid precipitants: Sleep deprivation, Alcohol CNS depressants	Enhancing sleep hygiene ensuring optimal sleep duration Psychotherapy and stress management comorbid mood or anxiety	Avoid precipitants: sleep deprivation Lithium, Non-benzodiazepines receptor agonists.		Reassurance of benign nature, relaxation therapy, hypnosis/autogenic training psychotherapy
Pharmacological management	Imipramine Clomipramine Clonazepam	Benzodiazepines: -clonazepam Antidepressants: -sertraline GABAergic agents: -lamotrigine -valproic acid. serotonin reuptake inhibitor	Benzodiazepines Clonazepam (0.5 -1mg) Diazepam (10 mg) Triazolam (0.25 mg) Imipramine (50-300 mg) Melatonin Paroxetine	Dopamine agonists, selective serotonin reuptake inhibitors, and topiramate (*) (*) Side effects include weight loss, cognitive impairment, paresthesias, visual symptoms, and less frequently, renal calculi	Paroxetine (20 to 40 mg) Clonazepam (0.5 – 1 mg) Trazodone Hydroxytryptophan Imipramine/ clomipramine

*Autogenic training is a special relaxation technique similar to meditation.
† Side effects include weight loss, cognitive impairment, paresthesias, visual symptoms, and less frequently, renal calculi. CBT = cognitive-behavioral therapy; MBSR: mindfulness-based stress reduction, CNS, central nervous system; GABAergic, gamma-aminobutyric acidergic; SRED, sleep-related eating disorder.

providing the safest possible sleeping environment, on the ground floor rather than upstairs and the lower rather than upper deck of a bunk bed. Frequent travelers with somnambulism may be advised to book hotel rooms on the ground floor and to reserve rooms without balconies or those without access to a swimming pool/beachfront. Behavioral intervention using *scheduled awakenings* can successfully ameliorate sleepwalking episodes and, compared with pharmacologic treatment modalities, has the added advantage of avoidance of CNS-acting medications.[48]

In adults with somnambulism, sleep disorder–focused psychotherapy and hypnosis constitute an effective alternative to pharmacotherapy.[77,123] Definitive pharmacotherapy with tricyclic antidepressants (TCA) or benzodiazepines is sometimes deemed necessary when the episodes are refractory to behavioral/environmental modifications and when frequent, severe, or associated with injury.[6,123]

Sleep Terrors

Treatment focuses on the safety of the patient. If the episodes are rare, treatment may be conservative on the behavioral approaches previously suggested for CA and SW. However, when ST are pervasive, more aggressive therapy is indicated, particularly when events are intense, frequent, disruptive to the patient's sleep, or when they place the patient or others at risk for harm. An essential first step is to facilitate safety measures because these are paramount in protecting the patient from injury. As with sleepwalking, security and protection of the patient from harm in the external environment are paramount. Typical measures include: (1) ensuring that the patient's sleeping area is on the ground floor; (2) avoiding the upper deck

Box 19.1 Summary of NREM Parasomnias

Identification: DOA may place patients at high risk for sleep-related injuries and can adversely affect their quality of life. Accordingly, clinicians and healthcare providers need to adequately screen for, correctly classify, and appropriately manage these disorders.[23,29]

Predisposition: Family history and genetics play a significant role in priming patients with an autosomal-dominant pattern of inheritance, whereas sleep fragmentation (due to OSA), and CNS depression are considered priming/precipitating factors (Figure 19.7)

Investigation: Evaluation of nocturnal events can be challenging to even the most ardent clinician and requires careful attention to detail. Formal evaluation with nocturnal polysomnography is essential, particularly in the pediatric epilepsy setting, where prolonged video EEG in patient monitoring during the course of their disease is required to help differentiate between parasomnias, other sleep events, SRE, and other non-epileptic events, ideally utilizing video EEG and polysomnography.[29,98] Polysomnographic fingerprints of DOA include the hypersynchronous slow waves but also EEG abnormalities within the K-complexes in N2 sleep.[124] Unique genetic markers for DOA include chromosome 20q12-q13.12, HLA DQB1*05:01, DQB1*05:01.[79,125,126]

Management: Essential to any degree of therapeutic success are identification and elimination/treatment of predisposing factors, including environmental issues, provoking medications and other substances, and concomitant sleep disorders.[25] Minimization of stimuli in the bedroom, including extraneous sounds and lights, may limit the occurrence of events. Alcohol remains a known precipitant for some arousal disorders, but its role in provoking somnambulism is controversial.[25,127] Formal evaluation and treatment of other sleep disorders are key to successful management. One of the largest studies to date, of over 500 mostly adult patients from Europe with DOA over 7.5 years, highlights the value of improving sleep hygiene advice as the first step and proceeding with the management of comorbid sleep disorders and treatment of priming factors such as anxiety, and finally resorting to pharmacotherapy, which has efficacy in up to 60% of patients.[79]

Current data support conservative non-medication modalities with the efficacy of up to a third of patients.[125] Clonazepam was universally effective in almost two-thirds of patients and may be considered as first-line therapy in the setting of NREM parasomnias, which results in injury. Only melatonin shares similar attributes and may be preferred to the latter considering its safety profile.

of a bunk bed; (3) removing sharp furniture close to the bed area; (4) blocking windows; (5) providing special bolts for windows and doors; and (6) using door alarms and bells to alert the family members should the child leave the room.[97] The parents and the patient need to be educated and reassured that these episodes are transient and self-limiting and typically will be outgrown with time. Additional measures should focus on maintaining a regular sleep-wake schedule and reducing or eliminating caffeinated beverages. As with the other arousal disorders considered here, it is best not to confront, restrain, or awaken the patient during the episodes because such interventions may prolong, intensify, or worsen the behaviors.[97]

Hypnosis is another practical, inexpensive, and effective treatment, especially when post-hypnotic suggestions are used to help decrease awareness of the unpleasant nocturnal sensory experience.[76,98–101] Adult sufferers with a history of a psychiatric disorder may benefit from psychotherapy and stress reduction as well as reassurance.[6,103–105] Pharmacotherapy should be reserved for patients with severe, frequent, and refractory sleep terror episodes. Treatment options consist of clonazepam and tricyclic antidepressants (TCA). Low-dose benzodiazepines (clonazepam, diazepam) may be effective when administered close to bedtime[106] (Table 19.2).

SUMMARY

The NREM parasomnias are a unique group of sleep disorders that share similar characteristics and have a common underlying pathophysiology. Successful amelioration of disturbing arousals will depend on accurate diagnosis, focusing on key distinguishing features and appropriate treatment strategies. Often reassurance, addressing safety issues, and education are important for the less dramatic parasomnias. Safety precautions and good general sleep hygiene measures are vital recommendations, because such disorders can be exacerbated by sleep deprivation and various other factors. When the nocturnal episodes are frequent or involve aggressive or dramatic behaviors, pharmacotherapy with a benzodiazepine, particularly clonazepam, at night is the preferred approach with most NREM parasomnias. Another therapy relies on the use of short-acting benzodiazepines, such as diazepam and alprazolam, or TCA in the case of sleep terrors. Relaxation training and guided imagery may be helpful strategies for some patients, especially those with NREM parasomnias.

REFERENCES

1. American Academy of Sleep Medicine. *International Classification of Sleep Disorders, Revised: Diagnostic and Coding Manual*. 3rd ed. American Academy of Sleep Medicine; 2023.
2. Howell MJ. Parasomnias: an updated review. *Neurotherapeutics*. 2012;9(4):753–775. doi:10.1007/s13311-012-0143-8.
3. Kotagal S. Sleep-wake disorders of childhood. *Continuum (Minneap Minn)*. 2017;23(4, Sleep Neurology):1132–1150. doi:10.1212/CON.0000000000000504.
4. Irfan M, Schenck CH, Howell MJ. Non-rapid eye movement sleep and overlap parasomnias. *Continuum (Minneap Minn)*. 2017;23(4, Sleep Neurology):1035–1050. doi:10.1212/CON.0000000000000503.
5. Brooks S, Kushida CA. Behavioral parasomnias. *Curr Psychiatry Rep*. 2002;4(5):363–368.
6. Broughton R. *Behavioral Parasomnias*. Butterworth-Heinemann; 1998.
7. Fleetham JA, Fleming JA. Parasomnias. *CMAJ*. 2014;186(8):E273–E280. doi:10.1503/cmaj.120808.
8. Mahowald MW, Bornemann MC, Schenck CH. Parasomnias. *Semin Neurol*. 2004;24(3):283–292.
9. Mahowald MW, Ettinger MG. Things that go bump in the night: The parasomnias revisited. *J Clin Neurophysiol*. 1990;7(1):119–143.
10. Avidan AY, Kaplish N. The parasomnias: Epidemiology, clinical features, and diagnostic approach. *Clin Chest Med*. 2010;31(2):353–370. doi:S0272-5231(10)00038-9 [pii]10.1016/j.ccm.2010.02.015.
11. Mahowald MW, Schenck CH. Non-rapid eye movement sleep parasomnias. *Neurol Clin*. 2005;23(4):1077–1106, vii. doi:10.1016/j.ncl.2005.06.001.
12. Ekambaram V, Maski K. Non-rapid eye movement arousal parasomnias in children. *Pediatric Ann*. 2017;46(9):e327–e331. doi:10.3928/19382359-20170814-01.
13. Derry CP, Harvey AS, Walker MC, et al. NREM arousal parasomnias and their distinction from nocturnal frontal lobe epilepsy: A video EEG analysis. *Sleep*. 2009;32(12):1637–1644.
14. Pressman MR. Hypersynchronous delta sleep EEG activity and sudden arousals from slow-wave sleep in adults without a history of parasomnias: Clinical and forensic implications. *Sleep*. 2004;27(4):706–710.
15. Kotagal S. Parasomnias of childhood. *Curr Opin Pediatr*. 2008;20(6):659–665. doi:10.1097/MOP.0b013e328316bd9d00008480-200812000-00009 [pii].
16. Guilleminault C, Palombini L, Pelayo R, et al. Sleepwalking and sleep terrors in prepubertal children: What triggers them? *Pediatrics*. 2003;111(1):e17–e25.

17. Baldini T, Loddo G, Sessagesimi E, et al. Clinical features and pathophysiology of disorders of arousal in adults: A window into the sleeping brain. *Front Neurol*. 2019;10:526. doi:10.3389/fneur.2019.00526.
18. Januszko P, Niemcewicz S, Gajda T, et al. Sleepwalking episodes are preceded by arousal-related activation in the cingulate motor area: EEG current density imaging. *Clin Neurophysiol*. 2016;127(1):530–536. doi:10.1016/j.clinph.2015.01.014.
19. Paquet V, Strul J, Servais L, et al. Sleep-related eating disorder induced by olanzapine. *J Clin Psychiatry*. 2002;63(7):597.
20. Owens J, Spirito A, Nobile C, et al. Incidence of parasomnias in children with obstructive sleep apnea. *Sleep*. 1997;20(12):1193–1196.
21. Ohayon MM, Mahowald MW, Leger D. Are confusional arousals pathological? *Neurology*. 2014;83(9):834–841. doi:10.1212/WNL.0000000000000727.
22. Ohayon MM, Priest RG, Zulley J, et al. The place of confusional arousals in sleep and mental disorders: Findings in a general population sample of 13,057 subjects. *J Nerv Ment Dis*. 2000;188(6):340–348.
23. Zadra A, Pilon M. NREM parasomnias. *Handb Clin Neurol*. 2011;99:851–868. doi:10.1016/B978-0-444-52007-4.00011-4.
24. Zergham AS, Chauhan Z. *Somnambulism (Sleep Walking)*. StatPearls; 2020.
25. Arnulf I. Sleepwalking. *Curr Biol*. 2018;28(22):R1288–R1289. doi:10.1016/j.cub.2018.09.062.
26. Rodriguez CL, Foldvary-Schaefer N. Clinical neurophysiology of NREM parasomnias. In: Levin KH, Chauvel P, eds. *Handbook of Clinical Neurology*. Elsevier; 2019:397–410.
27. Hilditch CJ, McHill AW. Sleep inertia: Current insights. *Nat Sci Sleep*. 2019;11:155–165. doi:10.2147/NSS.S188911.
28. Tassi P, Muzet A. Sleep inertia. *Sleep Med Rev*. 2000;4(4):341–353.
29. Lopez R, Shen Y, Chenini S, et al. Diagnostic criteria for disorders of arousal: A video-polysomnographic assessment. *Ann Neurol*. 2018;83(2):341–351. doi:10.1002/ana.25153.
30. Zaiwalla Z. Parasomnias. *Clin Med*. 2005;5(2):109–112.
31. Hopkins B, Glaze D. Disorders of arousal in children. *Pediatr Ann*. 2008;37(7):481–487. doi: 10.3928/00904481-20080701-08.
32. Tinuper P, Bisulli F, Provini F. The parasomnias: Mechanisms and treatment. *Epilepsia*. 2012;53 Suppl 7:12–19. doi:10.1111/j.1528-1167.2012.03710.x.
33. Castelnovo A, Amacker J, Maiolo M, et al. High-density EEG power topography and connectivity during confusional arousal. *Cortex*. 2022;155:62–74. doi:10.1016/j.cortex.2022.05.021.
34. Bejot Y, Juenet N, Garrouty R, et al. Sexsomnia: An uncommon variety of parasomnia. *Clin Neurol Neurosurg*. 2010;112(1):72–75. doi:10.1016/j.clineuro.2009.08.026.
35. Underwood A. It's called "sexsomnia." *Newsweek* 2007;149(24):53.
36. Andersen ML, Poyares D, Alves RS, et al. Sexsomnia: Abnormal sexual behavior during sleep. *Brain Res Rev*. 2007;56(2):271–282. doi:10.1016/j.brainresrev.2007.06.005.
37. Shapiro CM, Trajanovic NN, Fedoroff JP. Sexsomnia: A new parasomnia? *Can J Psychiatry*. 2003;48(5):311–317.
38. Schenck CH, Arnulf I, Mahowald MW. Sleep and sex: What can go wrong? A review of the literature on sleep related disorders and abnormal sexual behaviors and experiences. *Sleep*. 2007;30(6):683–702.
39. Arino H, Iranzo A, Gaig C, et al. Sexsomnia: Parasomnia associated with sexual behaviour during sleep. *Neurologia*. 2014;29(3):146–152. doi:10.1016/j.nrl.2013.01.013.
40. Avidan AY, Hasan R, Badami V, Schenck CH. Hand dominance shift during sleep in sexsomnia: A clue to pathophysiology? *J Clin Sleep Med*. 2025 Jan 16. doi:10.5664/jcsm.11554. Epub ahead of print. PMID: 39815730.
41. Mahowald MW, Schenck CH. NREM sleep parasomnias. *Neurol Clin*. 1996;14(4):675–696.
42. Boursoulian LJ, Schenck CH, Mahowald MW, et al. Differentiating parasomnias from nocturnal seizures. *J Clin Sleep Med*. 2012;8(1):108–112. doi:10.5664/jcsm.1676.
43. Tinuper P, Provini F, Bisulli F, et al. Movement disorders in sleep: Guidelines for differentiating epileptic from non-epileptic motor phenomena arising from sleep. *Sleep Med Rev*. 2007;11(4):255–267. doi:S1087-0792(07)00019-6 [pii]10.1016/j.smrv.2007.01.001.
44. Arnulf I, Groos E, Dodet P. Kleine–Levin syndrome: A neuropsychiatric disorder. *Rev Neurologique*. 2018;174(4):216–227. doi:https://doi.org/10.1016/j.neurol.2018.03.005.
45. Arnulf I, Rico TJ, Mignot E. Diagnosis, disease course, and management of patients with Kleine-Levin syndrome. *Lancet Neurol*. 2012;11(10):918–928. doi:10.1016/S1474-4422(12)70187-4.
46. Mukaddes NM, Alyanak B, Kora ME, et al. The psychiatric symptomatology in Kleine-Levin syndrome. *Child Psychiatr Human Dev*. 1999;29(3):253–258.
47. Schenck CH, Boyd JL, Mahowald MW. A parasomnia overlap disorder involving sleepwalking, sleep terrors, and REM sleep behavior disorder in 33 polysomnographically confirmed cases. *Sleep*. 1997;20:972–981.
48. Frank NC, Spirito A, Stark L, et al. The use of scheduled awakenings to eliminate childhood sleepwalking. *J Pediatr Psychol*. 1997;22(3):345–353.
49. Stallman HM, Bari A. A biopsychosocial model of violence when sleepwalking: Review and reconceptualisation. *Bjpsych Open*. 2017;3(2):96–101. doi:10.1192/bjpo.bp.116.004390.
50. Hunter E. The Noctambuli: Tales of sleepwalkers and secrets of the body in seventeenth-century England. *Seventeenth Century*. 2022;37(1):99–124. doi:10.1080/0268117X.2020.1855235.
51. Mahowald MW, Ettinger MG. Things that go bump in the night: The parasomnias revisited. *J Clin Neurophysiol*. 1990;7:119–143.
52. Mahowald MW, Schenck CH, Goldner M, et al. Parasomnia pseudo-suicide. *J Forensic Sci*. 2003;48(5):1158–1162.
53. Amouzadeh-Ghadikolai O, Pascale-Scharmuller L, Baranyi A, et al. [Strangulation as scenic behavior: A case report of a pseudosuicide in the course of a NREM-parasomnia]. *Neuropsychiatr*. 2019;33(3):165–169. doi:10.1007/s40211-018-0280-3.
54. Lopez R, Jaussent I, Scholz S, et al. Functional impairment in adult sleepwalkers: A case-control study. *Sleep*. 2013;36(3):345–351. doi:10.5665/sleep.2446.

55. Ohayon MM, Mahowald MW, Dauvilliers Y, et al. Prevalence and comorbidity of nocturnal wandering in the U.S. adult general population. *Neurology*. 2012;78(20):1583–1589. doi:10.1212/WNL.0b013e3182563be5.
56. Pilon M, Montplaisir J, Zadra A. Precipitating factors of somnambulism: Impact of sleep deprivation and forced arousals. *Neurology*. 2008;70(24):2284–2290. doi:10.1212/01.wnl.0000304082.49839.86.
57. Lam SP, Fong SY, Ho CK, et al. Parasomnia among psychiatric outpatients: A clinical, epidemiologic, cross-sectional study. *J Clin Psychiatry*. 2008;69(9):1374–1382. doi:ej08m03938 [pii].
58. Ott GE, Rao U, Lin KM, et al. Effect of treatment with bupropion on EEG sleep: Relationship to antidepressant response. *Int J Neuropsychopharmacol*. 2004;7(3):275–281. doi:10.1017/S1461145704004298.
59. Oulis P, Kokras N, Papadimitriou GN, et al. Bupropion-induced sleepwalking. *J Clin Psychopharmacol*. 2010;30(1):83–84. doi:10.1097/JCP.0b013e3181c9c8a2.
60. Yeh YW, Chen CH, Feng HM, et al. New onset somnambulism associated with different dosage of mirtazapine: A case report. *Clin Neuropharmacol*. 2009;32(4):232–233. doi:10.1097/WNF.0b013e318187bafc00002826-200907000-00012 [pii].
61. Kawashima T, Yamada S. Paroxetine-induced somnambulism. *J Clin Psychiatry*. 2003;64(4):483.
62. Kunzel HE, Schuld A, Pollmacher T. Sleepwalking associated with reboxetine in a young female patient with major depression: A case report. *Pharmacopsychiatry*. 2004;37(6):307–308. doi:10.1055/s-2004-832692.
63. Chopra A, Patel RS, Baliga N, et al. Sleepwalking and sleep-related eating associated with atypical antipsychotic medications: Case series and systematic review of literature. *Gen Hosp Psychiatry*. 2020;65:74–81. doi:10.1016/j.genhosppsych.2020.05.014.
64. Juszczak GR. Desensitization of GABAergic receptors as a mechanism of zolpidem-induced somnambulism. *Med Hypotheses*. 2011;77(2):230–233. doi:10.1016/j.mehy.2011.04.019.
65. Klackenberg G. Somnambulism in childhood: Prevalence, course and behavior correlates. A prospective longitudinal study (6–16 years). *Acta Paediatr Scan*. 1982;71:495–499.
66. Ohayon M, Guilleminault C, Priest RG. Night terrors, sleepwalking, and confusional arousal in the general population: Their frequency and relationship to other sleep and mental disorders. *J Clin Psychiatry*. 1999;60:268–276.
67. Bixler EO, Kales A, Soldatos CR, et al. Prevalence of sleep disorders in the Los Angeles metropolitan area. *Am J Psychiatry*. 1979;136(10):1257–1262.
68. Wajiha, Hasan Z, Afridi R, et al. A preliminary survey on prevalence and knowledge about different aspects of somnambulism in Buner District of Khyber Pakhtunkhwa, Pakistan. *Sleep Breath*. 2018;22(4):973–979. doi:10.1007/s11325-018-1629-3.
69. Neveus T, Cnattingius S, Olsson U, et al. Sleep habits and sleep problems among a community sample of schoolchildren. *Acta Paediatr*. 2001;90(12):1450–1455.
70. Wise MS. Parasomnias in children. *Pediatric Ann*. 1997;26(7):427–433.
71. Klackenberg G. *Incidence of Parasomnias in Children in a General Population*. Raven Press; 1987.
72. Lecendreux M, Bassetti C, Dauvilliers Y, et al. HLA and genetic susceptibility to sleepwalking. *Mol Psychiatry*. 2003;8(1):114–117. doi:10.1038/sj.mp.40012034001203 [pii]
73. Guilleminault C, Kirisoglu C, Bao G, et al. Adult chronic sleepwalking and its treatment based on polysomnography. *Brain*. 2005;128(Pt 5):1062–1069. doi:10.1093/brain/awh481.
74. Zadra A, Pilon M, Montplaisir J. Polysomnographic diagnosis of sleepwalking: Effects of sleep deprivation. *Ann Neurol*. 2008;63(4):513–519. doi:10.1002/ana.21339.
75. Pressman MR. Factors that predispose, prime and precipitate NREM parasomnias in adults: clinical and forensic implications. *Sleep Med Rev*. 2007;11(1):5–30; discussion 31–3. doi:10.1016/j.smrv.2006.06.003.
76. Pilon M, Zadra A, Joncas S, et al. Hypersynchronous delta waves and somnambulism: brain topography and effect of sleep deprivation. *Sleep*. 2006;29(1):77–84.
77. Pressman MR, Mahowald M, Schenck C, et al. Spectral EEG analysis and sleepwalking defense: unreliable scientific evidence. *J Clin Sleep* Med. 2014;10(1):111–112. doi:10.5664/jcsm.3380.
78. Guilleminault C, Moscovitch A, Leger D. Forensic sleep medicine: Nocturnal wandering and violence. *Sleep*. 1995;18(9):740–748.
79. Drakatos P, Marples L, Muza R, et al. NREM parasomnias: A treatment approach based upon a retrospective case series of 512 patients. *Sleep Med*. 2019;53:181–188. doi:https://doi.org/10.1016/j.sleep.2018.03.021.
80. Zhang X, Molsberry SA, Pavlova M, et al. Association of sleepwalking and REM sleep behavior disorder with Parkinson disease in men. *JAMA Netw Open*. 2021;4(4):e215713. doi:10.1001/jamanetworkopen.2021.5713.
81. Huang YZ, Chu NS. Episodic nocturnal wandering and complex visual hallucination: A case with long-term follow-up. *Seizure*. 1998;7(1):67–71.
82. Montagna P. Nocturnal paroxysmal dystonia and nocturnal wandering. *Neurology*. 1992;42(7 Suppl 6):61–67.
83. Morgenthaler TI, Silber MH. Amnestic sleep-related eating disorder associated with zolpidem. *Sleep Med*. 2002;3(4):323–327.
84. Najjar M. Zolpidem and amnestic sleep related eating disorder. *J Clin Sleep Med*. 2007;3(6):637–638.
85. Cho J, Lee JH, Hong SC. Sleep-related eating disorder and nocturnal eating syndrome. *Sleep Med Res*. 2020;11(2):65–69. doi:10.17241/smr.2020.00780.
86. Matsui K, Komada Y, Nishimura K, et al. Prevalence and associated factors of nocturnal eating behavior and sleep-related eating disorder-like behavior in Japanese young adults: Results of an internet survey using Munich Parasomnia Screening. *J Clin Med*. 2020;9(4) doi:10.3390/jcm9041243.
87. Mahowald MW, Rosen GM. Parasomnias in children. *Pediatrician*. 1990;17:21–31.
88. Mahowald MW, Ettinger MG. Things that go bump in the night: The parasomnias revisited. *J Clinical Neurophysiol*. 1990;7:119–143.
89. Kahn E, Fisher C, Edwards A. Night terrors and anxiety dreams. In: Ellman SD, Antrobus JS, eds. *The*

Mind in Sleep Psychology and Psychophysiology. 2nd ed. John Wiley & Sons; 1991:437–447.

90. Hurwitz TD, Mahowald MW, Schenck CH, et al. A retrospective outcome study and review of hypnosis as treatment of adults with sleepwalking and sleep terror. *J Nerv Ment Dis*. 1991;179(4):228–233.
91. Mahowald MW, Bundlie SR, Hurwitz TD, et al. Sleep violence-forensic science implications: Polygraphic and video documentation. *J Forensic Sci*. 1990;35:413–432.
92. Mahowald Mw, Schenck CH, Goldner M, et al. Parasomnia pseudo-suicide. *J Forensic Sci*. 2003;48:1158–1162.
93. Leung AKC, Leung AAM, Wong AHC, et al. Sleep terrors: An updated review. *Curr Pediatr Rev*. 2020;16(3):176–182. doi:10.2174/1573396315666191014152136
94. Fisher C, Kahn E, Edwards A, et al. A psychophysiological study of nightmares and night terrors. I. Physiological aspects of the stage 4 night terror. *J Nerv Ment Dis*. 1973;157:75–98.
95. Fisher C, Kahn E, Edwards A, et al. A psychophysiological study of nightmares and night terrors. III. Mental content and recall of stage 4 night terrors. *J Nerv Ment Dis*. 1974;158:174–188.
96. Provini F, Tinuper P, Bisulli F, et al. Arousal disorders. *Sleep Med* 2011;12 Suppl 2:S22–S26. doi:10.1016/j.sleep.2011.10.007
97. Tinuper P, Bisulli F, Cross JH, et al. Definition and diagnostic criteria of sleep-related hypermotor epilepsy. *Neurology*. 2016;86(19):1834–1842. doi:10.1212/WNL.0000000000002666.
98. Jain SV, Dye T, Kedia P. Value of combined video EEG and polysomnography in clinical management of children with epilepsy and daytime or nocturnal spells. *Seizure*. 2019;65:1–5. doi:10.1016/j.seizure.2018.12.009.
99. Zucconi M. Sleep-related epilepsy. *Handbk Clin Neurol*. 2011;99:1109–1137. doi:10.1016/B978-0-444-52007-4.00024-2.
100. Yaranagula SD, Asranna A, Nagappa M, et al. Sleep profile and polysomnography in patients with drug-resistant temporal lobe epilepsy (TLE) due to hippocampal sclerosis (HS) and the effect of epilepsy surgery on sleep-a prospective cohort study. *Sleep Med*. 2021;80:176–183. doi:10.1016/j.sleep.2020.12.016.
101. Stowe RC, Glaze DG. Electroencephalographic patterns during routine polysomnography in childhood and association with future epilepsy diagnosis. *J Clin Sleep Med*. 2019;15(4):553–562. doi:10.5664/jcsm.7712.
102. Jaseja B, Jaseja H. Replacement of electroencephalography with polysomnography in epilepsy for improved assessment: Need of the hour. *Epilepsy Behav*. 2013;29(2):422–423. doi:10.1016/j.yebeh.2013.07.030.
103. Phillips MC, Costello CA, White EJ, et al. Routine polysomnography in an epilepsy monitoring unit. *Epilepsy Res*. 2013;105(3):401–404. doi:10.1016/j.eplepsyres.2013.02.015.
104. Malow BA, Fromes GA, Aldrich MS. Usefulness of polysomnography in epilepsy patients. *Neurology*. 1997;48(5):1389–1394. doi:10.1212/wnl.48.5.1389.
105. Hrozanova M, Morrison I, Riha RL. Adult NREM parasomnias: An update. *Clocks Sleep*. 2019;1(1):87–104. doi:10.3390/clockssleep1010009.
106. Zucconi M, Ferini-Strambi L. NREM parasomnias: Arousal disorders and differentiation from nocturnal frontal lobe epilepsy. *Clin Neurophysiol*. 2000;111(Suppl 2):S129–S135.
107. Zucconi M, Manconi M, Bizzozero D, et al. EEG synchronisation during sleep-related epileptic seizures as a new tool to discriminate confusional arousals from paroxysmal arousals: preliminary findings. *Neurol Sci*. 2005;26(Suppl 3):s199–s204. doi:10.1007/s10072-005-0487-5.
108. Porter VR, Avidan AY. Clinical overview of REM sleep behavior disorder. *Semin Neurol*. 2017;37(4):461–470. doi:10.1055/s-0037-1605595.
109. Schenck CH, Hurwitz TD, Mahowald MW. REM sleep behavior disorder. *Am J Psychiatry*. 1988;145(5):652.
110. Boeve BF. REM sleep behavior disorder: Updated review of the core features, the REM sleep behavior disorder-neurodegenerative disease association, evolving concepts, controversies, and future directions. *Ann N Y Acad Sci*. 2010;1184:15–54. doi:10.1111/j.1749-6632.2009.05115.x.
111. White C, Hill EA, Morrison I, et al. Diagnostic delay in REM sleep behavior disorder (RBD). *J Clin Sleep Med*. 2012;8(2):133–136. doi:10.5664/jcsm.1762.
112. Shukla G, Gupta A, Chakravarty K, et al. Rapid eye movement (REM) sleep behavior disorder and REM sleep without atonia in the young. *Can J Neurol Sci*. 2019:1–9. doi:10.1017/cjn.2019.302.
113. Lam SP, Li SX, Mok V, et al. Young-onset REM sleep behavior disorder: Beyond the antidepressant effect. *Sleep Med*. 2012;13(2):211. doi:10.1016/j.sleep.2011.04.018.
114. Somboon T, Grigg-Damberger MM, Foldvary-Schaefer N. Epilepsy and sleep-related breathing disturbances. *Chest*. 2019;156(1):172–181. doi:10.1016/j.chest.2019.01.016.
115. Carreño M, Fernández S. Sleep-related epilepsy. *Curr Treat Options Neurol*. 2016;18(5):23. doi:10.1007/s11940-016-0402-9.
116. Meltzer LJ, Crabtree VM; American Psychological Association. *Pediatric Sleep Problems: A Clinician's Guide to Behavioral Interventions*. 1st ed. American Psychological Association; 2015.
117. Tobin JD Jr. Treatment of somnambulism with anticipatory awakening. *J Pediatr*. 1993;122(3):426–427. doi:10.1016/s0022-3476(05)83433-x.
118. Simon SL, Byars KC. Behavioral treatments for non-rapid eye movement parasomnias in children. *Curr Sleep Med Rep*. 2016;2(3):152–157. doi:10.1007/s40675-016-0049-9.
119. Frank NC, Spirito A, Stark L, et al. The use of scheduled awakenings to eliminate childhood sleepwalking. *J Pediatr Psychol*. 1997;22(3):345–353. doi:10.1093/jpepsy/22.3.345.
120. Kuhn BR, Elliott AJ. Treatment efficacy in behavioral pediatric sleep medicine. *J Psychosom Res*. 2003;54(6):587–597.
121. Wills L, Garcia J. Parasomnias: Epidemiology and management. *CNS Drugs*. 2002;16(12):803–810.
122. Remulla A, Guilleminault C. Somnambulism (sleepwalking). *Expert Opin Pharmacother*. 2004;5(10):2069–2074.

123. Reid WH, Ahmed I, Levie CA. Treatmeant of sleepwalking: A controlled study. *Am J Psychother.* 1981;35:27–37.
124. Sarilar AC, Ismailogullari S, Yilmaz R, et al. Electroencephalogram abnormalities in patients with NREM parasomnias. *Sleep Med.* 2021;77:256–260. doi:10.1016/j.sleep.2019.05.009.
125. Drakatos P, Marples L, Muza R, et al. NREM parasomnias: A treatment approach based upon a retrospective case series of 512 patients. *Sleep Med.* 2019;53:181–188. doi:10.1016/j.sleep.2018.03.021.
126. Erickson J, Vaughn BV. Non-REM parasomnia: The promise of precision medicine. *Sleep Med Clin.* 2019;14(3):363–370. doi:10.1016/j.jsmc.2019.05.002.
127. Pressman MR, Mahowald MW, Schenck CH, et al. Alcohol, sleepwalking and violence: Lack of reliable scientific evidence. *Brain.* 2013;136(Pt 2):e229. doi:10.1093/brain/aws248.
128. Mundt JM, Baron KG. Integrative behavioral treatment for NREM parasomnias: A case series. *J Clin Sleep Med.* 2021;17(6):1313–1316. doi:10.5664/jcsm.9186.

Chapter 20

Rapid Eye Movement Parasomnias

Michael Howell

INTRODUCTION

Rapid eye movement (REM) sleep is a fascinating state characterized by vivid dream mentation, quick saccadic eye movements, skeletal muscle paralysis, and autonomic arousal. Abnormal behaviors and experiential phenomena emanating from REM sleep, the REM parasomnias, can be mesmerizing and terrifying. These REM-related experiences include nightmares, isolated sleep paralysis, and the dream enactment of REM sleep behavior disorder (RBD). They have frightened patients over the eons, inspired artists, incited supernatural belief, and been leveraged by scientists to better understand the nature of sleep and consciousness. Their terror emanates from a combination of intense emotional mentation along with the persistence (in sleep paralysis) or absence (in RBD) of skeletal muscle paralysis.[1]

REM parasomnias only rarely happen in isolation and are typically signs of a separate underlying disorder. Narcolepsy, sleep deprivation, sedative drugs, or sleep-fragmentating disorders such as obstructive sleep apnea often underlie nightmares and isolated sleep paralysis (the term *isolated* being a misnomer). Relief for patients is typically found by addressing these primary conditions.[2] The dream enactment of RBD usually emerges during middle age and is a syndrome of alpha-synuclein neurodegeneration in the majority of cases. Alpha-synuclein pathology spreads through the brainstem and disrupts REM sleep-related neurons prior to the onset of Parkinson disease (PD) or dementia with Lewy bodies (DLB).[3] Understandably, patients are often distressed to learn that their nighttime thrashing, punching, and kicking behaviors indicate an increased risk of dementing illness. Fortunately, RBD has several therapeutic options, and a growing body of investigators are seeking disease-modifying therapies to delay or reverse alpha-synuclein neurodegeneration.[4]

PARADOXICAL SLEEP

Prior to 1953, sleep was considered a period of idling brain inactivity, and the origin of dreams was a mystery. Early electroencephalographic

(EEG) studies identified high-amplitude low-frequency oscillations that we now refer to as the slow wave sleep of N3.[5] When awoken out of these slow waves, individuals described minimal dream mentation. REM sleep was easy to miss because of its intermittent nature, and the low-frequency fast activity on EEG could be mistaken for wakefulness.

Nathanial Kleitman and Eugene Aserinksky identified REM sleep as the origin of dream sleep in 1953 at the University of Chicago. Their recordings demonstrated recurrent periods of low-amplitude high-frequency (wake-like) cortical activity combined with the behavioral quiescence of sleep. Patients awoken from this state described the "remarkably vivid visual imagery" of dreams, and the presence of hyperkinetic saccades led to its designation as rapid eye movement sleep.[6,7] The term *REM sleep* has often been used interchangeably with *paradoxical sleep*, a term that captures the combination of wake-like EEG activity with the behavioral quiescence induced by skeletal atonia.[8]

During REM sleep, intense cholinergic activity from the basal forebrain and pontine nuclei activates cortical and deep brain regions. A combination of limbic and hippocampal activity during REM sleep appears to serve the important function of consolidating emotionally salient memories.[9] These processes are dependent upon skeletal paralysis to prevent the manifestation of emotional experiences. For example, if someone is dreaming of being chased by an animal, their motor circuits will activate central pattern generators for sprinting; yet, the individuals remain behaviorally quiescent in order to allow their brain circuits to safely activate "offline."

NIGHTMARES AND SLEEP PARALYSIS

As it is characterized by a low threshold for arousal and is often the last stage of sleep before waking, most people will at least occasionally recall the bizarre imagery of REM sleep. This is what the vast majority of individuals refer to when they describe a dream. In addition, they will also occasionally perceive their own paralysis. An individual dreaming they are running away from an attacking dog, for example, will sense that they either are stuck or are moving agonizingly slowly. This perception may then heighten the terror and intensity of the dream itself[1] (see Table 20.1).

Nightmares and sleep paralysis exist upon a spectrum of REM mentation and the perception of REM atonia. While most individuals will occasionally, often vaguely, recall intermittent paralysis during a dream, the experiences evolve into recurrent isolated sleep paralysis disorder when there is frequent, often nightly, preservation of REM atonia after complete arousals. When this occurs, the terrified individual feels locked in, they will try to shout but are unable to vocalize, they will attempt to move but are frozen in place.[1] Dream mentation frequently coexists with sleep paralysis, resulting in frightening hypnogogic or

Table 20.1 **ICSD-3 Diagnostic Criteria for REM-Related Parasomnias**

Nightmare disorder	A. Repeated occurrences of extended, extremely dysphoric, and well-remembered dreams that usually involve threats to survival, security, or physical integrity.
	B. On awakening from the dysphoric dreams, the person rapidly becomes oriented and alert.
	C. The experience causes significant distress or impairment.
Recurrent isolated sleep paralysis	A. A recurrent inability to move in the sleep-wake transition.
	B. Each episode lasts seconds to a few minutes.
	C. The episodes cause significant distress.
	D. The disturbance is not better explained by another disorder (especially narcolepsy) or substance use.
REM sleep behavior disorder	A. Repeated episodes of sleep-related vocalization and/or complex motor behaviors.
	B. These behaviors are documented by PSG to occur during REM sleep, or based upon history of dream enactment, are presumed to occur during REM sleep.
	C. PSG demonstrates REM sleep without atonia.
	D. The disturbance is not better explained by another disorder or substance use.

hypnopompic hallucinations. Many patients will assign a paranormal or religious interpretation to the events. Patients without history of psychosis will describe fantastical incidents, such as alien abduction or demonic possession, in vivid detail. Despite lasting for only a few seconds, these concentrated disturbing experiences may be vividly recalled years later.[10]

Hypnopompic hallucinations and sleep paralysis represent a transition failure from REM sleep to wakefulness; the cortex partially awakens yet dream mentation and atonia persist. They occur most commonly in childhood, as children have the most REM sleep in the life cycle, but they can persist into adulthood. Sleep-related hallucinations (both hypnogogic as well as hypnopompic) and sleep paralysis are part of the diagnostic pentad of narcolepsy along with hypersomnolence, sleep fragmentation, and cataplexy.[1] Yet other disorders that disrupt healthy sleep consolidation, such as obstructive sleep apnea, can also lead to REM-wake transition failure. Interestingly, patients typically describe recurrent isolated sleep paralysis when supine, possibly indicating underlying airway obstruction.[11] In addition to sleep-disordered breathing, restless legs syndrome, sleep deprivation, and circadian misalignment can all lead to sleep paralysis and sleep-related hallucinations.[12,13]

Episodes of sleep paralysis last seconds to minutes and either spontaneously resolve or can be terminated by the tactile/auditory stimulation from a bed partner which arousals the patient's brainstem, disrupts REM atonia, and abolishes dream mentation.[2]

PARADOX LOST

Soon after the discovery of REM sleep, Michel Jouvet at the University of Lyon explored the brainstem circuitry responsible for REM paralysis. Using a feline model, he demonstrated that selective lesions in the pons resulted in REM sleep without skeletal paralysis. These otherwise normal, by day, cats would, at night, intermittently and suddenly stalk imaginary prey, swipe out with their paws, as well as bite and hiss at perceived enemies. The other features of REM sleep, activated EEG, autonomic instability, and rapid saccadic eye movements, persisted.[14]

As nonfatal focused lesions could release REM motor activity in animal models, a question was raised as to whether there were any medical (human) cases of "Jouvet's cats," caused by brainstem pathology.

Intriguingly, a review of classical literature reveals numerous examples of fictionalized RBD-like behaviors, suggesting that authors, and presumable the larger public, had a contemporary familiarity with dream enactment. In 1605, Miguel de Cervantes wrote about a sleeping man in Don Quixote[15p97]:

> he was thrusting his sword in all directions, speaking out loud as if he were actually fighting a giant. And the strange thing was that he did not have his eyes open, because he was asleep and dreaming that he was battling the giant. . . . He had stabbed the wine skins, believing that he was stabbing the giant, that the entire room was filled with wine.

In the decade prior to 1982, there were several descriptions of agitated nighttime behaviors among patients with narcolepsy; however, they were not recognized as dream enactment, nor was the loss of REM atonia demonstrated.[16]

In 1982, Carlos Schenck and Mark Mahowald, along with the astute technologist Andrea Patterson, met a 68-year-old male with history of thrashing, punching, and kicking at night. Dreaming he was a professional football (North American rules) player, he had recently jumped out of bed with the intention of tackling a ball carrier. Close scrutiny of the electroencephalographic and electrooculographic activity revealed that the behaviors were emanating from REM sleep. His paradox had been lost.[17]

The first 4 patients were collected over 4 years and reported in the journal *Sleep* in 1986. Then, once dream enactment was reported as a legitimate medical condition, a surge of patients presented to Schenck and Mahowald. Within a year they had 10 subjects (29 the year after) and the condition was named REM sleep behavior disorder (RBD).[18]

Considered a rare disorder, RBD was informally referred to as the Minnesota Sleep Disorder due to initial reports from the University of Minnesota and the Mayo Clinic. Over the decades, however, its recognized prevalence has grown. RBD is, in fact, common, occurring in approximately 1% of the general population (75 million individuals worldwide) and >5% among individuals older than 60.[19,20]

The presentation is typically thrashing, punching, and kicking during the second half of the sleep period. When awoken, RBD patients will describe dream mentation that matches with observed behaviors. Some examples: dreaming of kicking a soccer ball but kicking a bed partner, dreaming of jumping out of a moving car to escape an abduction but leaping out of bed, and dreaming of punching an attacker but fracturing the 5th metacarpal by punching the wall.[3] The dream enactment is so characteristic it can often be diagnosed by asking bed partners just one question. "Have you ever seen the patient appear to 'act out his/her dreams' while sleeping? (punched or flailed arms in the air, shouted or screamed)."[19] This question has been demonstrated to have a sensitivity of 100% and a specificity of 95%, especially when combined with an absence of symptoms suggestive of sleep-disordered breathing.

However, the vast majority of RBD cases pass without a diagnosis. The reasons include misdiagnosis, along with cultural taboos regarding bedroom behaviors. RBD has been falsely attributed to depression, psychosis, or some Freudian subconscious psychological conflict. In addition, many cases of RBD are characterized by subtle, non-injurious dream enactment occurring in the absence of an attentive bed partner.[21]

Dream enactment is underdiagnosed in women. Prior investigations reported that nearly all (>90%) of RBD subjects were men; however, more recent studies demonstrated that at least one-third are women.[22,23] This is most notable among RBD populations younger than 50, those with narcolepsy, and those who present after starting an antidepressant medication.[22]

The most common RBD behaviors are non-injurious subtle pantomiming (pointing, typing, writing) hand movements, that are often referred to as "hand babbling" and are yoked to the phasic eye movements of REM sleep.[24] Unlikely nocturnal epilepsy, the actions are not typically stereotyped, as they will vary from night to night. Unlike sleepwalking, most RBD behaviors occur in bed and do not involve prolonged nighttime ambulation (see Figure 20.1).[2]

As RBD emanates from REM sleep, a light stage of sleep with a low threshold for arousal, most patients can be pacified by a light touch and calming phrase from a bed partner. The ability of bed partners to soothe RBD patients is a common reason why they are often hesitant to sleep separately.[25]

Unfortunately, violent injurious activity can happen suddenly and unpredictably. Many of the most violent RBD episodes occur after a prolonged period of relative quiescence. Injuries can be life-threatening. They include: fractures of long bones and cervical vertebrae, subdural hematomas, lacerations, and internal bleeding. Bed partners have been punched, kicked, and choked. It is particularly dangerous when a firearm or knife is available at the bedside; however, even items such as clocks and phones have been wielded as weapons during

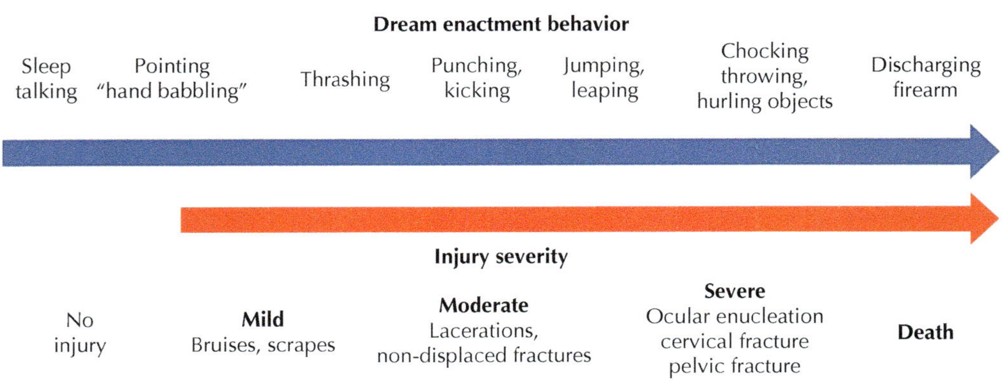

Figure 20.1. Spectrum of dream enactment behavior and injury.

RBD episodes. This violence can be terrifying to bed partners and shameful to patients. Many patients and bed partners are uncertain how to explain the activities without alarming medical providers or involving law enforcement.[21]

The following is an email the author received from a patient's wife:

> I have woken to my very tall, muscular husband kneeling over me, choking me—thankfully I could get in a scream. . . . There have been other incidents where he has punched me in the face, etc.—we have even discussed what would happen if he hurt me badly in his sleep, how he would be able to explain it to the police that he did it in his sleep—PLEASE ANY information would be greatly appreciated—I have loved this man since high school.

A HARBINGER OF BRAIN PATHOLOGY

RBD is caused by brainstem lesions to REM sleep circuitry. The complicated network involves a series of REM-on-related neurons (lateraldorsal, pedunculopontine tegmentum and sublateral dorsal [SLD]) whose activation promotes REM sleep and are counterbalanced by REM-off-related neurons (locus coeruleus) whose activation suppresses REM sleep.[26] Skeletal muscle activity is blocked during REM sleep by the magnocellular reticular formation in the medulla whose descending fibers ultimately inhibit spinal motor neurons[27] (see Table 20.2).

Orexin, a small neuropeptide secreted from the lateral hypothalamus, is critical for stabilizing the transition between states of wakefulness and sleep, NREM and REM. When deficient, as in narcolepsy, state transition is incomplete, resulting in non-stable sleep stages and admixtures of sleep and wakefulness. The consequences include: excessive daytime sleepiness as an intrusion of NREM sleep into wake; sleep paralysis along with sleep-related hallucinations (hypnogogic and hypnopompic) as a persistence of REM into wakefulness; sleep fragmentation as an intrusion of wake into NREM and REM sleep; and cataplexy as an intrusion of REM atonia into wakefulness.

Table 20.2 Etiologies of RBD

Neurodegeneration	Alpha-synuclein pathology 1. Dementia with Lewy bodies 2. Parkinson disease 3. Multiple system atrophy Non-alpha synuclein pathology 1. Amyotrophic lateral sclerosis 2. Alzheimer disease
Trinucleotide repeat disorders	1. Huntington's disease 2. Spinal cerebellar ataxia type 3
Lesional	Brainstem lesions 1. Stroke 2. Demyelinating disease 3. Malignancy
Orexin	Narcolepsy
Medication*	SSRIs 1. Citalopram 2. Escitalopram 3. Fluoxetine 4. Fluvoxamine 5. Paroxetine 6. Sertraline

* Recent evidence suggests that SSRI-induced RBD (5-HT RBD) may also be related to underlying alpha-synuclein neurodegeneration.

Notably, during REM sleep, they have an intrusion of wakeful motor tone, leading to the dream enactment of RBD.[28]

RBD is common in narcolepsy type 1, with over half of patients having RBD symptoms. Compared to other RBD etiologies, narcoleptics are younger, predominantly female, and have less injurious behaviors. In addition, as narcoleptics have sleep-onset REM, one distinguishing feature of narcolepsy associated with RBD is the presence of dream enactment during naps.[29]

The preponderance of RBD cases are caused by alpha-synuclein neurodegeneration, most notably the Lewy body pathological disorders of DLB and PD.[3] These disorders are the second most common class of neurodegenerative disease worldwide and are characterized by the slow accumulation of phosphorylated alpha-synuclein protein aggregates in neurons of the peripheral and central nervous systems. This Lewy body pathology, evolving over years to decades, results in a long prodromal syndrome which is only rarely recognized early as part of a neurodegenerative disorder. Early symptoms may include constipation and hyposmia (impaired sense of smell) as early pathology localizes to the enteric plexus of the gut and the olfactory bulb. These symptoms are subtle and, if considered by a clinician at all, typically are minimized or treated symptomatically. However, from these nidus alpha-synuclein pathology spreads from the gut through the vagus nerve, and from the olfactory bulb through limbic circuitry. Pathology extends to adjacent neurons "prion-like," inducing protein misfolding and slowly accumulating throughout the brainstem, diencephalon, and later, the cortex.[30]

As degeneration spreads through the central nervous system (CNS), cognitive and motor functions are often retained due to compensatory neuroplasticity.[31] This adaptation of brain networks is a hallmark of early-stage disease. For example, in PD, up to 70% of nigrostriatal dopaminergic neurons are lost by the time of diagnosis, yet most patients manifest only subtle motor signs.[32]

Conversely, RBD is a robust and clear indicator of Lewy body pathology. In contrast to subtle symptoms (constipation, hyposmia) and cortical signs masked by compensatory neuroplasticity (cognitive and motor deficits), individuals with Lewy body disorders often unequivocally and dramatically present with dream enactment as misfolding proteins travel through the pons, lurching from neuron to neuron in the circuitry that controls REM sleep.[33]

If RBD is diagnosed in the absence of another condition (such as DLB, PD, or narcolepsy) or precipitating agent (such as a serotonergic antidepressant medication), it is termed isolated RBD (iRBD). Recent investigations have demonstrated that iRBD is highly predictive of the eventual progression to a neurodegenerative disorder, with 74% of individuals phenoconverting (typically to DLB or PD) over 12 years.[34] Even among iRBD patients who do not phenoconvert before death, CNS Lewy body pathology has been demonstrated on post-mortem examination.[3]

Recent studies suggest that individuals with iRBD are at least as likely to develop DLB as they are PD.[35,36] DLB is characterized by progressive cognitive impairment in attention, visuoperceptual ability, and executive function, with profound day-to-day fluctuations in alertness.[37] They also have visual hallucinations and parkinsonism without a sustained response to levodopa. RBD is common, seen in 76% of DLB cases, and is considered a core clinical feature for DLB diagnosis.[38]

Among PD patients, dream enactment has been noted for over two centuries, since James Parkinson's description of the condition that would later bear his name. In his seminal monograph, *The Shaking Palsy*, published in 1817, he described one patient with a compelling history of behaviors suggestive of RBD[39p7]:

> the sleep becomes much disturbed. The tremulous motion of the limbs occur during sleep, and augment until they awaken the patient, and frequently with much agitation and alarm . . . even when exhausted nature seizes a small portion of sleep, the motion becomes so violent as not only to shake the bed-hangings, but even the floor and sashes of the room.

A sizable minority, estimated between 20%–40%, of PD patients have RBD. RBD in PD predicts a non-tremor predominant subtype, along with an aggressive clinical course with more severe bradykinesia, cognitive decline, autonomic instability, and hallucinations.[21] PD patients with RBD are at high risk of falling as they have frequent postural instability and freezing of gait (FOG).[40] FOG is defined as brief, episode absences of forward gait progression despite the intention to walk. Individuals with FOG will describe that "my feet are glued to the floor." Unfortunately, postural instability and FOG are unresponsive to conventional PD dopaminergic therapies.

Remarkably, James Parkinson in 1817 also reported an association between dream enactment and FOG. The same patient who suffered from behaviors consistent with RBD also reported the peculiar and distressing gait impairment[41p17-18]:

> It being asked, if whilst walking he felt much apprehension from the difficulty of raising his feet, if he saw a rising pebble in his path? He avowed in a strong manner, his alarm on such occasions; and it was observed by his wife that she believed, that in walking across the room, he would consider as difficulty the having to step over a pin.

Multiple system atrophy (MSA), another disorder of alpha-synuclein pathology with a predominance of autonomic features, has a very high prevalence of RBD, with over 90% of cases having dream enactment and REM sleep without atonia on polysomnography. Patients with MSA may have profound, disabling, autonomic instability, most notably orthostasis, urinary incontinence, and sexual dysfunction. Other MSA features may include cerebellar ataxia, peripheral neuropathy, and parkinsonism, which, like DLB, does not respond to levodopa therapy.[3]

Less often, RBD will be associated with non-alpha-synuclein neurodegeneration including Alzheimer disease, amyotrophic lateral sclerosis, and frontotemporal dementia, along with some trinucleotide repeat disorders (Huntington's disease and spinocerebellar ataxia type 3[SCA3]).[3,41] However, with the exception of SCA3, RBD has a much lower prevalence in these conditions compared to the Lewy body disorders. Further, these non-synuclein pathologies are not typically preceded by RBD but instead develop RBD coincidently or after the presentation of other neurological deficits.[3]

Prior to the development of an overt neurodegenerative disorder, clinical markers of early Lewy body pathology are found among individuals with iRBD.[3] Subliminal cognitive impairments (visual-pereceptual and executive deficits) along with parkinsonian changes in motor function (alterations in gait, muscle tone, muscle activation patterns) have been well characterized in iRBD.[42] Patients with iRBD also have autonomic dysfunction manifesting in urinary incontinence, erectile dysfunction, sweating abnormalities, and postural orthostasis,[43] as well as quantitative abnormalities in the vocal characteristics of speech.[44] On skin biopsy, abnormally phosphorylated alpha-synuclein deposits have been demonstrated in the cutaneous nerve fibers of iRBD and provide direct histopathological confirmation of underlying neurodegeneration.[45]

Approximately half of RBD patients, usually younger, develop dream enactment after starting a serotonergic antidepressant (5-HT RBD), most commonly a selective serotonin reuptake inhibitor (SSRI).[21,46,47] The emergence of dream enactment after starting an SSRI was until recently assumed to be caused by a toxic effect of serotonin upon REM sleep circuitry. However, careful scrutiny of patients with 5-HT RBD reveals neurodegenerative findings, such as olfactory deficits and constipation, not explained by serotonergic mechanisms.[48] In addition, there is further evidence to suggest that patients with 5-HT RBD are at an increased neurodegenerative risk based upon the presence of other early indicators of neurodegeneration: impaired color vision and orthostatic blood pressures, erectile dysfunction, mild cognitive impairment, and subclinical motor deficits in the timed up-and-go test, alternate tap test, Purdue Pegboard, and Unified Parkinson's Disease Rating Scale (UPDRS) II and III.[48] These insights suggest that SSRI antidepressants do not induce RBD but instead unmask RBD in an individual who is already burdened by early alpha-synuclein pathology.

CALMING THE FURIES

REM parasomnias are intense, distressing, and often difficult for patients to explain. As such, it is critically important for clinicians to first acknowledge the reality of these experiences and their widespread prevalence. It is not unusual for patients with nightmares and sleep paralysis to conclude that they are losing their sanity, or for those with RBD to deduce that they must harbor a malignant and violent personality. On the contrary, the ideation of REM sleep is universally intense and bizarre, but for most individuals it is buried in blissful unconsciousness. Patients are acutely aware of frightening and alien mentation, because dreams and atonia linger into wakefulness among those with nightmares and sleep paralysis, and because atonia is lost in RBD.

The essential role of sleep physicians in REM parasomnias, as with the management of all sleep disorders, is knowledge transfer. Helping patients understand the nature of REM sleep, and how it can become disrupted, is the critical step. Insight helps patients target their causative, and often cryptic, ancillary sleep disorders, or discontinue medications such as beta-blockers, notorious for causing nightmares. For RBD, patients must maintain treatment even when dangerous dream enactment is sporadic, and must understand the importance of returning year after year for neurological disease monitoring. Improving sleep requires often difficult behavioral change, such as addressing sleep deprivation and minimizing alcohol. Without effective knowledge transfer, patients are unlikely to maintain a treatment plan, whether or not a correct diagnosis was made.

An accurate diagnosis requires a detailed, 24-hour (whole day, not just nighttime) review of sleep-wake symptoms, followed by a neuropsychiatric history and examination. Bed partner reports, if available, are very helpful as most patients are unable to accurately recall nocturnal events. Abnormal behaviors occurring in the second half of the sleep period, followed by complete alertness and orientation upon awakening, are features that help distinguish REM parasomnias. Disorders of arousal from NREM sleep, such as sleepwalking, are characterized by a history of prolonged, complex, nonviolent activity emanating from the first half of the sleep period with residual confusion.[1]

In-laboratory video polysomnography (PSG) is useful for the workup of REM parasomnias. Its primary utilities are to rule out mimicking or exacerbating conditions, such as sleep-disordered breathing and periodic limb movement disorder, as well as to confirm the elevation of REM motor tone in RBD. During nightmares, tachycardia is noted and sleep paralysis can be visualized during testing with a persistence of REM atonia despite a wakeful EEG. After fully arousing from these events, sleep technologists should immediately ask patients to recall dream mentation.[2]

Sleep-related epilepsy is distinguished by spells that are stereotyped and repetitive; identical behaviors may occur dozens of times at night, and primarily in NREM. When seizures are suspected, the addition of an extended 32-lead EEG recording is helpful; however, deep frontal seizures elude scalp electrodes. Thus, clinicians should have a low threshold for initiating empiric therapy and may need to enlist the aid of specialty epilepsy programs for further in-depth testing.[2]

PSG is helpful in an RBD investigation even if dramatically abnormal behaviors are not captured during the overnight study. Careful review of the video recording can identify subtle motor activity in the hands with repetitive pointing, picking, and fidgeting movements. In males, penile tumescence, a REM sleep phenomenon, is present during RBD episodes. PSG criteria for RBD have been developed by the American Academy of Sleep Medicine. RBD is defined as either excessive bursts of transient motor activity in chin and/or limb leads (at least half of all 3-second mini epochs) or sustained elevation of chin EMG activity alone (limb leads are not used to identify tonic EMG activity) for at least 50% of 30-second epochs. As subtle dream enactment may only involve forearm musculature, EMG leads should be added to the upper extremities for any PSG performed to investigate abnormal nocturnal behaviors.[2]

Nightmares and sleep paralysis are treated by addressing underlying sleep disorders, optimizing the duration and circadian timing of sleep, and eliminating exacerbating medications or substances (see Table 20.3).

While nightmares are common in post-traumatic sleep disorder (PTSD), patients should be reassured that nightmares and sleep paralysis in isolation of mental illness do not indicate an underlying thought disorder.

When managing patients with nightmares, it is important to carefully explore whether the patient is ingesting any substances that can exacerbate vivid dreams. Common agents include: beta-blockers (atenolol, metoprolol, propranolol), dopaminergics (levodopa, pramipexole, ropinirole), selective serotonin receptor reuptake inhibitors (sertraline, fluoxetine, and most notably paroxetine), serotonin modulators (vilazodone), and corticosteroids (prednisone and methylprednisolone). In addition, alcohol, even in moderation, can lead to vivid

Table 20.3 **Treatable Comorbid Disorders/Conditions in Nightmares and Sleep Paralysis**

Medications	Beta-blockers Dopaminergics SSRIs Serotonin modulators Corticosteroids
Drug withdrawal	Alcohol
Sleep disordered breathing	1. Obstructive sleep apnea 2. Sleep-related hypoventilation
Sleep length and timing disorders	1. Sleep restriction 2. Circadian misalignment

distressing dreams, as its withdrawal causes REM rebound and sleep fragmentation.[2]

When nightmares persist, there are psychological and pharmacological treatment options; however, strong evidence for these interventions is still lacking. Dream rehearsal therapy, in which an individual with nightmares practices, while awake, redirecting the mental course of a dream, has been demonstrated to be effective in some cases.[49,50] The most commonly prescribed medication for nightmares has historically been prazosin, based upon its use in patients with PTSD. A meta-analysis of primarily small studies indicated that prazosin was superior to placebo in safety and efficacy in the treatment of PTSD-related nightmares.[51] Later, however, in a more definitive larger controlled study of military veterans with chronic PTSD, prazosin did not demonstrate efficacy in alleviating nightmares.[52] Numerous other medications, including risperidone, olanzapine, and trazodone, have all been tried for nightmare disorder with mixed results.[53,54] More recently, investigators have explored the potential for cannabinoids, in particular the analog nabilone, as a possible treatment for nightmares.[55]

Most episodes of sleep paralysis (in the absence of narcolepsy) are infrequent and do not require intervention. The events typically resolve by addressing any underlying sleep disorder, aligning circadian rhythms and minimizing sleep restriction.[2] When persistent, escitalopram can be considered.[56] The treatment of sleep paralysis and sleep-related hallucinations in the setting of narcolepsy is described in Chapter 16.

PARADOX FOUND

Sleeping safely is challenging as even well-controlled RBD patients can intermittently explode with violence. It is important to modify the bedroom environment. Seemingly benign objects, such as bedside lamps, can be weaponized during dream enactment as patients may ferociously swing or hurl them across the room. Of paramount importance is the removal of loaded firearms and in particular handguns as they can be easily discharged upon a sleeping bed partner by a patient with RBD. Lowering the height of the bed and sleeping in sleeping bags are two practical strategies found to decrease a patient's risk for injury.[21]

While advised to sleep separately, partners are often hesitant to leave the intimacy of a shared bed and have noticed that they can calm patients down with a gentle touch and phrase, such as, "Darryl its OK, you're having a dream." These interventions work because REM sleep is characterized by a low threshold for arousal, along with complex auditory processing. This is in contrast to NREM disorders of arousal, where the threshold for arousal is high and attempts to talk to or redirect a sleepwalker are futile or counterproductive. This combination, low arousal threshold and complex auditory processing, can be leveraged to prevent an RBD patient from leaving a bed with a pressure-sensitive bed alarm. When they arise from bed during dream enactment, a pre-recorded family member sends a calming message, "Jenny, you are dreaming, lay back down," returning them down to the bed and to somnolence.[25]

Aggravating agents, such as SSRIs, and comorbid sleep disorders, in particular obstructive sleep apnea, should be addressed. Decreasing or removing an SSRI may improve, but often does not fully eliminate, a patient's dream enactment. Among patients with 5-HT RBD who still require antidepressant therapy, many do well on an agent with a lower serotonergic profile such as bupropion. Obstructive sleep apnea is common among patients with RBD. At the time of diagnosis, it is often uncertain whether obstructive events during REM sleep are leading to pseudo-RBD or whether the 2 diagnoses are independent. Close scrutiny of the PSG recording can be helpful as patients with both OSA and RBD may have a clear persistence of increased REM motor activity in the absence of a respiratory events. However, many patients with severe OSA may have events continuously throughout REM sleep, and ultimately an empiric trial of positive airway pressure therapy during PSG is necessary to confirm the presence, or absence, of REM atonia.[21]

When violent dream enactment persists despite these interventions, or in situations with a high risk for injury, pharmacotherapy should be considered (see Table 20.4). As only a few small placebo-controlled trials have been conducted, a consensus has arisen, with the most commonly prescribed RBD medications

Table 20.4 **Pharmacological Treatment Options for Potentially Injurious RBD**

Agent	Notes
Melatonin	Available over the counter in the United States and Canada. Minimally sedating. First-line therapy in the majority of cases.
Clonazepam	Long-standing use as an RBD treatment over 40 years. Concerns with morning sedation, cognitive impairment, and imbalance, especially among elderly and those with dementia.
Rivastigmine	Cholinesterase inhibitor used in patients with cognitive impairment. Good option for patients with DLB and PD dementia.
Pramipexole	Limited efficacy primarily in the setting of patients who also have increased periodic limb movements on PSG.
Sodium oxybate	Reasonable treatment option in the setting of narcolepsy with associated RBD.

being melatonin and/or clonazepam.[57] More recently, however, there has been a growth in controlled clinical trials. The cholinesterase inhibitors, in particular rivastigmine, already frequently used to improve cognition in DLB and PD dementia, may also be an appropriate therapy in RBD.[58]

Melatonin

The mechanism by which melatonin may be effective for the treatment of RBD is unknown, but it suggests that a possible and intriguing circadian mechanism may underlie RBD. Melatonin binds to the M1 and M2 receptors, suppressing REM motor tone as well as renormalizing other circadian features of REM sleep. Under normal physiological conditions, the duration of REM sleep episodes and the rate of rapid eye movements (REMs index) increase over the sleep period. Both of the findings are lost in RBD, as patients show no evolution of REM sleep duration, nor in the REMs index.[59] These markers of REM sleep desynchrony are improved with exogenous melatonin in RBD patients, along with a decrease in REM motor activity and dream enactment. Consistent with melatonin's treatment of known circadian rhythm disorders, such as delayed sleep phase syndrome and jet lag, these improvements in REM sleep persist for several days after melatonin is discontinued but then gradually re-emerge over the next several weeks.[2,59]

Starting dose of melatonin in RBD is usually 3, taken at bedtime. The dose may be titrated up to address dream enactment by 3 mg increments to 6 mg, 9 mg, 12 mg, 15 mg, and 18 mg. Melatonin is available over the counter in the United States and Canada but requires a prescription in the European Union and the United Kingdom. Melatonin is an intriguing option for elderly patients as it is only mildly sedating. Other side effects include vivid dreams and sleep fragmentation, which only rarely result in patients stopping therapy.

Clonazepam

As a long-acting benzodiazepine, clonazepam promotes GABAergic inhibition by increasing the frequency of chloride channel opening. It has been the most commonly prescribed medication for RBD since its efficacy was described in the original 1986 report. Most patients initially respond well to low doses (0.25–1.0mg) administered at bedtime. Clonazepam reduces dream enactment, with only minimal reduction in of REM motor tone on PSG. Concerning side effects include morning sedation, gait imbalance, depression, and cognitive disturbances.[60] As most RBD patients ultimately develop a neurodegenerative disorder, progressive cognitive decline combined with age-related impairments in drug metabolism may explain the gradual intolerance of this agent seen in many patients.[2]

Rivastigmine

Acetylcholinesterase inhibitors, such as donepezil and rivastigmine, which increase cholinergic effects by blocking the metabolism of acetylcholine, are commonly employed in the treatment of DLB and PD dementia.

Donepezil has been used as a third-line agent in the treatment of RBD with observational studies reporting that the agent decreases the frequency dream enactment episodes. Subsequently, 2 placebo-controlled trials explored the benefits of the rivastigmine transdermal patch on RBD in patients with PD and in those with mild cognitive impairment alone. In both investigations, rivastigmine decreased the frequency and intensity of dream enactment with only mild adverse effects, most notably orthostatic hypotension, nausea, and excessive daytime sleepiness.[58,61] Considering its indication among patients with dementia, rivastigmine appears to be a good choice for RBD patients with cognitive impairment.

Other Treatments

The combination of melatonin, clonazepam, and rivastigmine provides the majority of RBD patients with effective therapy. If these agents are either ineffective or poorly tolerated, treatment options include: dopaminergics (pramipexole), other benzodiazepines (temazepam, diazepam), melatonin agonists (ramelteon), alpha-2 delta ligands (gabapentin, pregabalin) and a gamma hydroxybutyric acid salt (sodium oxybate). These therapies, based upon case reports or small case series, appear to be most effective when targeted to a relevant comorbid condition: for example, pramipexole in the setting of periodic limb movement disorder, pregabalin in patients with peripheral neuropathy, and sodium oxybate in narcolepsy.[27] Presumably, these treatments address dream enactment by addressing the patient's underlying sleep fragmenting condition.[2,57]

Establishing Expectations

Bed partners and family members should know that, among RBD patients, even those on medical treatment, some degree of dream enactment, along with some degree of vocalization, is inevitable. Unfortunately, these behaviors can disrupt the sleep of loved ones, and sleep-talking can quickly escalate to shouting expletives. However, as long as dream enactment is non-injurious, then conservative management is often warranted, as more aggressive pharmacotherapy is often futile and dangerous, increasing the risk of nighttime falls and daytime sleepiness. Ongoing conversations are thus important to monitor treatment efficacy, assess the severity of dream enactment, and explore whether bed partners should sleep separately.[21]

PROGNOSIS AND COUNSELING

One of the unique medical challenges of the 21st century is helping patients adapt to the ever-expanding discovery of preclinical and prodromal syndromes. After a diagnosis of RBD, a patient is only an internet search away from discovering the link between their disorder and diseases associated with dementia. This discovery can be anguishing for patients, and thus physicians should tactfully and expeditiously discuss the link as soon as the diagnosis is known, as well as promptly provide patients with a customized risk assessment.

Inquiring about ancillary, non-sleep symptoms linked to alpha-synuclein pathology, such as hyposmia (difficulty smelling), slowed bowel motility, and orthostasis, may provide historical clues helpful for stratifying patient risk. When these chronic symptoms coexist with RBD, they are strong predictors of phenoconversion in less than 5 years. Conversely, the absence of these symptoms, along with the presence of a serotonergic antidepressant, decrease the risk of developing a Lewy body disorder in the next 5 years.[62,63]

Sleep physicians can help patients view their disorder with a degree of cautious, useful optimism. After a grieving process, the vast majority of RBD patients handle their new prognosis well. The diagnosis itself can be a catalyst for patients to embrace life's joys and have a newfound appreciation for their remaining brain function.

CONCLUSION

REM sleep and its disorders are fascinating. Nightmares and sleep paralysis are common, yet terrifying, experiences which usually resolve with the correction of comorbid sleep phenomena. The dream enactment of RBD can be injurious to patients and bed partners. When violent, the patient is sometimes assumed to be harboring a malignant underlying personality. This assumption is wrong.

Alpha-synuclein pathology is the underlying etiology in the majority of RBD cases, with many individuals ultimately progressing to DLB or PD. As the dream enactment of RBD is a prodromal neurodegenerative syndrome, RBD research provides a unique opportunity to develop disease-modifying therapies. Many patients find that volunteering for clinical trials is a meaningful experience even if they do not personally benefit, for their actions help develop cures for future generations. The North American Prodromal Synucleinopathy Consortium is currently recruiting RBD subjects for neuroprotective clinical trials. Interested patients and clinicians can visit www.naps-rbd.org for more details.

RBD management is focused on injury prevention by creating a safe bedroom space and utilizing targeted pharmacotherapy. The most efficacious agents appear to be melatonin, clonazepam, and rivastigmine. Sleep physicians can help patients understand their risk for dementia by inquiring about the presence of ancillary symptoms such as hyposmia, constipation, and orthostasis. Regardless of prognosis, patients need to recognize their enduring ability to create meaning and experience joy. RBD offers all of us a valuable perspective—that we should have great and continuous appreciation for our mind's ability to ponder, contemplate, create, and love. Our brains are marvelous but ultimately short-lived wonders.

REFERENCES

1. American Academy of Sleep Medicine. *International Classification of Sleep Disorders: Diagnostic and Coding Manual*. 3rd ed. American Academy of Sleep Medicine; 2014.
2. Howell MJ. Parasomnias: An updated review. *Neurotherapeutics*. 2012;Oct;9(4):753–775. doi:10.1007/s13311-012-0143-8.
3. Boeve BF. REM sleep behavior disorder: Updated review of the core features, the REM sleep behavior disorder-neurodegenerative disease association, evolving concepts, controversies, and future directions. *Ann N Y Acad Sci*. 2010;1184:15–54.
4. Schenck CH, Montplaisir JY, Frauscher B, et al. Rapid eye movement sleep behavior disorder: devising controlled active treatment studies for symptomatic and neuroprotective therapy: A consensus statement from the International Rapid Eye Movement Sleep Behavior Disorder Study Group. *Sleep Med*. 2013;14(8):795–806.
5. Stone JL, Hughes JR. Early history of electroencephalography and establishment of the American Clinical Neurophysiology Society. *J Clin Neurophysiol*. 2013 Feb;30(1):28–44. doi:10.1097/WNP.0b013e31827edb2d.
6. Aserinsky E, Kleitman N. Regularly occurring periods of eye motility, and concomitant phenomena, during sleep. *Science*. 1953 Sept 4;118(3062):273–274.
7. Kleitman N. Basic rest-activity cycle—22 years later. *Sleep*. 1982;5(4):311–317.
8. Jouvet M. Paradoxical sleep mechanisms. *Sleep*. 1994 Dec;17:77–83.
9. Abel T, Havekes R, Saletin JM, Walker MP. Sleep, plasticity and memory from molecules to whole-brain networks. *Curr Biol*. 2013;23:774–788.
10. McNally RJ, Clancy SA. Sleep paralysis, sexual abuse, and space alien abduction. *Transcult Psychiatry*. 2005 Mar;42(1):113–122.
11. Cheyne JA. Situational factors affecting sleep paralysis and associated hallucinations: Position and timing effects. *J Sleep Res*. 2002;11:169–177.
12. Snyder S. Isolated sleep paralysis after rapid time-zone change ("jet-lag") syndrome. *Chronobiologia*. 1983;10:377–379.
13. Munezawa T, Kaneita Y, Osaki Y, et al. Nightmare and sleep paralysis among Japanese adolescents: A nationwide representative survey. *Sleep Med*. 2011;12:56–64.
14. Jouvet M. Paradoxical sleep: A study of its nature and mechanisms. *Prog Brain Res*. 1965;18:20–62.
15. Iranzo A, Santamaria J, de Requer M. Sleep and sleep disorders in Don Quixote. *Sleep Med*. 2004 Jan;5(1):97–100.
16. Guilleminault C, Raynal D, Takahashi S, Carskadon M, Dement W. Evaluation of short-term and long-term treatment of the narcolepsy syndrome with clomipramine hydrochloride. *Acta Neurol Scand*. 1976;54(1):71–87.
17. Schenck CH, Bundlie SR, Ettinger MG, Mahowald MW. Chronic behavioral disorders of human REM sleep: a new category of parasomnia. *Sleep*. 1986;9(2):293–308.
18. Schenck CH, Bundlie SR, Patterson AL, Mahowald MW. Rapid eye movement sleep behavior disorder: A treatable parasomnia affecting older adults. *JAMA*. 1987 Apr 3;257(13):1786–1789.
19. Boeve BF, Molano JR, Ferman TJ, et al. Validation of the Mayo Sleep Questionnaire to screen for REM sleep behavior disorder in a community-based sample. *JCSM*. 2013 May 15;12(5):445–53. doi:10.5664/jcsm.2670.
20. Haba-Rubio J, Frauscher B, Marques-Vidal P, et al. Prevalence and determinant of REM sleep behavior disorder in the general population. *Sleep*. 2018 Feb 1;41(2):zsx197. doi:10.1093/sleep/zsx197.
21. Howell MJ. Rapid eye movement sleep behavior disorder and other rapid eye movement parasomnias. *Continuum (Minneap Minn)*. 2020;26(4):929–945.
22. Ju Y, Larson-Prior L, Duntley S. Changing demographics in REM sleep behavior disorder: Possible effect of autoimmunity and antidepressants. *Sleep Med*. 2011;12:278–283.

23. Haba-Rubio J, Frauscher B, Marques-Vidal P, et al. Prevalence and determinants of rapid eye movement sleep behavior disorder in the general population. *Sleep*. 2018;41:zsx197.
24. Oudiette D, Leu-Semenescu S, Roze E, et al. A motor signature of REM sleep behavior disorder. *Mov Disord*. 2012;27(3):428–431.
25. Howell MJ, Arneson PA, Schenck CH. A novel therapy for REM sleep behavior disorder (RBD). *J Clin Sleep Med*. 2011;7(6):639–644A.
26. Luppi PH, Clement O, Sapin E, et al. The neuronal network responsible for paradoxical sleep and its dyfunctions causing narcolepsy and rapid eye movement (REM) behavior disorder. *Sleep Med Rev*. 2011 Jun;15(3):153–163. doi:10.1016/j.smrv.2010.08.002.
27. Valencia Garcia S, Libourel PA, Lazarus M, Grassi D, Luppi PH, Fort P. Genetic inactivation of glutamate neurons in the rat sublateraldorsal tegmental nucleus recapitulates REM sleep behaviour disorder. *Brain*. 2017 Feb;140(2):414–428. doi:10.1093/brain/aww310.
28. Schneider L, Mignot E. Diagnosis and management of narcolepsy. *Semin Neurol*. 2017 Aug;37(4):446–460. doi:10.1055/s-0037-1605554.
29. Dauvilliers Y, Jennum P, Plazzi G. Rapid eye movement sleep behavior disorder and rapid eye movement sleep without atonia in narcolepsy. *Sleep Med*. 2013;14(8):775–781.
30. Rietdijk CD, Perez-Pardo P, Garssen J, van Wezel RJ, Kraneveld AD. Exploring Braak's hypothesis of Parkinson's disease. *Front Neurol*. 2017 Feb 13;8:37.
31. Blesa J, Trigo-Damas I, Dileone M, Del Rey NL, Hernandez LF, Obeso JA. Compensatory mechanisms in Parkinson's disease: Circuits adaptations and role in disease modification. *Exper Neurol*. 2017;298:148–161.
32. Cheng HC, Ulane CM, Burke RE. Clinical progression in Parkinson disease and the neurobiology of axons. *Ann Neurol*. 2010;67:715–725.
33. Dauvilliers Y, Schenck CH, Postuma RB, et al. REM sleep behaviour disorder. *Nat Rev Dis Primers*. 2018;4:19.
34. Postuma RB, Iranzo A, Hu M, et al. Risk and predictors of dementia and parkinsonism in idiopathic REM sleep behaviour disorder: A multicentre study. *Brain*. 2019 Mar;142(3):744–759. doi:10.1093/brain/awz030.
35. Boot BP, Boeve BF, Roberts RO, et al. Probable rapid eye movement sleep behavior disorder increases risk for mild cognitive impairment and Parkinson disease: A population-based study. *Ann Neurol*. 2012 71(1):49–56.
36. Jung Y, Boot BP, Mielke MM, et al. Phenoconversion from probable rapid eye movement sleep behavior disorder to mild cognitive impairment to dementia in a population-based sample. *Alzheimers Dement (Amst)*. 2017;8:127–130.
37. McKeith IG, Boeve BF, Dickson DW, et al. Diagnosis and management of dementia with Lewy bodies: Fourth consensus report of the DLB Consortium. *Neurology*. 2017;89:88–100.
38. Chan P, Lee H, Hong C, Hu C, Wu D. REM sleep behavior disorder (RBD) in dementia with Lewy bodies (DLB). *Behav Neurol*. 2018:9421098.
39. Parkinson J. *An Essay on the Shaking Palsy*. Whittingham and Rowland; 1817.
40. Videnovic A, Marlin C, Alibiglou L, Planetta PJ, Vaillancourt De, Mackinnon CD. Increased REM sleep without atonia in Parkinson disease with freezing of gait. *Neurology*. 2013 Sep 17;81(12):1030–1035.
41. Arnulf I, Nielsen J, Lohmann E, et al. Rapid eye movement sleep disturbances in Huntington disease. *Arch Neurol*. 2008;65:482–488.
42. Fereshtehnejad SM, Yao C, Pelletier A, Montplaisir JY, Gagnon JF, Postuma RB. Evolution of prodromal Parkinson's disease and dementia with Lewy bodies: A prospective study. *Brain*. 2019;142:2051–2067.
43. Chiaro G, Calandra-Buonaura G, Cecere A, et al. REM sleep behavior disorder, autonomic dysfunction and synuclein-related neurodegeneration: Where do we stand? *Clin Auton Res*. 2018;28:519–533.
44. Rusz J, Hlavnicka J, Tykalova T, et al. Quantitative assessment of motor speech abnormalities in idiopathic rapid eye movement sleep behaviour disorder. *Sleep Med*. 2016;19:141–147.
45. Antelmi E, Pizza F, Donadio V, et al. Biomarkers for REM sleep behavior disorder in idiopathic and narcoleptic patients. *Ann Clin Transl Neurol*. 2019;6(9):1872–1876.
46. Temen PT, Tippmann-Peikert M, Silber MH, Slocumb NL, Auger RR. Idiopathic rapid-eye-movement sleep disorder: Associations with antidepressants, psychiatric diagnoses, and other factors, in relation to age of onset. *Sleep Med*. 2009;10:60–65.
47. McCarter SJ, St Louis EK, Sandness DJ, et al. Antidepressants increase REM sleep muscle tone in patients with and without REM sleep behavior disorder. *Sleep*. 2015;38(6):907–917.
48. Postuma RB, Gagnon JF, Tuineaig M, et al. Antidepressants and REM sleep behavior disorder: Isolated side effect or neurodegenerative signal? *Sleep*. 2013;36:1579–1585.
49. Hansen K, Hofling V, Kroner-Borowik T, Stangier U, Steil R. Efficacy of psychological interventions aiming to reduce chronic nightmares: A meta-analysis. *Clin Psychol Rev*. 2013;33(1):146–155.
50. vanSchagen A, Lancee J, de Groot I, Spoormaker V, van den Boot J. Imagery rehearsal therapy in addition to treatment as usual for patients with diverse psychiatric diagnoses suffering from nightmares: a randomized controlled trial. *J Clin Psychiatry*. 2015;76(9):e1105–e1113.
51. George KC, Kebejian L, Ruth LJ, Miller CWT, Himelhoch S. Meta-analysis of the efficacy and safety of prazosin versus placebo for the treatment of nightmares and sleep disturbances in adults with posttraumatic stress disorder. *J Trauma Dissociation*. 2016;17(4):494–510.
52. Raskind MA, Peskind ER, Chow B, et al. Trial of prazosin for post-traumatic stress disorder in military veterans. *N Engl J Med*. 2018;378(6):507–517.
53. Li TC, Su PY, Chiu HW, Peng CH. Trazodone ameliorates nightmares in major depressive disorder. *J Neuropsychiatry Clin Neurosci*. 2011(Winter);23(1):E4.
54. Malhotra S, Arnold RM, Patterson K. Nightmares, second edition #88. *J Palliat Med*. 2009;12(3):259–261.
55. Mamelak M. Nightmares and cannabinoids. *Curr Neuropharmacol*. 2020;18(8):754–768.
56. Hintze JP, Gault D. Escitalopram for recurrent isolated sleep paralysis. *J Sleep Res*. 2020;29(6):e13027.

57. Aurora RN, Zak RS, Maganti RK, et al. Best practice guide for the treatment of REM sleep behavior disorder (RBD). *JCSM*. 2010 Feb 15;6(1):85–95.
58. Brunetti V, Losurdo A, Testani E, et al. Rivastigmine for refractory REM behavior disorder in mild cognitive impairment. *Curr Alzheimer Res*. 2014;11(3):267–273.
59. Arnaldi D, Latimer A, Leu-Semenescu S, Vidailhet M, Arnulf I. Loss of REM sleep features across nighttime in REM sleep behavior disorder. *Sleep Med*. 2016 Jan;17:134–137. doi:10.1016/j.sleep.2015.10.019.
60. Anderson KN, Shneerson JM. Drug treatment of REM sleep behavior disorder: The use of drug therapies other than clonazepam. *J Clin Sleep Med*. 2009;5(3):235–239.
61. Di Giacopo R, Fasano A, Quaranta D, Marca GD, Bove F, Bentivoglio AR. Rivastigmine as alternative treatment for refractory REM behavior disorder in Parkinson's disease. *Mov Disord*. 2012;27(4):559–561.
62. Howell MJ, Schenck CH. Rapid eye movement sleep behavior disorder and neurodegenerative disease. *JAMA Neurol*. 2015;72(6):707–712.
63. Postuma RB, Iranzo A, Hu M, et al. Risk and predictors of dementia and parkinsonism in idiopathic REM sleep behaviour disorder: A multicentre study. *Brain*. 2019 Mar;142(3):744–759. doi:10.1093/brain/awz030.

SECTION V

The Adult Sleep Patient in the Clinic and Laboratory

Chapter 21

Approach in Sleep Medicine Clinic

Sheila C. Tsai

THE SLEEP HISTORY

When evaluating the sleep medicine patient, the clinician should approach the patient's issues with compassion and care. Poor sleep contributes to poor health outcomes and can negatively impact mood and quality of life. Not infrequently, patients have tried to manage the symptoms on their own for some time with varying success and can be quite frustrated.

As with much of the practice of medicine, the majority of sleep disorders can be diagnosed or suspected based on history alone. For example, the diagnosis of restless legs syndrome is based on meeting certain clinical symptom criteria without the need for further confirmatory testing. Therefore, a thorough sleep history, taken in the context of the patient's underlying medical conditions, age, and gender, can narrow the diagnosis for a patient's sleep disorder.

Eliciting the primary sleep complaint helps guide the history and evaluation of the patient. Often, based on the chief complaint alone, a path of questioning can open up to help focus on the diagnosis. Duration of symptoms, alleviating and exacerbating factors, and any precipitating events should be explored. Inquiring about age of symptom onset can help distinguish certain sleep disorders. For example, in adolescence, symptoms of narcolepsy and delayed sleep-wake phase disorder commonly start to manifest. One should use caution, however, in coming to a diagnosis too quickly lest the primary or other key diagnoses be overlooked. For example, although a patient may note insomnia issues, sometimes insomnia is not the sole underlying problem but rather a symptom resulting from another primary sleep disorder, such as a circadian rhythm abnormality. Therefore, a more extensive history ensures that diagnoses are not missed.

It is imperative to discuss the patient's sleep habits and factors that impact the sleep schedule, such as school and work. The sleep schedule should be explored: the clinician should determine whether there are established sleep routines; quantify how much sleep is obtained nightly; assess whether napping is occurring, intentionally or unintentionally; and evaluate weekday versus weekend or vacation sleep schedules. These details can help identify unintentional sleep restriction, inadequate sleep

Table 21.1 **Relevant Questions in the Assessment of Sleep Patterns**

Questions to help determine sleep patterns:	• What is the typical weekday bedtime and wake time? • What is the typical weekend bedtime and wake time? • What is the work and/or school schedule? • What other factors influence their sleep schedule? • What is the typical sleep schedule when on vacation? • Do they consider themselves a night owl or early bird? • How long does it usually take to fall asleep? • How many awakenings occur during the sleep period? What causes these awakenings? • Are they able to fall back asleep after awakening? • What are they doing while trying to fall asleep? • How much sleep do they get during their major sleep period? • Is there intentional or unintentional napping during the day? • What is the duration of the naps?

habits, and circadian rhythm issues. Poor sleep habits can contribute to insufficient night-time sleep and can perpetuate poor-quality sleep. Inquire about the bedroom environment—a cool, quiet, dark sleep environment tends to be more conducive to sleep. Determining how long it takes to fall asleep and whether sleep disruption occurs once asleep can help in the evaluation of insomnia in addition to hypersomnia. (Table 21.1 lists relevant questions that aid in the assessment of sleep patterns.)

It is important to understand the motivation behind the evaluation, whether driven by daytime consequences, encouragement by family, employment requirements, or based on other comorbid conditions. Furthermore, clinicians should assess the impact of the sleep symptoms on the patient's life, such as marital discord, sleepiness, motor vehicle accidents, or depressed mood. Reviewing medications, substances, and techniques that have been trialed, whether successfully or unsuccessfully, can provide further insight into evaluating and managing the sleep issues. Input from the bed partner can be helpful in describing patient symptoms or abnormal events occurring during sleep, in understanding effects of the sleep problems, and can be particularly helpful if the patient does not notice or minimizes symptoms.

As the sleep evaluation continues, the interview should progress around the salient complaints and features, which will help determine the underlying etiology for the sleep issues. In addition, specific disorders are more common at different stages in life and are related to certain disease states. For example, irregular sleep-wake rhythm disorder is more common in patients with neurodegenerative disorders. Therefore, questions assessing for the more common disorders relative to patient age and underlying medical conditions are recommended in addition to exploring other possible sleep disorders (Table 21.2 provides key relevant questions in the exploration of sleep disorders). It is particularly helpful to divide the patient's sleep issues into broad categories to help in the evaluation of sleep symptoms. These categories are listed in the *International Classification of Sleep Disorders*, 3rd edition, and include: insomnia, sleep-related breathing disorders, central disorders of hypersomnolence, circadian rhythm sleep-wake disorders, parasomnias, and sleep-related movement disorders.[1]

INSOMNIA

Insomnia is a common complaint. It may be either a primary sleep issue or a symptom of another sleep disorder. Often, patients with insomnia note prominent issues with fatigue. Here, it is important to mention that when classifying sleep complaints, one should distinguish between fatigue/tiredness and sleepiness. Although patients will often use these interchangeably, they can indicate different sleep disorders or underlying conditions. Fatigue generally describes a lack of energy and can be a common symptom of other underlying medical conditions, including depression, endocrine abnormalities, and neuromuscular disease. However, sleepiness defines the desire or need to sleep, often at inopportune times. Therefore, potential underlying medical conditions contributing to the fatigue or sleepiness should be considered. In the case of insomnia, it is important to understand events that may

Table 21.2 **Key Relevant Questions in the Evaluation of Sleep Disorders**

Any sleep concern	• When did the symptoms begin? • What are exacerbating and alleviating factors? • What are the current medications, substances, and timing of these? • Why are they seeking evaluation?
Insomnia	• What triggers, worsens, or contributes to the insomnia? • Is it predominantly difficulty falling asleep or staying asleep, or both? • What techniques have been tried to help with the insomnia? • What medications or supplements have been tried? Were they effective? • What are the daytime consequences or impact of the insomnia? • Is there sleepiness, fatigue, or both? • What is the sleep/wake schedule? • Is there napping during the day?
Sleep apnea	• Is there loud snoring? What makes the snoring worse? • Do they choke or gasp awake from sleep? • Has anyone witnessed pauses in the breathing during sleep? • Does there seem to be a positional component? • Is there sleepiness? • Are there other associated symptoms, such as daytime sleepiness, morning headaches, excessive sweating, reflux, palpitations? • Are there comorbid medical conditions such as: cardio-metabolic disease, cardiac arrhythmias, mood disorders? • What worsens symptoms, such as weight gain, alcohol, medications?
Hypersomnia	• What is the sleep schedule and duration? • Is there napping? If so, when, for how long, and are the naps refreshing? • Does the sleepiness persist or does it come and go? • What is the impact on work, school, social life? • Have there been acc the most frequently encountered insomnia issues idents related to sleepiness? • What has been tried to combat the sleepiness? • Are there associated symptoms such as hallucinations, paralysis, and cataplexy? (*narcolepsy tetrad*) • What medications and substances have been tried to help with the symptoms?
Circadian rhythm sleep-wake disorders	• What is the typical sleep schedule on weekdays and weekends? • Is there napping? If so, when and for how long? • What is the typical sleep and wake schedule when on holiday? • Is there difficulty falling asleep, daytime sleepiness, or both? • What is the work and school schedule? • Do they consider themselves an "early bird" or a "night owl"? • Are there other family members with similar sleep patterns?
Parasomnias	• What are the behaviors? • Are there triggers or exacerbating factors? • Do the behaviors occur during the beginning portion or later portion of the sleep period? • Is there recall for the events? • Is there dream enactment behavior?
Sleep-related movement disorders	• Is there an uncomfortable sensation and desire to move the legs and/or body? Is it improved with movement? Is it worse when sedentary? Does it prevent sleep onset? Is it worse in the evening or at bedtime? (*restless legs syndrome*) • What is the impact of these movements on sleep and daytime functioning?

have triggered the insomnia and the duration of symptoms. Knowing what techniques, substances, or medications have been successful or have failed in the past also can direct treatment options.

Exploring sleep habits is helpful as one teases out the insomnia complaints. Poor or inadequate sleep habits can perpetuate the insomnia. Insomnia can also lead to poor sleep habits as the person attempts to compensate for the lack of sleep. Timing of medications and substances, use of electronics prior to bed, and an uncomfortable bedroom environment may all contribute to difficulty sleeping. Insomnia may also be a prominent symptom in underlying medical conditions. Thyroid disorders, congestive heart failure, and chronic pain can all impact sleep and result in insomnia complaints. Other sleep disorders may also present with significant insomnia complaints. For example, sleep-disordered breathing may cause significant sleep disruption and the symptom of difficulty maintaining sleep.

In young children, the most frequently encountered insomnia issues are insomnia limit-setting type or insomnia due to inappropriate sleep associations. These are behavioral sleep issues and are distinguished by characteristic clinical presentation. In limit-setting type, there is a delay or refusal to go to sleep; whereas in sleep-onset association, certain conditions, such as rocking or a bottle, must be met for sleep to occur. Idiopathic chronic insomnia usually begins in childhood. Of course, potential sleep disruptors should be explored, such as restless legs syndrome or sleep-related breathing disorders.

In adults, underlying medical conditions, stress, and anxiety can play a greater role in insomnia. Evaluating potential underlying conditions that may be causing insomnia is important. Stressors and precipitating events can often lead to or exacerbate underlying insomnia. Anxiety and negative thoughts around sleep and insomnia should be explored, as these can fuel the insomnia and lead to poor sleep habits, such as spending prolonged amounts of time in bed not sleeping and worrying about sleep.

SLEEP-RELATED BREATHING DISORDERS

Sleep-disordered breathing should be considered when a patient notes snoring, breathing issues during sleep, or is specifically referred for this evaluation. Due to the high prevalence of obstructive sleep apnea (OSA) in the population, clinicians should consider asking all their patients about symptoms suggestive of sleep-related breathing disorders, such as snoring, awakening gasping or with a choking sensation, or having witnessed pauses in breathing during sleep. Daytime sleepiness and disrupted sleep can result from the breathing abnormalities occurring during sleep. Potential contributors, such as alcohol or neuromuscular disease, should be considered, along with the consequences of the abnormal respiration during sleep, such as its role in mood disorders, cardiovascular disease, insomnia, and sleepiness. Other symptoms that have been reported with sleep apnea include nocturnal reflux, nocturnal hyperhidrosis, and morning headaches. Associated comorbid medical conditions frequently include mood disorders, hypertension and other cardiovascular issues, obesity, metabolic syndrome, insomnia, and hypersomnia. Given the increased prevalence of sleep apnea in patients who have hypertension, atrial fibrillation, and chronic obstructive pulmonary disease (COPD), inquiring about OSA symptoms should occur in patients suffering from these conditions.

In other sleep-related breathing disorders such as central sleep apnea and hypoventilation, gathering additional information on underlying medical conditions and medications is necessary. Hypoventilation should be considered in patients who present with hypoxia, significant obesity, neuromuscular disease, restrictive chest wall abnormalities, or severe chronic respiratory disease such as COPD. Similarly, central sleep apnea may be suspected based on underlying neurologic or cardiovascular conditions or the use of certain medications, such as opiates.

CENTRAL DISORDERS OF HYPERSOMNOLENCE

Hypersomnia is a common symptom associated with various sleep and other medical disorders. One of the most common contributors to sleepiness is chronic insufficient sleep. The inadequate amount of sleep obtained may be intentional or unintentional, recognized or under-recognized. Sleepiness that improves on vacations may be due to chronic insufficient sleep or a circadian rhythm issue. Therefore, when evaluating sleepiness, it is important to assess the amount of sleep obtained and also to understand the duration of symptoms. For example, sleepiness that has been present since adolescence can suggest narcolepsy. However, hypersomnolence can be a symptom resulting from a number of sleep disorders; not all patients with sleepiness have narcolepsy. Important questions to discern primary hypersomnias from other sleep disorders include the presence of narcolepsy symptoms—cataplexy, hypnogogic or hypnopompic hallucinations—and sleep paralysis, which along with daytime sleepiness encompass the narcolepsy tetrad. It is also helpful to explore the urgency for naps, their duration, and whether they are refreshing. In patients with narcolepsy, the naps tend to result from a sleep attack, tend to be shorter in duration, and tend to be refreshing.

In exploring hypersomnia, it is particularly important to consider underlying medical conditions. For example, people who have experienced significant central nervous system (CNS) injury, such as from stroke or traumatic brain injury, can have resultant sleepiness or secondary narcolepsy. In addition, some patients with underlying mood disorders may have issues with sleepiness or amotivation, resulting in their spending significant amounts of time in bed.

As with the other disorders, understanding sleep habits and sleep schedule is crucial to investigating sleepiness. The coexistence of insomnia and sleepiness suggests the possibility of another unifying sleep disorder, such as sleep apnea or a circadian rhythm issue related to the timing of the sleep period versus the patient's internal clock.

In the assessment of sleepiness, it is helpful to determine the severity of symptoms. Sleepiness scales can help objectively quantify subjective symptoms. Scales such as the Epworth Sleepiness Scale [2] and the Stanford Sleepiness Scale[3] have been developed to grade and attempt to measure the sleepiness. The consequences of the symptoms are also important. For example, investigate whether the sleepiness has led to poor school or work performance or if it has contributed to motor vehicle accidents.

It is useful to determine whether the symptoms are persistent or whether they wax and wane. For example, in patients with non-24-hour sleep-wake rhythm disorder, there are times when the individual's sleep cycle aligns with the external environment and therefore they may have a few days when their sleep schedule feels normal or when their sleep symptoms are less severe. In addition, rare hypersomnia disorders, such as Kleine Levin syndrome, are associated with occasional episodes of hypersomnia punctuated with periods of normalcy.

CIRCADIAN RHYTHM SLEEP-WAKE DISORDERS

Circadian rhythm sleep-wake disorders (CRSD) may present with hypersomnia, insomnia, or both as a primary complaint. Generally, if symptoms of both sleep-onset insomnia and hypersomnia present in the same person, a CRSD should be suspected. This disorder results from a shift in the person's internal circadian sleep-wake timing versus the required patterns based on external factors such as school or work schedules. For example, a person with delayed sleep-wake phase disorder (DSWPD) will tend to note difficulty falling asleep, sometimes prolonged, when attempting to sleep at a more conventional time. They then often have difficulty waking up and/or may feel excessively sleepy when they need to awaken at a conventional, but earlier than circadian-preferred, time. Often, a person with DSPD functions better in the latter part of the day. The opposite trend will occur in a patient with advanced sleep-wake phase disorder (ASWPD), where they are unable to work late in the evening, but will often wake early, regardless of their bedtime. It may be especially helpful in diagnosing a CRSD to ask if a person would describe themselves as an "early bird," suggesting ASWPD, or as a "night owl," supporting DSWPD.

Determining sleep habits is critical since there may be behavioral components perpetuating or complicating the CRSDs. For example, late afternoon or evening caffeine usage, prolonged daytime napping and/or napping later in the day, and late-night use of electronics can all perpetuate DSWPD. The age of symptom onset and a family history of CRSD can also suggest this diagnosis. For example, DSWPD tends to develop in adolescence and young adulthood, while ASWPD increases in prevalence in the elderly population. Both have familial tendencies. Furthermore, the work schedule is important to understand, as it can create difficulties when it misaligns with the circadian rhythm. And, clearly, understanding the work schedule is crucial in determining shift work sleep disorder.

Consider the medical and psychiatric history relative to potential CRSD. For example, non-24-hour sleep-wake rhythm disorder is associated with blindness. Neurodegenerative and neurodevelopmental issues are associated with irregular sleep-wake rhythm disorder. Furthermore, dementia can be associated with dampening of the circadian rhythm with irregular sleep-wake schedule or other circadian sleep-wake issues. And, an increased incidence of mood disturbances can be associated with DSWPD.

PARASOMNIAS

Parasomnias are abnormal behaviors or activity occurring during sleep. Duration of symptoms and family history are helpful when evaluating these symptoms. It is important to ask about potential triggers to the events, timing of the events during the sleep period, and consequences of these behaviors. The timing in the sleep period when these events typically occur helps distinguish non-rapid eye movement (NREM) from REM-related parasomnias. NREM parasomnias tend to occur during the initial portion of sleep period and the patient tends to have less recall of the episodes. They may be associated with an abrupt awakening from sleep, such as a confusional arousal.

Associated symptoms, dream content, dream enactment, and recall of events also help categorize the parasomnias into either REM-related or NREM-related parasomnias. REM-related parasomnias are usually associated with abnormal or vivid dream content and tend to occur in the second half of the sleep period. The presence of dream recall is helpful in distinguishing these parasomnias. Dream content may be helpful. For example, in REM behavior sleep disorder, the dreams have commonly been described as defensive dreams—ones in which the patient is defending themselves or others—and the patient may find themselves physically acting out these scenarios while asleep. If dream content is recurrent or is the re-experiencing of a traumatic event, post-traumatic stress disorder may be suspected.

Parasomnias may be precipitated by disorders causing arousals from sleep, such as sleep apnea or periodic limb movement disorder; therefore, it is important to inquire about additional symptoms that could suggest these underlying contributors to or exacerbators of the parasomnias.

SLEEP-RELATED MOVEMENT DISORDERS

The sleep history is vital in evaluating sleep-related movement disorders. It is important to ask about impact of these symptoms on the patient's life—either sleep disruption, daytime sleepiness, or fatigue. Many of the movement disorders are diagnosed clinically without need for further confirmatory testing, emphasizing the importance of a thorough evaluation of the symptoms. For example, as mentioned previously, the diagnostic criteria for restless legs syndrome (RLS) are based on characteristic clinical symptomatology, timing of symptoms, exacerbating and alleviating factors, and resultant distress. These symptoms may overlap with other disorders, so assessing for other disorders that may mimic the movement disorders (e.g., neuropathy in the case of RLS) is necessary.

OTHER IMPORTANT ELEMENTS OF THE HISTORY

Other elements of the history can help uncover or solidify suspected sleep disorders. A comprehensive review of other organ systems helps uncover underlying medical problems or can provide support for a diagnosis. Table 21.3 outlines the key elements of the sleep history.

Reviewing medications and substance use is crucial in the evaluation of sleep symptoms. Medications can have desired or undesirable effects on sleep. Timing of medications during the day can also contribute to (or hide the presence of) sleep issues. Furthermore, the potential association between the initiation of medications and the development of symptoms should be examined. For example, selective serotonin reuptake inhibitors have been associated with the development or exacerbation of restless legs symptoms.

Furthermore, substances, including caffeine, alcohol, and recreational drugs, can all impact sleep. And withdrawal from the medications and substances can also cause significant sleep-related symptoms. Recognizing this, one should inquire about all these substances,

Table 21.3 **Key Elements of the Sleep History**

Chief complaint	• What are the primary sleep issues they would like to address?
Details of the current sleep issue	(see Table 21.2) • Symptom onset • Consequences of the sleep disorder • Exacerbating and alleviating factors • Reasons for seeking care
Past medical history	• Cardiovascular diseases • Endocrine and metabolic disorders • Neurologic disorders • Psychiatric disorders
Past surgical history	• Upper airway surgeries • CNS surgeries • Cardiovascular procedures • Orthopedic surgeries
Medications	• OTC: allergy medication, pain meds, melatonin, herbal supplements, vitamins, supplements • Pain: opiates • Sedatives: benzodiazepines, hypnotics, prescription sleep aides • sedatives/hyponotics • Psychiatric medications: antidepressants, anxiolytics, antipsychotics • Cardiovascular drugs • Respiratory medications • Hormonal therapies • Gastrointestinal medications • CNS medications
Family history	• Sleep disorders • Neurologic disorders • Psychiatric disorders • Cardiovascular diseases
Social history	• Is there a bed partner? • Do they co-sleep with children or pets? • Caffeine usage: form, amount, and timing • Tobacco usage • Recreational drug use: form, amount, timing • Alcohol consumption: amount and timing • Work and school schedule

amounts of use, and timing of use during the waking hours.

The past and active medical history may certainly impact sleep disorders, as the presence of these underlying medical disorders increases the probability of having certain sleep disorders. For example, the presence of symptomatic congestive heart failure increases the likelihood of central sleep apnea. Therefore, it is important to understand the patient's coexisting medical conditions since a number have been associated with sleep disorders, such as hypertension, obesity, hypothyroidism, and mood disorders.

The prevalence of many sleep disorders is increased in family members. These disorders include, but are not limited to, restless legs syndrome, circadian rhythm sleep-wake disorders, and non-REM parasomnias. Obtaining information about familial sleep issues can provide further evidence in support of a sleep disorder diagnosis.

The social history is especially important in evaluating sleep complaints. Psychosocial stressors, substance use or abuse, caffeine amount and timing, and work schedules can all impact the sleep-wake schedule and sleep symptoms. Occupational hazards and potential shift work should be explored in light of the negative impact that poor sleep and irregular sleep-wake schedules can have on job performance.

PHYSICAL EXAMINATION

After obtaining a detailed sleep history, the physical examination can provide clues in the evaluation of sleep disorders. Starting with a general overview of the patient, along with vital signs, can be helpful. The presence of morbid obesity should lead one to suspect a sleep-related breathing disorder such as OSA and/or obesity hypoventilation. Metrics such as body mass index and elevated blood pressure can help stratify risk for OSA. Pulse oximetry helps in assessing daytime oxygenation, potential issues with nocturnal oxygenation, and may suggest underlying cardiopulmonary disease.

The head, ears, eyes, nose, and throat examination is particularly helpful, noting craniofacial abnormalities, lid lag, nasal obstruction or deviated septum, and upper airway findings including modified Mallampati score.[4] Though none of these findings alone is diagnostic of a specific sleep disorder, a constellation of findings can be supportive of the diagnosis of OSA. Dental abnormalities, such as malocclusion or the wearing down of biting surfaces, can suggest sleep apnea or bruxism, respectively.

The neck and back examination should include measurement of neck circumference and palpation for thyroid abnormalities. A larger neck circumference and a large goiter have been independently associated with an increased risk of obstructive sleep apnea.[5] Significant scoliosis can contribute to restrictive lung disease and hypoventilation.

The lung exam evaluates for asymmetric breathing or respiratory difficulties that could suggest neuromuscular weakness, restrictive abnormalities, or underlying pulmonary issues, all of which may be exacerbating the sleep complaints. The presence of rales can point to an underlying pulmonary or cardiovascular issue. Wheezes may indicate airway obstruction. The presence of an underlying pulmonary disease plus the presence of OSA is considered an overlap syndrome and carries higher risk for poor outcomes if the sleep apnea is untreated. This information helps in counseling patients regarding their sleep disorders.

The cardiac exam includes assessing regularity of rhythm and extra heart sounds. Cardiac arrhythmias, particularly atrial fibrillation, have been associated with sleep apnea. Abnormal cardiac sounds could suggest other diagnoses, such as pulmonary hypertension or congestive heart failure.

The abdominal exam is important in assessing work of breathing and potential respiratory issues that could impact sleep.

Examine the extremities, looking for clubbing, cyanosis, or edema, which could point to other underlying issues with oxygenation and/or coexisting cardiopulmonary disease.

The neurologic exam should identify sensory and motor deficits and evaluate mental status. Sensory issues may suggest a neuropathy, a common mimic of restless legs syndrome. Dementia, suggested by certain mental status changes, can be associated with CRSDs. Neurologic findings such as cogwheel rigidity suggest Parkinson disease, which is associated with REM sleep behavior disorder. Localized deficits can be sequelae from prior neurologic insults such as stroke and increase the likelihood for sleep disorders.

The psychiatric examination should include an assessment of mental status, thought content, orientation, and signs of anxiety or depression. Mood and anxiety disorders are commonly associated with symptoms of insomnia and fatigue.

QUESTIONNAIRES

Pre-completed intake questionnaires can help guide the interview and make it more efficient. They can serve as a tool to ensure that key questions are not overlooked. Some more validated questionnaires may be used to attempt to assess a patient's risk for a sleep disorder (for example, the STOP-BANG questionnaire and OSA risk[6]) or to objectively quantify subjective symptoms, such as the Epworth Sleepiness Scale score[2] and the International Restless Legs Syndrome score.[7]

FURTHER TESTING

Once a sleep disorder is provisionally diagnosed, confirmatory testing may be available.

Despite a very high clinical suspicion for OSA, the standard of care is confirmatory testing via a sleep study. In-laboratory and at-home sleep testing are both acceptable means of diagnosing sleep apnea, depending on the clinical scenario. Actigraphy testing may assist in evaluating patients suspected of CRSDs or those from whom it is difficult to ascertain the sleep schedule and sleep-wake patterns. Multiple sleep latency testing helps in the assessment of sleepiness by comparing the patient's mean sleep latency to validated values in order to evaluate complaints of hypersomnia.[8]

Ancillary testing, including blood work to evaluate potential thyroid abnormalities or anemia, arterial blood gases to determine hypoventilation, or iron studies in patients with restless legs syndrome, can be helpful.

SUMMARY

Given the high prevalence and variety of sleep disorders, the approach to the sleep medicine patient is necessarily both broad and detailed. It entails tying in underlying medical conditions, psychosocial factors, sleep habits, medication and substance use, and subjective and objective complaints with a head-to-toe physical examination to determine a cause for the sleep complaints. This thorough approach ensures that contributing details are not missed, helps in broadly categorizing the sleep issues, and leads to a more accurate assessment of the patient's sleep complaints.

REFERENCES

1. American Academy of Sleep Medicine. *International Classification of Sleep Disorders*. 3rd ed. American Academy of Sleep Medicine; 2014.
2. John MW. A new method for measuring daytime sleepiness: The Epworth sleepiness scale. *Sleep*. 1991;14(6):540–545.
3. Hoddes E, Zarcone V, Smythe H, Phillips R, Dement WC. Quantification of sleepiness: A new approach. *Psychophysiology*. 1973;10(4):431–436.
4. Nuckton TJ, Glidden DV, Browner WS, Claman DM. Physical examination: Mallampati score as an independent predictor of obstructive sleep apnea. *Sleep*. 2006;29(7):903–908.
5. Davies RJ, Ali NJ, Stradling JR. Neck circumference and other clinical features in the diagnosis of the obstructive sleep apnoea syndrome. *Thorax*. 1992;47(2):101–105.
6. Chung F, Subramanyam R, Liao P, Sasaki E, Shapiro C, Sun Y. High STOP-Bang score indicates a high probability of obstructive sleep apneoa. *Br J Anaesth*. 2012;108(5):768–775.
7. Walters AS, LeBrocq C, Dhar A, et al.; International Restless Legs Syndrome Study Group. Validation of the International Restless Legs Syndrome Study Group rating scale for restless legs syndrome. *Sleep Med*. 2003;4(2):121–132.
8. Richardson GS, Carskadon MA, Flagg W, Van den Hoed J, Dement WC, Mitler MM. Excessive daytime sleepiness in man: Multiple sleep latency measurement in narcoleptic and control subjects. *Electroencephalogr Clin Neurophysiol*. 1978;45(5):621–627.

Chapter 22

Common Survey Tools/Questionnaires Used in Clinical Sleep Settings

Shakira King, Sara Benjamin, and Charlene Gamaldo

INTRODUCTION

The chapter opens with a clinical vignette to provide a contextual framework for discussing the utility, application and limitations of the commonly used sleep questionnaires available to providers caring for patients with sleep concerns. It contains high-yield content related to the validation studies surrounding these tools. Subsections labeled as "Context/Considerations" are also included to provide information on the relevant application or interpretation of these questionnaires from a clinical, health care profession/wellness, and public health context.

It is also important to note that the list of sleep assessment tools discussed in this chapter is neither exhaustive nor fully comprehensive. The focus is on some common tools that have appeared in sleep medicine and research in more recent years and have been studied in diverse populations.

Clinical Vignette

W.N. is a 48-year-old woman with a history of hypertension. She recently saw her primary care doctor for her annual wellness visit. Her blood pressure was 152/88 and she mentioned having readings above 150 systolic when she checked her pressure at home. Her blood pressure had previously been well controlled on amlodipine 5 mg per day. Vital signs were also significant for a 20 pound weight gain in the past year, with her current body mass index (BMI) now 35.

Her primary care doctor asked about diet, sleep, exercise, as well as her overall health and that of her family. W.N. became tearful, as she discussed multiple stressors, and admitted to sleeping poorly and feeling overwhelmed with family and work responsibilities. She felt tired all the time, had trouble sleeping, and often slept on the couch after being elbowed by her partner due to her loud snoring.

Clinical Question

How might the various sleep questionnaires be used to enhance this patient's diagnostic and workup regimen?

Sleep deprivation and disruption can have several negative effects on health and well-being; for example, lack of sleep contributes to about 3%–5% of the overall percentage of obesity in adults.[1] The short-term consequences of sleep disruption also include emotional distress, mood disorders, increased stress responsivity, reduced quality of life, behavioral issues, and cognitive/memory deficits.[2] The long-term consequences include increased risk for diseases, such as hypertension, metabolic syndrome, type 2 diabetes, colorectal cancer, dyslipidemia, and cardiovascular disease.[2]

Sleep deprivation can directly lead to death; for instance, drowsy driving results in an estimated 1,550 deaths and 40,000 non-fatal injuries yearly in the United States.[1] Insufficient sleep is potentially another contributor to disparities in healthcare and health outcomes. Lack of sleep has also been implicated as a contributor to medical errors that result in 100,000 deaths annually in U.S. hospitals.[1]

Given the negative impacts that sleep disorders have on health, it is important to have validated tools for assessment. Such questionnaires allow for the evaluation of sleep behavior and diagnosis of sleep disorders in order to provide effective treatments. By managing these conditions, their impact on the health and well-being of many individuals can be mitigated.

SLEEPINESS AND FATIGUE

Inadequate quality and/or quantity sleep, regardless of the underlying cause, typically manifests in the clinic as concerns with sleepiness and/or fatigue. For this reason, inventories to assess the symptoms of fatigue and sleepiness are essential when caring for patients with sleep care needs.

Epworth Sleepiness Scale (ESS)

The Epworth Sleepiness Scale (ESS) is a common questionnaire used to assess daytime sleepiness.[4] It consists of 8 self-rated questions that measure an individual's likelihood of "dozing" during certain activities (e.g., sitting and reading).[4] The questions are rated on a scale of 0–4 with higher values indicating an increased likelihood of dozing off.[4] The ratings are then combined into a total score that estimates an individual's general level of sleepiness.[4] The ESS scores are typically interpreted as[4]:

- 0–5: lower normal daytime sleepiness
- 6–10: higher normal daytime sleepiness
- 11–12: mild excessive daytime sleepiness (EDS)
- 13–15: moderate EDS
- 16–24: severe EDS.

CONTEXT/CONSIDERATIONS: REVIEW OF ESS VALIDATION STUDIES

The ESS has been validated among older Black and white women and obstetric patients in the United States.[5,6] It has been validated among OSA patients and studied in many high-risk OSA populations (e.g., patients with coronary artery disease, obesity, or COPD).[7] Studies have shown that the ESS is also useful longitudinally when measuring treatment response among patients with sleep disorders.[8] For example, the reduction in ESS scores indicated improved wakefulness after treatment with a new medication among narcolepsy patients.[8] However, the ESS has shown poor test-retest reliability in some studies, potentially limiting its accuracy in evaluating treatment response.[9]

CONTEXT/CONSIDERATIONS: USE OF ESS IN SPECIFIC POPULATIONS

The original designation for ESS pathology scores (Table 22.1) were obtained before the implementation of resident work-hour restrictions in 2003.[10] A more recent study (2018) investigated sleepiness among Arabic-speaking medical residents in the West Bank and found that about 40% of them had ESS scores of ≥10.[11] EDS had a significantly negative impact on quality of life among these residents.[11]

The ESS has also been studied among U.S. military personnel with and without sleep disorders (e.g., insomnia and OSA); the majority

Table 22.1 **Typical ESS Scores**

Population	~ESS Score
Normal	6
Insomnia	2
Obstructive sleep apnea	12
Narcolepsy	17
Medical residents (emergency/ internal/family medicine, pediatrics, surgery, and OB/GYN)	12–16

Adapted from Papp KK, Stoller EP, Sage P, et al. The effects of sleep loss and fatigue on resident-physicians: A multi-institutional, mixed-method study. *Acad Med.* 2004;79(5):394–406.

of them had EDS based on their ESS score (>10).[12] Studies have also identified sex and race differences in ESS scores.[13] For example, in a 2021 study, female patients had significantly higher total ESS scores than males.[13] Moreover, whereas African American males had significantly higher total ESS scores than white males, African American females had lower total ESS scores than white females.[13] The ESS has also been used to identify a high risk of EDS among commercial drivers in Nigeria.[14]

The ESS has also been translated from English into several languages and modified to be more appropriate for different cultures.[15,16] For example, the Arabic version has been validated among healthy adults and the Spanish version among patients with various sleep disorders (e.g., OSA, narcolepsy, and insomnia).[15,16]

Brief Fatigue Inventory (BFI)

The Brief Fatigue Inventory (BFI) is used for the rapid assessment of fatigue severity and its impact on daily functioning within the past 24 hours or week.[17] The questionnaire consists of 9 items rated on a scale of 0–10 (i.e., from no fatigue or interference to extreme fatigue or interference with daily functioning).[17] The first 3 questions measure the level of fatigue and the last 6 questions assess how fatigue impacts various aspects of daily life: general activity, mood, walking ability, normal work, relations with other people, and enjoyment of life.[17] The ratings are averaged into a global fatigue score: 1–3 (mild), 4–7 (moderate), or 8–10 (severe).[18]

CONTEXT/CONSIDERATIONS: REVIEW OF BFI VALIDATION STUDIES

The BFI is a reliable and valid way of assessing fatigue in several patient populations, including those with OSA and cancer-related fatigue.[7] For example, the questionnaire has shown good internal consistency and reliability among cancer patients hospitalized for chemotherapy in Brazil.[19] The BFI has also shown strong internal consistency and test-retest reliability among patients with chronic obstructive pulmonary disease (COPD) in Canada.[20]

CONTEXT/CONSIDERATIONS: USE OF BFI IN SPECIFIC POPULATIONS

One study found that night-shift nurses had higher BFI mean scores and experienced significantly more fatigue than day-shift nurses.[21] Such fatigue can have many consequences, such as medical errors, social difficulties, and impaired performance.[21]

The BFI has been studied among community-dwelling elderly individuals in the United States, showing that the 2 subscales (fatigue severity and interference) are individually valid and useful in addition to the global score.[22] The questionnaire has been translated and validated in several languages.[23,24] For example, the BFI has been validated among adults and cancer patients from Chinese- and Arabic-speaking populations.[23,24]

SLEEP QUALITY AND DAILY FUNCTIONING

Sleep disorders often lead to sleep deprivation and disruption in which individuals do not obtain an adequate amount or quality of sleep.[2] In fact, about 35% of non-Hispanic white adults in the United States report <7 hours of sleep daily, even though 7–9 hours of sleep are optimal.[1,3] This lack of sleep is more profound for non-Hispanic Blacks and individuals of other races with ~48% and ~39%, respectively, reporting <7 hours of sleep.[3]In this section, we discuss questionnaires often utilized as a screener for overall sleep quality and impacts on daily functioning.

PITTSBURGH SLEEP QUALITY INDEX (PSQI)

The Pittsburgh Sleep Quality Index (PSQI) measures sleep quality and disturbances during a 1-month period.[25] It consists of 19 self-rated questions that assess 7 sleep domains: quality, latency, duration, disturbances, use of sleep medications, daytime dysfunction, and habitual sleep efficiency (i.e. proportion of time in bed that is spent sleeping).[25] Each question is weighted on a 0–3 scale (i.e., from no difficulty to severe difficulty), yielding 7 component scores that are then combined into a global PSQI score.[25] The score ranges from 0 to 21, with a higher value indicating worse sleep quality.[25] Scores >5 represent "Bad Sleepers" whereas <5 represent "Good Sleepers."[25] There are 5 additional questions answered by a roommate or bed partner, which are used solely for clinical information (i.e., not included in the PSQI score).[25]

CONTEXT/CONSIDERATIONS: REVIEW OF PSQI VALIDATION STUDIES

The PSQI has been shown to have strong test-retest reliability and internal consistency among healthy adults and patients with sleep disorders.[25] Furthermore, a global score >5 had a sensitivity of 98.7% and specificity of 84.4% in measuring sleep disturbances among primary insomnia patients versus controls.[26] The questionnaire was also found to have high diagnostic accuracy in detecting insomnia among younger populations in the United States.[27] Moreover, it has shown good validity and internal consistency among the elderly (including Black and white women) in measuring sleep quality and disturbances.[5]

CONTEXT/CONSIDERATIONS: USE OF PSQI IN SPECIFIC POPULATIONS

Night-shift nurses have been shown to have significantly higher PSQI mean scores and poorer sleep quality than day-shift nurses.[21] The PSQI has also been studied among undergraduate medical students and residents, with the latter experiencing poorer sleep quality.[28] More recently (2020), the PSQI demonstrated that frontline healthcare workers had worse sleep quality than non-healthcare workers in Spain during the COVID-19 pandemic.[29]

The PSQI was able to distinguish between elderly subjects with no sleep disorder versus those with sleep disturbances, like restless legs syndrome, insomnia, and sleep apnea.[5] The questionnaire has also been translated and validated in several languages, making it accessible to diverse patient populations.[30,31] For example, the Korean and Italian versions have been validated among patients with sleep disorders, such as primary insomnia, narcolepsy, and sleep apnea syndrome.[30,31]

Functional Outcomes of Sleep Questionnaire (FOSQ) and FOSQ-10

The Functional Outcomes of Sleep Questionnaire (FOSQ) assesses the impact of excessive sleepiness (ES) on activities of daily living.[32] It also evaluates the effectiveness of treatments for functional impairment caused by ES.[32] The FOSQ consists of 30 questions divided into the following subscales: activity level (9 questions), vigilance (7), intimacy and sexual relationships (4), general productivity (8), and social outcome (2).[32] Individuals rate the difficulty of completing a certain activity on a scale of 1–4 (i.e., extreme difficulty to no difficulty).[32] A value of 0 indicates that they do not typically perform the activity.[32] Each subscale score is calculated by averaging the points from questions within that subscale (excluding questions with a "0" or missing response) and thus the subscale scores range from 1 to 4.[32] The subscale scores are then combined into a total score that ranges from 5 to 20.[32] A higher score suggests less functional impairment due to excessive sleepiness.[32]

The FOSQ-10 is a shorter version of this questionnaire that has been developed to measure the impact of excessive sleepiness more quickly and easily.[33] It consists of 10 questions that encompass each of the 5 subscales and were carefully selected to ensure an adequate evaluation of daily functioning that is comparable to the longer FOSQ.[33]

CONTEXT/CONSIDERATIONS: REVIEW OF FOSQ VALIDATION STUDIES

Both versions of the FOSQ have been studied and validated in several patient populations. For example, the FOSQ was first validated among patients with sleep disorders (e.g., OSA) and healthy adults; it displayed strong internal consistency and test-retest reliability.[32] It also effectively distinguished between individuals with and without sleep problems.[32] Moreover, both versions have been shown to be valid, reliable, and sensitive to treatment response among OSA patients undergoing continuous positive airway pressure therapy (CPAP).[33,34]

CONTEXT/CONSIDERATIONS: USE OF FOSQ IN SPECIFIC POPULATIONS

In a cohort of healthcare workers in a pediatric intensive care unit (PICU) in Spain, it was found that nurse assistants had worse sleep quality and lower FOSQ-10 than nurses and doctors.[35] Moreover, the night-shift nurses had poorer sleep quality and more functional impairment than those working mornings or evenings.[35] Overall, there was a weak correlation between perceived sleep quality and FOSQ-10 scores.[35] Many workers who believed they had good sleep quality actually had poor FOSQ-10 scores, suggesting a sleep quality misperception.[35]

The FOSQ and FOSQ-10 have also been translated and validated in other languages. For example, the FOSQ has been shown to be valid and reliable among OSA patients and healthy adults from Spanish- and Swedish-speaking populations.[36,37] FOSQ-10 has been validated among Farsi-speaking Iranian and Spanish-speaking Peruvian OSA patients undergoing CPAP treatment.[38,39] Additionally, the FOSQ has been studied among U.S. veterans undergoing CPAP treatment.[40] A positive correlation between CPAP adherence and FOSQ subscales (social and intimacy) was found among Black veterans; however, there was no significant correlation between CPAP and FOSQ among whites and Hispanics.[40]

Morningness-Eveningness Questionnaire (MEQ)

The Morningness-Eveningness Questionnaire (MEQ) assesses an individual's chronotype, which is their preference for being optimally active during the morning or evening.[41] Intermediate chronotypes reach their peak functioning some time in between the morning and evening.[41] The MEQ consists of 19 items that ask about daily experiences and behaviors and preferences for morning versus evening.[41] For example, one item asks, "At what time of the day do you think that you reach your 'feeling best' peak?"[41] The questions are rated on a 4- or 5-point scale and are combined into a total score that indicates the chronotype[41]:

- 16–30 = definitely evening type
- 31–41 = moderately evening type
- 42–58 = neither type
- 59–69 = moderately morning type
- 70–86 = definitely morning type.

Different variations of the MEQ have been developed, including the reduced MEQ (rMEQ).[42] The rMEQ consists of only 5 items from the MEQ, making it shorter and easier to complete.[42] The total score ranges from 4 to 26: <12 (eveningness), 12–17 (intermediate), and >17 (morningness).[42]

CONTEXT/CONSIDERATIONS: REVIEW OF MEQ VALIDATION STUDIES

The MEQ's validity has been supported through studies in varied clinical populations, including patients with psychiatric conditions and sleep disorders (e.g., OSA and insomnia).[43,44] It has demonstrated high internal consistency among bipolar disorder and insomnia patients.[43] Moreover, eveningness correlated with insomnia, whereas most OSA patients were found to be morning or intermediate types.[43, 44]

CONTEXT/CONSIDERATIONS: USE OF MEQ IN SPECIFIC POPULATIONS

The MEQ has been studied among nurses, allied health professionals, and midwives in different countries.[45,46] For example, among Indian healthcare professionals, a greater proportion of the intermediate types experienced poor sleep quality compared to the morning types.[45] Among Italian midwives, perception of risk of medication errors was associated with intermediate types.[46]

In one study, it was found that adults classified as morning types by the MEQ had a significantly earlier peak in their circadian rhythm than evening types, which further supports the MEQ's validity.[41] Studies have also shown that a preference for morningness increases with age (adulthood) while adolescents tend to be evening types.[47] Furthermore, the chronotype of adults has been shown to be independent of external factors like socioeconomic status, ethnicity, and gender.[48]

The MEQ has been translated and validated in several languages. For example, the MEQ demonstrated adequate internal consistency and good test-retest reliability among Korean young adults.[49] Moreover, the MEQ has been studied among French middle-aged adults, yielding new cutoffs for this age group: <53 (eveningness) and >64 (morningness).[50] The rMEQ has also been used and studied in different countries, displaying good validity and correlation with the MEQ, as well as good test-retest reliability.[42]

SLEEP DISORDERS (GENERAL)

Sleep disorders affect about 50–70 million adults in the United States.[1] The impact is not limited to the United States; for example, in Europe, about 45 million people have a chronic sleep disorder. The next section presents tools that can be used to assist in general sleep disorder screening and that have been utilized in diverse and specific patient populations.

Sleep Disorders Questionnaire (SDQ)

The Sleep Disorders Questionnaire (SDQ) assesses sleep quality and behavior as well as several other factors associated with common sleep disorders.[51] It consists of 175 items that can be divided into separate scales for conditions like narcolepsy, sleep apnea, periodic limb movement disorder, and psychiatric sleep disorder.[51] For example, the sleep apnea scale consists of questions about hypertension, snoring, and apneas during the night, whereas the narcolepsy scale includes questions about paralysis, hallucinations, and excessive daytime sleepiness.[51] Each question is rated on a 5-point Likert scale from never or strongly disagree to always or strongly agree.[51] BMI is also measured primarily to screen for OSA.[51] The length of the full SDQ may limit its full implementation in a clinical setting; thus, it may be more practical to use the subscales for different sleep disorders.

CONTEXT/CONSIDERATIONS: REVIEW OF SDQ VALIDATION STUDIES

The SDQ has been studied and validated among healthy adults and sleep disorder patients.[51] It has also shown adequate test-retest reliability over a 2-week period.[51] Moreover, the sleep apnea and narcolepsy scales have displayed good diagnostic sensitivities and specificities.[51] Given the high prevalence of OSA among epilepsy patients, the sleep apnea scale of the SDQ has also been validated among males and females with epilepsy.[52] It showed good diagnostic sensitivity and specificity for OSA, with a cutoff value of 25.[52]

CONTEXT/CONSIDERATIONS: USE OF SDQ IN SPECIFIC POPULATIONS

The SDQ has also been translated into languages such as French, Dutch, and Spanish.[7,53] It has been validated among Dutch-speaking individuals with sleep disorders.[53]

SLEEP APNEA

About 25 million U.S. adults have obstructive sleep apnea (OSA), which includes 9%–21% of women and 24%–31% of men.[1] OSA is the most common sleep disorder concern patients present in a health care setting. The following section presents some of the most common and well-studied questionnaires to screen and monitor sleep apnea presence and severity.

Berlin Questionnaire (BQ)

The Berlin Questionnaire (BQ) assesses for risk of OSA.[54] It consists of 10 questions with 3 categories: snoring severity, excessive daytime sleepiness, and history of hypertension or obesity.[54] Each question is assigned a score of 0 (no, less severe, or occurs less often) or 1 (yes, severe, or occurs very often).[54] The scores are combined based on their category, and each category is assessed according to the following criteria[54]:

- Category 1: positive if ≥2 points
- Category 2: positive if ≥2 points
- Category 3: positive if the individual has hypertension or BMI >30 kg/m^2.

Individuals are considered low risk for OSA if ≤1 category is positive, or high risk if ≥2 categories are positive.[54]

CONTEXT/CONSIDERATIONS: REVIEW OF BQ VALIDATION STUDIES

The BQ has been studied and validated among various populations, including OSA patients.[7] The BQ has shown good internal consistency and diagnostic sensitivity and specificity among primary care patients.[55] It has also been validated among sleep clinic and surgical patients.[56,57] Additionally, it has been useful in ruling out OSA among patients with treatment-resistant depression, which can be a comorbidity of OSA.[58]

CONTEXT/CONSIDERATIONS: USE OF BQ IN SPECIFIC POPULATIONS

The BQ has been shown to be valid and reliable among Serbian commercial drivers.[59] In Thailand, about 30% of a cohort of male healthcare workers were deemed as high risk for OSA based on their BQ scores.[60] The BQ was administered in a group of Turkish healthcare professionals (e.g., nurses, physicians, and medical students), among which about 15% were high risk for OSA.[61]

The BQ has been translated and validated among adults and sleep clinic patients from Arabic- and Portuguese-speaking populations.[62,63] It has also shown good diagnostic sensitivity but low specificity among the elderly in France.[64]

STOP Questionnaires

The STOP questionnaire is a quick and simple assessment tool for risk of OSA.[65] It consists of four yes/no questions about OSA symptoms, such as **s**noring, daytime *t*iredness, *o*bserved apnea during sleep, and high blood *p*ressure (STOP).[65] Additional questions about *B*MI, *a*ge, *n*eck circumference, and *g*ender were added to create two other versions: STOP-Bag and STOP-Bang.[65] These elements have been shown to significantly increase the questionnaire's sensitivity in detecting patients with moderate to severe OSA.[65]

The scoring of each question is binary (e.g., "yes" = 1; "no" = 0), yielding a total score that ranges from 0 to 8 for the STOP-Bang questionnaire.[66] The STOP-Bang scores are divided into ranges that represent increasing levels of risk for moderate to severe OSA[66]:

- Low risk = 0–2
- Intermediate risk = 3–4
- High risk = 5–8 or one of the following:
  - ≥2 and BMI >35 kg/m^2
  - ≥2 and neck circumference >40 cm
  - ≥2 and male gender.

Context/Considerations: Review of STOP Validation Studies The total STOP-Bang score has a positive correlation with the probability of moderate to severe OSA, which further supports the questionnaire's utility as an OSA screening tool.[66] In fact, the STOP-Bang has been shown to be the more accurate tool for detecting OSA in comparison to the STOP and Berlin questionnaires and Epworth Sleepiness Scale.[67] Moreover, the STOP-Bang has been reported to have a higher predictive value for OSA among male patients aged >50 years with a BMI >35 kg/m^2 and neck circumference >40 cm.[65] However, it does have some limitations; for example, it can be difficult to obtain accurate and consistent neck circumference measurements, and it can be difficult to obtain a score without the patient physically present.[66]

All of the STOP questionnaires have been studied and validated among OSA patients and several other populations, demonstrating high sensitivity as screening tools.[7,65] STOP-Bang has been studied in and validated among patients with multiple sclerosis and high-risk OSA populations, including patients with hypertension, obesity, and type 2 diabetes.[7] STOP-Bang has shown a strong sensitivity in detecting OSA among surgical patients, making it a particularly useful tool given the high prevalence of OSA among this population and its association with perioperative complication risk.[68] All three questionnaires have been studied in patients who have had strokes[7]; however, the STOP-Bag was shown to be the most useful in identifying patients after having had a stroke who have a higher risk of OSA.[69]

CONTEXT/CONSIDERATIONS: USE OF STOP IN SPECIFIC POPULATIONS

In a cohort of U.S. healthcare workers, about 37% were identified as high risk for OSA based on STOP scores.[70] The STOP-Bang has also been used to reveal a high risk of OSA among commercial drivers in Nigeria.[14]

The STOP and STOP-Bang questionnaires have been translated and validated in several languages and validated among the general population.[7] For example, the STOP-Bang has been validated among sleep clinic and OSA syndrome patients from Arabic- and Spanish-speaking populations.[71,72] Moreover, both the STOP and STOP-Bang have been validated among patients with suspected OSA in Hong Kong.[73]

Calgary Sleep Apnea Quality of Life Index (SAQLI)

The Calgary Sleep Apnea Quality of Life Index (SAQLI) is used to assess quality of life (QoL) components among patients with OSA.[74] It includes over 30 items that are divided into 4 core domains: (A) daily functioning, (B) social interactions, (C) emotional functioning, and (D) symptoms.[74] A 5th domain, treatment-related symptoms (E), can be used to assess the negative side effects of OSA treatment.[74] A trained interviewer obtains answers to these questions based on the subject's experiences during the previous 4 weeks.[74] Each item is rated on a scale from 1 to 7 in terms of problem severity (i.e., major problem to no problem) or frequency (i.e., all the time to not at all).[74] For domains D and E, individuals only rate the 5 most important symptoms they experience.[74] The averaged domain scores (A–D) are combined to yield a total (average) score between 1 and 7; higher scores indicate better quality of life.[75] If used, the 5th domain averaged score (adjusted by a weighting factor) should be subtracted from the other 4 domain scores to calculate the total score[75] (see Table 22.2 for sample scores from a cohort of OSA patients).[74]

Table 22.2 **Sample SAQLI Scores**

SAQLI Domain	Average Score
A	4.7
B	5.3
C	4.9
D	3.5
Total	4.6

Adapted from Flemons WW, Reimer MA. Development of a disease-specific health-related quality of life questionnaire for sleep apnea. *Am J Respir Crit Care Med.* 1998;158(2):494–503, table 5.

CONTEXT/CONSIDERATIONS: REVIEW OF SAQLI VALIDATION STUDIES

The SAQLI has been studied among snorers and sleep apnea patients, demonstrating high internal consistency and test-retest reliability across 2 weeks.[74,75] It also showed excellent responsiveness to treatment-related QoL changes among patients who underwent 4 weeks of CPAP.[75] Based on these results, a study recommended a minimal clinically important difference of ~1 point in the total score.[75] The SAQLI has also been shown to effectively measure QoL improvement after 6 months of CPAP treatment (≥4 hours per night).[76]

CONTEXT/CONSIDERATIONS: USE OF SAQLI IN SPECIFIC POPULATIONS

The SAQLI has been translated and validated in several other languages.[77,78] For example, the SAQLI demonstrated good internal consistency and test-retest reliability among Spanish and Persian-speaking patients with OSA.[77,78]

INSOMNIA

Insomnia is the most common sleep disorder: 30% of U.S. adults have short-term concerns with falling asleep and 10% report chronic insomnia.[1] Insomnia, specifically in the setting of chronically short sleep duration, has been associated with higher morbidity and mortality risk. As a result, health care providers should be familiar with useful insomnia screening and severity inventory scales.

Insomnia Severity Index (ISI)

The Insomnia Severity Index (ISI) measures insomnia severity and evaluates insomnia treatment response.[79] It includes 7 questions that address several insomnia symptoms: difficulty falling asleep, difficulty staying asleep, early morning awakenings, sleep dissatisfaction, noticeability of sleep difficulties by others, worry over sleep problems, and interference with daily functioning.[79] The items are rated on a scale from 0 to 4 (i.e., no problem to very severe problem) and combined into a final score[79]:

- 0–7 = no clinically significant insomnia
- 8–14 = subthreshold insomnia
- 15–21 = clinical insomnia (moderate severity)
- 22–28 = clinical insomnia (severe).

CONTEXT/CONSIDERATIONS: REVIEW OF ISI VALIDATION STUDIES

The ISI has shown sensitivity to treatment response among insomnia patients.[80,81] Furthermore, it has displayed good diagnostic sensitivity and specificity in assessing for insomnia among primary care patients.[82] The ISI has shown adequate internal consistency among sleep clinic patients.[81] The questionnaire has also been studied among psychiatric inpatients, revealing a high prevalence of insomnia, and among patients with rheumatologic diseases.[83,84]

While the ISI is very useful in insomnia evaluation, it has some limitations; for example, it cannot distinguish between different causes of insomnia.[84] Moreover, the guidelines for using the ISI to measure treatment response need further validation with different types of therapies and patient populations.[84] Nonetheless, studies have recommended at least a 6–9-point change in pre–post-treatment scores to be considered "clinically relevant."[80,84]

CONTEXT/CONSIDERATIONS: USE OF ISI IN SPECIFIC POPULATIONS

The ISI has been studied among healthcare professionals and commercial drivers in countries such as Jordan, Spain, and South Korea.[29,85,86] One study found a high prevalence of insomnia among medical students in Jordan; higher ISI scores were significantly associated with poor sleep quality and academic performance.[85] During the COVID-19 pandemic, ISI scores showed that insomnia was more prevalent among frontline healthcare workers than non-healthcare workers in Spain.[29] The prevalence of insomnia among South Korean commercial drivers is also higher than that of the general population.[86]

The ISI has been validated in the general population in Canada and studied among U.S. veterans, revealing that Black veterans have experienced more severe insomnia symptoms than whites and Hispanics.[40] The ISI has also been translated into several languages and validated among different cultural groups. For example, it was found to be reliable and valid among Italian-speaking insomnia patients undergoing cognitive behavioral therapy.[87] In addition, it has been validated among Hindi-speaking insomnia patients with comorbidities, such as depression and restless legs syndrome.[88]

NARCOLEPSY

Narcolepsy represents the most clinically defined and distinct conditions under the central hypersomnia classification. Although narcolepsy is less common, with an incidence of about 0.05% in the United States[1] as compared to sleep apnea and insomnia, individuals with narcolepsy report some of the highest morbidity rates. Moreover, in many cases patients may suffer with symptoms well beyond a decade before diagnosis, suggesting the need for greater awareness of symptom phenomenology and the available tools to assist in identification.

Swiss Narcolepsy Scale (SNS)

The Swiss Narcolepsy Scale (SNS) is a 5-item questionnaire that screens for narcolepsy.[89] It measures the frequency of the following excessive daytime sleepiness (EDS) and cataplexy symptoms: inability to fall asleep, feeling unrested in the morning, daytime napping, and weak/buckling knees and jaw sagging during emotions (e.g., laughing, happiness, or anger).[89] Items are rated on a 1–5 scale (i.e., from never to almost always) and the total score is calculated according to the following formula[89]:

$$6 \times Q_1 + 9 \times Q_2 - 5 \times Q_3 - 11 \times Q_4 - 13 \times Q_5 + 20$$

A total score of <0 indicates narcolepsy with cataplexy (NT1).[89]

CONTEXT/CONSIDERATIONS: REVIEW OF SNS VALIDATION STUDIES

In Switzerland and the Netherlands, the SNS displayed high diagnostic sensitivity and specificity among patients with narcolepsy type 1 (NT1) and even in the subgroup of NT1 patients with CSF hypocretin-1 deficiency.[90] It was also able to distinguish between those with EDS due to narcolepsy versus other causes (e.g., sleep-disordered breathing).[90] In fact, the SNS was more accurate than the ESS in screening for narcolepsy.[90]

The short-form SNS (sSNS) has been developed as an assessment tool that is easier to complete and score.[91] The sSNS consists of 2 questions from the SNS that were the most accurate at identifying NT1 patients.[91] It had significant correlation with the SNS, further supporting its validity.[91] However, both questionnaires poorly identified narcolepsy type 2 patients, suggesting that they may not be as useful for this narcolepsy subgroup.[91]

OTHER QUESTIONNAIRES

Sleep disorders, both untreated and undertreated, have been associated with several co-morbidities including several cardiovascular, metabolic, and endocrinological issues. In fact, affective disorders (depression and anxiety) and sleep disorders have a bidirectional relationship in serving as both a primary and secondary risk factor for developing one when the other is present and untreated. For this reason, basic knowledge on the questionnaires used to identify symptoms of anxiety and depression are also useful in the clinical sleep setting. Tools like the Beck Anxiety Inventory (BAI) and Beck Depression Inventory (BDI) help identify comorbidities (i.e., anxiety and depression) that can be treated to improve quality of life among patients with sleep disorders.

Beck Anxiety Inventory (BAI)

The Beck Anxiety Inventory (BAI) consists of a list of 21 anxiety symptoms.[92] Each symptom is rated on a scale from 0 to 3 (i.e., from not being bothered by the symptom at all to being severely bothered by it).[92] The ratings are then combined into a final score[92]:

- 0–21 = low anxiety
- 22–35 = moderate anxiety
- 36 and above = potentially concerning levels of anxiety.

CONTEXT/CONSIDERATIONS: REVIEW OF BAI VALIDATION STUDIES

The BAI can be used to determine if insomnia is present in the context of an untreated psychological condition, which if concomitantly addressed, could improve the sleep problem. Moreover, it has been studied and validated among patients with OSA who also have a higher risk for anxiety and depression.[7,93]

The BAI has been shown to have strong internal consistency and test-retest reliability over 1 week among psychiatric outpatients with depression or anxiety.[92]

CONTEXT/CONSIDERATIONS: USE OF BAI IN SPECIFIC POPULATIONS

In a study among Taiwanese female nurses with poor sleep quality, BAI scores revealed that over 20% of them had severe anxiety levels.[94] During the COVID-19 pandemic, 33% of frontline healthcare workers in Turkey had clinically significant anxiety; BAI scores were also positively correlated with PSQI scores (i.e., higher anxiety levels associated with worse sleep quality).[95]

The BAI has been translated and validated in several other languages, such as Chinese, Spanish, and French.[7] For example, in a Spanish study, the BAI demonstrated high internal consistency in the general population.[96]

Beck Depression Inventory (BDI)

The Beck Depression Inventory (BDI) measures depression severity through 21 items that address common attitudes and symptoms of depression.[97] Each item is rated on a 0–3 scale (i.e., from not present to severe) and combined into a final score[97]:

- 1–10: ups and downs are considered normal
- 11–16: mild mood disturbance
- 17–20: borderline clinical depression
- 21–30: moderate depression
- 31–40: severe depression.
- Over 40: Extreme depression

There are also other versions of the BDI, including a 13-item short form and the updated BDI-II.[97] The BDI-II is more compatible with the DSM-IV criteria for depression; for instance, the questions are answered based on the past 2 weeks rather than just 1 week as in the BDI.[98] The BDI and BDI-II have been shown to have strong internal consistency and test-retest reliability.[97,99]

CONTEXT/CONSIDERATIONS: REVIEW OF BDI VALIDATION STUDIES

The BDI can be used to determine if hypersomnia is occurring in the presence of untreated depression. Similarly to the BAI, the BDI can also be used to detect and address depression among patients with sleep apnea, who are at greater risk for psychopathology.[93]

Both versions have been studied and validated in several patient populations. For example, the BDI has demonstrated high internal consistency and validity among depressed patients.[100] Moreover, BDI scores revealed a higher prevalence of depression among OSA patients compared to controls.[101]

CONTEXT/CONSIDERATIONS: USE OF BDI IN SPECIFIC POPULATIONS

The BDI has been studied among healthcare workers and commercial drivers in several countries. For example, among Taiwanese female nurses, sleep disturbances were positively correlated with depression severity as measured by the BDI-II.[94] Using the BDI short form, Brazilian truck drivers were found to be at greater risk for depression compared to the general population.[102]

Both the BDI and BDI-II have been validated across several demographics, including age, gender, and nationality.[7,99] Translated versions of the BDI-II have been validated among depressed adolescents and adults from countries such as the Dominican Republic and Korea.[103,104]

Clinical Global Impressions Scale (CGI)

The Clinical Global Impressions Scale (CGI) is a general measure of disease severity and treatment response that can be used and adapted for various diseases.[105] It has 3 components: severity of illness (CGI-S), global improvement (CGI-I), and efficacy index (CGI-E).[105] The CGI-S and CGI-I are most often used together to establish the baseline condition and monitor changes after treatment.[106] Each consists of a single question rated by a clinician on a scale from 0 to 7 (Table 22.3).[106] The CGI-S asks: "Considering your total clinical experience with this particular population, how ill is the patient at this time?" (based on the past week).[106] The CGI-I asks: "Compared to the patient's condition [prior to treatment], how has their illness changed?"[106]

The CGI-E compares the patient's baseline condition to a ratio of the treatment benefits and side effects.[107] When using these scales, clinicians should consider: patient's history, family/caregiver input, symptoms and their impact on functioning, psychosocial circumstances, behavior, and any other relevant information.[106] The rating should also be made irrespective of symptom etiology and whether or not the clinician believes the changes are due to the treatment.[106]

CONTEXT/CONSIDERATIONS: REVIEW OF CGI VALIDATION STUDIES

The CGI's validity has been supported by correlations with longer clinical assessments across

Table 22.3 **CGI Rating Scale**

Score	CGI-S	CGI-I
0	Not assessed	Not assessed
1	Normal, not at all ill	Very much improved
2	Borderline ill	Much improved
3	Mildly ill	Minimally improved
4	Moderately ill	No change
5	Markedly ill	Minimally worse
6	Severely ill	Much worse
7	Among the most extremely ill	Very much worse

Adapted from Busner J, Targum SD. The clinical global impressions scale: Applying a research tool in clinical practice. *Psychiatry (Edgmont)*. 2007;4(7):28–37, tables 1, 2.

different psychiatric illnesses.[106] The CGI has also been studied within an OSA patient population in which over 50% of individuals had mild or worse CGI-S ratings.[108] Additionally, at a similar OSA severity, the elderly had worse CGI scores than adults aged ≤65 years, and women had worse CGI ratings than men.[108] There was also a higher prevalence of OSA comorbidities (e.g., metabolic and cardiovascular diseases) among patients with higher CGI ratings.[108] The CGI-I was sensitive to treatment response (e.g., CPAP, oral appliance, and surgery) and a better predictor of CPAP adherence than OSA severity and ESS scores at baseline.[108]

While the CGI can be very useful in evaluating disease severity and following patient progress, it does have limitations.[107] For example, the CGI-I rating can be impacted by memory errors and patient-reported events or symptoms irrelevant to the disease.[107] CGI improvements might include: using an average rating from several clinicians and creating more versions for different diseases.[107] Additionally, it could be helpful to have patients complete the Patient Global Impression Scale (PGI), which is similar to CGI but provides the patient's perspective instead.[107,109] The PGI has been shown to strongly correlate with the CGI, providing support for their joint use.[109]

CLINICAL VIGNETTE ANSWER

How might the various sleep-related questionnaires be used to enhance diagnostic and workup regimen?

The primary care doctor administered a *STOP questionnaire* that included the following questions and answers:

- Do you snore loudly? Yes
- Do you often feel tired, fatigued, or sleepy during the daytime? Yes
- Has anyone observed you stop breathing during sleep? Yes
- Do you have (or are you being treated for) high blood pressure? Yes

Based on this screening tool, W.N. was referred for a sleep medicine consult.

As a part of her sleep medicine assessment, W.N. completed an *Epworth Sleepiness Scale (ESS)*; her score was 8/24.

She had a home sleep test that revealed moderate sleep apnea, and she was started on auto-CPAP.

Two months later, she was seen for a sleep medicine follow-up, where her CPAP compliance data demonstrated adequate time using CPAP and good resolution of her sleep-disordered breathing. However, she still complained of sleep fragmentation and non-restorative sleep. She said that it felt like half the time she was wearing CPAP, she was just lying in her bed awake and staring at the ceiling.

The sleep medicine physician told the patient to continue CPAP use and referred her to behavioral sleep medicine for further evaluation and treatment.

The sleep psychologist took a careful history and included the *Beck Anxiety Index (BAI) and Beck Depression Index (BDI)* in the assessment. Her Beck Anxiety Index was 21 and Beck Depression index was 17 at the time of her initial assessment. Over the next 6 weeks, W.N. worked with the psychologist on sleep scheduling, bedtime routine, and sleep-restriction therapy. Her BAI scores reduced to 15 and the BDI to 10. She was able to continue wearing her CPAP nightly and reported subjectively more hours of sleep. Her ESS score was reduced to 4/24. As her sleep quality improved, she was able to be more consistent with her exercise routine and to prepare more homemade meals. She lost 4 pounds and hoped to continue to lose more weight.

CONCLUSION

This chapter has presented utility and validation metrics for several tools and questionnaires that can aid in the diagnosis of various sleep disorders. Certain questionnaires screen for specific sleep disorders (e.g., insomnia and OSA), while others more generally assess for several sleep conditions and associated symptoms (Table 22.4). Tools like the BAI and BDI help identify comorbidities, such as anxiety and depression, that can be treated to improve quality of life among sleep disorder patients.

Table 22.4 **Sleep Tool Functionality**

Sleep Tool	Permission Required for Clinical or Research Use	Platforms (in addition to paper)		Information Source (in addition to patient)		Grade Readability	Completion Time
		Electronic	Face-to-Face	Caregiver or Observer	Provider or Staff		
ESS	YES	X	X			6.9	1 min
BFI	YES	X	X			7.9	5 min
PSQI	YES	X	X			7.0	5 min
FOSQ	YES	X	X	X	X	Short: 8.5 Long: 7.7	Short: 5 min
SDQ	YES					8	30 min
STOP	Unknown		X	X	X	4.0	1 min
STOP-BAG	Unknown	X	X	X	X	3.7	1 min
STOP-BANG	Unknown	X	X	X	X	3.9	1–3 min
BQ	Unknown		X		X	2.9	5 min
SAQLI	YES		X	X(short)	X (long)	Long: 6.5 Short: 7.1	Long: 10–15 min Short: 7 min
ISI	YES		X	X	X	Unknown	<5 min
SNS	YES	X	X			Unknown	Few min
BAI	YES	X	X			8.3	Unknown
BDI	YES					3.5	10 min
CGI	NO					10.6	Unknown
MEQ	NO	X	X			Unknown	5–10 min

Gamaldo C, Buenaver L, Chernyshev O, et al.; OSA Assessment Tools Task Force of the American Academy of Sleep Medicine. Evaluation of clinical tools to screen and assess for obstructive sleep apnea. *J Clin Sleep Med*. 2018;14(7):1239–1244, tables S5, S13.

Table 22.5 **Demographics Studied by Sleep Tools**

Sleep Tool	General Population	Minorities	Various Nations (including U.S.)	Age		
				Young Adult (18–44 years)	Middle Age (45–65 years)	Elderly (65+ years)
ESS	X	X	X	X	X	X
BFI	X	X	X	X	X	X
PSQI	X	X	X	X	X	X
FOSQ	X	X	X	X	X	X
SDQ	X		X	X	X	
STOP	X		X	X	X	X
STOP-BAG	X	X	X		X	X
STOP-BANG	X	X	X		X	X
BQ	X		X		X	X
SAQLI		X	X	X	X	
ISI	X	X	X	X	X	X
SNS			X	X	X	
BAI	X	X		X	X	X
BDI			X	X	X	X
CGI	X		X		X	
MEQ	X	X	X	X	X	X

° All questionnaires have been studied among females and males.
Gamaldo C, Buenaver L, Chernyshev O, et al.; OSA Assessment Tools Task Force of the American Academy of Sleep Medicine. Evaluation of clinical tools to screen and assess for obstructive sleep apnea. *J Clin Sleep Med.* 2018;14(7):1239–1244, tables S4, S12.

Each tool has been studied and validated in different patient populations within and/or outside of the United States. Translated versions in several languages have also been validated, demonstrating that these questionnaires are useful in diverse geographic, ethnic, and cultural groups. While each tool has its benefits, there are also limitations; one overarching limitation is that all serve as screening and not diagnostic tools (Table 22.5). Thus, they should be used in conjunction with other diagnostic measures (e.g., clinical history, polysomnography, and MSLT) to accurately identify individuals with sleep disorders.

Whether used separately or together, these questionnaires can help patients receive a more expeditious and accurate diagnosis as a key step in receiving optimal treatment and achieving ideal outcomes.

REFERENCES

1. American Sleep Association. Sleep and Sleep Disorder Statistics. https://www.sleepassociation.org/about-sleep/sleep-statistics/. Accessed May 12, 2021.
2. Medic G, Wille M, Hemels ME. Short- and long-term health consequences of sleep disruption. *Nat Sci Sleep*. 2017;9:151–161. doi:10.2147/NSS.S134864.
3. Centers for Disease Control and Prevention (CDC). Unhealthy sleep-related behaviors: 12 states, 2009. *MMWR*. 2011;60(8):233–238.
4. Johns, MW. The Epworth Sleepiness Scale. https://epworthsleepinessscale.com/.
5. Beaudreau SA, Spira AP, Stewart A, et al. Validation of the Pittsburgh Sleep Quality Index and the Epworth Sleepiness Scale in older black and white women. *Sleep Med.* 2012;13(1):36–42. doi:10.1016/j.sleep.2011.04.005.
6. Baumgartel KL, Terhorst L, Conley YP, Roberts JM. Psychometric evaluation of the Epworth sleepiness scale in an obstetric population. *Sleep Med.* 2013;14(1):116–121. doi:10.1016/j.sleep.2012.10.007.
7. Gamaldo C, Buenaver L, Chernyshev O, et al.; OSA Assessment Tools Task Force of the American Academy of Sleep Medicine. Evaluation of clinical tools to screen and assess for obstructive sleep apnea. *J Clin Sleep Med.* 2018;14(7):1239–1244. https://doi.org/10.5664/jcsm.7232.
8. Thorpy MJ, Shapiro C, Mayer G, et al. A randomized study of solriamfetol for excessive sleepiness in narcolepsy [published correction appears in *Ann Neurol.* 2020 Jan;87(1):157]. *Ann Neurol.* 2019;85(3):359–370. doi:10.1002/ana.25423.
9. Taylor E, Zeng I, O'Dochartaigh C. The reliability of the Epworth Sleepiness Score in a sleep clinic population. *J Sleep Res.* 2019;28(2):e12687. doi:10.1111/jsr.12687.
10. Papp KK, Stoller EP, Sage P, et al. The effects of sleep loss and fatigue on resident-physicians: a multi-institutional, mixed-method study. *Acad Med.* 2004;79(5):394–406. doi:10.1097/00001888-200405000-00007.
11. Alami YZ, Ghanim BT, Zyoud SH. Epworth Sleepiness Scale in medical residents: Quality of sleep and its

relationship to quality of life. *J Occup Med Toxicol*. 2018;13:21. doi:10.1186/s12995-018-0203-z.

12. Hurlston A, Foster SN, Creamer J, et al. The Epworth Sleepiness Scale in service members with sleep disorders. *Mil Med*. 2019;184(11-12):e701–e707. doi:10.1093/milmed/usz066.
13. Packard A, Bautista R, Smotherman C, Gautham S. Gender differences in Epworth Sleepiness Scale revealed by paired patient-spouse scoring. *Epilepsy Behav*. 2021;114(Pt A):107272. doi:10.1016/j.yebeh.2020.107272.
14. Ozoh OB, Okubadejo NU, Akanbi MO, Dania MG. High-risk of obstructive sleep apnea and excessive daytime sleepiness among commercial intra-city drivers in Lagos metropolis. *Niger Med J*. 2013;54(4):224–229. doi:10.4103/0300-1652.119607.
15. Ahmed AE, Fatani A, Al-Harbi A, et al. Validation of the Arabic version of the Epworth Sleepiness Scale. *J Epidemiol Glob Health*. 2014;4(4):297–302. doi:10.1016/j.jegh.2014.04.004.
16. Sandoval-Rincón M, Alcalá-Lozano R, Herrera-Jiménez I, Jiménez-Genchi A. Validación de la escala de somnolencia de Epworth en población mexicana [Validation of the Epworth Sleepiness Scale in Mexican population]. *Gac Med Mex*. 2013;149(4):409–416.
17. Mendoza TR, Wang XS, Cleeland CS, et al. The rapid assessment of fatigue severity in cancer patients: Use of the Brief Fatigue Inventory. *Cancer*. 1999;85(5):1186–1196. doi:10.1002/(sici)1097-0142(19990301)85:5<1186::aid-cncr24>3.0.co;2-n.
18. Chang YJ, Lee JS, Lee CG, et al. Assessment of clinical relevant fatigue level in cancer. *Support Care Cancer*. 2007;15(7):891–896. doi:10.1007/s00520-007-0219-x.
19. Nunes AF, Bezerra CO, Custódio JDS, Friedrich CF, Oliveira IS, Lunardi AC. Clinimetric properties of the Brief Fatigue Inventory applied to oncological patients hospitalized for chemotherapy. *J Pain Symptom Manage*. 2019;57(2):297–303. doi:10.1016/j.jpainsymman.2018.10.508.
20. Chen YW, Coxson HO, Reid WD. Reliability and validity of the Brief Fatigue Inventory and Dyspnea Inventory in people with chronic obstructive pulmonary disease. *J Pain Symptom Manage*. 2016;52(2):298–304. doi:10.1016/j.jpainsymman.2016.02.018.
21. Kunert K, King ML, Kolkhorst FW. Fatigue and sleep quality in nurses. *J Psychosoc Nurs Ment Health Serv*. 2007;45(8):30–37. doi:10.3928/02793695-20070801-07.
22. Shuman-Paretsky MJ, Belser-Ehrlich J, Holtzer R. Psychometric properties of the Brief Fatigue Inventory in community-dwelling older adults. *Arch Phys Med Rehabil*. 2014;95(8):1533–1539. doi:10.1016/j.apmr.2014.03.026.
23. Wang XS, Hao XS, Wang Y, et al. Validation study of the Chinese version of the Brief Fatigue Inventory (BFI-C). *J Pain Symptom Manage*. 2004;27(4):322–332. doi:10.1016/j.jpainsymman.2003.09.008.
24. Suleiman K, Al Kalaldeh M, AbuSharour L, et al. Validation study of the Arabic version of the Brief Fatigue Inventory (BFI-A). *East Mediterr Health J*. 2019;25(11):784–790. Published 2019 Nov 25. doi:10.26719/emhj.19.032.
25. Buysse DJ, Reynolds CF 3III Monk TH, Berman SR, Kupfer DJ. The Pittsburgh Sleep Quality Index: A new instrument for psychiatric practice and research. *Psychiatry Res*. 1989;28(2):193–213. doi:10.1016/0165-1781(89)90047-4.
26. Backhaus J, Junghanns K, Broocks A, Riemann D, Hohagen F. Test-retest reliability and validity of the Pittsburgh Sleep Quality Index in primary insomnia. *J Psychosom Res*. 2002;53(3):737–740. doi:10.1016/s0022-3999(02)00330-6.
27. Dietch JR, Taylor DJ, Sethi K, Kelly K, Bramoweth AD, Roane BM. Psychometric evaluation of the PSQI in U.S. college students. *J Clin Sleep Med*. 2016;12(8):1121–1129. doi:10.5664/jcsm.6050.
28. Purim KS, Guimarães AT, Titski AC, Leite N. Sleep deprivation and drowsiness of medical residents and medical students. *Rev Col Bras Cir*. 2016;43(6):438–444. doi:10.1590/0100-69912016006005.
29. Herrero San Martin A, Parra Serrano J, Diaz Cambriles T, et al. Sleep characteristics in health workers exposed to the COVID-19 pandemic. *Sleep Med*. 2020;75:388–394. doi:10.1016/j.sleep.2020.08.013.
30. Sohn SI, Kim DH, Lee MY, Cho YW. The reliability and validity of the Korean version of the Pittsburgh Sleep Quality Index. *Sleep Breath*. 2012;16(3):803–812. doi:10.1007/s11325-011-0579-9.
31. Curcio G, Tempesta D, Scarlata S, et al. Validity of the Italian version of the Pittsburgh Sleep Quality Index (PSQI). *Neurol Sci*. 2013;34(4):511–519. doi:10.1007/s10072-012-1085-y.
32. Weaver TE, Laizner AM, Evans LK, et al. An instrument to measure functional status outcomes for disorders of excessive sleepiness. *Sleep*. 1997;20(10):835–843.
33. Chasens ER, Ratcliffe SJ, Weaver TE. Development of the FOSQ-10: A short version of the Functional Outcomes of Sleep Questionnaire. *Sleep*. 2009;32(7):915–919. doi:10.1093/sleep/32.7.915.
34. Billings ME, Rosen CL, Auckley D, et al. Psychometric performance and responsiveness of the functional outcomes of sleep questionnaire and sleep apnea quality of life instrument in a randomized trial: The HomePAP study. *Sleep*. 2014;37(12):2017–2024. doi:10.5665/sleep.4262.
35. Puerta Y, García M, Heras E, et al. Sleep characteristics of the staff working in a pediatric intensive care unit based on a survey [published correction appears in *Front Pediatr*. 2018 Oct 10;6:287]. *Front Pediatr*. 2017;5:288. doi:10.3389/fped.2017.00288.
36. Vidal S, Ferrer M, Masuet C, Somoza M, Martínez Ballarín JI, Monasterio C. Valores de la versión española del Cuestionario del Impacto Funcional del Sueño (FOSQ) en sujetos sanos y en pacientes con apnea obstructiva del sueño [Spanish version of the Functional Outcomes of Sleep Questionnaire: Scores of healthy individuals and of patients with sleep apnea-hypopnea syndrome]. *Arch Bronconeumol*. 2007;43(5):256–261. doi:10.1016/s1579-2129(07)60063-9.
37. Korpe L, Lundgren J, Dahlström L. Psychometric evaluation of a Swedish version of the Functional Outcomes of Sleep Questionnaire, FOSQ. *Acta Odontol Scand*. 2013;71(5):1077–1084. doi:10.3109/00016357.2012.741708.
38. Rahavi-Ezabadi S, Amali A, Sadeghniiat-Haghighi K, Montazeri A. Adaptation of the 10-item Functional Outcomes of Sleep Questionnaire to Iranian patients with obstructive sleep apnea. *Qual Life Res*. 2016;25(2):337–341. doi:10.1007/s11136-015-1081-9.
39. Rey de Castro J, Rosales-Mayor E, Weaver TE. Reliability and validity of the Functional Outcomes of Sleep Questionnaire–Spanish Short Version (FOSQ-10SV) in Peruvian patients with obstructive sleep apnea. *J Clin Sleep Med*. 2018;14(4):615–621. doi:10.5664/jcsm.7056.

40. Wallace DM, Wohlgemuth WK. Does race-ethnicity moderate the relationship between CPAP adherence and functional outcomes of sleep in US veterans with obstructive sleep apnea syndrome? *J Clin Sleep Med*. 2014;10(10):1083–1091. doi:10.5664/jcsm.4106.
41. Horne JA, Ostberg O. A self-assessment questionnaire to determine morningness-eveningness in human circadian rhythms. *Int J Chronobiol*. 1976;4(2):97–110.
42. Danielsson K, Sakarya A, Jansson-Fröjmark M. The reduced Morningness-Eveningness Questionnaire: Psychometric properties and related factors in a young Swedish population. *Chronobiol Int*. 2019;36(4):530–540. doi:10.1080/07420528.2018.1564322.
43. Kanagarajan K, Gou K, Antinora C, et al. Morningness-Eveningness Questionnaire in bipolar disorder. *Psychiatry Res*. 2018;262:102–107. doi:10.1016/j.psychres.2018.02.004.
44. Kim LJ, Coelho FM, Hirotsu C, Bittencourt L, Tufik S, Andersen ML. Is the chronotype associated with obstructive sleep apnea? *Sleep Breath*. 2015;19(2):645–651. doi:10.1007/s11325-014-1070-1.
45. Palanichamy, PT. Morningness, eveningness chronotype traits and sleep quality among healthcare workers in shift work-a cross-sectional study from a tertiary care hospital in Kerala. *Int J Commun Med Public Health*. 2021;8(1):417-423. 10.18203/2394-6040.ijcmph20205732.
46. Cappadona R, Di Simone E, De Giorgi A, et al. Individual circadian preference, shift work, and risk of medication errors: A cross-sectional web survey among Italian midwives. *Int J Environ Res Public Health*. 2020;17(16):5810. doi:10.3390/ijerph17165810.
47. Díaz-Morales JF, Gutiérrez Sorroche M. Morningness-eveningness in adolescents. *Span J Psychol*. 2008;11(1):201–206. doi:10.1017/s1138741600004248.
48. Paine SJ, Gander PH, Travier N. The epidemiology of morningness/eveningness: Influence of age, gender, ethnicity, and socioeconomic factors in adults (30–49 years). *J Biol Rhythms*. 2006;21(1):68–76. doi:10.1177/0748730405283154.
49. Lee JH, Kim SJ, Lee SY, Jang KH, Kim IS, Duffy JF. Reliability and validity of the Korean version of Morningness-Eveningness Questionnaire in adults aged 20–39 years. *Chronobiol Int*. 2014;31(4):479–486. doi:10.3109/07420528.2013.867864.
50. Taillard J, Philip P, Chastang JF, Bioulac B. Validation of Horne and Ostberg Morningness-Eveningness Questionnaire in a middle-aged population of French workers. *J Biol Rhythms*. 2004;19(1):76–86. doi:10.1177/0748730403259849.
51. Douglass AB, Bornstein R, Nino-Murcia G, et al. The Sleep Disorders Questionnaire. I: Creation and multivariate structure of SDQ. *Sleep*. 1994;17(2):160–167. doi:10.1093/sleep/17.2.160.
52. Economou NT, Dikeos D, Andrews N, Foldvary-Schaefer N. Use of the Sleep Apnea Scale of the Sleep Disorders Questionnaire (SA-SDQ) in adults with epilepsy. *Epilepsy Behav*. 2014;31:123–126. doi:10.1016/j.yebeh.2013.12.006.
53. Sweere Y, Kerkhof GA, De Weerd AW, Kamphuisen HA, Kemp B, Schimsheimer RJ. The validity of the Dutch Sleep Disorders Questionnaire (SDQ). *J Psychosom Res*. 1998;45(6):549–555. doi:10.1016/s0022-3999(98)00030-0.
54. Tan A, Yin JD, Tan LW, van Dam RM, Cheung YY, Lee CH. Using the Berlin Questionnaire to predict obstructive sleep apnea in the general population. *J Clin Sleep Med*. 2017;13(3):427–432. doi:10.5664/jcsm.6496.
55. Netzer NC, Stoohs RA, Netzer CM, Clark K, Strohl KP. Using the Berlin Questionnaire to identify patients at risk for the sleep apnea syndrome. *Ann Intern Med*. 1999;131(7):485–491. doi:10.7326/0003-4819-131-7-199910050-00002.
56. Senaratna CV, Perret JL, Matheson MC, et al. Validity of the Berlin Questionnaire in detecting obstructive sleep apnea: A systematic review and meta-analysis. *Sleep Med Rev*. 2017;36:116–124. doi:10.1016/j.smrv.2017.04.001.
57. Chung F, Yegneswaran B, Liao P, et al. Validation of the Berlin Questionnaire and American Society of Anesthesiologists checklist as screening tools for obstructive sleep apnea in surgical patients. *Anesthesiology*. 2008;108(5):822–830. doi:10.1097/ALN.0b013e31816d91b5.
58. Best MW, Fitzpatrick M, Milev R, Bowie CR, Jokic R. Utility of the Berlin Questionnaire for predicting obstructive sleep apnea in individuals with treatment-resistant depression. *Sleep Breath*. 2013;17(4):1221–1227. doi:10.1007/s11325-013-0827-2.
59. Popević MB, Milovanović A, Nagorni-Obradović L, Nešić D, Milovanović J, Milovanović APS. Screening commercial drivers for obstructive sleep apnea: translation and validation of Serbian version of Berlin Questionnaire. *Qual Life Res*. 2016;25(2):343–349. doi:10.1007/s11136-015-1087-3.
60. Arunsurat I, Luengyosluechakul S, Prateephoungrat K, et al. Simplified Berlin Questionnaire for screening of high risk for obstructive sleep apnea among Thai male healthcare workers. *J UOEH*. 2016;38(3):199–206. doi:10.7888/juoeh.38.199.
61. Aydın Güçlü Ö, Karadağ M, İntepe YS, Acıcan T, Arslan S, Sertoğullarından B. Assessment of the risk of obstructive sleep apnoea syndrome among healthcare workers. Sağlık çalışanlarında obstrüktif uyku apne sendromu riskinin değerlendirilmesi. *Tuberk Toraks*. 2019;67(1):47–54. doi:10.5578/tt.68166.
62. Saleh AB, Ahmad MA, Awadalla NJ. Development of Arabic version of Berlin Questionnaire to identify obstructive sleep apnea at risk patients. *Ann Thorac Med*. 2011;6(4):212–216. doi:10.4103/1817-1737.84775.
63. Andrechuk CRS, Netzer N, Zancanella E, Almeida AR, Ceolim MF. Cultural adaptation and evaluation of the measurement properties of the Berlin Questionnaire for Brazil. *Sleep Med*. 2019;60:182–187. doi:10.1016/j.sleep.2019.03.022.
64. Sforza E, Chouchou F, Pichot V, Herrmann F, Barthélémy JC, Roche F. Is the Berlin Questionnaire a useful tool to diagnose obstructive sleep apnea in the elderly?. *Sleep Med*. 2011;12(2):142–146. doi:10.1016/j.sleep.2010.09.004.
65. Chung F, Yegneswaran B, Liao P, et al. STOP questionnaire: A tool to screen patients for obstructive sleep apnea. *Anesthesiology*. 2008;108(5):812–821. doi:10.1097/ALN.0b013e31816d83e4.
66. Chung F, Abdullah HR, Liao P. STOP-Bang Questionnaire: A practical approach to screen for obstructive sleep apnea. *Chest*. 2016;149(3):631–638. doi:10.1378/chest.15-0903.

67. Chiu HY, Chen PY, Chuang LP, et al. Diagnostic accuracy of the Berlin Questionnaire, STOP-BANG, STOP, and Epworth Sleepiness Scale in detecting obstructive sleep apnea: A bivariate meta-analysis. *Sleep Med Rev*. 2017;36:57–70. doi:10.1016/j.smrv.2016.10.004.
68. Nagappa M, Liao P, Wong J, et al. Validation of the STOP-Bang Questionnaire as a screening tool for obstructive sleep apnea among different populations: A systematic review and meta-analysis. *PLoS One*. 2015;10(12):e0143697. doi:10.1371/journal.pone.0143697.
69. Katzan IL, Thompson NR, Uchino K, Foldvary-Schaefer N. A screening tool for obstructive sleep apnea in cerebrovascular patients. *Sleep Med*. 2016;21:70–76. doi:10.1016/j.sleep.2016.02.001.
70. Pascoe M, Alberts J, Wang L, et al. Feasibility of electronic sleep disorder screening in healthcare workers of a large healthcare system. *Sleep Med*. 2020;73:181–186. doi:10.1016/j.sleep.2020.07.028.
71. BaHammam AS, Al-Aqeel AM, Alhedyani AA, Al-Obaid GI, Al-Owais MM, Olaish AH. The validity and reliability of an Arabic version of the STOP-Bang Questionnaire for identifying obstructive sleep apnea. *Open Respir Med J*. 2015;9:22–29. doi:10.2174/1874306401509010022.
72. Delgado-Vargas B, Acle-Cervera L, Narciso López G. Validation of the Spanish Version of the STOP-Bang Questionnaire: Usefulness as a screening tool for obstructive sleep apnea in adults. *Ear Nose Throat J*. 2021;100(10_suppl). doi:10.1177/0145561320932334.
73. Ha SC, Lee DL, Abdullah VJ, van Hasselt CA. Evaluation and validation of four translated Chinese questionnaires for obstructive sleep apnea patients in Hong Kong. *Sleep Breath*. 2014;18(4):715–721. doi:10.1007/s11325-013-0889-1.
74. Flemons WW, Reimer MA. Development of a disease-specific health-related quality of life questionnaire for sleep apnea. *Am J Respir Crit Care Med*. 1998;158(2):494–503. doi:10.1164/ajrccm.158.2.9712036.
75. Flemons WW, Reimer MA. Measurement properties of the Calgary Sleep Apnea Quality of Life Index. *Am J Respir Crit Care Med*. 2002;165(2):159–164. doi:10.1164/ajrccm.165.2.2010008.
76. Batool-Anwar S, Goodwin JL, Kushida CA, et al. Impact of continuous positive airway pressure (CPAP) on quality of life in patients with obstructive sleep apnea (OSA). *J Sleep Res*. 2016;25(6):731–738. doi:10.1111/jsr.12430.
77. Catalán P, Martínez A, Herrejón A, et al. Internal consistency and validity of the Spanish version of the Quality of Life Questionnaire specific for obstructive sleep apnea: Sleep Apnea Quality of Life Index. *Arch Bronconeumol*. 2012;48(12):431–442. doi:10.1016/j.arbres.2012.05.004.
78. Rahavi-Ezabadi S, Amali A, Sadeghniiat-Haghighi K, Montazeri A, Nedjat S. Translation, cultural adaptation, and validation of the Sleep Apnea Quality of Life Index (SAQLI) in Persian-speaking patients with obstructive sleep apnea. *Sleep Breath*. 2016;20(2):523–528. doi:10.1007/s11325-015-1228-5.
79. U.S. Department of Veterans Affairs. Insomnia Severity Index. https://www.myhealth.va.gov/mhv-portal-web/insomnia-severity-index.
80. Morin CM, Belleville G, Bélanger L, Ivers H. The Insomnia Severity Index: Psychometric indicators to detect insomnia cases and evaluate treatment response. *Sleep*. 2011;34(5):601–608. doi:10.1093/sleep/34.5.601.
81. Bastien CH, Vallières A, Morin CM. Validation of the Insomnia Severity Index as an outcome measure for insomnia research. *Sleep Med*. 2001;2(4):297–307. doi:10.1016/s1389-9457(00)00065-4.
82. Gagnon C, Bélanger L, Ivers H, Morin CM. Validation of the Insomnia Severity Index in primary care. *J Am Board Fam Med*. 2013;26(6):701–710. doi:10.3122/jabfm.2013.06.130064.
83. Doghramji K, Tanielian M, Certa K, Zhan T. Severity, prevalence, predictors, and rate of identification of insomnia symptoms in a sample of hospitalized psychiatric patients. *J Nerv Ment Dis*. 2018 Oct;206(10):765-769. doi:10.1097/NMD.0000000000000888. PMID: 30273272.
84. Omachi TA. Measures of sleep in rheumatologic diseases: Epworth Sleepiness Scale (ESS), Functional Outcome of Sleep Questionnaire (FOSQ), Insomnia Severity Index (ISI), and Pittsburgh Sleep Quality Index (PSQI). *Arthritis Care Res (Hoboken)*. 2011;63(Suppl 11):S287–S296. doi:10.1002/acr.20544.
85. Alqudah M, Balousha SAM, Al-Shboul O, Al-Dwairi A, Alfaqih MA, Alzoubi KH. Insomnia among medical and paramedical students in Jordan: Impact on academic performance. *Biomed Res Int*. 2019;2019:7136906. doi:10.1155/2019/7136906.
86. Sunwoo JS, Shin DS, Hwangbo Y, et al. High risk of obstructive sleep apnea, insomnia, and daytime sleepiness among commercial motor vehicle drivers. *Sleep Breath*. 2019;23(3):979–985. doi:10.1007/s11325-019-01805-7.
87. Castronovo V, Galbiati A, Marelli S, et al. Validation study of the Italian version of the Insomnia Severity Index (ISI). *Neurol Sci*. 2016;37(9):1517–1524. doi:10.1007/s10072-016-2620-z.
88. Lahan V, Gupta R. Translation and validation of the insomnia severity index in hindi language. *Indian J Psychol Med*. 2011;33(2):172–176. doi:10.4103/0253-7176.92060.
89. Narcolepsy Link. Swiss Narcolepsy Scale. https://www.narcolepsylink.com/screening-and-diagnosis/swiss-narcolepsy-scale/. Accessed May 12, 2021.
90. Sturzenegger C, Baumann CR, Lammers GJ, Kallweit U, van der Zande WLM, Bassetti CL. Swiss Narcolepsy Scale. *Clin Transl Neurosci*. 2018;2(2):1–5. doi:10.1177/2514183x18794175.
91. Bargiotas P, Dietmann A, Haynes AG, et al. The Swiss Narcolepsy Scale (SNS) and its short form (sSNS) for the discrimination of narcolepsy in patients with hypersomnolence: A cohort study based on the Bern Sleep-Wake Database. *J Neurol*. 2019;266(9):2137–2143. doi:10.1007/s00415-019-09365-2.
92. Beck AT, Epstein N, Brown G, Steer RA. An inventory for measuring clinical anxiety: Psychometric properties. *J Consult Clin Psychol*. 1988;56:893–897.
93. Kaufmann CN, Susukida R, Depp CA. Sleep apnea, psychopathology, and mental health care. *Sleep Health*. 2017;3(4):244–249. doi:10.1016/j.sleh.2017.04.003.
94. Chueh KH, Chen KR, Lin YH. Psychological distress and sleep disturbance among female nurses: Anxiety

or depression? *J Transcult Nurs*. 2021;32(1):14–20. doi:10.1177/1043659619881491.

95. Korkmaz S, Kazgan A, Çekiç S, Tartar AS, Balcı HN, Atmaca M. The anxiety levels, quality of sleep and life and problem-solving skills in healthcare workers employed in COVID-19 services. *J Clin Neurosci*. 2020;80:131–136. doi:10.1016/j.jocn.2020.07.073.
96. Magán I, Sanz J, García-Vera MP. Psychometric properties of a Spanish version of the Beck Anxiety Inventory (BAI) in general population. *Span J Psychol*. 2008;11(2):626–640.
97. American Psychology Association. Beck Depression Inventory (BDI). https://www.apa.org/pi/about/publications/caregivers/practice-settings/assessment/tools/beck-depression. January 2011.
98. Beck AT, Steer RA, Brown G. Beck Depression Inventory–II [Database record]. *APA PsycTests*. 1996. https://www.thoracic.org/members/assemblies/assemblies/srn/questionaires/bdi-ii.php. Accessed April 29, 2025.
99. American Thoracic Society. Beck Depression Inventory-II (BDI-II). https://www.thoracic.org/members/assemblies/assemblies/srn/questionaires/bdi-ii.php. Accessed May 12, 2021.
100. Richter P, Werner J, Heerlein A, Kraus A, Sauer H. On the validity of the Beck Depression Inventory. A review. *Psychopathology*. 1998;31(3):160–168. doi:10.1159/000066239.
101. Karamanlı H, Kayhan F, Akgedik R. Depressive symptoms in patients with obstructive sleep apnea. *Turk Thorac J*. 2016;17(3):109–113. doi:10.5578/ttj.30506.
102. da Silva-Júnior FP, de Pinho RS, de Mello MT, de Bruin VM, de Bruin PF. Risk factors for depression in truck drivers. *Soc Psychiatry Psychiatr Epidemiol*. 2009;44(2):125-129. doi:10.1007/s00127-008-0412-3.
103. García-Batista ZE, Guerra-Peña K, Cano-Vindel A, Herrera-Martínez SX, Medrano LA. Validity and reliability of the Beck Depression Inventory (BDI-II) in general and hospital population of Dominican Republic. *PLoS One*. 2018;13(6):e0199750. doi:10.1371/journal.pone.0199750.
104. Lee EH, Lee SJ, Hwang ST, Hong SH, Kim JH. Reliability and validity of the Beck Depression Inventory-II among Kor.ean adolescents. *Psychiatry Investig*. 2017;14(1):30–36. doi:10.4306/pi.2017.14.1.30
105. Mapi Research Trust. Clinical Global Impressions Scale: Improvement, Severity, Change and Efficacy (CGI-I, CGI-S, CGI-C and CGI-E). https://eprovide.mapi-trust.org/instruments/clinical-global-impressions-scale-improvement-severity-change-and-efficacy#need_this_questionnaire. Accessed May 12, 2021.
106. Busner J, Targum SD. The Clinical Global Impressions Scale: Applying a research tool in clinical practice. *Psychiatry (Edgmont)*. 2007;4(7):28–37.
107. Forkmann T, Scherer A, Boecker M, Pawelzik M, Jostes R, Gauggel S. The Clinical Global Impression Scale and the influence of patient or staff perspective on outcome. *BMC Psychiatry*. 2011;11:83. doi:10.1186/1471-244X-11-83.
108. Dieltjens M, Verbraecken JA, Hedner J, et al. Use of the Clinical Global Impression Scale in sleep apnea patients: Results from the ESADA database. *Sleep Med*. 2019;59:56–65. doi:10.1016/j.sleep.2018.10.028.
109. Mohebbi M, Dodd S, Dean OM, Berk M. Patient centric measures for a patient centric era: Agreement and convergent between ratings on The Patient Global Impression of Improvement (PGI-I) Scale and the Clinical Global Impressions-Improvement (CGI-S) Scale in bipolar and major depressive disorder. *Eur Psychiatry*. 2018;53:17–22. doi:10.1016/j.eurpsy.2018.05.006.

Chapter 23

Laboratory and Non-Laboratory Sleep Testing

David Kuhlmann

INTRODUCTION

Polysomnography is singularly responsible for the development of sleep medicine as a scientific discipline. Before the objective measures that polysomnography provided, sleep was unable to be studied. It is therefore not surprising that the history of polysomnography is also the history of modern-day sleep medicine. Well into the 20th century, the predominant view of sleep was that it was a time of mental inactivity, prompting the eminent Irish surgeon, Robert J. Graves, to state that sleep was "the daily rehearsal of our death."[1p377] Even the grandfather of the electroencephalogram (EEG), Hans Berger, was hesitant to disclose his findings of electrical activity in the brain during sleep for fear of being scientifically dismissed. The chapter begins by exploring how a man trying to harness "psychic energy"[2] created the EEG, and then turns to how the early researchers in sleep medicine expanded on this tool to be able to stage sleep and create what is now known as polysomnography. The chapter will give historical background on some of the disorders that polysomnography has come to diagnose. The chapter will conclude by giving a history of home sleep apnea testing and providing possible future directions for sleep testing.

HISTORY OF POLYSOMNOGRAPHY

Englishman Richard Caton was the first to view electrical activity in the brains of animals. Caton had hypothesized that because recordable action potentials had recently been documented in peripheral nerves, the brain might produce electrical signals as well.[3] Using a mirror galvanometer, Caton placed electrodes on the exposed brains of rabbits and monkeys and detected electrical current. In the abstract of his presentation to the British Medical Association in 1875, Caton wrote, "Feeble currents of varying direction pass through the multiplier when the electrodes are placed on two points of the external surface, or one electrode on the gray matter, and one on the surface of the skull."[4p278] Two years later, he would prove that these signals could be detected through surface electrodes. He also noted that these electrical currents changed with sleep.[5] Despite being the first to detect electrical activity in the brain, these accomplishments were largely unrecognized in his academic life, and were not mentioned in obituaries upon his death in 1926.[6]

Caton's work was taken up by the most unlikely of champions. Whereas the physiologist Caton was renowned for his life of science and public service, culminating in his becoming lord major of Liverpool,[7] German psychiatrist Hans Berger was more socially awkward and solitary, performing decades of research with minimal assistance.[8] Berger's initial interest in the electrical activity of the brain may have stemmed from an equestrian accident.

At the age of 18 years, on maneuvers with the German army, Berger had a near fatal accident and, at the same time, hundreds of miles away, his sister told their father that Hans was in grave danger and the father sent him a telegram. Berger then became a firm believer in psychic phenomena or telepathy, providing his great motivation to record from the human brain.[9]

Like Caton before him, Berger initially worked to detect the brainwaves of animals. However, in 1924, Berger began to look at human beings with skull defects, hypothesizing that he could better detect the brain's electrical current with more direct access. After noticing faint electrical activity, Berger spent the subsequent 5 years refining his tools and methods, culminating in his seminal work, Über das Elektroenkephalogramm des Menschen.[5] Berger would go on to write over a dozen articles on the subject of EEG, continuing to use his own notes as reference after his lab was disassembled by the Nazis in 1935.[9] Berger is credited for coining the term *electroencephalogram*, and with discovering both sleep spindles[10] and alpha (or Berger) waves, which were present when the subject relaxed with his eyes closed and disappeared with sleep onset.

Berger's discovery of electrical activity in the brain was initially viewed with much skepticism among his contemporaries. "The nearby Berlin-Buch neurophysiology group, who likely possessed the finest recording instrumentation in the world, considered Berger a misguided, nonphysiologist with limited technical knowledge and support."[9] However, when Berger's findings were confirmed by Nobel Prize–winner Lord Edgar Adrian of England in 1933, there soon was a keen interest in the new EEG technology.

In the United States, a postgraduate student of Adrian's, Hallowell Davis, was among the notable electrophysiologists to confirm Berger's alpha waves while at Harvard Medical School.[11]

> I went with them to the lab and Bill stuck needles into Howard's scalp. Howard sat in the shielded room and closed his eyes. The spot wobbled unsteadily across the scope. That's what I thought, I said, but three heads are better than two. Put the electrodes on my head. They did, and I sat in the room and closed my eyes. Immediately there were shouts outside: There it is! There it is! It was indeed the Berger rhythm. It seems that I have very strong alpha waves. Bill's and Howard's are weaker, and they were excited, anxious, and perhaps more uncomfortable than I was. . . . We were convinced Berger was right. It was some time later that we learned that Adrian had already confirmed him; but at least my alpha rhythm was the first to be recognized as such in the Western Hemisphere.[9p33]

The work on EEG by Davis at Harvard Medical School caught the attention of Alfred Loomis, who had combined his interest in science with his vast fortune to create a state-of-the-art sleep laboratory in Tuxedo Park, New York, in the 1920s. Rivaling the technology of any university labs of the day, the room had "adequate sleeping space, infrared photography, microphones, and a large drum—three-channel ink-writing oscillograph for prolonged recordings."[9p37] Loomis and colleagues most notable accomplishments to Sleep Medicine were the identification of EEG waveforms during sleep, and developing a staging system for sleep.

A new type of push-pull amplifier system, especially designed to record accurately the large slow potentials, was used to study the potential patterns of sleep. Five states of sleep characterized by marked differences in potential could be recognized. They are A, alpha; B, low voltage; C, spindle; D, spindle and random; E, random; in order of appearance and in order of resistance to change by disturbances.[12]

The Loomis Laboratory in Tuxedo Park hosted intellectual greats of the time, such as Albert Einstein, Niels Bohr, and Enrico Fermi. The Conference on the Electrical Potentials of the Brain, which was surely the first gathering of neurophysiologists, also took place at Tuxedo Park in 1935. Like Berger, Loomis's work on the EEG was cut short by World War II. However, unlike Berger who was forced to stop his experiments, Loomis donated his EEG equipment to Harvard Medical School, and created the Massachusetts Institute of Technology's Radiation Laboratory. It is believed that Loomis's work with radar, long-range navigation, and ground-controlled approach (allowing planes to land in bad weather) was instrumental in shortening World War II.[13]

The Discovery of Rapid Eye Movement (REM) Sleep

> As normal blinking is involuntary, it might be expected that blinking would proceed at its normal or at a somewhat reduced rate during sleep, as with breathing and the heart-beat. This is not so, however, though little seems to have been published on the subject, especially on the quantitative side. Whereas many of the muscles are relaxed during sleep, "the muscular tone of the muscles which keep the eyes closed is undoubtedly increased."[14p81]

Thus begins the article written in the journal *Nature* in 1950 that gave Nathaniel Kleitman the idea to look at the role of eye movements in sleep onset.[15] Kleitman, who created the first sleep research lab at the University of Chicago in the 1920s and wrote the first authoritative text on sleep, *Sleep and Wakefulness*, in the 1930s, asked his graduate student, Eugene Aserinsky, to study the relationship between blinking rate and sleep. Through his research, Aserinsky learned about the difference in electrical potential between the cornea and the retina. He was able to obtain an Offner Dynograph (a type of oscilloscope that can graph electric current over time)[16] to measure both eye movements with electrooculography (EOG) and brainwaves with electroencephalography (EEG). Unfortunately, because of the significant artifact associated with using the oscillograph to measure the voltage from both EOG and EEG leads, he was unable to conclusively show what happens to the eyes when the eyelids were shut during sleep. It nearly doomed his research. Then he had an idea:

> By comparing the phase and amplitude of two channels simultaneously I would surely eliminate certain artifacts. Comparing the left and right eye channels should identify the horizontal component of binocular movements, while a comparison of the frontal EEG with the vertical component of the EOG on the same side would identify a vertical movement.[15]

Having now invented an EOG capable of detecting eye movements during sleep with significantly less artifact, Aserinsky returned to studying the sleep of his 8-year-old son, Armond. He was the first to be able to notice the saccadic-like eye movement during REM sleep.[17] Initially wanting to call it "Jerky Eye Movement periods," he settled on "Rapid Eye Movement periods" because of negative connotations of the word "jerk."[15] The discovery of REM sleep was monumental to sleep research, as it confirmed both that sleep is an active brain process, and that it has two distinct states: REM and non-rapid eye movement (NREM) sleep.

In the autumn of 1952, a medical student by the name of William Dement joined Kleitman's sleep lab to assist Aserinsky with his research on REM sleep. An aspiring Freudian psychoanalyst, Dement was hooked by the possibility that this newly discovered stage of sleep may lead to the ability to interpret dreams.[18] Like many of his day, Dement believed that by analyzing the dream content from REM sleep, psychoanalysts might be able to better treat patients with mental disorders. In fact, the pervasiveness of this belief among early sleep researchers led to the formation of the Association for the Psychophysiological Study of Sleep (APSS), the first sleep medicine society, in 1964. While Dement's theory that selective REM sleep deprivation would lead to psychosis was ultimately disproven,[19] Dement nevertheless contributed significantly to polysomnographic research. His most significant research contribution was the discovery that REM sleep had an ultradian rhythm.[20] He also created a new sleep staging system for EEG that, unlike the Loomis staging system, incorporated REM sleep.

POLYSOMNOGRAPHY FOR THE DIAGNOSIS OF SLEEP DISORDERS

It was not only for his research prowess that Dement became recognized as "the father of sleep medicine." Dement understood that this new tool of polysomnography had more than just research applications.

Narcolepsy

Before the advent of polysomnography, narcolepsy was already a well-known syndrome. Sleepiness attributed to this syndrome was first described by Thomas Willis in 1672,[21] while Jean Baptiste Edouard Gellineau coined the term "narcolepsy" and described the "astasisa," or cataplexy associated with the syndrome in 1880.[22] Robert Yoss and David Daly of the Mayo Clinic completed the clinical tetrad in 1960 by incorporating previous findings that hypnagogic hallucinations and sleep paralysis were linked to the condition.[23],[24]

The presence of potential polysomnographic changes associated with narcolepsy were first noted by Gerald Vogel.[25] Vogel noted that patients with narcolepsy, unlike those without narcolepsy, would not always go through a full 90-minute NREM sleep cycle before entering REM sleep. "Narcoleptics also showed more body movements, the presence of 9-11 c/sec. activity in anterior EEG leads, and a tendency to have less than a normal amount of large slow wave activity."[26] Dement, who opened his Narcolepsy Clinic at Stanford in 1964, would perform a single nap study looking for a sleep-onset REM period (SOREMP).[27] Because this was viewed as an experimental procedure, it was not reimbursed by insurance, causing the narcolepsy clinic to fold. When Dement re-established the Sleep Research Center at Stanford in 1970, he followed insomnia as well as narcolepsy patients. All patients had an overnight sleep study and a single nap period in the daytime, looking for a SOREMP. With the help of Mary Carskadon, the Multiple Sleep Latency Test (MSLT) was subsequently standardized in 1976[28] and became the primary test used to diagnose patients with narcolepsy.[29,30]

Because the MSLT looks at a patient's tendency to fall asleep rather than their ability to stay awake, researchers created 2 offshoots of the MSLT in attempts to standardize a scale for vigilance. The Repeated Test of Sustained Wakefulness (RTSW)[31] and Maintenance of Wakefulness Test (MWT)[32] consisted of a series of "nap opportunities" in dimly lit conditions, with the patient laying in a bed or sitting up in a recliner, respectively. The conditions of the MWT were later standardized to having the patient lay propped up in bed.[33] The MWT never enjoyed as widespread usage as the MSLT, in part because the MWT is not required for any clinical diagnosis. There also continues to be some discrepancy with how the test should be performed, with sleep-latencies of MWTs being used in research but any sleep on an MWT being considered a failed test in clinical settings. In addition, there continues to be some disagreement as to whether a polysomnogram should be performed prior to MWT.[34]

Impotence

In 1944, Paul Ohlmeyer and colleagues noted that during sleep, men tended to have an erection approximately once every 85 minutes that would last for about 25 minutes.[35] Recognizing that REM sleep follows a similar pattern, Ian Oswald,[36] Charles Fisher, and others[37] began in the 1960s to look into the relationship of sleep-related erections (SRE) to dreaming. They noted that generally an SRE tended to occur a few minutes before or after the onset of atonia during REM sleep. In 1970, Ishmet Karacan suggested that the nocturnal penile tumescence (NPT) test could provide an objective measure of impotence.[38] Karacan's theory was that if the patient could have erections during REM sleep, then the underlying impotence is likely psychogenic in nature. This led to the NPT being performed frequently during polysomnography the 1970s and 1980s, to help determine if a patient was a candidate for a penile implant.

The NPT test consisted of fitting mercury strain gauges around the shaft and corona of the penis. The gauges worked as a plethysmograph as blood filled the area. "An episode of NPT was defined as a gradual increase in base circumference corresponding to a change in pen deflection of ~3 mm over a 60-s period and persisting for at least 5 minutes."[39p369] The SREs could be referenced to the hypnogram and were measured in millimeters both by the gauges and on the actual polysomnogram. Measurements included *Tup* (onset of tumescence), time of maximal circumference increase, *Tdown* (time of onset of detumescence), and *Tzero* (ending time of detumescence). The number of episodes, total tumescence time, and index of *Tmax* (period of maximum circumference) to REM sleep could also be calculated. Multiple nights were frequently needed, as the first night was often used for adaptation to the equipment. NPT research was helpful in gaining a better understanding of the sexuality of aging in men, with the number of episodes and size of the SRE remaining relatively constant, but the minutes of the SRE and the rigidity gradually decreasing with age.[40p816]

There were several problems with the NPT testing, including subjectivity in scoring[41] and lack of normative data.[39] The NPT test measured rigidity, but did not always measure buckling force, which is required for penetration.[42] Other non-organic causes of impotence could impact the NPT test, particularly major depression. Finally, the very premise that if an erection occurs during sleep then the cause of impotence must be psychogenic has been questioned.[43,44] Ultimately, with medications to treat impotence such as papaverine and sildenafil becoming available in the 1990s, the demand for penile implants, and subsequently NPT testing, diminished.

REM Sleep Behavior Disorder (RBD)

REM sleep is named after its characteristic eye movements, first discovered on EOG by Aserinsky and Kleitman. However, the 2 other polysomnographic findings of REM sleep—a desynchronized brainwave pattern on EEG, and muscle atonia on electromyography (EMG)—were discovered by the French neurosurgeon Louis Jouvet. Jouvet, who had trained in the laboratory of Horace Magoun,[45] was working on decorticate cats in hopes of disproving the era's prevailing belief that sleep was a passive process caused by a lack of sensory input. In his experiments, Jouvet noticed that the decorticate cats had a significant decrease in nuchal tone on EMG despite having an EEG that was more like wakefulness.[46] In addition to the muscle atonia, Jouvet noted that behavioral arousals required more stimulation compared to the other sleep states. For this reason, he described REM sleep as paradoxical sleep. Over the next decade, Jouvet would work on delineating areas of the brain responsible for sleep and wakefulness. He discovered that the pons was entirely responsible for paradoxical sleep, and that lesions to the pontine tegmentum could cause paradoxical sleep without atonia.[47]

Jouvet's model of REM sleep without atonia was confirmed clinically by Carlos Schenk and Mark Mahowald in 1986:

> Polysomnography did not detect seizures but did document REM sleep pathology with variable loss of chin atonia, extraordinarily increased limb-twitch activity, and increased REM ocular activity and density. A broad range of REM sleep behaviors was recorded on videotape, including stereotypical hand motions, reaching and searching gestures, punches, kicks, and verified dream movements.[48p293]

The disorder, which came to be known as REM sleep behavior disorder (RBD), has since become intertwined with the progression of synucleinopathies such as Parkinson disease and Lewy body dementia,[49] and raises the importance of the diagnosis of sleep disorders in neurologic disease.

Obstructive Sleep Apnea (OSA)

In 1836, Charles Dickens wrote his first novel, *The Posthumous Papers of the Pickwick Club*. In the novel, Dickens describes "Fat Joe," a boy with classical symptoms of obstructive sleep apnea (OSA), including snoring and daytime sleepiness.[50] The father of modern medicine, Sir William Osler, referenced Dicken's description of the boy in *The Principles and Practice of Medicine*, "An extraordinary phenomenon in excessively fat young persons is an uncontrollable tendency to sleep—like the fat boy in Pickwick. It is quite possible that this narcolepsy is also a manifestation of disturbed internal secretions."[51p451] Charles Sydney Burwell, a cardiologist and former dean of Harvard Medical School, later popularized the term "Pickwickian syndrome," but falsely attributed the sleepiness to obesity hypoventilation syndrome rather than OSA.[52] Ironically, Burwell, who got the assessment of sleepiness in the morbidly obese half-right, was also famously quoted as saying to incoming medical students, "Half of what we are going to teach you is wrong, and half of it is right. Our problem is that we don't know which half is which."[53]

Early researchers in polysomnography tried to reconcile the sleepiness experienced in the morbidly obese with the carbon dioxide retention of obesity hypoventilation syndrome.[54,55] In 1965, two European studies, one by the renowned French epileptologist Henri Gastaut,[56] and the other by German neurologists Richard Jung and Wolfgang Kuhlo,[57] hypothesized that it was interruptions from sleep, not carbon dioxide retention, that was responsible for sleepiness.[58] Both groups are credited with discovering OSA.[59]

During the 1960s and early 1970s, OSA went largely overlooked in the United States, as sleep labs, predominantly focused on dream research, used only EEG and EOG. They did not incorporate signals for measuring respiratory effort. That all changed in 1972 when Frenchman Christian Guilleminault joined Stanford as a visiting professor. He suggested that the Stanford lab add respiratory channels, including an ear oximeter, a buccal thermistor, and thoracic and abdominal belts.[60] Guilleminault would go on to coin the term "obstructive sleep apnea" and create the apnea hypopnea index (AHI) to measure sleep-disordered breathing.

HOME SLEEP TESTING

The artificial environment of sleep laboratories was not lost on the early practitioners of polysomnography. Because of both the artificial surroundings and the significant amount of equipment required for patient hook-up, sleep laboratories would often have patients stay at least 2 nights in the sleep lab to account for "first night effect." In attempts to try to get a better sense of a patient's sleep in their home setting, some laboratories equipped recreational vehicles with polysomnographic equipment and would string the wires from their vehicles into the patient's bedroom.[61] Telephone transmission of EEG signal from home to lab was utilized,[62] but was limited by the quality of the land line. As the incidence of sleep disorders became apparent, practitioners began looking for other ways to evaluate sleep disorders outside of the laboratory.

Actigraphy

One of the earliest devices used in home sleep research was the actigraph.[63] Historically worn on the non-dominant wrist,[64] the actigraph is a multi-directional accelerometer capable of discerning between sleep and wakefulness based on movement. Daniel Kripke, who first referred to the device as an actigraph, utilized a piezoelectric transducer, which can convert the pressure from movement into measurable voltage. While the initial output of an actigraph was on a tape recorder,[65] digitalization allowed for the computer display of raw data from actigraphs beginning in the 1990s.[66]

Home Sleep Apnea Testing

Recognizing both the high prevalence of OSA and the cost of diagnosis with polysomnography, Sonia Ancoli-Israel, Kripke, and colleagues created one of the first home sleep apnea tests (HSAT) in 1980.[67] They fitted their 4-channel Medilog™ portable analog recorder with actigraphy, tibialis EMG, and two Respitrace™ respiratory inductance plethysmography (RIP) belts. Their device compared favorably to polysomnography for diagnosing OSA, with a sensitivity in the home setting of 78%.

There were significant technical impediments for early HSAT devices. They had limited internal and external memory, which impacted how much data could be collected. Suboptimal amplification technology limited the quality of the recording. Finally, difficulty converting analog signal to digital output and long retrieval times limited the utility of the early HSAT devices.[68] However, the combination of improving microprocessing technology and more widespread availability of continuous positive airway pressure (CPAP) in the late 1980s and early 1990s led to a significant increase in the number of HSAT devices on the market.

By 1994, there were at least 27 devices that could be used in an off-site setting.[69] Since many of these HSAT devices utilized different numbers and types of sensors, the American Sleep Disorders Association (ASDA, later to be called the American Academy of Sleep Medicine [AASM]) created a practice guideline for the emerging use of portable recording. They grouped sleep apnea evaluation studies into 1 of 4 categories. Type I was attended polysomnography with at least 7 channels; type II was unattended polysomnography with at least 7 channels; type III was unattended portable sleep apnea test with at least 4 channels, including to respiratory channels; and type IV was at least 1 bioparameter recording. The task force determined that while attended type III studies had high sensitivity and specificity for OSA, there was not sufficient peer-reviewed, validated studies for the use of type III and type IV studies in the unattended setting. A second ASDA Polysomnography Task Force,[70] the Agency for Healthcare Research and Quality,[71] and a collaboration between the AASM, American College of Chest Physicians, and the American Thoracic Society[72,73] all came up with similar findings, resulting in the Centers for Medicare & Medicaid Services (CMS) denying coverage for HSAT in 2005.[74]

However, throughout the 1990s, technology for both polysomnography and HSAT devices improved significantly, resulting in increased storage and decreased processing times. The output of sleep testing shifted from paper to computer based. The inputs also improved as nasal pressure transducers began to replace nasal thermistors and RIP belts began to replace piezo electric belts. With increased technological advances came more studies on HSAT devices, including a new type of HSAT device that showed promise in diagnosing OSA through a novel mechanism. The WatchPAT™ plethysmograph purported to be able to diagnose OSA by measuring the pulsatile blood flow pressure changes through a probe on the fingertip.[75] The 2 major problems with the device were that it had output that was much more difficult to interpret, and it only met the classification as a type IV device since it had less than 4 channels.

With the changes in technology that had taken place, the American Academy of Otolaryngology-Head and Neck Surgery requested that CMS resurvey the coverage determination for CPAP to include HSAT.[76] Also motivating a CMS resurvey of HSAT was a 2006 Institute of Medicine report highlighting the scarcity of sleep medicine resources.[77] The resulting CMS National Coverage Determination (NCD) in 20007 allowed for the use of HSAT so long as the study was performed by an accredited sleep center.[78]

In anticipation of the changes, the AASM put together a portable monitoring task force to determine the appropriate indications for HSAT and devices that could be used.[79] At that time, they determined that HSAT should not be utilized in patients with comorbid sleep disorders, or with moderate to severe pulmonary disease, neuromuscular disease, or congestive heart failure. They also concluded, "At a minimum, the PMs (portable monitors) must record airflow, respiratory effort, and blood oxygenation." Since the WatchPAT™ neither had these channels, nor had the ability to manually score raw data, it was not included in the initial list of recommended devices.

Recognizing that new scoring and classification systems for HSAT devices were needed, the AASM assembled another task force to devise a way to categorize both current and future technology.[80] In addition to introducing the term "respiratory event index (REI)," which divided total apneas and hypopneas by total recording time, the committee developed a system for categorizing HSAT devices based on how they measure Sleep, Cardiovascular, Oximetry, Position, Effort and Respiratory (SCOPER) parameters. While the system proved to be much more inclusive for all HSAT devices, it was also more complicated for the clinician to navigate.[81] As a result, the older terminology of type I–IV devices continues to be utilized.

FUTURE DIRECTIONS

With a better understanding in the general population of how sleep can impact health, there has been an explosion of interest in sleep and activity monitoring. Gaining an understanding of how emerging technologies work may allow for sleep testing to provide value added services, better patient experiences, or even new discoveries for the field.

An example of a technology that could potentially be applied to sleep testing is the photoplethysmograph (PPG). A plethysmograph measures changes in volume in the body. Respiratory inductance plethysmography (RIP) belts, which indirectly measure respiratory ventilation through changes in the anterior poster (AP) diameter of the chest and abdomen during breathing, is a plethysmograph already utilized in polysomnography. As the name would suggest, a photoplethysmograph uses optics to measures blood volume changes by emitting low intensity light through the skin.[82] As blood can absorb light better than the surrounding tissue, the photoplethysmograph is able to sense changes in blood volume. This application could potentially measure blood pressure, cardiac output, heart rate variability, endothelial function, and more.[65,83] A new wireless sternal biopatch has a microchip that contains PPG as well as a seismocardiogram (recording of body vibrations induced by beat), electrocardiogram, and accelerometer. The device, which researchers state meet all SCOPER criteria for home sleep apnea testing, uses deep learning (a type of artificial intelligence that uses neural networks to "learn" from responses to computer algorithms) to score an AHI.[84]

PPG technology is also being used in many of the new wearable technologies such as the Fitbit™ and Apple Watch.™ In addition to PPG technology, the devices have a triaxial accelerometer for activity and sleep measurements. The Oura™ ring uses PPG and skin temperature, and was found to be sensitive for detecting sleep stage, but not specific for detecting wake episodes, compared to polysomnography.[85]

Another sensor that may be capable of differentiating sleep from wakefulness is impulse radio ultra-wideband (IR-UWB) radar sensors.[86] Placed under a mattress, nearby the patient, or embedded on the ceiling, IR-UWB sensors send and receive brief (sub-nanosecond)[87] low-energy radio waves to discern body position. Unlike actigraphy, IR-UWB does not have to be worn on the wrist and can be continuously monitored. In addition to detecting large body movements, IR-UWB may be able to detect small body movements such as breathing and heart rate. IR-UWB may even potentially be used in the future to diagnose obstructive sleep apnea[88,89] and Cheyne Stokes respirations.[90]

A potentially new ways of diagnosing OSA in the home setting is the cardiopulmonary coupling (CPC) device,[91] which uses a PPG or ECG sensors to determine heart and breathing rates. The device then uses an algorithm to assess the relationship between the autonomic and respiratory oscillations. Normally, heart rate will increase or decrease based on rate of breathing. The 2 become less synchronized in times of breathing instability. Whereas NREM sleep and deeper sleep tend to have more breathing stability (high-frequency coupling), REM sleep and wakefulness are more unstable (low-frequency coupling). If a patient exhibits excessive low frequency coupling, it could be an indicator of sleep fragmentation or events of sleep-disordered breathing.

CONCLUSION

Breakthroughs in technology in the 20th century such as EEG and EOG led to the realization that sleep was not a passive process. With the discovery of polysomnography, we have gained a better understanding of sleep and its clinical disorders. However, while technology continues to evolve, polysomnography has remained mostly unchanged in the past 50 years. Advancements in technology have the potential to improve diagnostic capabilities and provide value-added services during testing. By embracing emerging technologies, we may be able to further our understanding of sleep as a physiological process and provide a better patient experience.

REFERENCES

1. Graves RJ. On Sleep and sleeplessness. *J Psychol Med Ment Pathol*. 1849;2(7):377.
2. Millett D. Hans Berger: from psychic energy to the EEG. *Perspect Biol Med*. 2001 Fall;44(4):522–542. doi:10.1353/pbm.2001.0070. PMID: 11600799.
3. Brazier MAB. *A History of Neurophysiology in the 19th Century*. Raven Press; 1988
4. Caton R. The electric currents of the brain. *Br Med J*. 1875;2:278.
5. Berger H. Über das Elektroenkephalogramm des Menschen. *Arch Psychiatr*. 1929;87:527–570. doi:10.1007/BF01797193.

6. Cohen, Henry, Richard Caton. (1842–1926). Pioneer electrophysiologist. *Proc Royal Soc Med*. 1959;52(8):645–651. doi:10.1177/003591575905200816.
7. Caton R. C.B.E., M.D., F.R.C.P. *Br Med J*. 1926; 1(3393):71–72. doi:10.1136/bmj.1.3393.71.
8. La Vaque J. The History of EEG Hans Berger: Psychophysiologist. A Historical Vignette. *J Neurother: Investigations in Neuromodulation, Neurofeedback and Applied Neuroscience*. 1999;3(2):1–9. doi:10.1300/J184v03n02_01
9. Stone JL, Hughes JR. Early history of electroencephalography and establishment of the American Clinical Neurophysiology Society. *J Clin Neurophysiol*. 2013 Feb;30(1):28–44. doi:10.1097/WNP.0b013e31827edb2d. PMID: 23377440.
10. Subasi A. *Practical Guide for Biomedical Signals Analysis Using Machine Learning Techniques*. 2019. 10.1016/B978-0-12-817444-9.00001-5.
11. https://beckerarchives.wustl.edu/VC091.
12. Loomis AL, Harvey N, Hobart GA. Cerebral states during sleep, as studied by human brain potentials. *J Exp Psychol*. 1937;21:127.
13. Alvarez LW. *Alfred Lee Loomis*. National Academy of Sciences. Biographical memoirs. 51. National Academies Press; 1980:308–341.
14. Lawson, R. Blinking and sleep. *Nature*. 1950;165:81. https://doi.org/10.1038/165081b0.
15. Aserinsky E. The discovery of REM sleep. *J Hist Neurosci*. 1996 Dec;5(3):213–227. doi:10.1080/09647049609525671. PMID: 11618742.
16. https://worldradiohistory.com/hd2/IDX-Site-Technical/Engineering-General/Archive-Electronics-IDX/IDX/50s/Electronics-1954-0749.pdf.
17. Aserinsky E, Kleitman N. Regularly occurring periods of eye motility, and concomitant phenomena, during sleep. *Science*. 1953 Sep 4;118(3062):273–274. doi:10.1126/science.118.3062.273. PMID: 13089671.
18. Dement W, Vaughan C. *The Promise of Sleep: A Pioneer in Sleep Medicine Explores the Vital Connection Between Health, Happiness, and a Good Night's Sleep*. Dell Publishing; 1999.
19. Foulkes D, Pivik T, Ahrens JB, Swanson EM. Effects of "dream deprivation" on dream content: An attempted cross-night replication. *J Abnorm Psychol*. 1968 Oct;73(5):403–415. doi:10.1037/h0026151. PMID: 4301890.
20. Dement W, Kleitman N. Cyclic variations in EEG during sleep and their relation to eye movements, body motility, and dreaming. *Electroencephalogr Clin Neurophysiol*. 1957 Nov;9(4):673–960. doi:10.1016/0013-4694(57)90088-3. PMID: 13480240.
21. Lennox WG. Thomas Wills on narcolepsy. *Arch NeurPsych*. 1939;41(2):348–351. doi:10.1001/archneurpsyc.1939.02270140134010.
22. Schenck CH, Bassetti CL, Arnulf I, Mignot E. English translations of the first clinical reports on narcolepsy and cataplexy by Westphal and Gélineau in the late 19th century, with commentary. *J Clin Sleep Med*. 2007;3(3):301–311.
23. Yoss RE, Daly DD. Narcolepsy. *Arch Intern Med*. 1960;106(2):168–171. doi:10.1001/archinte.1960.03820020008003.
24. Kinnier Wilson SA, The narcolepsies. *Brain*. 1928 Mar;51(1):63–109. https://doi.org/10.1093/brain/51.1.63.
25. Vogel G. Studies in psychophysiology of dreams. III. The dream of narcolepsy. *Arch Gen Psychiatry*. 1960 Oct;3:421–428. doi:10.1001/archpsyc.1960.01710040091011. PMID: 13781811.
26. Rechtschaffen A, Wolpert E, Dement W, et al. Nocturnal Sleep of Narocleptics. *Electroencephalogr Clin Neurophysiol*. 1963 Aug;15:599. doi: 10.1016/0013-4694(63)90032-4. PMID: 14161512.
27. Dement WC. History of sleep medicine. *Neurol Clin*. 2005 Nov;23(4):945–965, v. doi:10.1016/j.ncl.2005.07.001. PMID: 16243610.
28. Carskadon MA, Dement WC. Sleep tendency: An objective measure of sleep loss. *Sleep Res*. 1977;6:200.
29. Richardson GS, Carskadon MA, Flagg W, Van den Hoed J, Dement WC, Mitler MM. Excessive daytime sleepiness in man: Multiple sleep latency measurement in narcoleptic and control subjects. *Electroencephalogr Clin Neurophysiol*. 1978 Nov;45(5):621–627. doi:10.1016/0013-4694(78)90162-1. PMID: 81764; PMCID: PMC2391074.
30. Carskadon MA, Dement WC, Mitler MM, Roth T, Westbrook PR, Keenan S. Guidelines for the multiple sleep latency test (MSLT): A standard measure of sleepiness. *Sleep*. 1986 Dec;9(4):519–524. doi:10.1093/sleep/9.4.519. PMID: 3809866.
31. Hartse KM, Roth T, Zorick FJ. Daytime sleepiness and daytime wakefulness: The effect of instruction. *Sleep*. 1982;5(Suppl 2):S107–S118. doi:10.1093/sleep/5.s2.s107. PMID: 7156646.
32. Mitler MM, Gujavarty KS, Browman CP. Maintenance of wakefulness test: A polysomnographic technique for evaluation treatment efficacy in patients with excessive somnolence. *Electroencephalogr Clin Neurophysiol*. 1982 Jun;53(6):658–661. doi:10.1016/0013-4694(82)90142-0. PMID: 6177511; PMCID: PMC2480525.
33. Littner MR, Kushida C, Wise M, et al.; Standards of Practice Committee of the American Academy of Sleep Medicine. Practice parameters for clinical use of the multiple sleep latency test and the maintenance of wakefulness test. *Sleep*. 2005 Jan;28(1):113–121. doi:10.1093/sleep/28.1.113. PMID: 15700727.
34. Krahn LE, Arand DL, Avidan AY, et al. Recommended protocols for the Multiple Sleep Latency Test and the Maintenance of Wakefulness Test in adults: Guidance from the American Academy of Sleep Medicine. *J Clin Sleep Med*. 2021;17(12):2489–2498.
35. Ohlmeyer P, Brilmayer H, Hüllstrung H. Periodische Vorgänge im Schlaf. *Pflügers Arch*. 1944;248:559–560. https://doi.org/10.1007/BF01764449.
36. Oswald I. *Sleeping and Waking: Physiology and Psychology*. Amsterdam: Elsevier; 1962.
37. Fisher C, Gross J, Zuch J. Cycle of penile erection synchronous with dreaming (REM) sleep: Preliminary report. *Arch Gen Psychiatry*. 1965;12(1):29–45. doi:10.1001/archpsyc.1965.01720310031005.
38. Karacan I. Clinical value of nocturnal erection in the prognosis and diagnosis of impotence. *Med Aspect Human Sexuality*. 1970;4:27–34.
39. Reynolds CF III, Thase ME, Jennings JR, et al. Nocturnal penile tumescence in healthy 20- to 59-year-olds: A revisit. *Sleep*. 1989 Aug;12(4):368–373. PMID: 2762691.
40. Barnhoorn P, Gianotten W, Van Driel M. Sleep-related painful erections following sexual intercourse.

Arch Sexual Behav. 2018;47:816. doi:10.1007/s10508-017-1132-0.
41. Campbell PI, Reynolds CF III, Jennings JR, et al. Reliability of NPT scoring and visual estimates of erectile fullness. *Sleep*. 1987 Oct;10(5):480–485. doi:10.1093/sleep/10.5.480. PMID: 3685756.
42. Nofzinger EA, Fasiczka AL, Thase ME, et al. Are buckling force measurements reliable in nocturnal penile tumescence studies? *Sleep*. 1993 Feb;16(2):156–162. PMID: 8446836.
43. Aldrich MS. *Sleep Medicine*. Oxford University Press; 1999.
44. Cho JW, Duffy JF. Sleep, sleep disorders, and sexual dysfunction. *World J Mens Health*. 2019;37(3):261–275. doi:10.5534/wjmh.180045.
45. Cespuglio R. In memoriam: Michel Jouvet (1925–2017). *Sleep Vigil*. 2017;1:119–122. https://doi.org/10.1007/s41782-017-0022-9.
46. Jouvet M, Michel F, Courjon J. Sur la mise en jeu de deux méchanismes àexpression électro-encéphalographique différente au cours du sommeilphysiologique chez le chat. *C R Acad Sci*. 1959;248:3043–3045.
47. Jouvet M. Research on the neural structures and responsible mechanisms in different phases of physiological sleep. *Arch Ital Biol*. 196;100:125–206.
48. Schenck CH, Bundlie SR, Ettinger MG, Mahowald MW. Chronic behavioral disorders of human REM sleep: A new category of parasomnia. *Sleep*. 1986 Jun;9(2):293. doi:10.1093/sleep/9.2.293. PMID: 3505730.
49. St Louis EK, Boeve BF. REM sleep behavior disorder: Diagnosis, clinical implications, and future directions. *Mayo Clin Proc (Rev)*. 2017 Nov;92(11):1723–1736. doi:10.1016/j.mayocp.2017.09.007. PMC 6095693. PMID 29101940.
50. Dickens C. *The Posthumous Papers of the Pickwick Club*. Chapman & Hall; 1837.
51. Osler W, McCrae T. *Principles and practice of medicine: Designed for the use of practitioners and students of medicine*. 8th. edition, largely rewritten and thoroughly revised with the assistance of Thomas McCrae. New York: Appleton; 1912.
52. Bickelmann AG, Burwell CS, Robin ED, et. al. Extreme obesity associated with alveolar hypoventilation: a Pickwickian syndrome. *Am J Med*. 1956 Nov;21(5):811–818. doi:10.1016/0002-9343(56)90094-8. PMID: 13362309.
53. https://hms.harvard.edu/about-hms/office-dean/past-deans-faculty-medicine.
54. Gerardy W, Herberg D, Kuhn HM. Vergleichende Untersuchungen der Lungenfunktion und des Elektroencephalogramms bei zwei Patienten mit Pickwickian-Syndrom, Z. *Klin Med*. 1960;156:362–380.
55. Drachman DB, Gumnit RJ. Periodic alteration of consciousness in the "pickwickian" syndrome. *Arch Neurol*. 1962 Jun;6:471–477. doi:10.1001/archneur.1962.00450240049006. PMID: 13887682.
56. Gastaut H. Etude polygraphique des manifestations episodiques (hypniques et respiratorires) diurnes et nocturnes du syndromes de Pickwick. *Ev Neurol*. 1965;112:568.
57. Jung R, Kuhlo W. Neurophysiological studies of abnormal night sleep and the pickwickian syndrome. *Prog Brain Res*. 1965;18:140–159. doi:10.1016/s0079-6123(08)63590-6. PMID: 14329033.
58. Gastaut H, Tassinari CA, Duron B. Polygraphic study of the episodic diurnal and nocturnal (hypnic and respiratory) manifestations of the pickwick syndrome. *Brain Res*. 1966;1(2):167–186. ISSN 0006-8993. https://doi.org/10.1016/0006-8993(66)90117-X.
59. Chesson AL, Ferber RA, Fry JM, et al. Practice parameters for the indications for polysomnography and related procedures. *Sleep*. 1997 Jun;20(6):406–422. https://doi.org/10.1093/sleep/20.6.406.
60. Guilleminault C, Eldridge FL, Dement WC. Insomnia with sleep apnea: A new syndrome. *Science*. 1973 Aug 31;181(4102):856–858. doi:10.1126/science.181.4102.856. PMID: 4353301.
61. Hirshkowitz M, Moore C. Computers in Sleep Medicine. In: Kryger M, Roth T, Dement C, eds. *Principles and Practice of Sleep Medicine*. WB Saunders; 2000:1302–1307.
62. Rosekind MR, Coates TJ, Thoresen CE. Telephone transmission of all-night polysomnographic data from subjects' homes. *J Nerv Ment Dis*. 1978 Jun;166(6):438–441. doi:10.1097/00005053-197806000-00008. PMID: 660178.
63. Kripke DF, Mullaney DJ, Messin S, Wyborney VG. Wrist actigraphic measures of sleep and rhythms. *Electroencephalogr Clin Neurophysiol*. 1978 May;44(5):674–676. doi:10.1016/0013-4694(78)90133-5. PMID: 77772.
64. Driller MW, O'Donnell S, Tavares F. What wrist should you wear your actigraphy device on? Analysis of dominant vs. non-dominant wrist actigraphy for measuring sleep in healthy adults. *Sleep Sci*. 2017;10(3):132–135. doi:10.5935/1984-0063.20170023.
65. Lujan MR, Perez-Pozuelo I, Grandner MA. Past, present, and future of multisensory wearable technology to monitor sleep and circadian rhythms. *Front Digit Health*. 2021;3:721919. doi:10.3389/fdgth.2021.721919.
66. Sadeh A, Sharkey M, Carskadon MA. Activity-based sleep-wake identification: an empirical test of methodological issues. *Sleep*. 1994 May;17(3):201–207. https://doi.org/10.1093/sleep/17.3.201.
67. Ancoli-Israel S, Kripke DF, Mason W, Messin S. Comparisons of home sleep recordings and polysomnograms in older adults with sleep disorders. *Sleep*. 1981 Sep;4(3):283–291. https://doi.org/10.1093/sleep/4.3.283.
68. Penzel T, Peter JH. Ambulatory diagnosis of sleep-related breathing disorders. *Sleep*. 1992 Dec;15(Suppl 6):S9–S12. https://doi.org/10.1093/sleep/15.suppl_6.S9.
69. Ferber R, Millman R, Coppola M, et al. Portable recording in the assessment of obstructive sleep apnea. *Sleep*. 1994 Jun;17(4):378–392. https://doi.org/10.1093/sleep/17.4.378.
70. Polysomnography Task Force, American Sleep Disorders Association Standards of Practice Committee. Practice parameters for the indications for polysomnography and related procedures. *Sleep*. 1997 Jun;20(6):406–422. PMID: 9302725.
71. Ross SD, Sheinhait IA, Harrison KJ, et al. Systematic review and meta-analysis of the literature regarding the diagnosis of sleep apnea. *Sleep*. 2000 Jun 15;23(4):519–532. PMID: 10875559.

72. Chesson AL Jr, Berry RB, Pack A; American Academy of Sleep Medicine; American Thoracic Society; American College of Chest Physicians. Practice parameters for the use of portable monitoring devices in the investigation of suspected obstructive sleep apnea in adults. *Sleep*. 2003 Nov 1;26(7):907–913. doi:10.1093/sleep/26.7.907. PMID: 14655928.
73. Flemons WW, Littner MR, Rowley JA, et al. Home diagnosis of sleep apnea: A systematic review of the literature. An evidence review cosponsored by the American Academy of Sleep Medicine, the American College of Chest Physicians, and the American Thoracic Society. *Chest*. 2003 Oct;124(4):1543–1579. doi:10.1378/chest.124.4.1543. PMID: 14555592.
74. Decision Memo for Continuous Positive Airway Pressure (CPAP) Therapy for Obstructive Sleep Apnea (OSA) (CAG-00093R). 2005. https://www.cms.gov/medicare-coverage-database/view/ncacal-decision-memo.aspx?proposed=N&ncaid=204
75. Schnall RP, Shlitner A, Sheffy J, Kedar R, Lavie P. Periodic, profound peripheral vasoconstriction: A new marker of obstructive sleep apnea. *Sleep*. 1999 Nov 1;22(7):939–946. PMID:10566912.
76. Chediak AD. Why CMS approved home sleep testing for CPAP coverage. *J Clin Sleep Med*. 2008;4(1):16–18.
77. Institute of Medicine (US) Committee on Sleep Medicine and Research; Colten HR, Altevogt BM, eds. *Sleep Disorders and Sleep Deprivation: An Unmet Public Health Problem*. National Academies Press; 2006. PMID: 20669438.
78. Centers for Medicare & Medicaid Services. Decision Memo for Continuous Positive Airway Pressure (CPAP) Therapy for Obstructive Sleep Apnea (OSA). 2007. https://www.cms.hhs.gov/mcd/viewdraftdecisionmemo.asp?id=204.
79. Collop NA, Anderson WM, Boehlecke B, et al.; Portable Monitoring Task Force of the American Academy of Sleep Medicine. Clinical guidelines for the use of unattended portable monitors in the diagnosis of obstructive sleep apnea in adult patients. *J Clin Sleep Med*. 2007 Dec 15;3(7):737–747. PMID: 18198809; PMCID: PMC2556918.
80. Collop NA, Tracy SL, Kapur V, et al. Obstructive sleep apnea devices for out-of-center (OOC) testing: Technology evaluation. *J Clin Sleep Med*. 2011 Oct 15;7(5):531–548. doi:10.5664/JCSM.1328. PMID: 22003351; PMCID: PMC3190855.
81. Kapur VK, Auckley DH, Chowdhuri S, et al. Clinical practice guideline for diagnostic testing for adult obstructive sleep apnea: An American Academy of Sleep Medicine clinical practice guideline. *J Clin Sleep Med*. 2017 Mar 15;13(3):479–504. doi:10.5664/jcsm.6506. PMID: 28162150; PMCID: PMC5337595.
82. Tamura T. Current progress of photoplethysmography and SPO2 for health monitoring. *Biomed Eng Lett*. 2019;9(1):21–36. doi:10.1007/s13534-019-00097-w.
83. Fonseca P, Weysen T, Goelema MS, et al. Validation of photoplethysmography-based sleep staging compared with polysomnography in healthy middle-aged adults. *Sleep*. 2017 Jul;40(7):zsx097. https://doi.org/10.1093/sleep/zsx097.
84. Zavanelli N, Kim H, Kim J, et al. At-home wireless monitoring of acute hemodynamic disturbances to detect sleep apnea and sleep stages via a soft sternal patch. *Sci Adv*. 2021 Dec 24;7(52):eabl4146. doi:10.1126/sciadv.abl4146. PMID: 34936438.
85. de Zambotti M, Rosas L, Colrain IM, Baker FC. The sleep of the ring: Comparison of the ŌURA sleep tracker against polysomnography. *Behav Sleep Med*. 2019;17(2):124–136. doi:10.1080/15402002.2017.1300587.
86. Heglum HSA, Kallestad H, Vethe D, Langsrud K, Sand T, Engstrøm M. Distinguishing sleep from wake with a radar sensor: a contact-free real-time sleep monitor. *Sleep*. 2021 Aug 13;44(8):zsab060. doi:10.1093/sleep/zsab060. PMID: 33705555; PMCID: PMC8361351.
87. Khan F, Ghaffar A, Khan N, Cho SH. An overview of signal processing techniques for remote health monitoring using impulse radio UWB transceiver. *Sensors*. 2020;20(9):2479. https://doi.org/10.3390/s20092479.
88. Kang S, Kim DK, Lee Y, et al. Non-contact diagnosis of obstructive sleep apnea using impulse-radio ultra-wideband radar. *Sci Rep*. 2020;10:5261. https://doi.org/10.1038/s41598-020-62061-4.
89. Chavoshan B, Dungan G, Liu PY. Contact-free screening for obstructive sleep apnea: comfort, especially in a physically distanced brave new world. *J Clin Sleep Med*. 2021 May 1;17(5):873–874. doi:10.5664/jcsm.9238. PMID: 33688825; PMCID: PMC8320497.
90. Penzel T, Schöbel C, Fietze I. New technology to assess sleep apnea: Wearables, smartphones, and accessories. *F1000Res*. 2018;7:413. doi:10.12688/f1000research.13010.1.
91. Thomas RJ, Wood C, Bianchi MT. Cardiopulmonary coupling spectrogram as an ambulatory clinical biomarker of sleep stability and quality in health, sleep apnea, and insomnia. *Sleep*. 2018;41(2):zsx196. doi:10.1093/sleep/zsx196.

Chapter 24

Clinical Use of Actigraphy and Consumer Technology for Assessment of Sleep

Cathy Goldstein

INTRODUCTION: WHY TRACK SLEEP?

A paradox exists in the field of sleep medicine. Sleep deprivation and sleep disorders are problematic, not due to singular exposure, but in the context of nightly disturbances in sleep quality and duration. However, our gold standard objective measurement of sleep is the polysomnogram (PSG). The PSG, which relies on the monitoring of various physiological parameters, a sleep laboratory, and trained experts for conduct and interpretation, is impractical over more than one night, not only for technical reasons (labor-intensive and expensive) but also for physiological reasons. Therefore, monitoring sleep over time requires methods that are less obtrusive and resource-intense. In the sections that follow, we will describe options for longitudinal objective sleep assessment.

ACTIGRAPHY

Here we will use the term *actigraphy* to describe the tracking of sleep with accepted, U.S. Food and Drug Administration (FDA) cleared actigraphs. Actigraphs are wrist-worn motion sensors that operate under the rationale that the sleep state is marked by reduced mobility compared to wakefulness. Some also include a light-sensor indicating when the user is exposed to light.

History of Actigraphy

The first described use of wearable motion recording to estimate sleep took place in the 1970s among patients with psychiatric conditions.[1] Early iterations of actigraphs were described as a telemetric mobility-sensing system, movement-activated recording monitor (MARM), and ambulatory activity monitor with solid-state memory.[2–4] The term *actigraphy* was first used by Kripke and colleagues in 1978,[5] and since that time, a number of actigraphs have emerged for clinical and research applications. However, actigraphy has not been universally deployed in sleep clinics due to cost and lack of consistent reimbursement.

Actigraphy Sensors

Actigraphs monitor motion with a piezoelectric accelerometer that consists of a piezoelectric element and a seismic mass. With acceleration, the piezoelectric element is deformed by the mass, and voltage is produced proportional to the amount of acceleration.[6]

Older actigraphs used piezoelectric accelerometers that measured acceleration in only one axis, and attempts to record in multiple axes increased the size.[7] The advent of accelerometers integrated into microelectromechanical systems (MEMS), which are used ubiquitously in portable electronic devices that monitor movement and position (i.e., smartphones), allowed for monitoring of triaxial data without increasing sensor size.[7]

Additionally, most older actigraphs used limited capacity, solid-state memory storage; therefore, to maintain a small size, the acceleration signal was summarized into a single activity count quantity for each epoch interval. The transformation of acceleration signal to activity counts uses methods such as the zero-crossing method (ZCM), time above threshold (TAT), and proportional integrating mode (PIM).[8] ZCM counts the number of times the activity reaches zero during the epoch. TAT determines the amount of time per epoch that the activity is above some defined threshold. PIM calculates the area under the curve. For the same amount of motion, different methods of signal processing can produce different activity counts.[9] Therefore, another benefit of MEMS accelerometers is the ability to sample and store high-resolution raw triaxial acceleration data as opposed to reduction to activity counts. The availability of raw acceleration data allows for standardization of activity count derivation and sleep-wake classification, and will ultimately allow for pooling of data acquired with devices from different manufacturers.[7]

Although sleep-estimation capabilities are based on movement, given the role of light in entraining the circadian timing system, FDA-cleared actigraphs often incorporate a sensor to measure ambient light levels.

Actigraphy Data Management and Analysis

After digitization and conversion into activity counts, motion data are extracted from the actigraphy device, which typically requires a dock or USB connection. Next, a software program applies an algorithm to differentiate sleep from wake. Initially, data required hand scoring, but automated algorithms were soon developed.[10] Sleep-estimation algorithms often apply a weighted sum to motion data, and if a certain threshold is exceeded, wake is scored. Otherwise, the time interval in consideration is scored as sleep. Figure 24.1 shows the different algorithms applied to activity count data to differentiate sleep from wake. More recently, machine learning algorithms have been applied to data collected by actigraphy.[11]

Once sleep and wake are classified and time in bed (TIB) is specified, sleep summary metrics are calculated and include total sleep time (TST), sleep onset latency (SOL), wake after sleep onset (WASO), and sleep efficiency (SE). However, identification of TIB is not always straightforward, and may utilize patient report (sleep diaries), use of event markers, appraisal of raw data, or algorithms that auto-detect TIB. Given the potential for incomplete self-report data and inconsistencies between different detection methods for a single TIB period, one group of investigators described a standardized hierarchical approach based on event marker, diary, light, and activity data.[12] Because the accuracy of computed sleep summary metrics is contingent (in part) on the correct designation of TIB, use of careful data-cleaning methods is required.

Actigraphy Performance

Actigraphy has been evaluated against gold-standard PSG to evaluate sleep estimation performance. The appraisal of statistics that reflect the performance of actigraphy in comparison

COLE-KRIPKE

Mean activity per minute

$D=0.001(106A_{-4}+54A_{-3}+58A_{-2}+76A_{1}+230A_{0}+74A_{+1}+67A_{+2})$

Maximum 30 second activity

$D=0.0001(50A_{-4}+30A_{-3}+14A_{-2}+28A_{-1}+121A_{0}+8A_{+1}+50A_{+2})$

$D<1$=Sleep, $D\geq 1$=Wake

Where A_0, A_{-1}, A_{+1} = activity in the present, previous, and subsequent minute respectively.

SADEH

PS=7.601-0.065·MeanW5 min-91.08·NAT - 0.056·SDlast 6 min - 0.703·LOGAct

PS (probability of sleep) ≥ 0 =Sleep, PS <0=Wake

Where...

MeanW5 min = the average number of activity counts during the scored epoch and the window of preceding and following five epochs

SDlast 6 min = the standard deviation of the activity counts during the scored epoch and the preceding five epochs

NAT = the number of epochs with 50 ≤activity counts<100 in a window of 11 minutes (the scored epoch and preceding and following five epochs)

LOGAct = natural logarithm of the number of activity counts during the scored epoch + 1

ACTIWARE

$A=0.04E_{-2}+0.2E_{-1}+1E_{0}+0.2E_{+1}+0.04E_{+2}$

A≤ T (threshold)=Sleep, A>T =Wake

High threshold = 80

Medium threshold =40

Low threshold =20

A=sum of activity counts for 30S scored epoch and surrounding epochs

E0=activity counts recorded during scored epoch

En=activity counts recorded during each preceding (−1, −2, −3, −4) or following (+1, +2, +3, +4) successive epoch

Figure 24.1. Commonly used algorithms that differentiate sleep from wakefulness when applied to activity count data acquired by actigraphs.

Cole RJ, Kripke DF, Gruen W, Mullaney DJ, Gillin JC. Automatic sleep/wake identification from wrist activity. *Sleep*. 1992;15(5):461–469.

Sadeh A, Sharkey KM, Carskadon MA. Activity-based sleep-wake identification: An empirical test of methodological issues. *Sleep*. 1994;17(3):201–207. doi:10.1093/sleep/17.3.201.

Kushida CA, Chang A, Gadkary C, Guilleminault C, Carrillo O, Dement WC. Comparison of actigraphic, polysomnographic, and subjective assessment of sleep parameters in sleep-disordered patients. *Sleep Med*. 2001;2(5):389–396. doi:10.1016/s1389-9457(00)00098-8.

to manually scored PSG should take into account that measured physiological parameters are different (e.g., accelerometry vs. electroencephalogram, electrooculogram, and electromyogram data) and that scoring is computer automated versus human. Furthermore, although scored PSG is considered ground truth, the agreement between expert scorers is imperfect (80% among registered PSG technologists).[13,14]

A comprehensive description of the methods behind actigraphy validation studies is beyond the scope of this chapter. However, in general, such studies simultaneously record PSG in an individual wearing an actigraph and time-synchronize the data collection. Methods are used to harmonize PSG data, viewed and scored at 30-second intervals, with actigraphy epochs, automatically scored in 60-second intervals in most cases.

The comparison of simultaneous intervals of scored PSG and actigraphy data is referred to as an epoch-by-epoch (EBE) comparison and allows for the calculation of sensitivity, specificity, and accuracy (see Figure 24.2). Sensitivity refers to the fraction of PSG sleep epochs

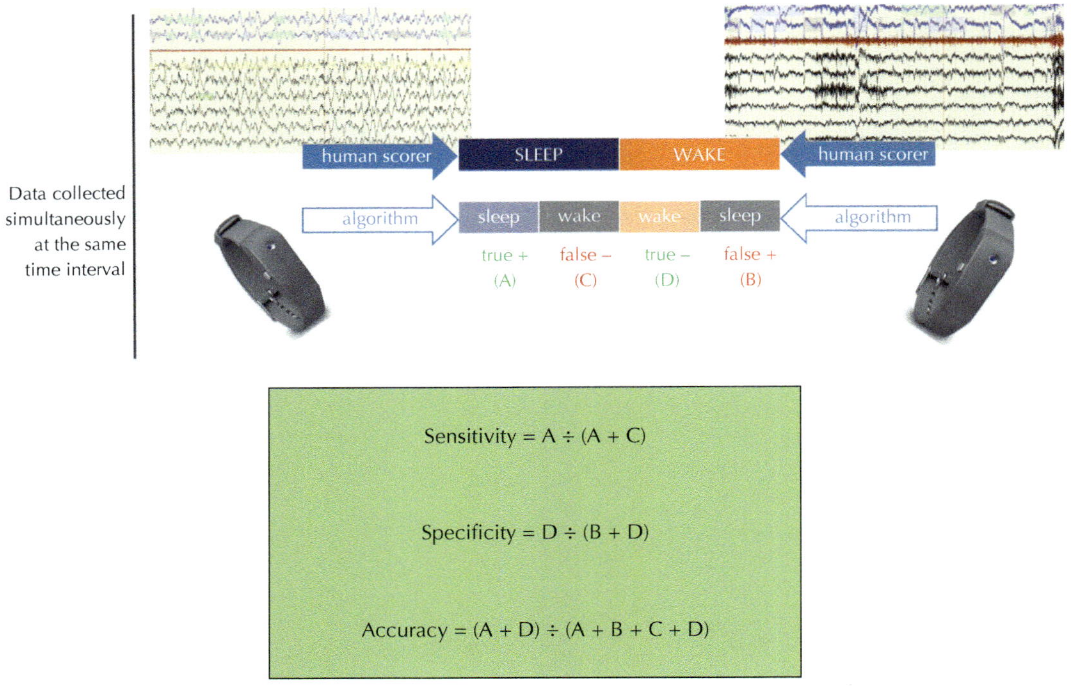

Figure 24.2. Comparison of scored sleep data from polysomnogram and actigraphy during an epoch-by-epoch analysis and derivation of sensitivity, specificity, and accuracy. In an epoch-by-epoch analysis, the state of interest is sleep and the population is epochs as opposed to disease and individuals in a traditional 4 × 4 table comparing a new test to gold-standard.

correctly designated as sleep by actigraphy. Specificity refers to the fraction of PSG wake epochs correctly designated as wake by actigraphy. Accuracy refers to the fraction of scored PSG epochs correctly designated as sleep or wake by actigraphy. Validation studies conducted overnight in healthy individuals may result in misleading accuracy values, given that most of the overnight period is spent asleep. Therefore, even if an algorithm arbitrarily scores every single 60-second epoch as sleep, if sleep efficiency is high, accuracy will also be deceptively high.

Similarly, analyses of summary sleep-wake metrics (TST, SOL, WASO, and SE) over the course of the night are not a sufficient sole measure of performance. In individuals with high SE, summary sleep metrics are often statistically similar between PSG and actigraphy. However, in individuals with more wakefulness during the TIB period, greater discrepancies are observed due to the actigraphy's tendency toward high sensitivity and low specificity (nonmoving wake misclassified as sleep). However, summary sleep parameters have clinical and research utility and therefore should be considered.

To evaluate the performance of actigraphy-derived TST, SOL, WASO, and SE summary metrics compared to PSG, first, individual- and group-level differences are quantified between the assessment methods. This allows for the identification of statistical differences between groups and calculation of bias and upper and lower limits of agreement, which can be visualized with a Bland-Altman plot to determine the magnitude and direction of discrepancy. A standardized and open-source framework was recently published to operationalize the performance assessment of actigraphy and other sleep-tracking devices.[15] It is important to recognize that because summary sleep measures are contingent on the TIB window, the accuracy of actigraphy in deriving these parameters is contingent not only on the performance of the sleep-wake classifier but also on appropriate identification of the TIB interval, as discussed previously.

Of note, the actigraphy scoring software version and any adjustable settings should be static during the evaluation process and documented.

SLEEP-WAKE, HEALTHY SUBJECTS

In studies of healthy subjects, compared to PSG, EBE analyses demonstrate that actigraphy has a sensitivity of approximately 90% and specificity of approximately 50%.[16–18] The misclassification of non-moving wakefulness as sleep generally leads to an overestimation of TST and SE and an underestimation of SOL and WASO.[16,18,19] Greater amounts of true wakefulness during the attempted sleep window (i.e., daytime sleep periods and administration of caffeine) augment the discrepancies between actigraphy and PSG-derived summary sleep metrics.[16] However, heterogeneity in performance has been observed, which may be explained in part by different manufacturer hardware and algorithms.[17–19]

SLEEP-WAKE, SLEEP DISORDERS

Given actigraphy's low specificity for wakefulness, it is not surprising that measures of performance are worse in sleep disorders than in healthy subjects. A task force of the American Academy of Sleep Medicine (AASM) performed meta-analyses of studies that compared sleep parameters derived from actigraphy to gold-standard PSG.[20] Mean differences between actigraphy and PSG were computed in individuals with sleep disorders. A priori clinically significant thresholds for the maximal allowable 95% confidence interval (CI) of the mean difference were determined.[20] For insomnia, the maximal allowable 95% CI for TST, sleep latency (SL), WASO, and SE were 40 minutes, 30 minutes, 30 minutes, and 5% respectively.[20] For both TST the night prior to multiple sleep latency test (pre-MSLT TST) and home sleep apnea test TST, the maximal allowable 95% CI was 40 minutes.[20] Additionally, for both pre-MSLT TST and home sleep apnea test TST, the task force set an absolute threshold for the mean difference (40 minutes).

Table 24.1 demonstrates the results of the meta-analyses that compared sleep parameter measurements between actigraphy and PSG in sleep disorders. For insomnia, actigraphy provides potentially reliable estimates of TST and SL but not WASO or SE.[20] For insomnia after intervention, actigraphy provides reliable estimates of SL only.[20] Actigraphy estimates were below the acceptable threshold for mean difference, but exceeded the maximally allowable 95% CI, for both pre-MSLT TST and home sleep apnea test TST.[20]

Table 24.1 **Actigraphy versus Polysomnogram in Sleep Disorders, Data from Meta-Analysis**

	Mean difference (95% CI)			
Clinical scenario	**TST (MIN)**	**SL (MIN)**	**WASO (MIN)**	**SE (%)**
Insomnia	10.14 (−8.07, 27.05)	6.1 (−2.29, −9.07)	1.5 (−13.68, 19.54)	1 (−4.9, 3.0)
Insomnia after intervention	4.6(−37.1, 46.3)	−16.60 (−18.66. −14.54)* −9.90 (21.07, 1.27)* 1.90 (−5.98, 9.69)* 2.80(−12.12,17.72)*	10.2 (−53.2, 32.8)	4.2 (0.2,8.1)
Sleep assessment in the context of sleep-disordered breathing	14.54 (−20.7, 49.8)	—	—	—
PSG before MSLT	−15.6 (−40.30, 9.10)	—	—	—

Green-filled cells indicate that the range (95% confidence interval) of discrepancy between actigraphy and PSG is narrow enough that actigraphy can be reliably used to provide an objective assessment of the sleep parameter of interest for the purpose of making clinical care decisions. Orange-filled cells indicate that the range of discrepancy between actigraphy and PSG is clinically significant and should not be used interchangeably. The small number of studies precluded pooling and therefore individual studies reported.

CIRCADIAN METRICS

After scoring of sleep and wake, appraisal of the derived actograms allows for visualization of the circadian rest-activity pattern. In addition to the visual depiction, quantifications of circadian properties of activity data are available. Cosinor analysis has long been applied to actigraphy to estimate acrophase, mesor, period, and amplitude of the rest-activity rhythm. A cosine curve with a period at or near 24 hours is fit to the data by the least-squares method and from that, acrophase (time to peak activity), amplitude (peak to nadir difference), and mean of the curve can be identified.[8] Transformation of the cosine curve provides a better fit to activity data, which is often non-sinusoidal.[8,21] The pseudo F statistic captures the extent that an individual's sleep-wake activity conforms to the extended cosine model and is a marker of the strength of the circadian rhythm.[8,21] Other promising circadian prediction methods include the limit oscillator model (and modifications) and demonstrate the ability to reasonably estimate objective circadian phase.[22]

Use Cases for Actigraphy

Longitudinal, passive, objective monitoring of sleep confers benefit of actigraphy use in a variety of scenarios.

CLINICAL

The International Classification of Sleep Disorders, 3rd edition, recommends actigraphy as part of the diagnostic evaluation in several disorders. For suspected central disorders of hypersomnolence, use of actigraphy is recommended for at least 7 days to ensure adequate sleep duration before in-laboratory assessment with PSG and MSLT, to document 24-hour sleep duration of longer than 660 minutes in certain cases of idiopathic hypersomnia, and to identify sleep restriction in insufficient sleep syndrome. Sleep estimation with actigraphy is also recommended to evaluate sleep-wake timing in suspected circadian rhythm sleep-wake disorders for at least 7 days (14 days for non-24-hour sleep-wake rhythm disorder).

Meta-analyses revealed significant differences that preclude the use of actigraphy and PSG interchangeably to measure some sleep parameters (see Table 24.1).[20] However, actigraphy was found to provide data that are distinct from sleep logs, which demonstrates the benefit of this objective information over self-report. Therefore, actigraphy was recommended by the AASM to estimate sleep parameters in insomnia disorder, circadian rhythm sleep-wake disorders, and suspected insufficient sleep syndrome.[20] Additionally, actigraphy is recommended to estimate TST prior to in laboratory testing with PSG and MSLT and integrated with home sleep apnea test devices.[20]

RESEARCH

In addition to the well-known impact of chronic sleep loss on day-to-day safety, performance, and quality of life,[23–25] investigations have revealed that both insufficient and (less frequently observed) prolonged sleep durations are associated with negative health consequences, including cardiovascular disease and unfavorable cardiovascular profiles,[26–29] immune system dysfunction,[30,31] and obesity,[32] diabetes, and metabolic syndrome.[33] Extremes in sleep duration have also been linked to increased mortality[34]; however, not all studies have reached this conclusion.[35]

The measurement of sleep with self-reported sleep duration introduces uncertainty into the contribution of sleep to health and disease, as self-reported sleep duration may be inaccurate. Demographics, the presence or absence of comorbid sleep disorders, the timing of the query, and how the question of sleep amount is asked are all known contributors to the accuracy of subjective sleep estimates.[36]

Additionally, a singular, cross-sectional assessment of sleep cannot be used as a proxy for nightly sleep duration in most cases, given the ubiquity of variable sleep timing and sleep duration between work/school days and weekend days.[37,38] A growing body of literature has associated these phenomena, known as social jet lag and social sleep restriction, with negative cardiometabolic, cognitive performance, and mental health outcomes.[39–43] Intraindividual variability (IIV) is another measure of sleep variability and quantifies the daily variation around the mean when sleep parameters are measured over multiple days.[44] Greater IIV and other measures of instability in sleep metrics, such as the composite phase deviation (CPD) and the sleep regularity index (SRI), have also been associated with worse well-being and cardiovascular, metabolic, and mental health conditions.[44–50] Regardless of the metric used to operationalize sleep variability, assessment of sleep over multiple days is required, which is best attained with passive, objective methods such as actigraphy to increase the completeness of data and reduce participant burden.

Additionally, sleep health is not encapsulated by 1 sleep parameter (such as sleep duration) considered in isolation. A 7-domain sleep definition has been proposed and includes measures of duration, quality, timing, continuity, circadian rhythmicity, regularity, and daytime sleepiness.[51] To easily quantify a variety of sleep measures simultaneously, passive and objective recording is required.

Actigraphy Limitations

Actigraphy is well-accepted by medical and research communities; however, significant inadequacies limit usefulness, such as expense, the requirement of a trained member of the sleep team to set up the device and recover the data, burdensome data-cleaning procedures, and lack of easy integration between actigraphy software and the electronic medical record or other digital health data sources.[52] Additionally, reimbursement for recording and interpretation is unlikely despite a current procedural technology (CPT) code. Further, actigraphs are owned by clinicians or research teams, not patients, and therefore, although small and unobtrusive, recording rarely exceeds 1 or 2 weeks before return.

Collectively, the shortcomings of actigraphy limit adoption in clinical sleep medicine. Consequently, sleep providers frequently rely on self-report sleep measures, which are often inaccurate or incomplete and may reduce the ability to accurately and efficiently manage sleep disorders. In research, actigraphy is used relatively commonly, but population size is limited and recording duration is only microlongitudinal.

CONSUMER SLEEP TECHNOLOGIES

Consumer sleep technologies may provide a solution to the need for longitudinal objective sleep recording that is inexpensive, patient and research participant accepted, and easy to use.

Emergence and Expansion of Consumer Sleep Technologies

The past decade has brought a proliferation in both the number of new consumer-facing sleep technologies (CST) as well as an increase in the breadth of data generated by these devices. Sleep-related technologies account for increasing market share (year-over-year) at the annual Consumer Electronics Show (CES). Sleep metrics have been incorporated into a variety of consumer-facing products that include fitness trackers, smartphone applications (apps), mattresses, and even voice assistants such as the Google Nest. In a 2017 assessment, 8% of adults reported current use of a sleep tracker, but 45% could imagine using a sleep tracker in the near future (https://www.statista.com/statistics/699422/us-adults-that-use-apps-to-track-sleep/).

The COVID-19 pandemic demonstrated the importance of our health, and sleep emerged as a top personal priority for many. Social media posts evangelized the importance of sleep. Pandemic-related searches emphasized the relevance of sleep in preventing infection and improving immune response to vaccination.[53] Additionally, consumer sleep-tracking technologies, given their concurrent heart rate (HR), HR variability (HRV), and activity metric tracking, combined with mobile app acquisition of self-report data, demonstrated the capacity for early detection of COVID-19.[54–57] Sales of over-the-counter pulse oximeters increased over 500% during early 2020 (https://qz.com/1832464/pulse-oximeters-for-coronavirus-unnecessary-but-selling-strong). Consumers were looking toward technology to assuage their fears and provide some measure of objective, actionable health data.

Consumer Sleep Technologies: The Basics

An understanding of the technology underlying consumer sleep technologies is crucial in identifying the strengths and weaknesses of this tool.

WHAT ARE CST?

According to a position statement released by the American Academy of Sleep Medicine (AASM) in 2018, CST are non-prescription devices marketed to consumers that may make an assertion to perform sleep tracking or sleep-related interventions.[58] These include fitness trackers, smartwatches, smart beds, insomnia apps, sleep coaching apps, headbands, smart pillows, sleep robots, and an ever-expanding list of other sleep-related technologies.

CST are grouped into 3 broad categories: wearables, nearables, and mobile apps. Notably, wearables and nearable devices are associated with their own app for data acquisition, analysis, and presentation to the user and often, for delivery of interventions.

WEARABLE SENSORS

A wearable is a device that is worn, such as a wrist-worn fitness tracker, headband, ring, or other smart accessories/clothing, that collects data. At minimum, most devices measure movement and heart rate, and some devices collect other metrics (oximetry, temperature, skin conductance).

Wrist-Worn (and Ring) Consumer Sleep Technologies

Wrist-worn devices dominate the consumer wearable technology market and were initially aimed at fitness tracking by monitoring motion to quantify steps and activity. However, many consumer wearable devices have progressed to also report sleep. With the addition of heart rate, consumer wearable devices became multisensory, which improved activity and sleep-tracking capabilities. More recently, oxygen saturation measurement has positioned consumer wearable devices to add sleep-disordered breathing to their list of reported metrics. For example, one smart ring focuses primarily on obstructive sleep apnea (OSA) detection.[59]

As detailed in the actigraphy section, the motion-recording capability of wrist-worn CST is conferred by an accelerometer. Acceleration is typically recorded by microelectromechanical system accelerometers which provide small, low-cost motion measurements in 3 axes (triaxial).[7]

Photoplethysmography (PPG) is an optical technique that measures HR (and derived features such as HRV and respiratory rate [RR]) and blood oxygen saturation.[60] Because blood absorbs light and increased blood volume is present in the periphery after systole, less light is reflected back to the PPG photodetector at that time and conversely, more light is reflected back just after diastole.[60] Therefore, changes in light absorption and reflection allow for the measurement of HR and the calculation of HRV.[60] Reflective PPG is used in current CST, as opposed to transmissive PPG used in medical pulse oximeters.[61]

Reflective PPG-derived HR and HRV are considered valuable surrogates for the same parameters measured by gold-standard electrocardiogram in different states (i.e., wake, sleep)[61] and health conditions (e.g., atrial fibrillation).[62] Therefore, these values are used as inputs to models to estimate sleep given the characteristic changes in HRV across sleep stages.[61] Additionally, PPG HR measurement allows for the quantification of RR and apnea hypopnea index (AHI) during sleep.[61]

Although less commonly encountered than wrist-worn, ring CST are also available and similarly use accelerometry to measure movement and PPG to measure HR and derived values as well as oximetry. One of the few ring devices available also measures temperature,[63] and others are novel given the ability to provide a vibratory stimulus (https://thim.io/) for the purpose of intensive sleep retraining for insomnia.[64,65]

Dry Electroencephalogram (EEG) Headbands

Even prior to the widespread adoption of wrist-worn CST, in 2009, a dry electroencephalogram (EEG) headband was introduced to track sleep and time an alarm to promote waking out of lighter sleep stages. Multiple studies regarding the device's performance were conducted; however, the company dissolved in 2013.[66] Dry EEG headbands remain available and are useful in the ambulatory state given that adhesive is not required to affix EEG sensors.

The claimed use of these devices typically goes beyond sleep estimation, as they also aim to improve sleep quality by generating more delta sleep.[67] Specifically, one device that is currently available provides audiotones based on sleep stage with the goal of promoting slow wave sleep in individuals who regularly sleep <6 hours per night (https://www.usa.philips.com/c-e/smartsleep/deep-sleep-headband.html).

EEG has also been incorporated into eye masks alongside accelerometers and PPG for sleep tracking and interventions and has been included in a forehead monitor that offers an evaluation for obstructive sleep apnea (eegsmart.com/en/UMindSleep.html). Earbuds have also been developed that incorporate EEG (https://clinicaltrials.gov/ct2/show/NCT05066009).

NEARABLE SENSORS

A nearable is a device that sits near the patient in the sleep environment but is not worn. Some examples include smart mattresses and bedside devices that record sleep without being attached to the user.

Bedside

Non-contact bedside CST use radiofrequency biomotion sensors to measure movement with ultralow power radiofrequency waves that estimate sleep and respiratory parameters.[68–70] Additionally, they collect information from the sleep environment, such as light, noise, and ambient temperature. From these signals, they can generate suggestions to improve the user's sleep that include environmental adjustments, such as reducing the room temperature.

Google's Nest Hub device uses Soli radar specifically to estimate sleep and respiratory patterns and has launched a partnership with the AASM that allows users to be automatically directed to vetted sleep educational content based on the readings taken by the Nest Hub (https://aasm.org/american-academy-of-sleep-medicine-google-help-people-improve-their-sleep/). Amazon's Alexa has also been granted permission by the Federal Communications Commission (FCC) to utilize this same radar technology.

Under (or Within) Mattress

CST that are used under or within an individual's bed are based on the static charge-sensitive bed, described over 40 years ago as a potential alternative to "very expensive and troublesome" sleep studies.[71] The static charge-sensitive bed used metal plates placed under a mattress to measure ballistocardiography (the visual representation of body movement owing to cardiac expulsion of blood into the arteries).[71,72] Current iterations of under-the-mattress CST use thin flexible force sensors to monitor ballistocardiography, breathing, and body movement, allowing the estimation of cardiac, respiratory, and sleep parameters.[72] This technology has also been embedded into smart mattresses such as the SleepIQ (sleepnumber.com/pages/sleep-science-smart-sensing).

MOBILE APPLICATIONS

Sleep-related applications rank among the top 10 of health-related mobile apps. They range from programs that play soft music to facilitate the initiation of sleep to more sophisticated algorithms that analyze noise and screen for OSA.

Mobile apps may use sensors native to the smartphone on which the app is downloaded to acquire sleep-related data, for example, the embedded accelerometer to monitor movement in bed or evaluate snoring through the microphone.[73,74] Direct user input or indirect analysis of smartphone usage metrics (i.e., touch screen use, tappigraphy) also can assist apps in tracking sleep parameters.[73–75] Tappigraphy is based on widespread, ubiquitous mobile device behaviors. Tappigraphy measures mobile device use right before sleep and immediately upon awakening. This has proven to be a more reliable measure of wakefulness in bed than actigraphy.[75] Apps can estimate total sleep time based on this metric, independent from a wearable.

Some sleep apps do not rely on sensors but query user symptoms to identify individuals at risk of sleep disorders or to tailor educational material. The choice of application is often telling—asking patients why they chose to download a particular app may provide insight into their sleep concerns. The vast number and rapid turnover of standalone sleep applications preclude a comprehensive index of apps in this chapter.

Data Processing and Management

The signal data derived from the sensors embedded in wearable and nearable devices and smartphones are managed by apps specific to the CST and cloud-based servers. Algorithms are applied to this data that distinguish sleep from wake, designate sleep stages, provide HR, HRV, oximetry readings, and more uncommonly, an AHI.

Initially, wearable devices monitored only motion, but the integration of PPG provided a surrogate measurement of HRV, which allowed for estimates of sleep stages.[76,77] As CST sensors and sleep classification algorithms become more sophisticated, other physiologic features and calculated parameters such as circadian estimates[78] and models of the sleep homeostat may continue to improve sleep-staging performance.

Like traditional actigraphy, the designation of TIB is highly relevant to the summary sleep metrics (e.g., sleep efficiency) reported by CST-associated apps.[79] Older iterations of CST required users to actively designate the window within which sleep was attempted, but to make sleep tracking completely passive, the TIB window is now automatically designated (with unclear accuracy and influence on reported sleep summary metrics).

Notably, signal processing and algorithms used by CST are proprietary; therefore, users are typically unable to visualize raw data or adjust algorithms to improve sleep-tracking performance in certain populations or scenarios. Because clinicians and researchers are provided only the processed, summarized data without the benefit of understanding the derivation of these results, hesitancy has surrounded the adoption of CST in medicine and research. There is also significant variability from one CST to another, thus making it difficult to compare across platforms in a meaningful way.

Performance

CST were previously considered inferior to research and clinical-grade, FDA-cleared actigraphy, primarily due to the lack of high-quality evidence that compared CST performance to gold-standard polysomnogram (PSG).[80] However, a growing body of literature now reports the performance of CST when compared to PSG, and in many studies, simultaneous comparison of actigraphy is reported. In considering the performance of CST, given the multiple reported measures, comparison of CST- and PSG-derived sleep-wake classification, sleep stages, and respiratory parameters is required.

Similar to actigraphy, when evaluating the performance statistics between CST and PSG measured sleep, the following should be considered: (1) CST-derived data are scored with automated algorithms, while PSGs are scored visually by humans; (2) agreement between technologists in scoring PSG is imperfect (approximately 80%)[13,14]; (3) different physiologic properties are recorded (i.e., heart rate and motion by CST vs. EEG, electrooculogram, and electromyogram by PSG).

The evaluation of CST performance is conducted as noted earlier in the section "Actigraphy Performance," and best practices are described by Depner, et al in 2019.[80] As noted for actigraphy, given that healthy subjects spend most of the nocturnal period asleep, simultaneous epoch-by-epoch (EBE) comparison between PSG and CST is considered superior to the comparison of summary metrics averaged over the course of the night in ascertaining the performance of CST.

The derivation of quantitative metrics that describe CST performance are also described in the section "Actigrapy Performance," and are visually depicted in Figure 24.2. Sleep staging is a newer output of CST (compared to actigraphy) and is a multi-class problem as opposed to the binary distinction between sleep and wake. Therefore, in addition to sensitivity, specificity, and accuracy, a confusion matrix is often constructed to both demonstrate agreement and identify sleep stages where misclassification occurs. Additionally, Cohen's kappa and prevalence and bias-adjusted kappa (PABAK) statistics are useful metrics to mitigate the possibility of agreement by chance and the unequal distribution of sleep stages over the night.[81] An open-source analytical framework was published by Menghini and colleagues in 2021 with the goal of standardizing and facilitating studies that evaluate the sleep-tracking capabilities of CST.[15]

A comprehensive review of the performance of specific CST is beyond the scope of this chapter; the reader is directed to de Zambotti (2019) and Lujan (2021).[82,83] Observed trends in performance are noted in the following. Please note that different devices, software versions, study protocols, patient populations, and reported statistics often preclude direct comparisons between studies. A recent study that simultaneously compared traditional actigraphy, 4 wrist-worn wearable devices, and 3 nearable devices to PSG is beneficial, in part, in mitigating some of the inherent problems of CST performance evaluations. [84]

SLEEP-WAKE CLASSIFICATION

The next section examines the performance of consumer sleep tracking devices in estimating sleep as defined by PSG.

Wrist-Worn (and Ring) CST

In regard to differentiation of sleep from wake, EBE comparisons of CST output to PSG usually demonstrate sensitivity around or exceeding 90%, but wider ranges of specificity (approximately 20%–80%) for multisensory wrist-worn (and ring) CST.[80,82,84] These values are similar to the historically cited performance of actigraphy,[8,85,86] and investigations that compare wrist-worn CST and actigraphy with PSG in the same population have demonstrated minimal differences.[80,84]

Dry Electroencephalogram (EEG) Headbands

Limited peer-reviewed publications are available that describe the capacity of dry EEG headbands to differentiate sleep from wake. The sensitivity and specificity of one dry EEG headband device was reported at 97.6% and 56.1%, with overall agreement of around 90%; however, this particular device is no longer available.[87,88] An industry-sponsored study of a currently available dry EEG headband device demonstrated specificity of 74% and less than 3-minute differences in TST, SE, SOL, and WASO between automatically scored sleep from the headband and the consensus PSG scoring among 5 different technologists.[89]

Bedside

Non-contact bedside nearable devices have demonstrated sensitivity that ranges from the high 80s up to 94%, whereas specificity ranged more widely at 50% to 73%.[68–70,84]

Under (or Within) Mattress

Although ballistocardiography is a well-verified method, the current consumer iterations that utilize this technology for under (or within) mattress sleep tracking has not always yielded optimal results. For example, one device significantly underestimated WASO and overestimated TST.[90] In line with these findings, another device demonstrated high sensitivity for sleep (96%) and low specificity for wake (47%).[84] However, an earlier investigation (and prior model) of that device demonstrated sensitivity and specificity of 92.5% and 80.4%, respectively, which highlights the difficulty in comparing the performance metrics between studies.[91]

SLEEP STAGING

In addition to sleep-wake differentiation, CST classify sleep as light, deep, and rapid eye movement (REM), comparable to the PSG scored equivalents of NREM1 + NREM2 (N1 + N2), NREM3 (N3), and stage R sleep, respectively. Of note, sleep stages are constructs primarily based on EEG activity; therefore, sleep stages derived from CST should be approached cautiously. Additionally, nightly, long-term recordings of sleep stages are of unclear clinical relevance. Newer publications typically demonstrate better agreement between PSG and CST derived sleep staging, which demonstrates improvement in algorithms over time.

Wrist-Worn (and Ring) CST

Overall accuracy in sleep staging has ranged widely, 60%–80% for N1 + N2, 40%–87% for N3, and 30%–89% for stage R sleep derived from wrist-worn (or ring) CST.[63,84,92–94]

Dry Electroencephalogram (EEG) Headbands

One available dry EEG headband predicted N3 sleep with 70% sensitivity and 90% specificity, although other sleep stages were not reported.[67] More recently, the current model of the same device was compared to a consensus of 5 scorers manually annotating PSG. Overall sleep staging accuracy of the headband compared to consensus was 83.5% ± 6.4%, while the average accuracy of individual human sleep scorers was only marginally better (86.4% ±

8.0%) when compared to consensus.[89] The headband-acquired EEG data, which was scored by a machine learning algorithm, correctly identified wake, N1, N2, N3, and stage R sleep in 74%, 47.7%, 82.9%, 82.6% and 84.5% of epochs.[89]

Bedside

The most recent evaluation of 2 different nearable devices compared to PSG demonstrated similar performance for light (sensitivity 67% and 68%, specificity 61% and 60%), deep (sensitivity of both 59%, specificity of both 88%), and REM sleep (sensitivity 50% and 49%, specificity of both 95%) staging,[84] similar to previously cited performance values.[68]

Under (or Within) Mattress

While one under-the-bed sensor demonstrated poor agreement with PSG staged sleep (Cohen's kappa 0.1),[90] a recent report demonstrated sensitivities of 57%, 68%, 64%, and specificities of 69%, 84%, 89% for light, deep, and stage REM sleep, respectively.

RESPIRATORY PARAMETERS

The cardiac parameters collected by CST also allow for computation of respiratory rate[95] and apnea hypopnea index (AHI). The ubiquity of PPG in wrist- (and ring)-worn CST provides an excellent substrate of cardiorespiratory data for machine learning algorithms. For example, a deep learning algorithm applied to wrist-worn PPG and accelerometry data approximated PSG AHI well, with a weighted Cohen's kappa = 0.51, and stratified individuals into OSA severity classes (area under the receiver operating characteristic curve of 0.84, 0.86, and 0.85 for mild, moderate, severe OSA, respectively).[96]

Recently, oximetry monitoring capabilities have been incorporated into the reflective PPG sensors used by wrist- and ring-worn CST, and may add to OSA prediction capabilities. For example, use of both cardiac and oximetry measurements from the PPG (along with accelerometry) of a wrist-worn CST allowed algorithm prediction of OSA (AHI ≥5) with accuracy, sensitivity, and specificity of 81.1%, 76.5%, and 100%.[97] A ring device that includes an FDA-cleared oximeter utilized a neural network applied to ring-acquired oximetry, pulse rate, HRV, accelerometry, and PPG waveform data to predict total sleep time and AHI.[98] The comparison of ring-estimated AHI correlated highly with AHI collected during PSG or home sleep apnea testing. Accuracy, sensitivity, and specificity in categorizing individuals with AHI ≥15 were 0.808 (95% CI, 0.703–0.888), 0.931 (95% CI, 0.772–0.992), and 0.735 (95% CI, 0.589–0.850), respectively.[98] The addition to oximetry to other PPG parameters is expected to increase the ability of CST to detect respiratory events and, combined with the capacity for simultaneous quantification of TST, may increase the ability of CST to approximate PSG AHI in the home.

Nearable devices do not use PPG, which requires contact with the user, and therefore cannot measure oximetry. However, given monitoring of ballistocardiography, under-the-mattress devices have demonstrated promise in detecting OSA. Using an AHI threshold of 15 per hour, different under-the-mattress CST were able to identify obstructive sleep apnea with sensitivities of 72%–89% and specificities of 70%–91%.[99–101] Bedside CST allows for an even more direct measurement of respiratory movement with radar technology, which lends this technology to OSA assessment. One noncontact bedside nearable appropriately classified OSA patients with a sensitivity of 90% and a specificity of 92%.[102]

LIMITATIONS OF PERFORMANCE ESTIMATES

Although the available literature that describes studies that compare CST to gold-standard PSG has expanded considerably, and algorithms used by CST have improved in parallel to artificial intelligence advances, cited performance must be carefully appraised when translating performance to home use (see Figure 24.3). Rapid changes in device models, firmware, and software may impede the translation of in-laboratory performance metrics to the field. Although this is also the case with actigraphy software, manufacturers of FDA-cleared actigraphs typically disclose sleep classifier algorithms (see Figure 24.1). Conversely, CST manufacturers use black box AI algorithms to stage sleep and do not typically provide details regarding algorithm development.

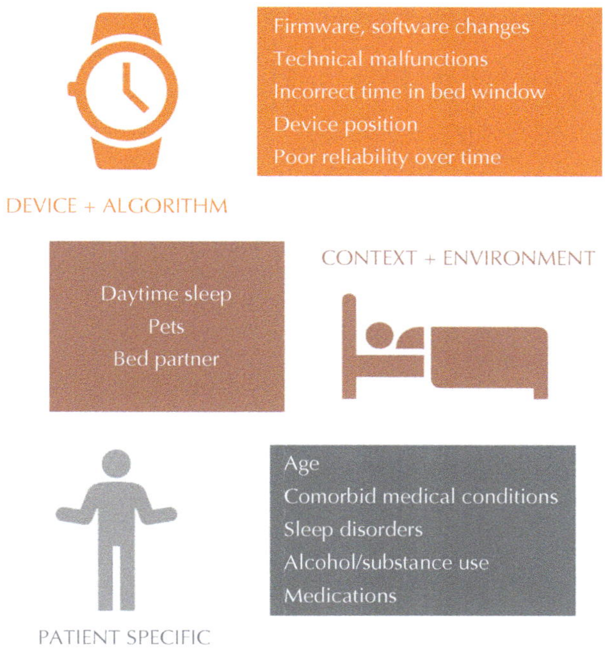

Figure 24.3. Factors limiting translation of CST performance outside of the laboratory.

In addition to heterogeneous study protocols, populations, and analyses methods, the in-lab context of CST performance evaluation may also interfere reproducibility and generalizability of cited performance metrics. In-laboratory CST performance evaluations artificially impose TIB, while use in the home environment utilizes passive detection to determine the periods in which sleep classifiers are deployed. Therefore, performance is influenced by not only the capabilities of the sensors and sleep (and AHI) scoring algorithms but also the designation of the correct TIB window.

Additionally, measures such as bedtime, wake-up time, TST, wake time, SE, light sleep, deep sleep, and REM sleep have gold-standard equivalents for comparison; however, proprietary scores or metrics such as "restless sleep," "sleep disturbances," or "readiness" may be impossible to harmonize with usual clinical and scientific terms.

Furthermore, device position, technical failures, bed partners, and pets could also prevent translation of CST performance to the home environment. Notably, CST comparison to PSG typically takes place over a single night of study; therefore, reliability night to night, during sleep outside of nighttime hours, and sleep periods outside of the main sleep bout (i.e., naps) remain unclear.[94,103]

Patient-specific factors like age, comorbid sleep disorders,[93,94,104–108] other health conditions, alcohol use, and age all may impact the real-life accuracy of CST.[80]

Regulation and Guidelines

By definition, CST devices have not been evaluated by the FDA and are typically categorized as "entertainment" devices. As the technology continues to improve, many are moving closer to what might be considered a diagnostic device. Devices that hope to surpass this threshold must submit validation/performance data to the FDA. Recently, a CST was identified by the FDA as a medical device and a request was made that the company either discontinue the device or apply for the appropriate FDA designation since it was providing clinically actionable data (https://www.usatoday.com/story/tech/2021/11/30/fda-warning-owlet-baby-monitor-socks/8805723002/). The company discontinued this device to comply with the FDA.

The FDA also specifies Software as a Medical Device (SaMD) (https://www.fda.gov/medical-devices/digital-health-center-excellence/software-medical-device-samd). This is defined by the International Medical Device Regulators Forum (IMDRF) as "software intended to be used for one or more medical purposes that perform these purposes without being part of a hardware medical device" (https://www.fda.gov/medical-devices/digital-health-center-excellence/software-medical-device-samd). These have already been deployed for use in sleep medicine, such as the Sleepimage device (https://www.accessdata.fda.gov/cdrh_docs/pdf18/K182618.pdf). While the algorithm has been FDA cleared, the actual hardware has not been cleared, thus adding a layer of both complexity and ambiguity for sleep clinicians. The IMDRF is composed of a group of medical device regulators who voluntarily work together to develop guidance regarding SaMD. As innovation continues to expand our field, guidelines are being developed to provide clarity and guardrails.

FDA clearance can be somewhat opaque—a device may have one component that has been cleared or approved by the FDA, such as an included pulse oximeter, but the entire device has not been FDA cleared. This can lead to confusion among consumers and clinicians. It also blurs the lines between consumer and clinical devices. Marketing may highlight the FDA clearance and allude to the entire device being FDA cleared when in reality, only one part of it may have been cleared. For example, a device with an FDA-cleared oximeter has not been cleared to screen for OSA, but the marketing may make this difficult to elucidate.

Use Cases

The most immediate applications for consumer sleep technologies in sleep medicine are likely to emulate actigraphy; however, unique features of consumer sleep technologies allow for novel uses.

ACTIGRAPHY AS A PRECEDENT

The Centers for Medicare & Medicaid Services (CMS) recently increased the reimbursement for remote patient and remote therapy monitoring (RPM and RTM, respectively) while simultaneously decreasing reimbursement for HSAT. This shift signals a change in the mindset of payors who are exploring the abundance of data contained within Patient-Generated-Health-Data (PGHD). Therefore, if a CST was deemed acceptable, a provider could consider its use for the existing clinical indications for actigraphy (i.e., in the evaluation and management of central disorders of hypersomnolence, insomnia, circadian rhythm sleep-wake disorders [CRSWD], and integrated into home sleep apnea tests [HSAT]), as detailed earlier in this chapter ("Use Cases for Actigraphy" section). Because CST may be used by patients long before the first sleep appointment and between visits, substitution for actigraphy for already established indications could streamline the sleep clinic workflow.

From a research standpoint, CST have already replaced traditional actigraphy in research studies across a variety of subject areas and have allowed for the study of sleep at scale. For example, gender and age differences in sleep were revealed in a study of 11 million nights of Fitbit data from nearly 70,000 subjects across 47 countries.[109]

NEW APPLICATIONS

CST are characterized by features distinct from FDA-cleared actigraphy, including widespread acceptance and use, lower cost, ownership by the patient or research participant, prolonged and continuous patterns of use, wireless and near real-time data transmission, and the capacity to interface with other apps and health technologies. These unique traits provide novel clinical and research applications.

Off-PAP Sleep Time

Concerns regarding the effectiveness of CPAP in preventing detrimental outcomes attributable to OSA has been raised in randomized controlled trials[110,111] and by the Agency for Healthcare Research and Quality (AHRQ; https://www.ahrq.gov/sites/default/files/wysiwyg/research/findings/ta/drafts-for-review/sleep-apnea-draftreport.pdf).

Though the acquisition of data from positive airway pressure (PAP) machines and data management through cloud-based platforms provides an easy assessment of PAP use and estimated efficacy, sleep that takes place without PAP or "Off-PAP sleep time" is not captured.[111] CST track sleep independent of PAP use and additionally, with the use of certain devices, can measure sleep-disordered breathing; therefore, sleep periods which were not previously considered (i.e., naps, sleep periods with partial PAP use) could be evaluated in OSA patients. This capability allows the assessment of the balance of sleep with and without PAP and the burden of sleep-disordered breathing on and off therapy in the ambulatory setting. In this use case, CST could reveal another underlying sleep disorder or suboptimal treatment of a patient's sleep-disordered breathing. Because patients may not recognize these sleep periods as abnormal and fail to mention them during a clinic visit, this is a medically novel and relevant application of CST.

Integration with Other Digital Health Tools and Care Models

The recording of sleep data with CST does not take place in isolation. For example, wearable CST also collect activity and exercise data across a 24-hour day, calculate energy expenditure, recovery, and detect heart arrhythmias.[112] Additionally, CST are not stand-alone hardware; they are associated with mobile apps for data analysis and management. Such apps confer the ability to collect self-report information about sleep and daytime function and can interface with other apps through application programming interfaces (APIs). This allows simultaneous collection of sleep metrics alongside other subjective and objective (e.g., connected scales, glucometers) digital health measures. Parallel access to the electronic health record and passive collection of metadata such as geolocation now provide an in-depth, multifaceted representation of health during and between interactions with a care provider or hospital. Apple HealthKit, ResearchKit, CareKit, and SensorKit demonstrate the ability of consumer-facing technology to comprehensively assess health in the ambulatory environment (https://developer.apple.com/documentation/healthkit; https://www.apple.com/lae/researchkit/, https://developer.apple.com/documentation/sensorkit).

From a research standpoint, the capabilities of multi-sensory CST and their interoperability with mobile applications to assess other information have allowed for large-scale longitudinal studies to identify the influence of sleep on other outcomes, such as mood assessed through an ecological momentary assessment app,[113] wearable measured resting heart rate,[114] and many others. The University of California, San Francisco, has harnessed these versatile capabilities with the Eureka platform, which integrates consumer-facing mobile technologies to seamlessly collect data from apps, devices, and other novel sources for research (https://info.eurekaplatform.org/).

Because the collection of digital data with tools owned entirely by the consumer circumvents any exchange of medical hardware, CST and other health technologies are easily integrated into a contactless telemedicine program with both synchronous and asynchronous possibilities. Synchronous telehealth visits might be enriched by view of the patient's CST data without ever meeting in a physical office. Asynchronous or store-and-forward telehealth could entail the review of electronic health record information and patient-generated data derived from a wearable CST (objectively tracked sleep parameters, sleep-disordered breathing indices) and mobile app (self-report digital questionnaires and even oropharyngeal imagery from the smartphone camera). Based on this information, recommendations regarding evaluation and treatment could be provided to the patient or a primary care physician seeking consultation.

Intervention

While CST can serve to track sleep and increase the awareness of the importance of sleep, they can also serve as a therapeutic tool for insomnia disorder, CRSWD, and can facilitate the treatment of OSA. For example, CST-tracked sleep parameters have provided input to a cognitive behavioral therapy for insomnia (CBT-I) mobile app.[105,115] CST use in insomnia therapy is likely to transcend CBT-I; for example, some devices incorporate intensive sleep retraining in an attempt to treat chronic insomnia. This is based on data from in-lab intensive sleep retraining.[64] Currently, this work is being translated to the home environment through the use of a device worn on the finger, which awakens the patient once they drift off to sleep in order to increase the homeostatic drive for sleep (Thim.io).

Another intervention already in use is the promotion of PAP use with patient-facing mobile apps. This patient-engagement technique could be harnessed further by the addition of wearable CST oximetry to identify when therapy is suboptimal.

Moving forward, CST has the potential to influence sleep in a positive way—to help reduce the use of mobile devices before bed by locking the apps at a predetermined time, to provide short educational content on demand, and to provide feedback on existing sleep durations and timing. These capabilities exist today and will likely continue to become more refined.

CST extend to our environment through connectivity to thermostats and smart lighting that will help to create ideal sleep conditions passively. Adjustments initially may be programmed but are expected to evolve so that environmental parameters (such as ambient light, room temperature, etc.) change based on CST-measured sleep duration, quality, timing, and metadata such as day of the week, season, and travel schedule. Behavioral nudges can be delivered based on patient-specific patterns revealed by CST to also improve sleep hygiene, sleep timing, and sleep duration.

As CST becomes smaller and touchless, utilization outside the home may increase in healthcare facilities such as nursing homes and hospitals. Touchless monitors may alert caregivers to apneas or desaturations, thus allowing for prompt evaluation and treatment. An aging population will also see benefit as ballistocardiography may identify the presence of an underlying cardiac abnormality during sleep passively and routinely as monitors are embedded into mattresses and headboards.

Innovation and creativity will allow for new methods of treatment for a myriad of sleep disorders while simultaneously increasing awareness and accessibility to sleep healthcare.

LIMITATIONS

While promising, CST are not without significant pitfalls. In addition to the previously described shortcomings regarding the translation of performance to real-world settings (Figure 24.3) and unclear regulation, implementation into clinical practice is another barrier that prevents the adoption of CST into clinical practice.

To successfully integrate patient-generated data, a device and manufacturer agnostic platform is required so that CST data can be collected, distilled in a meaningful way, and viewed by providers. If developed, a subsequent requirement is the ability to interface with the electronic health record. The development and maintenance of such a program, along with ensuring data security, will require significant information technology resources. Additionally, significant staff effort is required to enact workflows to manage this new data stream and provide patient education. To rationalize the cost of such resources, a robust reimbursement mechanism for utilization of CST data is needed.

The ownership of CST by the patient and the pattern of more long-term use will provide sleep information beyond the limited recording duration of actigraphy use cases (i.e., beyond the diagnostic period or brief assessment of treatment response). Additionally, as opposed to use in carefully selected individuals, patients may self-select. Therefore, the potential data from CST are actually novel and distinct, as opposed to the concept of CST as a replacement for actigraphy. The availability of such data may have undesirable consequences, such as over-reliance on CST sleep parameters, change in medical decision-making based on inaccurate parameters, or unnecessary diagnostic testing or referrals. Collection, but not expert viewing, of continuous cardiopulmonary and sleep metrics may have legal repercussions in the case of at-home cardiac events or motor vehicle accidents.

Already, investigators have revealed that the performance of pulse oximetry varies by skin tone, and the green LED lights used for PPG assessment of heart rate and oximetry in CST are much less accurate in individuals with dark skin.[116] Furthermore, convenience samples used to test the accuracy of CST often lack diversity and result in metrics that fail to translate to individuals in minority groups.[116] Therefore, the use of CST in diagnostic and treatment pathways could augment racial disparities in healthcare at scale.[116]

Data security is another concern among researchers and clinicians. For example, the location of undisclosed U.S. military bases was inadvertently uncovered and made public via geolocation data from a popular fitness app that utilizes wearables (https://www.theguardian.

com/world/2018/jan/28/fitness-tracking-app-gives-away-location-of-secret-us-army-bases).

CONCLUSIONS

CST has inarguably provided another dimension to the clinical practice of sleep medicine, in addition to sleep and circadian research, and may ultimately allow for more robust longitudinal assessment. Current barriers include opacity of the raw signals, proprietary algorithms, and no clear way to compare sleep metrics across devices and platforms. Additionally, EBE comparison to known HSAT or PSG signal is not usually performed. It is evident, however, that consumers are utilizing these technologies, and while they presently do not replace FDA-cleared sleep studies (either PSG and HSAT), it is clear that they do have the potential to provide additional information and may help to fill a void that currently exists in sleep medicine. Further research should not only improve the accuracy of sleep-wake detection but also establish if longitudinal sleep-stage analysis is truly helpful, as opposed to the ability to differentiate sleep from wakefulness, engage patients, and provide feedback and encouragement to establish better sleep-wake routines and demonstrate the essential nature of sleep.

REFERENCES

1. Kupfer DJ, Detre TP, Foster G, Tucker GJ, Delgado J. The application of Delgado's telemetric mobility recorder for human studies. *Behav Biol*. 1972;7(4):585–590.
2. Kupfer DJ, Weiss BL, Foster G, Detre TP, McPartland R. Psychomotor activity in affective states. *Arch Gen Psychiatry*. 1974;30(6):765–768.
3. McPartland RJ, Kupfer DJ, Gordon Foster F. The movement-activated recording monitor: A third-generation motor-activity monitoring system. *Behav Res Methods Instrumentation*. 1976;8(4):357–360.
4. Colburn TR, Smith BM, Guarini JJ, Simmons NN. An ambulatory activity monitor with solid state memory. *Biomed Sci Instrum*. 1976;12:117–122.
5. Kripke DF, Mullaney DJ, Messin S, Wyborney VG. Wrist actigraphic measures of sleep and rhythms. *Electroencephalogr Clin Neurophysiol*. 1978;44(5):674–676.
6. Chen KY, Bassett DR Jr. The technology of accelerometry-based activity monitors: Current and future. *Med Sci Sports Exerc*. 2005;37(11 Suppl):S490–S500.
7. te Lindert BHW, Van Someren EJW. Sleep estimates using microelectromechanical systems (MEMS). *Sleep*. 2013;36(5):781–789.
8. Ancoli-Israel S, Cole R, Alessi C, Chambers M, Moorcroft W, Pollak CP. The role of actigraphy in the study of sleep and circadian rhythms. *Sleep*. 2003;26(3):342–392.
9. Jean-Louis G, Kripke DF, Mason WJ, Elliott JA, Youngstedt SD. Sleep estimation from wrist movement quantified by different actigraphic modalities. *J Neurosci Methods*. 2001;105(2):185–191.
10. Webster JB, Kripke DF, Messin S, Mullaney DJ, Wyborney G. An activity-based sleep monitor system for ambulatory use. *Sleep*. 1982;5(4):389–399.
11. Li X, Zhang Y, Jiang F, Zhao H. A novel machine learning unsupervised algorithm for sleep/wake identification using actigraphy. *Chronobiol Int*. 2020;37(7):1002–1015.
12. Patel SR, Weng J, Rueschman M, et al. Reproducibility of a standardized actigraphy scoring algorithm for sleep in a US Hispanic/Latino population. *Sleep*. 2015;38(9):1497–1503.
13. Younes M, Raneri J, Hanly P. Staging sleep in polysomnograms: Analysis of inter-scorer variability. *J Clin Sleep Med*. 2016;12(6):885–894.
14. Danker-Hopfe H, Anderer P, Zeitlhofer J, et al. Interrater reliability for sleep scoring according to the Rechtschaffen & Kales and the new AASM standard. *J Sleep Res*. 2009;18(1):74–84.
15. Menghini L, Cellini N, Goldstone A, Baker FC, de Zambotti M. A standardized framework for testing the performance of sleep-tracking technology: Step-by-step guidelines and open-source code. *Sleep*. 2020;44(2). doi:10.1093/sleep/zsaa170.
16. Paquet J, Kawinska A, Carrier J. Wake detection capacity of actigraphy during sleep. *Sleep*. 2007;30(10):1362–1369.
17. Rupp TL, Balkin TJ. Comparison of Motionlogger Watch and Actiwatch actigraphs to polysomnography for sleep/wake estimation in healthy young adults. *Behav Res Methods*. 2011;43(4):1152–1160.
18. Quante M, Kaplan ER, Cailler M, et al. Actigraphy-based sleep estimation in adolescents and adults: A comparison with polysomnography using two scoring algorithms. *Nat Sci Sleep*. 2018;10:13–20.
19. Zinkhan M, Berger K, Hense S, et al. Agreement of different methods for assessing sleep characteristics: A comparison of two actigraphs, wrist and hip placement, and self-report with polysomnography. *Sleep Med*. 2014;15(9):1107–1114.
20. Smith MT, McCrae CS, Cheung J, et al. Use of actigraphy for the evaluation of sleep disorders and circadian rhythm sleep-wake disorders: An American Academy of Sleep Medicine systematic review, meta-analysis, and GRADE assessment. *J Clin Sleep Med*. 2018;14(07):1209–1230.
21. Marler MR, Gehrman P, Martin JL. The sigmoidally transformed cosine curve: A mathematical model for circadian rhythms with symmetric non-sinusoidal shapes. *Stat Med*. 2006;25(22):3893–3904.doi:10.1002/sim.2466.
22. Cheng P, Walch O, Huang Y, et al. Predicting circadian misalignment with wearable technology: Validation of wrist-worn actigraphy and photometry in night shift

workers. *Sleep*. 2021;44(2):zsaa180. doi:10.1093/sleep/zsaa180.
23. Gottlieb DJ, Ellenbogen JM, Bianchi MT, Czeisler CA. Sleep deficiency and motor vehicle crash risk in the general population: a prospective cohort study. *BMC Med*. 2018;16(1):44.
24. Barger LK, Ayas NT, Cade BE, et al. Impact of extended-duration shifts on medical errors, adverse events, and attentional failures. *PLoS Med*. 2006;3(12):e487.
25. Ayas NT, Barger LK, Cade BE, et al. Extended work duration and the risk of self-reported percutaneous injuries in interns. *JAMA*. 2006;296(9):1055–1062.
26. Lao XQ, Liu X, Deng HB, et al. Sleep quality, sleep duration, and the risk of coronary heart disease: A prospective cohort study with 60,586 adults. *J Clin Sleep Med*. 2018;14(01):109–117.
27. Kim CW, Chang Y, Kang JG, Ryu S. Changes in sleep duration and subsequent risk of hypertension in healthy adults. *Sleep*. 2018;41(11). doi:10.1093/sleep/zsy159.
28. Ai S, Zhang J, Zhao G, et al. Causal associations of short and long sleep durations with 12 cardiovascular diseases: linear and nonlinear Mendelian randomization analyses in UK Biobank. *Eur Heart J*. 2021;42(34):3349–3357.
29. St-Onge MP, Grandner MA, Brown D, et al. Sleep duration and quality: Impact on lifestyle behaviors and cardiometabolic health: A scientific statement from the American Heart Association. *Circulation*. 2016;134(18):e367–e386.
30. Spiegel K, Sheridan JF, Van Cauter E. Effect of sleep deprivation on response to immunizaton. *JAMA*. 2002;288(12):1471–1472.
31. Cohen S, Doyle WJ, Alper CM, Janicki-Deverts D, Turner RB. Sleep habits and susceptibility to the common cold. *Arch Intern Med*. 2009;169(1):62–67.
32. Cooper CB, Neufeld EV, Dolezal BA, Martin JL. Sleep deprivation and obesity in adults: A brief narrative review. *BMJ Open Sport Exerc Med*. 2018;4(1):e000392.
33. Wang Y, Qian YX, Liu JH, Miao YM, Ma QH, Pan CW. Longitudinal association between sleep and 5-year incident metabolic syndrome in older Chinese adults: A community-based cohort study. *Sleep Med*. 2021;81:1–7.
34. Cappuccio FP, D'Elia L, Strazzullo P, Miller MA. Sleep duration and all-cause mortality: A systematic review and meta-analysis of prospective studies. *Sleep*. 2010;33(5):585–592.
35. Kurina LM, McClintock MK, Chen JH, Waite LJ, Thisted RA, Lauderdale DS. Sleep duration and all-cause mortality: A critical review of measurement and associations. *Ann Epidemiol*. 2013;23(6):361–370.
36. Bianchi MT, Thomas RJ, Westover MB. An open request to epidemiologists: Please stop querying self-reported sleep duration. *Sleep Med*. 2017;35:92–93.
37. Wittmann M, Dinich J, Merrow M, Roenneberg T. Social jetlag: Misalignment of biological and social time. *Chronobiol Int*. 2006;23(1-2):497–509.
38. Roenneberg T, Pilz LK, Zerbini G, Winnebeck EC. Chronotype and social jetlag: A (self-) critical review. *Biology*. 2019;8(3):54. doi:10.3390/biology8030054.
39. Wong PM, Hasler BP, Kamarck TW, Muldoon MF, Manuck SB. Social jetlag, chronotype, and cardiometabolic risk. *J Clin Endocrinol Metab*. 2015;100(12):4612–4620.
40. Levandovski R, Dantas G, Fernandes LC, et al. Depression scores associate with chronotype and social jetlag in a rural population. *Chronobiol Int*. 2011;28(9):771–778.
41. Depner CM, Melanson EL, Eckel RH, et al. Ad libitum weekend recovery sleep fails to prevent metabolic dysregulation during a repeating pattern of insufficient sleep and weekend recovery sleep. *Curr Biol*. 2019;29(6):957–967.e4.
42. Ash T, Kang A, Hom C, Risica PM. Association between sleep duration and differences between weekday and weekend sleep with body mass index & waist circumference among Black women in Sistertalk II. *Sleep Health*. 2020;6(6):797–803.
43. Lv Y, Cai L, Zeng X, Gui Z, Lai L, Tan W. Association between weekend catch-up sleep and executive functions in Chinese school-aged children. *J Clin Sleep Med*. 2020;16(8):1285–1293. https://jcsm.aasm.org/doi/abs/10.5664/jcsm.8494
44. Bei B, Wiley JF, Trinder J, Manber R. Beyond the mean: A systematic review on the correlates of daily intraindividual variability of sleep/wake patterns. *Sleep Med Rev*. 2016;28:108–124.
45. Fischer D, Klerman EB, Phillips AJK. Measuring sleep regularity: Theoretical properties and practical usage of existing metrics. *Sleep*. 2021;44(10). doi:10.1093/sleep/zsab103
46. Huang T, Redline S. Cross-sectional and prospective associations of actigraphy-assessed sleep regularity with metabolic abnormalities: The multi-ethnic study of atherosclerosis. *Diabetes Care*. 2019;42(8):1422–1429.
47. Huang T, Mariani S, Redline S. Sleep irregularity and risk of cardiovascular events: The multi-ethnic study of atherosclerosis. *J Am Coll Cardiol*. 2020;75(9):991–999.
48. Slavish DC, Taylor DJ, Lichstein KL. Intraindividual variability in sleep and comorbid medical and mental health conditions. *Sleep*. 2019;42(6). doi:10.1093/sleep/zsz052.
49. Bernert RA, Hom MA, Iwata NG, Joiner TE. Objectively assessed sleep variability as an acute warning sign of suicidal ideation in a longitudinal evaluation of young adults at high suicide risk. *J Clin Psychiatry*. 2017;78(6):e678–e687.
50. Bei B, Manber R, Allen NB, Trinder J, Wiley JF. Too long, too short, or too variable? Sleep intraindividual variability and its associations with perceived sleep quality and mood in adolescents during naturalistically unconstrained sleep. *Sleep*. 2017;40(2). doi:10.1093/sleep/zsw067
51. Wallace ML, Stone K, Smagula SF, et al. Which sleep health characteristics predict all-cause mortality in older men? An application of flexible multivariable approaches. *Sleep*. 2018;41(1). doi:10.1093/sleep/zsx189.
52. Ancoli-Israel S, Martin JL, Blackwell T, et al. The SBSM guide to actigraphy monitoring: Clinical and research applications. *Behav Sleep Med*. 2015;13(Suppl 1):S4–S38.
53. Benedict C, Cedernaes J. Could a good night's sleep improve COVID-19 vaccine efficacy? *Lancet Respir Med*. 2021;9(5):447–448.

54. Radin JM, Quer G, Ramos E, et al. Assessment of prolonged physiological and behavioral changes associated with COVID-19 infection. *JAMA Netw Open*. 2021;4(7):e2115959.
55. Quer G, Radin JM, Gadaleta M, et al. Wearable sensor data and self-reported symptoms for COVID-19 detection. *Nat Med*. 2021;27(1):73–77.
56. Gadaleta M, Radin JM, Baca-Motes K, et al. Passive detection of COVID-19 with wearable sensors and explainable machine learning algorithms. *NPJ Digit Med*. 2021;4(1):166.
57. Alavi A, Bogu GK, Wang M, et al. Real-time alerting system for COVID-19 and other stress events using wearable data. *Nat Med*. 2022;28(1):175–184.
58. Khosla S, Deak MC, Gault D, et al. Consumer sleep technology: An American Academy of Sleep Medicine position statement. *J Clin Sleep Med*. 2018;14(5):877–880. doi:10.5664/jcsm.7128.
59. Gu W, Leung L, Kwok KC, Wu IC, Folz RJ, Chiang AA. Belun Ring Platform: A novel home sleep apnea testing system for assessment of obstructive sleep apnea. *J Clin Sleep Med*. 2020;16(9):1611–1617.
60. Allen J. Photoplethysmography and its application in clinical physiological measurement. *Physiol Meas*. 2007;28(3):R1–R39.
61. Vulcan RS, André S, Bruyneel M. Photoplethysmography in normal and pathological *sleep*. Sensors. 2021; 21(9):2928. doi:10.3390/s21092928.
62. Pereira T, Tran N, Gadhoumi K, et al. Photoplethysmography based atrial fibrillation detection: A review. *NPJ Digit Med*. 2020;3:3.
63. de Zambotti M, Rosas L, Colrain IM, Baker FC. The sleep of the ring: Comparison of the ŌURA Sleep Tracker against polysomnography. *Behav Sleep Med*. 2019;17(2):124–136.
64. Harris J, Lack L, Kemp K, Wright H, Bootzin R. A randomized controlled trial of intensive sleep retraining (ISR): A brief conditioning treatment for chronic insomnia. *Sleep*. 2012;35(1):49–60.
65. Scott H, Whitelaw A, Canty A, Lovato N, Lack L. The accuracy of the THIM wearable device for estimating sleep onset latency. *J Clin Sleep Med*. 2021;17(5):973–981.
66. Bianchi MT. Sleep devices: Wearables and nearables, informational and interventional, consumer and clinical. *Metabolism*. 2018;84:99–108.
67. Debellemaniere E, Chambon S, Pinaud C, et al. Performance of an ambulatory dry-EEG device for auditory closed-loop stimulation of sleep slow oscillations in the home environment. *Front Hum Neurosci*. 2018;12:88.
68. Schade MM, Bauer CE, Murray BR, et al. Sleep validity of a non-contact bedside movement and respiration-sensing device. *J Clin Sleep Med*. 2019;15(7):1051–1061.
69. De Chazal P, Fox N, O'Hare E, et al. Sleep/wake measurement using a non-contact biomotion sensor. *J Sleep Res*. 2011;20(2):356–366.
70. O'Hare E, Flanagan D, Penzel T, Garcia C, Frohberg D, Heneghan C. A comparison of radio-frequency biomotion sensors and actigraphy versus polysomnography for the assessment of sleep in normal subjects. *Sleep Breath*. 2015;19(1):91–98. doi:10.1007/s11325-014-0967-z.
71. Alihanka J, Vaahtoranta K, Saarikivi I. A new method for long-term monitoring of the ballistocardiogram, heart rate, and respiration. *Am J Physiol*. 1981;240(5):R384–R392.
72. Sadek I, Biswas J, Abdulrazak B. Ballistocardiogram signal processing: A review. *Health Inf Sci Syst*. 2019;7(1):10.
73. Choi YK, Demiris G, Lin SY, et al. Smartphone applications to support sleep self-management: Review and evaluation. *J Clin Sleep Med*. 2018;14(10):1783–1790.
74. Fino E, Mazzetti M. Monitoring healthy and disturbed sleep through smartphone applications: a review of experimental evidence. *Sleep Breath*. 2019;23(1):13–24.
75. Borger JN, Huber R, Ghosh A. Capturing sleep-wake cycles by using day-to-day smartphone touchscreen interactions. *NPJ Digital Med*. 2019;2(1):1–8.
76. Beattie Z, Oyang Y, Statan A, et al. Estimation of sleep stages in a healthy adult population from optical plethysmography and accelerometer signals. *Physiol Meas*. 2017;38(11):1968–1979.
77. Zhang X, Kou W, Chang EIC, Gao H, Fan Y, Xu Y. Sleep stage classification based on multi-level feature learning and recurrent neural networks via wearable device. *Comput Biol Med*. 2018;103:71–81.
78. Walch O, Huang Y, Forger D, Goldstein C. Sleep stage prediction with raw acceleration and photoplethysmography heart rate data derived from a consumer wearable device. *Sleep*. 2019;42(12):zsz180. doi:10.1093/sleep/zsz180.
79. van Hees VT, Sabia S, Jones SE, et al. Estimating sleep parameters using an accelerometer without sleep diary. *Sci Rep*. 2018;8(1):12975.
80. Depner CM, on behalf of the participants of the 2018 International Biomarkers Workshop on Wearables, Cheng PC, et al. Wearable technologies for developing sleep and circadian biomarkers: A summary of workshop discussions. *Sleep*. 2019;43(2). doi:10.1093/sleep/zsz254.
81. Byrt T, Bishop J, Carlin JB. Bias, prevalence and kappa. *J Clin Epidemiol*. 1993;46(5):423–429.
82. de Zambotti M, Cellini N, Goldstone A, Colrain IM, Baker FC. Wearable sleep technology in clinical and research settings. *Med Sci Sports Exerc*. 2019;51(7):1538–1557.
83. Lujan MR, Perez-Pozuelo I, Grandner MA. Past, present, and future of multisensory wearable technology to monitor sleep and circadian rhythms. *Front Digit Health*. 2021;3:721919.
84. Chinoy ED, Cuellar JA, Huwa KE, et al. Performance of seven consumer sleep-tracking devices compared with polysomnography. *Sleep*. 2021;44(5):zsaa291. doi:10.1093/sleep/zsaa291.
85. Sadeh A. The role and validity of actigraphy in sleep medicine: An update. *Sleep Med Rev*. 2011;15(4):259–267.
86. Van De Water ATM, Holmes A, Hurley DA. Objective measurements of sleep for non-laboratory settings as alternatives to polysomnography: A systematic review. *J Sleep Res*. 2011;20(1pt2):183–200.
87. Tonetti L, Cellini N, de Zambotti M, et al. Polysomnographic validation of a wireless dry headband technology for sleep monitoring in healthy young adults. *Physiol Behav*. 2013;118:185–188.

88. Shambroom JR, Fábregas SE, Johnstone J. Validation of an automated wireless system to monitor sleep in healthy adults. *J Sleep Res*. 2012;21(2):221–230. doi:10.1111/j.1365-2869.2011.00944.x.
89. Arnal PJ, Thorey V, Debellemaniere E, et al. The Dreem Headband compared to polysomnography for electroencephalographic signal acquisition and sleep staging. *Sleep*. 2020;43(11):zsaa097. doi:10.1093/sleep/zsaa097
90. Tuominen J, Peltola K, Saaresranta T, Valli K. Sleep parameter assessment accuracy of a consumer home sleep monitoring ballistocardiograph Beddit Sleep Tracker: A validation study. *J Clin Sleep Med*. 2019;15(3):483–487.
91. Tal A, Shinar Z, Shaki D, Codish S, Goldbart A. Validation of contact-free sleep monitoring device with comparison to polysomnography. *J Clin Sleep Med*. 2017;13(3):517–522.
92. de Zambotti M, Goldstone A, Claudatos S, Colrain IM, Baker FC. A validation study of Fitbit Charge 2™ compared with polysomnography in adults. *Chronobiol Int*. 2018;35(4):465–476. doi:10.1080/07420528.2017.1413578.
93. Cook JD, Eftekari SC, Dallmann E, Sippy M, Plante DT. Ability of the Fitbit Alta HR to quantify and classify sleep in patients with suspected central disorders of hypersomnolence: A comparison against polysomnography. *J Sleep Res*. 2019;28(4):e12789.
94. Cook JD, Prairie ML, Plante DT. Ability of the Multisensory Jawbone UP3 to quantify and classify sleep in patients with suspected central disorders of hypersomnolence: A comparison against polysomnography and actigraphy. *J Clin Sleep Med*. 2018;14(5):841–848.
95. Berryhill S, Morton CJ, Dean A, et al. Effect of wearables on sleep in healthy individuals: A randomized crossover trial and validation study. *J Clin Sleep Med*. 2020;16(5):775–783.
96. Papini GB, Fonseca P, van Gilst MM, Bergmans JWM, Vullings R, Overeem S. Wearable monitoring of sleep-disordered breathing: estimation of the apnea–hypopnea index using wrist-worn reflective photoplethysmography. *Sci Rep*. 2020;10(1):1–15.
97. Chen Y, Wang W, Guo Y, Zhang H, Chen Y, Xie L. A single-center validation of the accuracy of a photoplethysmography-based smartwatch for screening obstructive sleep apnea. *Nat Sci Sleep*. 2021;13:1533–1544.
98. Yeh E, Wong E, Tsai CW, et al. Detection of obstructive sleep apnea using Belun Sleep Platform wearable with neural network-based algorithm and its combined use with STOP-Bang questionnaire. *PLoS One*. 2021;16(10):e0258040.
99. Huysmans D, Borzée P, Testelmans D, et al. Evaluation of a commercial ballistocardiography sensor for sleep apnea screening and sleep monitoring. *Sensors*. 2019;19(9):2133. doi:10.3390/s19092133.
100. Agatsuma T, Fujimoto K, Komatsu Y, et al. A novel device (SD-101) with high accuracy for screening sleep apnoea-hypopnoea syndrome. *Respirology*. 2009;14(8):1143–1150.
101. Norman MB, Middleton S, Erskine O, Middleton PG, Wheatley JR, Sullivan CE. Validation of the Sonomat: A contactless monitoring system used for the diagnosis of sleep disordered breathing. *Sleep*. 2014;37(9):1477–1487.
102. Zaffaroni A, Kent B, O'Hare E, et al. Assessment of sleep-disordered breathing using a non-contact biomotion sensor. *J Sleep Res*. 2013;22(2):231–236.
103. Sargent C, Lastella M, Romyn G, Versey N, Miller DJ, Roach GD. How well does a commercially available wearable device measure sleep in young athletes? *Chronobiol Int*. 2018;35(6):754–758.
104. Toon E, Davey MJ, Hollis SL, Nixon GM, Horne RSC, Biggs SN. Comparison of commercial wrist-based and smartphone accelerometers, actigraphy, and PSG in a clinical cohort of children and adolescents. *J Clin Sleep Med*. 2016;12(3):343–350.
105. Kang SG, Kang JM, Ko KP, Park SC, Mariani S, Weng J. Validity of a commercial wearable sleep tracker in adult insomnia disorder patients and good sleepers. *J Psychosom Res*. 2017;97:38–44.
106. Meltzer LJ, Hiruma LS, Avis K, Montgomery-Downs H, Valentin J. Comparison of a commercial accelerometer with polysomnography and actigraphy in children and adolescents. *Sleep*. 2015;38(8):1323–1330.
107. Moreno-Pino F, Porras-Segovia A, López-Esteban P, Artés A, Baca-García E. Validation of Fitbit Charge 2 and Fitbit Alta HR against polysomnography for assessing sleep in adults with obstructive sleep apnea. *J Clin Sleep Med*. 2019;15(11):1645–1653.
108. Gruwez A, Bruyneel AV, Bruyneel M. The validity of two commercially-available sleep trackers and actigraphy for assessment of sleep parameters in obstructive sleep apnea patients. *PLoS One*. 2019;14(1):e0210569.
109. Jonasdottir SS, Minor K, Lehmann S. Gender differences in nighttime sleep patterns and variability across the adult lifespan: A global-scale wearables study. *Sleep*. 2021;44(2):zsaa169. doi:10.1093/sleep/zsaa169.
110. McEvoy RD, Antic NA, Heeley E, et al. CPAP for prevention of cardiovascular events in obstructive sleep apnea. *N Engl J Med*. 2016;375(10):919–931.
111. Thomas RJ, Bianchi MT. Urgent need to improve PAP management: The devil is in two (fixable) details. *J Clin Sleep Med*. 2017;13(5):657–664.
112. Topol EJ. A decade of digital medicine innovation. *Sci Transl Med*. 2019;11(498):eaaw7610. doi:10.1126/scitranslmed.aaw7610
113. Fang Y, Forger DB, Frank E, Sen S, Goldstein C. Day-to-day variability in sleep parameters and depression risk: A prospective cohort study of training physicians. *NPJ Digit Med*. 2021;4(1):28.
114. Faust L, Feldman K, Mattingly SM, Hachen D, Chawla NV. Deviations from normal bedtimes are associated with short-term increases in resting heart rate. *NPJ Digit Med*. 2020;3:39.
115. Luik AI, Farias Machado P, Espie CA. Delivering digital cognitive behavioral therapy for insomnia at scale: Does using a wearable device to estimate sleep influence therapy? *NPJ Digit Med*. 2018;1:3.
116. Colvonen PJ, DeYoung PN, Bosompra NOA, Owens RL. Limiting racial disparities and bias for wearable devices in health science research. *Sleep*. 2020;43(10):zsaa159. doi:10.1093/sleep/zsaa159.

SECTION VI

Sleep and Other Aspects of Medicine

Chapter 25

Sleep and Common Neurologic Conditions

Tiffany J. Braley and Subhendu Rath

INTRODUCTION

Although sleep disorders have become increasingly recognized for their adverse health consequences in the general population,[1,2] people with chronic neurological conditions may suffer disproportionately from their impact. In addition to their high prevalence in chronic neurological conditions,[3–5] sleep disorders and sleep disturbances have the potential to exacerbate the pathophysiological underpinnings of several neurological disorders, and share bidirectional ties with these conditions.[6–8] That said, sleep disorders in people with neurological conditions remain under-recognized.[9,10] Sleep disorders represent key treatable factors to consider in the management and prevention of these conditions, and a keen knowledge of their causes, consequences, presentations, and management are critical to providing optimal care.

This chapter focuses on several sleep disorders associated with 3 of the most common and impactful neurological conditions in the United States: stroke, epilepsy, and cognitive disorders/dementia, with an emphasis on Alzheimer disease. Here, we discuss the scope and impact of sleep disorders most frequently encountered in these conditions, as well as diagnostic and treatment considerations, including variables that may influence risk for these conditions or response to therapy.

ALZHEIMER DISEASE AND RELATED COGNITIVE DISORDERS

Sleep Disturbances: A Potential Risk Factor for Cognitive Decline and AD

Approximately 6.7 million Americans over age 65 have Alzheimer's dementia (AD), the most common dementia subtype.[11] This neurodegenerative disease is characterized by an excessive accumulation of extracellular amyloid-beta (Aβ) in the brain and intracellular formation of neurofibrillary tau tangles, which lead to neuronal injury and progressive decline in cognition. Following AD, vascular dementia, caused by cumulative small vessel occlusions and large-vessel strokes, represents the second most common dementia subtype and is responsible for approximately 10%–15% of dementia cases.[12] At least another 10% of those with dementia may suffer from "mixed dementia" subtype, which includes pathological features of both AD and vascular dementia.[13] Dementia may also arise from a set of less common neurodegenerative conditions related to abnormal buildup of α-synuclein in neurons (synucleinopathies), including dementia with Lewy bodies and Parkinson's dementia, or arise as a consequence of other central nervous system disorders (e.g., multiple sclerosis or traumatic brain injury).

Mild cognitive impairment (MCI), a term classified by the DSM-5 as "minor neurocognitive disorder," is a state of modest cognitive decline from a previous level of performance in one or more cognitive domains, that does *not* involve a change in daily function. Mild cognitive impairment affects 15%–20% of persons 60 years and older.[14,15] *Although the majority of MCI cases progress to AD, approximately 20% of persons with MCI may revert back to normal cognition in 5 years,*[16–18] *highlighting the importance of research to identify treatable risk factors for conversion of MCI to dementia.*

The growing prevalence and impact of dementia syndromes such as AD have galvanized the need to identify modifiable risk factors for these conditions. Although patients with AD may be at a higher risk for sleep disturbances, sleep disturbances including sleep fragmentation, sleep deprivation, and obstructive sleep apnea may contribute to cognitive decline, and the pathophysiological changes of AD that develop in the pre-clinical stages.

Sleep Deprivation/Sleep Fragmentation and Dementia Risk

Sleep fragmentation and deprivation are independently associated with increased risk for AD progression and all-cause cognitive decline.[19]

Recent evidence suggests that sleep deprivation or insufficient sleep may contribute to accumulation of pathological AD-associated biomarkers (Aβ42 and tau protein) in cognitively intact individuals,[20] and clinical dementia in late life.[21] In a small study of cognitively unimpaired older participants, each additional hour of nighttime sleep was associated with a statistically significant reduction of Aβ, measured with positron emission tomography.[22]

Sleep fragmentation may also independently increase the risk of cognitive decline.[23] In a prior study of 737 cognitively normal older adults, actigraphy-based measures of sleep fragmentation were associated with increased rate of AD. As the study was observational, a cause-and-effect relationship could not be determined. Further studies are still needed to determine whether causal relationships exist between dementia onset and sleep fragmentation or deprivation.

Obstructive Sleep Apnea and Dementia Risk

Sleep deprivation, sleep fragmentation, and *downstream inflammation* are salient features of obstructive sleep apnea (OSA). The prevalence of OSA increases with age, making this condition particularly germane when considering causal pathways to dementia in older adults.

Prior work has revealed compelling relationships between OSA and objective measures of cognitive performance outside of AD, and concerning measures of AD-associated biomarker signatures in the cerebrospinal fluid (CSF) and central nervous system.[24–26] Furthermore, recent data suggest associations between OSA and *incident* dementia diagnoses. In the Study of Osteoporotic Fractures,[27] women with evidence of moderate sleep apnea were 85% more likely to develop MCI or dementia.

Numerous studies have identified associations between OSA and immune-mediated changes that may contribute to AD pathogenesis. The immune system plays a key role in the onset and progression of AD. Under homeostatic circumstances, pro- and anti-inflammatory responses are balanced to provide efficient removal of pathogens and toxins in the brain, while minimizing "collateral" damage from chronic inflammation. Microglia—the principal effector cells of the immune system in the brain—rely upon these tightly regulated pro- and anti-inflammatory cues from the brain and the periphery to efficiently remove pathogens and toxins, as well as Aβ.[28] OSA is associated with chronic inflammation and sleep deprivation, which may each contribute to impairment in microglial function and to decreased clearance of Aβ.[29,30] Proinflammatory cytokines that are commonly elevated in the plasma of patients with OSA are linked to reductions in brain volume in AD and vascular dementia.[31,32]

The potentially shared pathways between OSA, dementia, and Apolipoprotein Eε4 (APOEε4) genotype also require further exploration. Obstructive sleep apnea may represent a critical yet poorly understood link between APOEε4 genotype and incident dementia. The APOEε4 allele is one of the strongest genetic risk factors for AD, with a dose-dependent effect. However, not all (47%) APOEε4 carriers develop dementia,[33] and the impact of OSA on the likelihood of conversion to dementia in APOEε4 carriers is not well understood. Prior research has demonstrated increased associations between OSA and cognitive impairment among carriers of at least one APOEε4 allele, relative to non-APOEε4 carriers.[34–36] A possibility exists that, even in the absence of a direct association between OSA and APOEε4 genotype, OSA could moderate the risk of dementia among APOEε4 carriers.[37]

Diagnostic Considerations

A systematic review and meta-analysis suggested that approximately 15% of AD cases may be attributable to sleep problems.[38] Despite this, sleep disorders remain under-recognized among older adults in clinical settings. Further, medical evaluations for conditions that may be worsened by sleep disorders (e.g., hypertension, falls) rarely include sleep evaluations. This under-recognition may lead to unnecessary delays in treatment that could impact neurological health outcomes.

Although prior work estimates OSA to affect >20% of adults over age 65, a substantially higher proportion of older adults may have undiagnosed OSA. In an analysis of the National Health and Aging Trends Study, more than half of Medicare beneficiaries were at risk for OSA, based on an adapted version of the STOP-Bang—a validated OSA screening tool.[39] Yet, only 8% of beneficiaries who were at risk received an overnight sleep study, suggesting a high degree of OSA under-recognition.[40] Among those beneficiaries who *did* receive a sleep study, >90% were diagnosed with OSA. This discrepancy highlights potentially missed opportunities to recognize OSA in older adults. Although traditional correlates of OSA (snoring, tiredness) are recognized triggers for sleep apnea testing in the general population, many of these characteristics are also attributed to "normal aging." Consequently, older adults who exhibit these characteristics may be more likely to escape sleep evaluations. This is a critical gap in care, as OSA is associated with attentional deficits and changes in executive function that can trigger costly dementia workups, and, as discussed earlier, OSA could independently increase the risk of future dementia.

Insomnia and sleep deprivation are similarly under-treated in older individuals. Older age is, in and of itself, associated with changes in sleep architecture. Decreases in stage N3 sleep, sleep efficiency, and to a lesser extent stage R sleep, are expected, and increases in WASO and nocturnal arousals are considered part of the aging process. That said, more extreme deviations in these same sleep parameters may signal another underlying sleep disorder, or a neurodegenerative process. As mentioned previously, pathological sleep and neurodegenerative conditions appear to have a bidirectional relationship. Although sleep disturbances are associated with increased risk of AD, the neuropathological changes associated with AD also predispose patients to more severe sleep fragmentation and circadian disruption.[41]

Keen discernment between sleep changes associated with normal aging, and changes that could signal an underlying sleep disorder, is critical, yet challenging. Such distinction requires a knowledge of the normal sleep architecture in an older adult,[42] and recognition of factors that may signal the presence of specific sleep disorders (including OSA), which may present differently in older adults. Up to half of older adults report at least one sleep problem, including disturbed or "light" sleep, frequent awakenings, early morning awakenings, and daytime sleepiness. For many, these symptoms are associated with impaired quality of life, excessive napping, and fatigue; however, sleep-wake disturbances are also associated with daytime symptoms, such as mood disturbances, cognitive complaints, and falls.[43–45]

Consensus regarding algorithms for sleep disorders screening in older adults has yet to be reached. However, given the emerging associations between sleep disturbances and cognitive decline, and the potential for atypical presentations for OSA in older adults, the authors recommend screening for excessive sleep deprivation, sleep fragmentation, and OSA symptoms in older adults who present with cognitive concerns, even if they do not endorse sleep complaints per se. The authors also suggest maintaining a low threshold for sleep apnea testing in older adults who present with cognitive issues.

Treatment Considerations

One key area that has received scant attention in AD or dementia research is the effect of OSA *treatment* on cognitive outcomes and dementia risk in older adults. Evidence summarized by a recent systematic review suggests a possible therapeutic benefit of positive airway pressure (PAP) therapy on MCI and AD incidence (e.g., delayed age at MCI onset, reduced MCI or AD incidence), slower cognitive decline, or progression to AD.[46]

Furthermore, the effect of OSA treatment on the incidence of specific neurodegenerative conditions including AD has not been sufficiently studied. Specifically, whether use of PAP in older persons with OSA mitigates the risk of development of MCI or dementia syndromes remains unknown, and longitudinal, population-level data are scant. A prior single-center study did not demonstrate a benefit of PAP on conversion from MCI to dementia.[47] However, in a recent analysis of a nationally representative dataset from 53321 Medicare beneficiaries with OSA, PAP use was associated with lower incident diagnoses of MCI, AD, and dementia not-otherwise-specified in older adults at 3 years. These data highlight a potentially protective role for PAP therapy on short-term dementia risk. Follow-on work using longer follow-up intervals is now underway.

Promoting Sleep Health in People with Dementia Syndromes

Disrupted sleep affects up to 70% of AD patients.[48] As neurodegeneration progresses, sleep-wake regulation processes are increasingly affected.[49,50] External factors, including reduced social interaction, inactivity, and medications, may compound these sleep disturbances. Experts recommend several environmental strategies to promote sleep regularity and minimize sundowning.[11]

Additionally, even among patients with existing AD, positive airway pressure (PAP) therapy for OSA may still offer some cognitive benefits. PAP has recently been shown to have beneficial effects on cognition in AD, with the possibility for sustained benefits.[51] The presence of AD should not preclude provision of PAP therapy if concomitant OSA is present.

STROKE

Stroke is defined as a focal neurological deficit that arises from acute injury to the central nervous system, due to disruption in the blood supply to the brain or spinal cord.[52]

Stroke can be ischemic or hemorrhagic. An ischemic stroke is the most common form of a cerebrovascular accident and occurs when there is obstruction of a blood vessel. Ischemic events that resolve within 24 hours are known as a transient ischemic attacks (TIAs). Hemorrhagic stroke occurs when an intracranial blood vessel ruptures, causing bleeding into the brain. Given the high morbidity, mortality, and societal costs associated with stroke, the identification and treatment of risk factors for the incidence or recurrence of stroke, including sleep disorders, are paramount.

Sleep-Related Risk Factors for Stroke

Obstructive sleep apnea is an independent risk factor for stroke. In an observational cohort study, OSA was independently associated with increased risk for *first* stroke or death from any cause,[53] a finding that has been replicated in other samples.[54]

Patients with OSA also have an increased prevalence of asymptomatic infarctions on brain imaging.[55] Several studies have demonstrated an increased prevalence of subcortical white matter changes in the brain in patients with OSA, which may be reduced with PAP therapy.[56]

Several mechanisms are thought to be responsible for these associations.[57] First, apneic episodes are associated with increased sympathetic nervous stimulation, with increased blood pressure during sleep.[58,59] Second, OSA is associated with hypoxia and subsequent increased levels of pro-inflammatory cytokines and vascular adhesion molecules in the periphery, which may contribute to endothelial damage and increased platelet aggregation.[60] Finally, OSA is associated with high blood pressure, dyslipidemia, and cardiac arrhythmias—known risk factors for stroke.

Presence of insomnia is also linked to an increased risk of ischemic stroke.[19] Insomnia in patients with subacute stroke has been associated with reduced recovery during the rehabilitation process.[61]

In addition to OSA and insomnia, changes in sleep duration and schedule have been associated with a higher risk of stroke. A J-shaped curve was noted in a meta-analysis, with a heightened risk of stroke being associated with both increased or decreased duration from a reference of 7 hours.[62] Reports of greater stroke risk in individuals who work non-standard work schedules also exist.[63]

Stroke as a Risk Factor for Sleep Disorders

Sleep disorders, and OSA in particular, share a bidirectional association with stroke. In a prior meta-analysis, greater than 70% of patients with stroke experienced subsequent sleep-disordered breathing. The majority of the patients with stroke and sleep-disordered breathing had OSA, while only 7% of the patients had primary central sleep apnea.[64] Although some reports suggest brainstem stroke as a neuroanatomical risk factor,[65] data are somewhat conflicting.[66] A meta-analysis suggested that OSA was associated with increased risk of mortality in patients with a history of stroke.[67]

Obstructive sleep apnea tends to persist in the chronic post-stroke stage, while central sleep apnea frequency decreases significantly, and could be considered an acute reaction to stroke. Stroke patients with OSA also have a worse prognosis, with longer hospitalization and rehabilitation stays.[68]

Secondary rapid eye movement (REM) sleep behavior disorder (RBD) can also develop in stroke patients, with an increased likelihood in patients with brainstem infarcts.[69] This relationship may also be bidirectional (Figure 25.1).[70]

The prevalence of restless legs syndrome (RLS) is itself common, occurring in about 8%–10% of patients with acute stroke.[71,72] Subcortical and brainstem infarcts are more commonly associated with post-stroke RLS.[71,73] There is also an increased prevalence of insomnia in post-stroke patients, with nearly half experiencing symptoms over 18 months.[74]

Diagnostic and Treatment Considerations

Despite the high prevalence of OSA post-stroke, screening for OSA is rare in the 90-day post-stroke period, and is not explained by a high pre-stroke testing frequency.[75] This suggests an important gap in care, when considering a 2014 American Heart/Stroke Association guideline that suggested consideration of a sleep study for patients with stroke or TIA given the high prevalence of post-stroke sleep apnea, and evidence that treatment of sleep apnea in general improves outcomes.[76]

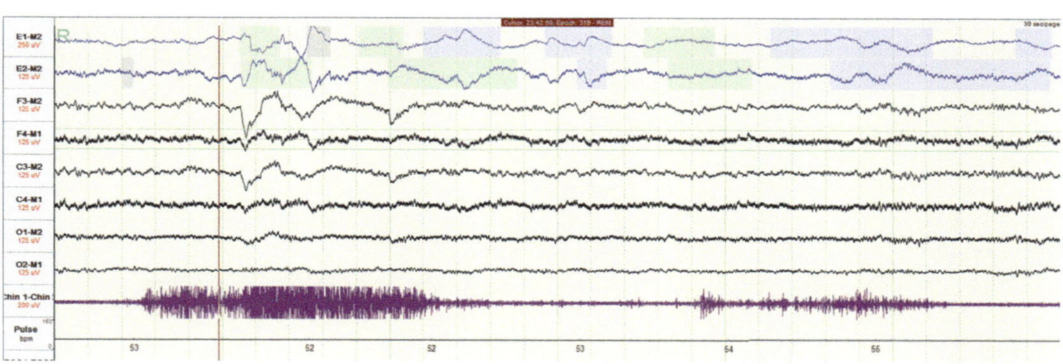

Figure 25.1. REM sleep without atonia (RSWA) is observed in patients with REM sleep behavior disorder (RBD).

Treatment of stroke patients with moderate and severe sleep OSA has been associated with reduced risk of stroke recurrence[77] and reduced mortality.[78] The use of PAP for treatment of OSA may lead to lower morbidity/better neurologic improvement following a stroke[79,80]; however, stroke-specific benefits of PAP treatment have yet to be definitively established. An NIH-funded multicenter trial (NCT03812653) is underway to determine if early intervention with PAP post-stroke reduces recurrent stroke and all-cause mortality.

EPILEPSY

An epileptic seizure is defined as a transient occurrence of signs and/or symptoms due to an abnormal excessive or synchronous neuronal activity in the brain. The diagnosis of epilepsy as a condition is characterized by an elevated risk of recurrent and unprovoked epileptic seizures. Etiologies and risk factors vary considerably across the life span, but include autoimmune, metabolic, structural, infectious, developmental, and genetic causes.[81]

Association of Epileptiform Discharges with Sleep

Multiple studies have demonstrated a reciprocal interaction between sleep and epilepsy. Slow wave sleep (SWS) in particular is associated with increased epileptiform activity in people with epilepsy. Activation of focal and generalized spikes are present in about one-third of patients with epilepsy (PWE) during sleep (Figure 25.2).[82] Increased neuronal synchronization during SWS causes activation of interictal spikes, with appearance of spikes in PWE who had none during wakefulness.[83] High-frequency oscillations in electrocorticography, which have some correlation with increased epileptogenic potential, are also most prevalent in non-rapid eye movement (NREM) sleep.[84]

Due to desynchronization, there is limited propagation of interictal epileptiform discharges in REM sleep, which allows more localizing value for primary epileptogenic focus.[85]

Sleep deprivation has also been shown to facilitate epileptiform discharges in patients with generalized epilepsy, during sleep as well as wakefulness on the following day.[86]

Association of Seizures with Sleep

Seizures often follow circadian rhythms. In general, sleep-related seizures are most common in stage N2 sleep, followed by stage N1 and then stage N3 sleep (Figure 25.3). Nocturnal seizures are least frequent during REM sleep.[87,88] Secondary generalization of focal seizures is more likely to occur during sleep rather than wakefulness.[88] The majority of seizures in patients with benign childhood epilepsy with

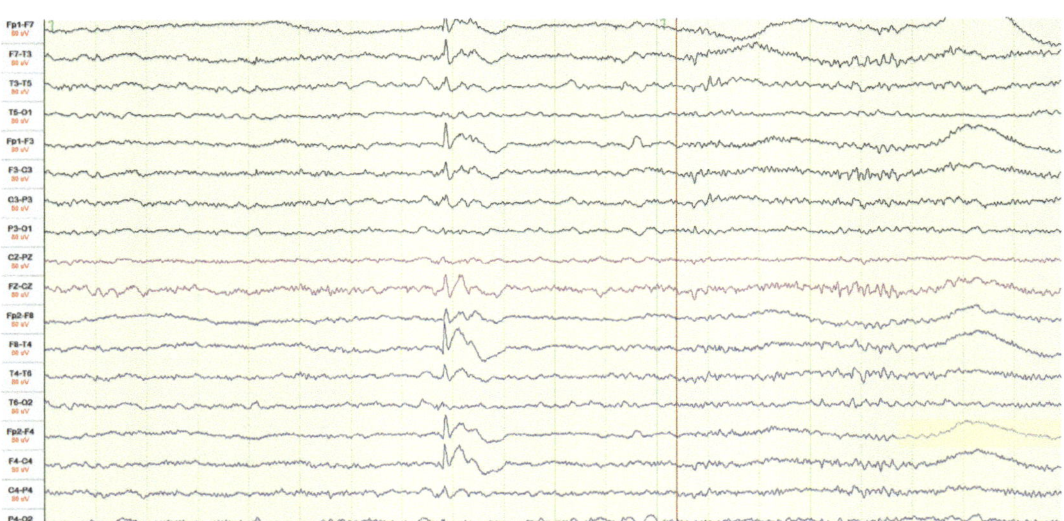

Figure 25.2. Bifrontal maximal diffuse interictal spike-waves.

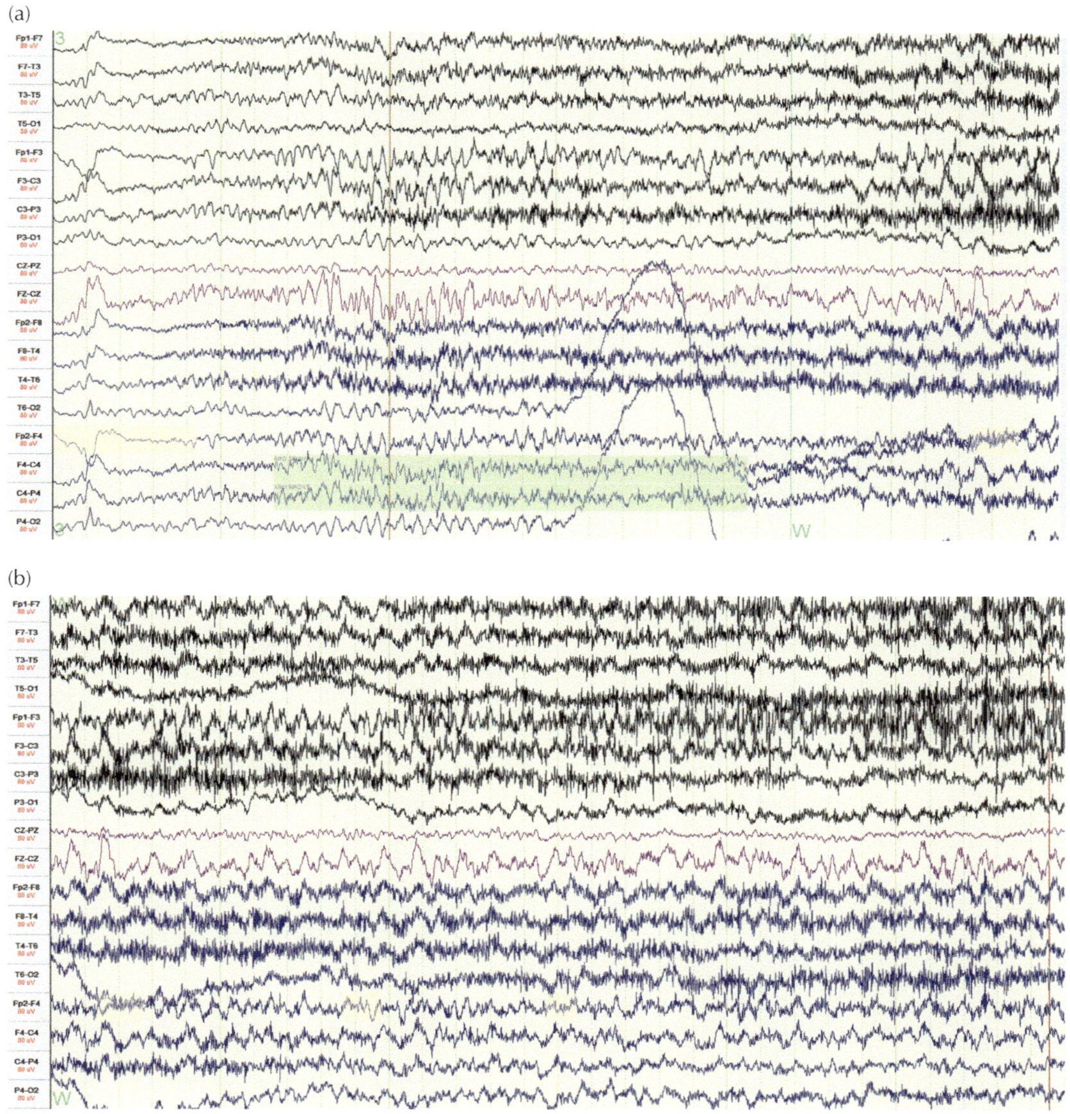

Figure 25.3. Electrographic seizure, with consecutive 15-second epochs showing onset over the right side (a) with evolution over the next 15 seconds (b).

centrotemporal spikes and benign childhood occipital epilepsy occur during sleep.[89,90]

Some specific epilepsy syndromes are characterized by the relative predominance or absence of nocturnal seizures. Seizures in autosomal dominant nocturnal frontal lobe epilepsy (ADNFLE) and nocturnal temporal lobe epilepsy (NTLE) occur nearly exclusively during sleep. Conversely, the majority of the patients with idiopathic generalized epilepsy, such as juvenile myoclonic epilepsy, have seizures upon wakefulness.[91]

Epilepsy with continuous spike waves during slow wave sleep (CSWS) and Landau–Kleffner syndrome are epileptic encephalopathy syndromes, which have nearly continuous interictal epileptiform discharges occurring during sleep.[92,93]

Effects of Seizures on Sleep

Seizures have been found to affect sleep architecture. Reduction in stage R sleep with increased REM latency is observed on nights with seizures. Reduced sleep efficiency and total sleep time are also observed, with increased sleep fragmentation and recurrent arousals.[93,94]

Daytime seizures can also cause reduced duration of REM and NREM sleep on the night following the seizure.[95]

Epilepsy and Sleep Disorders

When compared to the general population, people with epilepsy have higher prevalence of sleep disorders, which are associated with increased morbidity. Mood disorders in adults and behavioral problems in children with epilepsy are more common when sleep disorders are present.[96,97] Some reports of increased prevalence of moderate-severe RLS in adults with epilepsy also exist.[98] In adults with epilepsy, about 50% of patients have insomnia.[99] The majority of patients with epilepsy report increased daytime somnolence.[100–102] The sedating effect of anti-seizure medications could also contribute to daytime sleepiness, and is an important treatment consideration when evaluating PWE who report sleepiness.[103,104]

In PWE, the incidence of OSA in people with refractory epilepsy is reported to be as high as 33%.[105] It has been postulated that the sleep fragmentation associated with sleep apnea may contribute to seizures. Treatment of OSA with PAP has been shown to reduce excessive daytime sleepiness and seizure frequency, with improvement in quality of life.[106,107] Treatment of underlying OSA with adenotonsillectomy in children with epilepsy may also reduce seizure frequency.[108]

AEDs and Sleep/Treatment Considerations

Anti-epileptic drugs (AEDs) have independent effects on sleep and daytime symptoms, and these side effects (as well any concomitant sleep problems) should be considered when selecting the most appropriate agent(s) for an individual.

Among older AEDs, phenytoin is associated with reduced sleep latency, increased arousals, increased NREM sleep, and reduced stage R sleep.[109,110] Phenobarbital shortens latency to sleep and reduces arousals, while prolonging REM latency, decreasing stage R sleep, and increasing stage N2 NREM sleep.[109] Carbamazepine appears to consolidate sleep, reducing awakenings and arousals.[111,112] Valproic acid has no significant reported effect on sleep, with the exception of potential mild increases in SWS.[109,111]

The newer AEDs in general have fewer negative effects on sleep, and some have positive effects. Gabapentin has been associated with increased sleep consolidation and increased SWS.[113] Pregabalin may also significantly increase SWS.[114] Further work is needed to elucidate these causal pathways given the heterogeneity of these agents and the conditions they treat, which could serve as confounders or mediators. Lamotrigine appears to stabilize sleep and is infrequently associated with insomnia.[111,115] Levetiracetam has minimal effect on sleep architecture.[116]

In addition to AEDs, other treatment modalities may also affect sleep. Vagus nerve stimulation (VNS) has been noted to reduce sleep latency and increase of SWS.[117] It should be noted that VNS has been associated with worsening of sleep-related breathing disorders in some cases, and repeat PAP titration or changes to VNS settings may be necessary.[118,119] Temporal lobe epilepsy surgery has also been associated with improvements in REM sleep and total sleep duration.[120]

REFERENCES

1. Azarbarzin A, Sands SA, Stone KL, et al. The hypoxic burden of sleep apnoea predicts cardiovascular disease-related mortality: The Osteoporotic Fractures in Men Study and the Sleep Heart Health Study. *Eur Heart J*. 2019;40(14):1149–1157.
2. Javaheri S, Redline S. Insomnia and risk of cardiovascular disease. *Chest*. 2017;152(2):435–444.
3. Peter-Derex L, Yammine P, Bastuji H, Croisile B. Sleep and Alzheimer's disease. *Sleep Med Rev*. 2015;19:29–38.
4. Kataria L, Vaughn BV. Sleep and epilepsy. *Sleep Med Clin*. 2016;11(1):25–38.
5. Braley TJ, Chervin RD. A practical approach to the diagnosis and management of sleep disorders in patients with multiple sclerosis. *Ther Adv Neurol Disord*. 2015;8(6):294–310.
6. Brown DL, He K, Kim S, et al. Prediction of sleep-disordered breathing after stroke. *Sleep Med*. 2020;75:1–6.

7. Brown DL, Shafie-Khorassani F, Kim S, et al. Sleep-disordered breathing is associated with recurrent ischemic stroke. *Stroke*. 2019;50(3):571–576.
8. Wang C, Holtzman DM. Bidirectional relationship between sleep and Alzheimer's disease: Role of amyloid, tau, and other factors. *Neuropsychopharmacology*. 2020;45(1):104–120.
9. Dunietz GL, Chervin RD, Burke JF, Braley TJ. Obstructive sleep apnea treatment disparities among older adults with neurological disorders. *Sleep Health*. 2020;6(4):534–540.
10. Braley TJ, Segal BM, Chervin RD. Obstructive sleep apnea and fatigue in patients with multiple sclerosis. *J Clin Sleep Med*. 2014;10(2):155–162.
11. 2023 Alzheimer's disease facts and figures. *Alzheimers Dement*. 2023;19(4):1598–1695.
12. Marchant NL, Reed BR, Sanossian N, et al. The aging brain and cognition: Contribution of vascular injury and abeta to mild cognitive dysfunction. *JAMA Neurol*. 2013;70(4):488–495.
13. Jellinger K, Attems J. Neuropathological evaluation of mixed dementia. *J Neurol Sci*. 2007;257(1–2):80–87.
14. Albert MS, DeKosky ST, Dickson D, et al. The diagnosis of mild cognitive impairment due to Alzheimer's disease: Recommendations from the National Institute on Aging-Alzheimer's Association workgroups on diagnostic guidelines for Alzheimer's disease. *Alzheimers Dement*. 2011;7(3):270–279.
15. Plassman BL, Langa KM, McCammon RJ, et al. Incidence of dementia and cognitive impairment, not dementia in the United States. *Ann Neurol*. 2011;70(3):418–426.
16. Boyle PA, Wilson RS, Aggarwal NT, Tang Y, Bennett DA. Mild cognitive impairment: Risk of Alzheimer disease and rate of cognitive decline. *Neurology*. 2006;67(3):441–445.
17. Ganguli M, Dodge HH, Shen C, DeKosky ST. Mild cognitive impairment, amnestic type: An epidemiologic study. *Neurology*. 2004;63(1):115–121.
18. Lopez OL, Kuller LH, Becker JT, et al. Incidence of dementia in mild cognitive impairment in the cardiovascular health study cognition study. *Arch Neurol*. 2007;64(3):416–420.
19. Xu W, Tan CC, Zou JJ, Cao XP, Tan L. Sleep problems and risk of all-cause cognitive decline or dementia: An updated systematic review and meta-analysis. *J Neurol Neurosurg Psychiatry*. 2020;91(3):236–244.
20. Kam K, Parekh A, Sharma RA, et al. Sleep oscillation-specific associations with Alzheimer's disease CSF biomarkers: Novel roles for sleep spindles and tau. *Molecular Neurodegeneration*. 2019;14(1):10.
21. Sabia S, Fayosse A, Dumurgier J, et al. Association of sleep duration in middle and old age with incidence of dementia. *Nat Commun*. 2021;12(1):2289.
22. Insel PS, Mohlenhoff BS, Neylan TC, Krystal AD, Mackin RS. Association of sleep and beta-amyloid pathology among older cognitively unimpaired adults. *JAMA Netw Open*. 2021;4(7):e2117573.
23. Lim AS, Kowgier M, Yu L, Buchman AS, Bennett DA. Sleep fragmentation and the risk of incident Alzheimer's disease and cognitive decline in older persons. *Sleep*. 2013;36(7):1027–1032.
24. Elias A, Cummins T, Tyrrell R, et al. Risk of Alzheimer's disease in obstructive sleep apnea syndrome: Amyloid-beta and tau imaging. *J Alzheimers Dis*. 2018;66(2):733–741.
25. Liguori C, Mercuri NB, Izzi F, et al. Obstructive sleep apnea is associated with early but possibly modifiable Alzheimer's disease biomarkers changes. *Sleep*. 2017;40(5):zsx011.
26. Sharma RA, Varga AW, Bubu OM, et al. Obstructive sleep apnea severity affects amyloid burden in cognitively normal elderly: A longitudinal study. *Am J Respir Crit Care Med*. 2018;197(7):933–943.
27. Yaffe K, Laffan AM, Harrison SL, et al. Sleep-disordered breathing, hypoxia, and risk of mild cognitive impairment and dementia in older women. *JAMA*. 2011;306(6):613–619.
28. Lee CY, Landreth GE. The role of microglia in amyloid clearance from the AD brain. *J Neural Transm (Vienna)*. 2010;117(8):949–960.
29. Bergeron C, Kimoff J, Hamid Q. Obstructive sleep apnea syndrome and inflammation. *J Allergy Clin Immunol*. 2005;116(6):1393–1396.
30. Heneka MT, Golenbock DT, Latz E. Innate immunity in Alzheimer's disease. *Nat Immunol*. 2015;16(3):229–236.
31. Dearborn JL, Zhang Y, Qiao Y, et al. Intracranial atherosclerosis and dementia: The Atherosclerosis Risk in Communities (ARIC) Study. *Neurology*. 2017;88(16):1556–1563.
32. Jefferson AL, Massaro JM, Wolf PA, et al. Inflammatory biomarkers are associated with total brain volume: The Framingham Heart Study. *Neurology*. 2007;68(13):1032–1038.
33. Liu CC, Liu CC, Kanekiyo T, Xu H, Bu G. Apolipoprotein E and Alzheimer disease: Risk, mechanisms and therapy. *Nat Rev Neurol*. 2013;9(2):106–118.
34. O'Hara R, Schröder CM, Kraemer HC, et al. Nocturnal sleep apnea/hypopnea is associated with lower memory performance in APOE epsilon4 carriers. *Neurology*. 2005;65(4):642–644.
35. Spira AP, Blackwell T, Stone KL, et al. Sleep-disordered breathing and cognition in older women. *J Am Geriatr Soc*. 2008;56(1):45–50.
36. Nikodemova M, Finn L, Mignot E, Salzieder N, Peppard PE. Association of sleep disordered breathing and cognitive deficit in APOE ε4 carriers. *Sleep*. 2013;36(6):873–880.
37. Polsek D, Gildeh N, Cash D, et al. Obstructive sleep apnoea and Alzheimer's disease: In search of shared pathomechanisms. *Neurosci Biobehav Rev*. 2018;86:142–149.
38. Bubu OM, Brannick M, Mortimer J, et al. Sleep, cognitive impairment, and Alzheimer's disease: A systematic review and meta-analysis. *Sleep*. 2017;40(1):zsw032.
39. Chung F, Subramanyam R, Liao P, Sasaki E, Shapiro C, Sun Y. High STOP-Bang score indicates a high probability of obstructive sleep apnoea. *Br J Anaesth*. 2012;108(5):768–775.
40. Braley TJ, Dunietz GL, Chervin RD, Lisabeth LD, Skolarus LE, Burke JF. Recognition and diagnosis of obstructive sleep apnea in older Americans. *J Am Geriatr Soc*. 2018;66(7):1296–1302.
41. Crowley K, Sullivan EV, Adalsteinsson E, Pfefferbaum A, Colrain IM. Differentiating pathologic delta from healthy physiologic delta in patients with Alzheimer disease. *Sleep*. 2005;28(7):865–870.

42. Yaremchuk K. Sleep disorders in the elderly. *Clin Geriatr Med*. 2018;34(2):205–216.
43. Young T, Shahar E, Nieto FJ, et al. Predictors of sleep-disordered breathing in community-dwelling adults: The Sleep Heart Health Study. *Arch Intern Med*. 2002;162(8):893–900.
44. Cauley JA, Blackwell TL, Redline S, et al. Hypoxia during sleep and the risk of falls and fractures in older men: The Osteoporotic Fractures in Men Sleep Study. *J Am Geriatr Soc*. 2014;62(10):1853–1859.
45. Celle S, Annweiler C, Camicioli R, Barthelemy JC, Roche F, Beauchet O. Sleep-related breathing disorders and gait variability: A cross-sectional preliminary study. *BMC Pulm Med*. 2014;14:140.
46. Shieu MM, Zaheed A, Shannon C, et al. Positive airway pressure and cognitive disorders in adults with obstructive sleep apnea: A systematic review of the literature. *Neurology*. 2022;99(4):e334–346.
47. Skiba V, Novikova M, Suneja A, McLellan B, Schultz L. Use of positive airway pressure in mild cognitive impairment to delay progression to dementia. *J Clin Sleep Med*. 2020;16(6):863–870.
48. Webster L, Costafreda Gonzalez S, Stringer A, et al. Measuring the prevalence of sleep disturbances in people with dementia living in care homes: A systematic review and meta-analysis. *Sleep*. 2020;43(4):zsz251.
49. Wulff K, Gatti S, Wettstein JG, Foster RG. Sleep and circadian rhythm disruption in psychiatric and neurodegenerative disease. *Nat Rev Neurosci*. 2010;11(8):589–599.
50. Pat-Horenczyk R, Klauber MR, Shochat T, Ancoli-Israel S. Hourly profiles of sleep and wakefulness in severely versus mild-moderately demented nursing home patients. *Aging (Milano)*. 1998;10(4):308–315.
51. Cooke JR, Ayalon L, Palmer BW, et al. Sustained use of CPAP slows deterioration of cognition, sleep, and mood in patients with Alzheimer's disease and obstructive sleep apnea: a preliminary study. *J Clin Sleep Med*. 2009;5(4):305–309.
52. Sacco RL, Kasner SE, Broderick JP, et al. An updated definition of stroke for the 21st century: A statement for healthcare professionals from the American Heart Association/American Stroke Association. *Stroke*. 2013;44(7):2064–2089.
53. Yaggi HK, Concato J, Kernan WN, Lichtman JH, Brass LM, Mohsenin V. Obstructive sleep apnea as a risk factor for stroke and death. *N Engl J Med*. 2005;353(19):2034–2041.
54. Redline S, Yenokyan G, Gottlieb DJ, et al. Obstructive sleep apnea-hypopnea and incident stroke: The sleep heart health study. *Am J Respir Crit Care Med*. 2010;182(2):269–277.
55. Nishibayashi M, Miyamoto M, Miyamoto T, Suzuki K, Hirata K. Correlation between severity of obstructive sleep apnea and prevalence of silent cerebrovascular lesions. *J Clin Sleep Med*. 2008;4(3):242–247.
56. Salsone M, Caligiuri ME, Castronovo V, et al. Microstructural changes in normal-appearing white matter in male sleep apnea patients are reversible after treatment: A pilot study. *J Neurosci Res*. 2021;99(10):2646–2656.
57. Jehan S, Farag M, Zizi F, et al. Obstructive sleep apnea and stroke. *Sleep Med Disord*. 2018;2(5):120–125.
58. Shamsuzzaman AS, Gersh BJ, Somers VK. Obstructive sleep apnea: Implications for cardiac and vascular disease. *JAMA*. 2003;290(14):1906–1914.
59. Somers VK, Dyken ME, Mark AL, Abboud FM. Sympathetic-nerve activity during sleep in normal subjects. *N Engl J Med*. 1993;328(5):303–307.
60. Eisensehr I, Ehrenberg BL, Noachtar S, et al. Platelet activation, epinephrine, and blood pressure in obstructive sleep apnea syndrome. *Neurology*. 1998;51(1):188–195.
61. Huang RJ, Lai CH, Lee SD, et al. Objective sleep measures in inpatients with subacute stroke associated with levels and improvements in activities of daily living. *Arch Phys Med Rehabil*. 2018;99(4):699–706.
62. He Q, Sun H, Wu X, et al. Sleep duration and risk of stroke: A dose-response meta-analysis of prospective cohort studies. *Sleep Med*. 2017;32:66–74.
63. Brown DL, Feskanich D, Sanchez BN, Rexrode KM, Schernhammer ES, Lisabeth LD. Rotating night shift work and the risk of ischemic stroke. *Am J Epidemiol*. 2009;169(11):1370–1377.
64. Johnson KG, Johnson DC. Frequency of sleep apnea in stroke and TIA patients: A meta-analysis. *J Clin Sleep Med*. 2010;6(2):131–137.
65. Brown DL, McDermott M, Mowla A, et al. Brainstem infarction and sleep-disordered breathing in the BASIC sleep apnea study. *Sleep Med*. 2014;15(8):887–891.
66. Stevens D, Martins RT, Mukherjee S, Vakulin A. Post-stroke sleep-disordered breathing-pathophysiology and therapy options. *Front Surg*. 2018;5:9.
67. Xie W, Zheng F, Song X. Obstructive sleep apnea and serious adverse outcomes in patients with cardiovascular or cerebrovascular disease: A PRISMA-compliant systematic review and meta-analysis. *Medicine (Baltimore)*. 2014;93(29):e336.
68. Kaneko Y, Hajek VE, Zivanovic V, Raboud J, Bradley TD. Relationship of sleep apnea to functional capacity and length of hospitalization following stroke. *Sleep*. 2003;26(3):293–297.
69. Tang WK, Hermann DM, Chen YK, et al. Brainstem infarcts predict REM sleep behavior disorder in acute ischemic stroke. *BMC Neurol*. 2014;14:88.
70. Ma C, Pavlova M, Liu Y, et al. Probable REM sleep behavior disorder and risk of stroke: A prospective study. *Neurology*. 2017;88(19):1849–1855.
71. Chandan S, Shukla G, Gupta A, Srivastava A, Vibha D, Prasad K. Acute-onset restless legs syndrome in acute neurological conditions: A prospective study on patients with the Guillain-Barre syndrome and acute stroke. *Acta Neurol Scand*. 2018;137(5):488–499.
72. Shiina T, Suzuki K, Okamura M, Matsubara T, Hirata K. Restless legs syndrome and its variants in acute ischemic stroke. *Acta Neurol Scand*. 2019;139(3):260–268.
73. Woo HG, Lee D, Hwang KJ, Ahn TB. Post-stroke restless leg syndrome and periodic limb movements in sleep. *Acta Neurol Scand*. 2017;135(2):204–210.
74. Palomaki H, Berg A, Meririnne E, et al. Complaints of poststroke insomnia and its treatment with mianserin. *Cerebrovasc Dis*. 2003;15(1–2):56–62.
75. Brown DL, Jiang X, Li C, et al. Sleep apnea screening is uncommon after stroke. *Sleep Med*. 2019;59:90–93.
76. Kernan WN, Ovbiagele B, Black HR, et al. Guidelines for the prevention of stroke in patients with stroke and transient ischemic attack: A guideline for healthcare professionals from the American

Heart Association/American Stroke Association. *Stroke*. 2014;45(7):2160–2236.

77. Martinez-Garcia MA, Galiano-Blancart R, Roman-Sanchez P, Soler-Cataluna JJ, Cabero-Salt L, Salcedo-Maiques E. Continuous positive airway pressure treatment in sleep apnea prevents new vascular events after ischemic stroke. *Chest*. 2005;128(4):2123–2129.
78. Martinez-Garcia MA, Soler-Cataluna JJ, Ejarque-Martinez L, et al. Continuous positive airway pressure treatment reduces mortality in patients with ischemic stroke and obstructive sleep apnea: A 5-year follow-up study. *Am J Respir Crit Care Med*. 2009;180(1):36–41.
79. Bravata DM, Concato J, Fried T, et al. Continuous positive airway pressure: Evaluation of a novel therapy for patients with acute ischemic stroke. *Sleep*. 2011;34(9):1271–1277.
80. Parra O, Sanchez-Armengol A, Bonnin M, et al. Early treatment of obstructive apnoea and stroke outcome: A randomised controlled trial. *Eur Respir J*. 2011;37(5):1128–1136.
81. Wirrell E. Evaluation of first seizure and newly diagnosed epilepsy. *Continuum (Minneap Minn)*. 2022;28(2):230–260.
82. Kotagal P, Yardi N. The relationship between sleep and epilepsy. *Semin Pediatr Neurol*. 2008;15(2):42–49.
83. Malow BA, Lin X, Kushwaha R, Aldrich MS. Interictal spiking increases with sleep depth in temporal lobe epilepsy. *Epilepsia*. 1998;39(12):1309–1316.
84. Clemens Z, Molle M, Eross L, Barsi P, Halasz P, Born J. Temporal coupling of parahippocampal ripples, sleep spindles and slow oscillations in humans. *Brain*. 2007;130(Pt 11):2868–2878.
85. Kang X, Boly M, Findlay G, et al. Quantitative spatio-temporal characterization of epileptic spikes using high density EEG: Differences between NREM sleep and REM sleep. *Sci Rep*. 2020;10(1):1673.
86. Halasz P, Filakovszky J, Vargha A, Bagdy G. Effect of sleep deprivation on spike-wave discharges in idiopathic generalised epilepsy: A 4 x 24 h continuous long term EEG monitoring study. *Epilepsy Res*. 2002;51(1-2):123–132.
87. Terzano MG, Parrino L, Garofalo PG, Durisotti C, Filati-Roso C. Activation of partial seizures with motor signs during cyclic alternating pattern in human sleep. *Epilepsy Res*. 1991;10(2-3):166–173.
88. Bazil CW, Walczak TS. Effects of sleep and sleep stage on epileptic and nonepileptic seizures. *Epilepsia*. 1997;38(1):56–62.
89. Bazil CW. Sleep and epilepsy. *Semin Neurol*. 2002;22(3):321–327.
90. Koutroumanidis M. Panayiotopoulos syndrome. *BMJ*. 2002;324(7348):1228–1229.
91. Janz D. The grand mal epilepsies and the sleeping-waking cycle. *Epilepsia*. 1962;3:69–109.
92. St Louis EK. Sleep and epilepsy: Strange bedfellows no more. *Minerva Pneumol*. 2011;50(3):159–176.
93. Derry CP, Duncan S. Sleep and epilepsy. *Epilepsy Behav*. 2013;26(3):394–404.
94. Zanzmera P, Shukla G, Gupta A, et al. Markedly disturbed sleep in medically refractory compared to controlled epilepsy: A clinical and polysomnography study. *Seizure*. 2012;21(7):487–490.
95. Bazil CW, Castro LH, Walczak TS. Reduction of rapid eye movement sleep by diurnal and nocturnal seizures in temporal lobe epilepsy. *Arch Neurol*. 2000;57(3):363–368.
96. Tsai SY, Lee WT, Jeng SF, Lee CC, Weng WC. Sleep and behavior problems in children with epilepsy. *J Pediatr Health Care*. 2019;33(2):138–145.
97. Cilliler AE, Guven B. Sleep quality and related clinical features in patients with epilepsy: A preliminary report. *Epilepsy Behav*. 2020;102:106661.
98. Geyer JD, Geyer EE, Fetterman Z, Carney PR. Epilepsy and restless legs syndrome. *Epilepsy Behav*. 2017;68:41–44.
99. Khatami R, Zutter D, Siegel A, Mathis J, Donati F, Bassetti CL. Sleep-wake habits and disorders in a series of 100 adult epilepsy patients: A prospective study. *Seizure*. 2006;15(5):299–306.
100. de Weerd A, de Haas S, Otte A, et al. Subjective sleep disturbance in patients with partial epilepsy: A questionnaire-based study on prevalence and impact on quality of life. *Epilepsia*. 2004;45(11):1397–1404.
101. Malow BA, Bowes RJ, Lin X. Predictors of sleepiness in epilepsy patients. *Sleep*. 1997;20(12):1105–1110.
102. Giorelli AS, Passos P, Carnaval T, de Mata Gomes M. Excessive daytime sleepiness and epilepsy: A systematic review. *Epilepsy Res Treat*. 2013;2013:629469.
103. Mattson RH. Selection of drugs for the treatment of epilepsy. *Semin Neurol*. 1990;10(4):406–413.
104. Manni R, Tartara A. Evaluation of sleepiness in epilepsy. *Clin Neurophysiol*. 2000;111(Suppl 2):S111–S114.
105. Weatherwax KJ, Lin X, Marzec ML, Malow BA. Obstructive sleep apnea in epilepsy patients: The Sleep Apnea scale of the Sleep Disorders Questionnaire (SA-SDQ) is a useful screening instrument for obstructive sleep apnea in a disease-specific population. *Sleep Med*. 2003;4(6):517–521.
106. Hollinger P, Khatami R, Gugger M, Hess CW, Bassetti CL. Epilepsy and obstructive sleep apnea. *Eur Neurol*. 2006;55(2):74–79.
107. Malow BA, Fromes GA, Aldrich MS. Usefulness of polysomnography in epilepsy patients. *Neurology*. 1997;48(5):1389–1394.
108. Segal Z, Vincent P, Levitt A. Efficacy of combined, sequential and crossover psychotherapy and pharmacotherapy in improving outcomes in depression. *J Psychiatry Neurosci*. 2002;27(4):281–290.
109. Mendez M, Radtke RA. Interactions between sleep and epilepsy. *J Clin Neurophysiol*. 2001;18(2):106–127.
110. Declerck AC, Wauquier A. Influence of antiepileptic drugs on sleep patterns. *Epilepsy Res Suppl*. 1991;2:153–163.
111. Placidi F, Scalise A, Marciani MG, Romigi A, Diomedi M, Gigli GL. Effect of antiepileptic drugs on sleep. *Clin Neurophysiol*. 2000;111(Suppl 2):S115–119.
112. Gigli GL, Placidi F, Diomedi M, et al. Nocturnal sleep and daytime somnolence in untreated patients with temporal lobe epilepsy: Changes after treatment with controlled-release carbamazepine. *Epilepsia*. 1997;38(6):696–701.
113. Lo HS, Yang CM, Lo HG, Lee CY, Ting H, Tzang BS. Treatment effects of gabapentin for primary insomnia. *Clin Neuropharmacol*. 2010;33(2):84–90.
114. Bazil CW, Dave J, Cole J, Stalvey J, Drake E. Pregabalin increases slow-wave sleep and may improve attention in patients with partial epilepsy and insomnia. *Epilepsy Behav*. 2012;23(4):422–425.

115. Sadler M. Lamotrigine associated with insomnia. *Epilepsia*. 1999;40(3):322–325.
116. Bazil CW, Battista J, Basner RC. Effects of levetiracetam on sleep in normal volunteers. *Epilepsy Behav*. 2005;7(3):539–542.
117. Hallbook T, Lundgren J, Kohler S, Blennow G, Stromblad LG, Rosen I. Beneficial effects on sleep of vagus nerve stimulation in children with therapy resistant epilepsy. *Eur J Paediatr Neurol*. 2005;9(6):399–407.
118. Malow BA, Edwards J, Marzec M, Sagher O, Fromes G. Effects of vagus nerve stimulation on respiration during sleep: A pilot study. *Neurology*. 2000;55(10):1450–1454.
119. Marzec M, Edwards J, Sagher O, Fromes G, Malow BA. Effects of vagus nerve stimulation on sleep-related breathing in epilepsy patients. *Epilepsia*. 2003;44(7):930–935.
120. Serafini A, Kuate C, Gelisse P, et al. Sleep before and after temporal lobe epilepsy surgery. *Seizure*. 2012;21(4):260–265.

Chapter 26

Sleep and Emotion, Cognition, and Memory

Mohan Dutt

Sleep regulates the human body in multiple ways, and detriments in it may lead to clinically significant pathologies. As research is performed on the effects of sleep, we continue to find further areas in which sleep exerts its control, and this has led to a recent craze in which sleep is starting to be "bio-hacked" as a means to improve overall quality of life and reduce the risk of comorbid disease. In this chapter we will explore the effect that sleep plays on the processes surrounding emotion and memory, and also discuss the association between sleep and dementia.

SLEEP AND EMOTION

To begin our discussion of emotion, it will help us to separate the regulatory process into 3 distinct stages—emotion generation, emotional regulation, and emotional processing—though physiologically they are not separated, and likely occur in tandem. By making these distinctions we can discuss the role that sleep plays in each of these phases. The majority of studies exploring the associations between sleep and emotion involve sleep deprivation, either in the lab, or self-reported in the real world, and then comparing the results to individuals who received a "normal" night of sleep. We will use Gross's model and process models of emotion as a framework in which to discuss the emotion generation and emotional regulation. Emotions are generated when an individual encounters a situation, appraises it, and then generates an emotional response. The emotion which is generated is taken in context of an overarching goal, which gives the emotion meaning, for example, graduating medical school, or going to play tennis.[1] Generally speaking, the emotions which are generated can be separated into positive or negative. Neurobiologically, the emotional generative process starts at the amygdala, which is involved in the perception and encoding of stimuli, then to the ventral striatum, which is involved in learning which cues will give rewards. The third brain structure is the ventromedial prefrontal cortex, which serves to integrate the information received by the amygdala and ventral striatum; and the fourth structure involved is the insula, which integrates viscerosensory inputs from the body.[2] The process by which an individual can affect the emotions that they have is deemed *emotional regulation*. This can occur either intrinsically (self-regulating emotions), or extrinsically (regulating the emotions of others). Per the process model, emotions may be regulated anywhere along the timeline of emotion generation, using one of 5 different emotional regulation processes: situational selection, situation modification, attentional deployment, cognitive change, and response modulation. Depending on the desired outcome, the magnitude or valence of the emotion is impacted. Once an emotion has been generated and regulated, it is then stored into memory; this is termed as *emotional processing*, and determines how an individual recalls their emotional experience, and plays a role in empathy, fear conditioning, and threat generalization.[3] We will discuss the emotional processing aspect in the section on memory.

Sleep and Emotion Generation

The research to date demonstrates that individuals who are sleep deprived and or objectively have a poor night of sleep experience a greater number of negative emotions compared to positive ones. One hallmark study which demonstrates this connection occurred in medical residents in Israel. In this study, medical residents were monitored throughout their residencies using actigraphy, which helped to determine those who were sleep deprived, or those who had poor sleep quality as evidenced by sleep fragmentation. Residents who experienced objective sleep loss were found to have greater negative emotions in response to disruptive events, and fewer positive emotions in response to goal-enhancing events.[4] In one study using partial sleep deprivation (to mimic real-world situations), adults who were forced to experience 7 days of cumulative sleep deprivation reported a progressive worsening of mood via the POMS questionnaire. Furthermore, mood was observed to progressively recover in 2 nights of recovery sleep following sleep deprivation.[5] These findings correlate with neuroimaging studies in which sleep deprivation was found to cause an increase in amygdala activity of 60%, and a decrease in amygdala-medial prefrontal cortex connectivity in response to viewing negative images while undergoing functional magnetic resonance imaging (fMRI).[6] As the medial prefrontal cortex is known to exert inhibitory control on the amygdala, in a top-down fashion,[7] these findings suggest that a poor night of sleep is associated with a hyper-limbic response when negative stimuli are encountered.[6] Increases in pupil diameter—a sign of emotional reactivity—were also found to be increased in sleep-deprived subjects when viewing negative pictures.[8]

Sleep and Emotional Regulation

The process model of emotion lists 5 separate stages on the timeline of emotion generation in which emotions can be regulated. Emotional regulation can begin prior to the emotion being experienced (situational selection) so that individuals put themselves in a situation in which they will either experience or avoid an emotion. Next, the situation can be altered (situational modification) so that the emotional experience is either heightened or lessened, attention can either be focused or redirected (attentional deployment), the experience can be alternatively appraised (cognitive change), or the response to a situation may be altered (response modulation).[9] The first 2 methods may be considered to be regulatory, measured by changing things external to themselves, whereas the final 3 are more internal in nature.

There have not been many studies looking explicitly at sleep and situational selection; there is overwhelming evidence that suggests that poor sleepers, and those who are sleep deprived, avoid situations in which positive emotional reward may be experienced.[10] For example, in one study researchers divided college students into either good sleepers or poor sleepers based on a Pittsburgh sleep quality index (PSQI) cut-off of 5. In the 243 students evaluated, the study found that good sleepers were more likely to engage in daily activities than poor sleepers, and that poor sleepers particularly avoided activities involving social interactions.[11] These findings correlate with neurobiological studies that altered sleep leads to changes in the neural rewards circuitry, associated with a decrease in motivation for rewards. These studies must be used as surrogates for evaluation situational selection, as they do not test a subject's ability to remove themselves from a potentially negative situation, or place themselves in a positive one.

In situational modification, a person will attempt to alter a situation to change their experience of it; for instance, if a loud noise causes anxiety, then covering their ears would be an example of a modifying behavior. If we look at studies evaluating an individual's social and emotional interactions after a night of poor sleep, then we can gain knowledge on how sleep affects emotional regulation through situational modification. In a dyadic study examining 71 couples, researchers found that couples in which one partner experienced a poor night of sleep (as measured by the PSQI) there was an increase in conflict the following day. Furthermore, the study found that poor sleepers demonstrated a lack of empathetic accuracy, which is the ability to properly gauge their emotions, and more importantly an inaccuracy in identifying their partner's emotions.[12] Other studies have demonstrated that poor sleep is associated with difficulties in understanding nonverbal cues and with social interactions.[10] Taken together, the data demonstrated that poor sleep leads to a likely misunderstanding of a situation, and thus any response elicited in the situation is likely to be maladaptive.

Coming to the internal methods for emotional regulation, we will first discuss attentional deployment, of which distraction is one of the most common forms. In attentional deployment, an individual would shift attention away from a negative emotionally generating experience, or toward a positive one. In a study using fMRI examining the effects of attentional deployment on normal sleepers, researchers found that in response to unpleasant images, the amygdala was less activated when attention was paid to a stimulating portion of the image, and that the prefrontal and parietal regions of the brain were more active.[13] This finding is consistent with our working knowledge that the prefrontal cortex exhibits top-down control on the amygdala in regard to emotional processes and that poor sleep disrupts this control.[6] As there are no studies examining attentional deployment specifically in regard to sleep, we will have to use the information as a useful heuristic to interpret the potential effect that sleep has on attentional deployment.

Cognitive change is the process by which an individual can change the meaning or appraisal of an emotionally generating stimulus; it is a high-order cognitive process, akin to the methods that are employed in cognitive behavioral therapy (CBT).[10] In a meta-review analyzing the neurobiological effects of cognitive reappraisal in normal sleepers, researchers found that reappraisal activates the prefrontal cortex and that it also modulates the amygdala bilaterally.[14] This finding again is consistent with the top-down view of emotional regulation. Conversely, however, in a recent study 80 subjects were split into groups based on age (20–30 and 65–75) and the fMRI effects of cognitive appraisal were evaluated after nights of normal sleep and curtailed sleep (3 hours). Researchers found that while subjects self-reported that they felt that they were less successful in regulating emotions after shortened sleep, there were no associated fMRI findings of loss of prefrontal cortex to amygdala connectivity.[15] In another study which looked at the effects of cognitive reappraisal in adolescents aged 13–17 years, researchers found that after 1 night of sleep loss (4 hours) there was no loss of ability in using reappraisal in the face of negative stimuli.[16] The authors of both studies suggest that while the findings are contradictory to expected findings, it is possible that more than 1 night of poor sleep is needed to effect change, and that this is a potential future area of research.

The final stage of emotional regulation is termed *response modulation*, and occurs after an emotion has already been generated, the goal being to alter the emotional or physiological response to an emotional stimulus.[10] The most commonly used form is expressive suppression, in which an individual attempts to hide their emotional response. There is to date little research examining the direct association between poor sleep and expressive suppression. However, in a recent study examining the effects of 24 hours of sleep deprivation on various emotional regulatory techniques (distraction, reappraisal, and suppression) as measured by late positive potential (LPP) amplitudes, suppression was ineffective in reducing LPP amplitudes after a normal night of sleep and was not impacted by a night of sleep deprivation. The other methods were found to decrease LPP amplitude after normal sleep, and it was negatively impacted after sleep deprivation.[17]

While it is clear that poor sleep is associated with an inability to regulate emotions, the mechanism behind which this occurs still does not appear to be clear. The current working hypothesis is that there is a loss of top-down control of the amygdala by the prefrontal cortex; however, recent studies looking at functional neuroimaging during the emotional regulatory process do not necessarily yield this result. As there have not been many studies examining this phenomenon, this is an area in which future research may be directed. Furthermore, as we discuss later in the chapter, slow wave sleep (SWS) and rapid eye movement (REM) sleep may also exhibit a variable influence on the emotional regulatory process, as they do in the processing of emotions, and this likely needs to be further explored.

SLEEP AND MEMORY

Memory formation involves 3 processes: encoding, consolidation, and retrieval. Encoding and retrieval occur in the waking state, but consolidation is a sleep-dependent process in which in which memory traces are strengthened, stabilized, and integrated into preexisting knowledge networks. Memories are divided into 2 systems; they can be either declarative or non-declarative. Declarative memories are generally information that is easy to recall and information which the subject knows is stored and is being accessed. They can be further subdivided into either episodic—memories which are stored that have contextual clues such as timing and location—and semantic, which are memories that do not require any spatiotemporal cues. In contrast, non-declarative memories are not easily accessible to recall, and can be expressed implicitly; examples of this are memories for procedural and perceptual skills. Another distinction between declarative and non-declarative memories is that declarative memories require the medial temporal lobe structures to be accessed.[18]

The question of what role sleep plays in the consolidation of memories can be explained by the 2-stage memory formation mechanism which was proposed by Marr in 1971. This process states that memories are first encoded into fast-term storage, and then over time are transferred from fast-term storage to long-term storage. For declarative memories, the fast-term storage is the hippocampus, and the long-term storage system is the neocortex. This off-line process occurs during sleep, and there are myriad competing theories as to what specific role sleep plays in the process.[19] One model is the dual-process hypothesis of sleep, which dictates that SWS and REM sleep preferentially benefit declarative and non-declarative memory, respectively. This hypothesis is supported by the use of night-half paradigm, in which a memory task is followed by either early sleep, or late sleep. As it is known that SWS is more prevalent in the first half of the night, and REM sleep occurs in more frequency in the later half, we are able to study the effect that each stage of sleep plays in the consolidation of memory.[20] Another popular model is the active system consolidation hypothesis, which posits that memory encoding occurs via theta oscillations during wakefulness, and that consolidation occurs during non-rapid eye movement (NREM) sleep via hippocampal sharp-wave ripples (SWR).[21] There are numerous studies which support and contradict both theories, and therefore it is clear that a unified theory for memory consolidation does not exist. For the purposes of this chapter, we will use the active consolidation hypothesis within the framework of the dual-process hypothesis to define the specific processes which occur during NREM sleep during declarative memory consolidation.

SWS or N3 sleep is defined by an electroencephalogram demonstrating delta waves (0.5–4 Hz) which occur for 20% of an epoch. Delta rhythms in the ~1 Hz range are defined as slow oscillations (SO). They are generated in the medial prefrontal cortex and represent synchronous changes in membrane potential. Sleep spindles are rhythmic (12–16 Hz) wave forms usually lasting at least 0.5 seconds in duration. They can be further separated into slow (11–13.5 Hz) and fast (13.5–16 Hz) spindles, with differing functions and topographical locations.[22,23] Generally, sleep spindles are seen in N2 sleep; they also occur during SWS, but may be obscured by the predominant delta rhythm. Sharp wave ripples are 100–300 Hz waves that are generated in the hippocampus, and which occur during SWS. In the process of memory consolidation there is a carefully coordinated interaction between the aforementioned wave forms. Spindles occur during the upstate (depolarization) of the slow oscilllation, and SWRs occur during the spindle troughs. This pattern represents the transfer of memories from the hippocampus to the cortex, with the SO acting to synchronize transfer between the 2 different brain regions.[22,24]

Sleep and Declarative Memory

In one study Diekelmann et al.[25] compared the effects of 40 minutes of sleep and 90 minutes of sleep on the ability to retain information following a 2-D object-location task. In this study they demonstrated that after 90 minutes of sleep, study participants had improved recall performance when compared to the participants who slept for 40 minutes. Furthermore, the study also demonstrated that the amount of SWS was positively correlated with memory performance, and that recall performance was independent of REM sleep. In a study[26] examining the importance of hippocampal memory reactivation, researchers compared the participants with either temporal lobe epilepsy and unilateral hippocampal sclerosis, or temporal lobe epilepsy with bilateral hippocampal sclerosis, to a control group. The groups were trained to encode episodic memories using the process of cueing (a process by which memories can be reactivated using external stimuli), and the study demonstrated that strengthening of memories occurred only in the control group and unilateral hippocampal sclerosis group. In addition, the study found that hippocampal volume and spindle density during SWS were positively correlated with memory benefit. The importance of SWS was further elucidated in a study[27] using odor to cue memory reactivation from an object-location task (participants encoded the locations of card pairs) in SWS. The odor cue was presented to study participants either during wakefulness or during SWS and was followed by an interference task (the first object card was in the same location, but the second object card was not). The study found that SWS stabilized memories against interference; in addition, the study demonstrated that this stabilization was independent of REM sleep. There is further evidence to demonstrate the importance of sleep spindles in memory consolidation, in that patients with decreased spindle activity were found to exhibit memory deficits.[23] These studies serve to strengthen the association that declarative memories are formed in NREM sleep, and that slow wave activity (SWA) and sleep spindles play a key role in memory consolidation and neural plasticity. As sleep spindles are seen in both N2 and SWS, studies have been performed to elucidate whether the effect that spindles have on memory consolidation is truly specific to SWS, or if consolidation of declarative processes could also happen in N2, but the results are inconclusive.[20]

SLEEP AND NON-DECLARATIVE MEMORY

Non-declarative or procedural memories, in contrast to declarative ones, are those that are thought to be skill-based (e.g., playing a sport, driving a car, playing an instrument). Common forms of procedural memory tasks are finger-sequence tapping, mirror tracing, or other types of visuo-motor learning.[20] Formation of procedural memories does not typically require the hippocampus, but there is a likely interaction between the hippocampus and the skill-forming areas of the brain (motor cortex and striatal areas). Traditionally, according to the dual process hypothesis, these memories are consolidated selectively during REM sleep, and while there is some evidence which supports this theory, much of the recent research is not as supportive of this dichotomous view. In a study in which the fluvoxamine and reboxetine (REM-suppressing antidepressants) were administered prior to post-training sleep of procedural memory tasks (mirror tracing and finger tapping), investigators found that there was a strengthening of task performance the following day, and that REM suppression was associated with increased spindle density.[28] This finding correlated with those that selective serotonin reuptake inhibitor/selective norepinephrine reuptake inhibitor and monoamine oxidase inhibitor (SSRI/SNRI and MAO-I) use does not impair cognitive or memory function; however, amitriptyline, which is a tricyclic antidepressant (TCA) and also anticholinergic, was found have a deleterious effect.[29] These findings may suggest that procedural memory consolidation is associated with a cholinergic process, but not necessarily REM sleep.[20]

Studies supporting the importance of NREM sleep in procedural memory consolidation underline the importance of spindles and SWA in this process. In a study testing post-night visuomotor training, investigators introduced an SWA-suppressing tone during sleep, and on the following day found that performance on the same visuomotor task had decreased compared to the control group.[30] Spindles have been demonstrated to be increased in sleep, after both a finger-sequence tapping task or a simple motor task.[20]

While there remains evidence supporting the importance of REM sleep in the consolidation of procedural memories, these largely stem from the night-half paradigm, which we have described earlier in this section. One potential flaw in this paradigm is the finding that while REM sleep does predominate over SWS in the latter half of the night, N2 sleep and therefore sleep spindles remain present. Therefore it is possible that the strengthening effect that was previously ascribed to REM sleep is actually from N2 sleep in the later half of the night.[19]

SLEEP AND EMOTIONAL MEMORY

Emotional memories are episodic memories with an associated emotional valance attached to them. According to the memory modulation hypothesis, the consolidation of emotional memories are strengthened beyond that of neutral memories due to the activation of the amygdala by emotions, which serves to increase neural plasticity.[31] This additional stimulus, when compared to neutral memories, which do not activate the amygdala, lead emotional memories to be stored for a longer period of time.[32] While episodic in nature, and thus falling under the purview of the dual-process hypothesis, there has always been a suggestion that emotional REM sleep plays a salient role in the consolidation of memories. Much of this stems from the fact that during REM sleep the emotional centers of the brain, like the limbic system and amygdala, are active.[24] Compounding on this is that cholinergic activity is known to be increased during REM sleep.[19] In line with previous studies demonstrating the selective importance of NREM sleep in the encoding of episodic memories, a study performed by Kaida et al.[33] demonstrated that emotional memories followed this same pattern. The study compared the effects of total sleep deprivation and REM-specific sleep deprivation on neutral and emotional memories. As expected, neutral memories were found to deteriorate after a night of total sleep deprivation, but not of selective REM sleep deprivation; interestingly, the same was found to be true for emotional memories. The association continues to be seen in studies examining emotional memory consolidation. A study by Lehmann using cueing of emotional stimuli during both REM and NREM sleep found that it was during NREM sleep in which cueing demonstrated a strengthening of emotion memory. In addition, the valance of emotion attached to the memory served to strengthen the response, and was found to decrease with emotional memories with less valence.[32]

Despite these findings demonstrating that REM sleep is not preferentially selective, or necessary for the strengthening of emotional memories, there remains a contradictory view in which REM sleep remains a key modulator of the emotional experience; much of this stems from work on fear conditioning. Essentially, fear conditioning paradigms involve pairing a neutral item (sound) with a noxious event (pain stimulus) and then generating a response. Repeated pairing leads the neutral item to elicit an emotional response, or fear reaction, in the absence of the noxious stimuli.[34] One study demonstrated that sleep was shown to have a positive effect in helping to discriminate between fearful and non-fearful stimuli, and the magnitude of this discrimination was positively correlated with the amount of REM sleep.[35] It is believed that theta rhythm (4–7 Hz), which is one of the prominent rhythms during REM sleep,[23] is the carrier frequency for emotional memory encoding.[34]

These findings have led to the development of an alternate hypothesis of the purpose of REM sleep in the process of emotional memory generation. The "sleep to remember, sleep to forget" hypothesis states that not only does REM sleep serve to consolidate and strengthen emotional memories, but also recurrent reactivations strip away the emotional context of the memory, so that only memory of the event remains.[34]

We have presented a few of the myriad hypothesis regarding sleep's role in memory formation, and due to either contradictory or repeatable results, there exists no single governing theory. From the available data, it does seem to be certain that memories are encoded in a 2-step fashion: first, quickly to a short storage system, and then over time into long-term memory, and that this process is primarily governed by NREM sleep, specifically SWS, SOs, sleep spindles, and SWRs, and that REM may function to lessen the emotional impact of emotional memories over time.

INCREASING SLOW WAVE SLEEP

From a clinical perspective an obvious question arises: Can we improve memory by using exogenous methods to increase SWS? Thankfully, there has been a wealth of research performed to answer this clinically important question; they generally revolve around attempting to increase SWS by one of 3 different paradigms: (1) auditory stimulation; (2) transcranial direct current stimulation (tDCS); (3) pharmacological stimulation.

Auditory Stimulation

Auditory stimulation uses short bursts of pink noise to the amplitude or frequency of SOs during SWS. The bursts of sounds can be delivered with the goal of evoking SOs (open loop) and occur at any point during SWS. In comparison, closed-loop simulation serves to increase the amplitude of SOs by targeting the delivery of acoustic simulation to a certain phase of the SO. Studies have demonstrated that closed-loop simulation, when targeted to the SO up-state, increases the amplitude of SOs, and the power of both fast and slow spindles. These electroencephalogram (EEG) findings were also found to correlate with improvements in declarative memory tasks. In contrast, open-loop simulation studies were found to increase SWA; they were not found to improve performance on declarative memory tasks.[22,36]

Transcranial Direct Current Stimulation

Transcranial direct current stimulation (tDCS) involves placing electrodes bilaterally, either at frontal or central locations, and applying currents at 0.75 Hz with the intent of increasing the power and/or duration of SWA. The majority of studies employing tDCS have demonstrated that there is an increase in power of SO and delta frequency bands after stimulation. The effect on sleep spindles is varied, with studies reporting that tDCS can either increase, decrease, or have no effect on spindle density. From a cognitive standpoint, studies are also varied on the effect that tDCS has on declarative memories, but they are consistent in demonstrating that tDCS did not improve procedural memory tasks. There were potentially clinically relevant findings in some studies which demonstrated that tDCS improved memory in children with attention deficit hyperactivity disorder (ADHD), reduced forgetting in individuals with paranoid schizophrenia, and improved declarative verbal memory in patients with temporal lobe epilepsy.[22,36]

Pharmacological Stimulation

It is well documented that many pharmacological agents can increase the duration of SWS. One review looked at studies comparing the effects of tiagabine, gabodoxol, sodium oxybate, baclofen, olanzapine, and interleukin-6 on SWS and memory. The review demonstrated that while all medications could increase the duration of SWS, only sodium oxybate, tiagabine, and interleukin-6 had any positive effects on memory.[36]

SLEEP AND DEMENTIA

Per the *Diagnostic and Statistical Manual of Mental Disorders* (DSM-5) dementia is termed a major neurocognitive disorder and is defined as significant cognitive decline from a previous level of performance in one or more cognitive domains (complex attention, executive function, learning and memory, language, perceptual-motor, or social cognition). The deficit must interfere with daily function and independence, not occur solely with delirium, and must not be explained by other mental disorders.[37] From the World Health Organization fact sheet on dementia, the worldwide prevalence is approximately 50 million people, with an estimated 10 million new cases per year. Alzheimer disease (AD) is the most common cause of dementia and contributes to approximately 60%–70% of cases.[38] The prevalence is estimated to increase to 115.4 million by 2050.[39] In this chapter we have previously discussed the association between sleep and memory, illustrating how sleep is a fundamental process in all aspects of memory formation. We can build on this baseline to further expand upon the relationships between sleep and dementia.

In a meta-review by Shi and colleagues[40] reviewed 18 longitudinal studies with over 240000 subjects, to study the association between sleep disturbances (insomnia, sleep-disordered breathing, self-reported sleep disturbances, sleep-related movement disorder, and circadian rhythm sleep disturbances) and dementia. Results demonstrated that individuals with sleep disturbances (all types) had a 1.19 times higher chance to develop all-cause dementia and AD and vascular dementia subtypes when compared to those without sleep disturbances. In subgroup analysis it was determined that sleep-disordered breathing (obstructive sleep apnea, central sleep apnea) alone was a predictive risk factor for all-cause dementia, and both AD and vascular dementia subtypes. Interestingly, insomnia was found to increase the risk of AD, but not vascular dementia or all-cause dementia. Excessive daytime sleepiness and circadian rhythm disorders were also found to be associated with all-cause dementia. There was no such association elicited in regard to sleep-related movement disorders. A recent observational study yielded similar results; Sabia et al. followed studied the incidence of dementia in self-reported short sleepers in comparison to normal sleepers, and found that short sleepers in their 50s, 60s, and 70s demonstrated nearly a 30% greater incidence of all-cause dementia.[41] In a recent theoretical review of literature, Hwang et al.[42] postulate that orexin, a modulator of sleep and wakefulness, was a key mediator in the pathogenesis of behavioral variant frontotemporal dementia.

The finding that sleep-disordered breathing is predictive for both AD and vascular dementia subtypes, whereas insomnia is only associated with AD, is a good place to discuss the potential pathophysiological mechanisms by which sleep disturbances cause dementia.

Sleep-Disordered Breathing

Sleep-disordered breathing is characterized by repetitive obstruction or pause of air flow which induces a transient oxygen desaturation; this process is termed chronic intermittent hypoxemia (CIH) and sleep fragmentation. In studies performed on rats, it was found that hypoxemia increased the rate of amyloid beta (AB) plaques,[43] which is the hallmark of AD. Hypoxia has also been found to increase the production of tau protein, another influencer of AD. Increased apoptosis thought to be secondary to hypoxia-induced oxidative stress has also been reported.[40]

Vascular dementia is characterized by changes in white matter intensity which are caused small cerebral vessel lesions.[40] It is well documented that sleep-disordered breathing can promote vascular changes by inducing an inflammatory signaling cascade in response to chronic intermittent hypoxemia, which is mediated via hypoxia inducible factor 1 alpha and tumor necrosis factor and results in an increased production of endothelin-1, which promotes luminal endothelial cell proliferation and vasoconstriction. As insomnia is not associated with chronic intermittent hypoxemia, it does fit that it is not associated with an increased incidence of vascular dementia.

Insomnia

To discuss the potential causes that insomnia may play in the pathogenesis of dementia, let us first review the proposed mechanism by which sleep plays in neuroprotection, which have recently come to light through studies on AD, and are discussed in more depth in Chapter 25. Briefly, however, studies have demonstrated that there is an innate neurological metabolite clearance mechanism termed the *glymphatic system* which serves to clear toxins from the brain, and whose activity is driven by sleep; specifically, that interstitial fluid volume was greater during sleep, and that this drove more efficient clearance of AB. These findings were demonstrated as sleep deprivation was found to increase AB cerebrospinal fluid levels.[44] This finding may explain that sleep deprivation caused insomnia, and sleep fragmentation from sleep-disordered breathing may cause AD.

Circadian Rhythm Disturbances

Circadian rhythm sleep-wake disturbances (Chapter 15) encompass a set of disorders in which there exists a dysregulation between the endogenous body clock, which is controlled by the suprachiasmatic nuclei, and the exogenous clock. These disagreements between the 2 clocks can either be exogenous (jet lag, shift work disorder) or endogenous (non-24 sleep-wake disorder, irregular sleep-wake disorder). Studies in animals have used a forced "jet lag" paradigm to simulate the effects of circadian dysregulation. This was achieved by progressively advancing the animal to a phase advance (going to bed earlier) to simulate eastward travel. In one study performed on mice, researchers found that this resulted in an increase an inflammation, specifically in pro-inflammatory cytokines IL-1B, IL-2, and IL-13. The study also demonstrated that there was a decrease in the anti-inflammatory cytokine IL-10.[45] Another study using a forced "jet lag" paradigm demonstrated that in hamsters, circadian disruptions were associated with both a decrease in hippocampal cell proliferation and a decrease in hippocampal-dependent learning and memory.[46] These findings were corroborated in human studies with flight attendants after transatlantic flights. This study compared the salivary cortisol levels and temporal lobe volume of flight attendants who flew internationally and had different jet lag recovery periods (short recovery and long recovery). The findings demonstrated that the flight attendants in the short recovery group had elevated levels of salivary cortisol, and that this was thought to induce hippocampal atrophy, as evidenced by a decreased temporal lobe volume when measured by MRI.[47]

SUMMARY

In this chapter we have discussed the role that sleep plays in the processes surrounding emotional generation and regulation. It is evident that poor sleep is associated with more negative emotions, and an impaired ability when attempting to regulate them; though the exact mechanism by which this occurs has not been elucidated, it is thought to occur by control of the amygdala by the prefrontal cortex. The storage of emotions or processing of them into memory appears to occur as an interplay between NREM and REM sleep, in that NREM sleep is necessary for the formation of memory engrams, and the function of REM sleep is to strip away the emotional association behind them. Overall, the formation of memories occurs as a 2-step process in which memories are first stored in the hippocampus, and then transferred into long-term memory in the cortex during sleep in a process which is largely mediated by NREM sleep, specifically SWS, SOs, spindles, and hippocampal ripples. Studies clearly demonstrate that disrupted sleep is associated with impairment of all types of memories, and therefore may be one of the explanations behind the association between sleep and dementia; another being that poor sleep leads to an increase in neural plaque formation, due to a reduction in glymphatic flow.

REFERENCES

1. Gross JJ. Emotion regulation: Conceptual and empircal foundation. In: Gross JJ. *Handbook of Emotion Regulation*. 2nd ed. Guilford Press; 2013.
2. Ochsner KN, Silvers JA, Buhle JT. Functional imaging studies of emotion regulation: A synthetic review and evolving model of the cognitive control of emotion. *Ann N Y Acad Sci*. 2012;1251(1):E1–E24.
3. Tempesta D, Socci V, De Gennaro L, Ferrara M. Sleep and emotional processing. *Sleep Med Rev*. 2018;40:183–195.
4. Zohar D, Tzischinsky O, Epstein R, Lavie P. The effects of sleep loss on medical residents' emotional reactions to work events: A cognitive-energy model. *Sleep*. 2005;28(1):47–54.
5. Dinges DF, Pack F, Williams K, et al. Cumulative sleepiness, mood disturbance, and psychomotor vigilance performance decrements during a week of sleep restricted to 4–5 hours per night. *Sleep*. 1997;20(4):267–277.
6. Yoo S-S, Gujar N, Hu P, Jolesz FA, Walker MP. The human emotional brain without sleep: A prefrontal amygdala disconnect. *Curr Biol*. 2007;17(20):R877–R878.
7. Sotres-Bayon F, Bush DE, LeDoux JE. Emotional perseveration: An update on prefrontal-amygdala interactions in fear extinction. *Learn Mem*. 2004;11(5):525–535.
8. Franzen PL, Buysse DJ, Dahl RE, Thompson W, Siegle GJ. Sleep deprivation alters pupillary reactivity to emotional stimuli in healthy young adults. *Biol Psychol*. 2009;80(3):300–305.
9. Fairholme CP, Manber R. *Sleep, Emotions, and Emotion Regulation: Sleep and Affect*. Elsevier; 2015.
10. Palmer CA, Alfano CA. Sleep and emotion regulation: An organizing, integrative review. *Sleep Med Rev*. 2017;31:6–16.
11. Carney CE, Edinger JD, Meyer B, Lindman L, Istre T. Daily activities and sleep quality in college students. *Chronobiol Int*. 2006;23(3):623–637.
12. Gordon AM, Chen S. The role of sleep in interpersonal conflict. *Soc Psychol Personal Sci*. 2014;5(2):168–175.

13. Ferri J, Schmidt J, Hajcak G, Canli T. Neural correlates of attentional deployment within unpleasant pictures. *NeuroImage*. 2013;70:268–277.
14. Buhle JT, Silvers JA, Wager TD, et al. Cognitive reappraisal of emotion: A meta-analysis of human neuroimaging studies. *Cerebral Cortex*. 2014;24(11):2981–2990.
15. Tamm S, Nilsonne G, Schwarz J, et al. Sleep restriction caused impaired emotional regulation without detectable brain activation changes: A functional magnetic resonance imaging study. *Royal Soc Open Sci*. 2019;6(3):181704.
16. Reddy R, Palmer CA, Jackson C, Farris SG, Alfano CA. Impact of sleep restriction versus idealized sleep on emotional experience, reactivity and regulation in healthy adolescents. *J Sleep Res*. 2017;26(4):516–525.
17. Zhang J, Lau EYY, Hsiao JH-W. Using emotion regulation strategies after sleep deprivation: ERP and behavioral findings. *Cogn Affect Behav Neurosci*. 2019;19(2):283–295.
18. Squire LR, Zola SM. Structure and function of declarative and nondeclarative memory systems. *Proc Natl Acad Sci*. 1996;93(24):13515-13522.
19. Rasch B, Born J. About sleep's role in memory. *Physiolog Rev*. 2013;93(2):681–766.
20. Ackermann S, Rasch B. Differential effects of non-REM and REM sleep on memory consolidation? *Curr Neurol Neurosci Rep*. 2014;14(2):430.
21. Damien L, Eden D, Arnaud R, Virginie B, Karim B, Mounir C. Slow-wave sleep: From the cell to the clinic. *Sleep Med Rev*. 2018;41:113–132.
22. Roneil GM, Phyllis CZ. Brain stimulation for improving sleep and memory. *Sleep Med Clin*. 2020;15(1):101–115.
23. Peigneux P, Fogel S, Smith C. Memory processing in relation to sleep. In: Kryger M, Roth T, Dement WC, eds. *Principles and Practice of Sleep Medicine*. 6th ed. Elsevier; 2017.
24. Peigneux P. Neuroimaging studies of sleep and memory in humans. In: Meerlo P, Benca RM, Abel T, eds. *Sleep, Neuronal Plasticity and Brain Function*. Springer Berlin Heidelberg; 2015.
25. Susanne D, Simon B, Björn R, Jan B. Offline consolidation of memory varies with time in slow wave sleep and can be accelerated by cuing memory reactivations. *Neurobiol Learn Mem*. 2012;98(2):103–111.
26. Fuentemilla L, Miró J, Ripollés P, et al. Hippocampus-dependent strengthening of targeted memories via reactivation during sleep in humans. *Curr Biol*. 2013;23(18):1769–1775.
27. Diekelmann S, Büchel C, Born J, Rasch B. Labile or stable: Opposing consequences for memory when reactivated during waking and sleep. *Nat Neurosci*. 2011;14(3):381–386.
28. Rasch B, Pommer J, Diekelmann S, Born J. Pharmacological REM sleep suppression paradoxically improves rather than impairs skill memory. *Nat Neurosci*. 2009;12(4):396–397.
29. Vertes RP, Eastman KE. The case against memory consolidation in REM sleep. *Behav Brain Sci*. 2000;23(6):867–876; discussion 904–1121.
30. Landsness EC, Crupi D, Hulse BK, et al. Sleep-dependent improvement in visuomotor learning: a causal role for slow waves. *Sleep*. 2009;32(10): 1273–1284.
31. McGaugh JL. The amygdala modulates the consolidation of memories of emotionally arousing experiences. *Annu Rev Neurosci*. 2004;27:1–28.
32. Lehmann M, Schreiner T, Seifritz E, Rasch B. Emotional arousal modulates oscillatory correlates of targeted memory reactivation during NREM, but not REM sleep. *Sci Rep*. 2016;6(1):39229.
33. Kaida K, Niki K, Born J. Role of sleep for encoding of emotional memory. *Neurobiol Learn Mem*. 2015;121:72–79.
34. Goldstein AN, Walker MP. The role of sleep in emotional brain function. *Ann Rev Clin Psychol*. 2014;10(1):679–708.
35. Menz MM, Rihm JS, Salari N, et al. The role of sleep and sleep deprivation in consolidating fear memories. *NeuroImage*. 2013;75:87–96.
36. Zhang Y, Gruber R. Can slow-wave sleep enhancement improve memory? A review of current approaches and cognitive outcomes. *Yale J Biol Med*. 2019;92(1):63–80.
37. American Psychiatric Association. *Diagnostic and Statistical Manual of Mental Disorders*. 5th ed. American Psychiatric Association; 2013.
38. World Health Organization. Dementia. 2020; https://www.who.int/news-room/fact-sheets/detail/dementia.
39. Prince M, Bryce R, Albanese E, Wimo A, Ribeiro W, Ferri CP. The global prevalence of dementia: A systematic review and metaanalysis. *Alzheimer Dement*. 2013;9(1):63–75.e62.
40. Shi L, Chen S-J, Ma M-Y, et al. Sleep disturbances increase the risk of dementia: A systematic review and meta-analysis. *Sleep Med Rev*. 2018;40:4–16.
41. Sabia S, Fayosse A, Dumurgier J, et al. Association of sleep duration in middle and old age with incidence of dementia. *Nat Commun*. 2021;12(1).
42. Hwang YT, Piguet O, Hodges JR, Grunstein R, Burrell JR. Sleep and orexin: A new paradigm for understanding behavioural-variant frontotemporal dementia? *Sleep Med Rev*. 2020;54:101361.
43. Li L, Zhang X, Yang D, Luo G, Chen S, Le W. Hypoxia increases Aβ generation by altering β- and γ-cleavage of APP. *Neurobiol Aging*. 2009;30(7):1091–1098.
44. Van Egroo M, Narbutas J, Chylinski D, et al. Sleep-wake regulation and the hallmarks of the pathogenesis of Alzheimer's disease. *Sleep*. 2019;42(4).
45. Castanon-Cervantes O, Wu M, Ehlen JC, et al. Dysregulation of inflammatory responses by chronic circadian disruption. *J Immunol*. 2010;185(10): 5796–5805.
46. Gibson EM, Wang C, Tjho S, Khattar N, Kriegsfeld LJ. Experimental "jet lag" inhibits adult neurogenesis and produces long-term cognitive deficits in female hamsters. *PLoS One*. 2010;5(12):e15267.
47. Cho K. Chronic "jet lag" produces temporal lobe atrophy and spatial cognitive deficits. *Nat Neurosci*. 2001;4(6):567–568.

Chapter 27

Sleep and Psychiatry

Bhanu Prakash Kolla, Meghna P. Mansukhani, and Raphael Golebiowski

Psychiatric disorders are prevalent in the general population with estimates of 30.5%.[1] The majority of psychiatric disorders, as defined by the *Diagnostic and Statistical Manual of Mental Disorders*, 5th edition (DSM-5), include criteria for some type of sleep disturbance.[2] Insomnia, the most common sleep disorder, characterized by difficulty initiating or maintaining sleep occurring at least a few days a week for at least a month, has a 30% incidence rate in the general population.[3] Studies evaluating comorbidities in patients with insomnia have found a significantly elevated odds ratio for comorbid psychiatric illness of 5.04 for severe insomnia, 2.63 for moderate insomnia, and 1.7 for subthreshold insomnia.[4] Traditionally, sleep disturbances in psychiatric illnesses were considered as part of the disorder, but the emerging view is that this is a complex relationship, with bidirectional causality. In this chapter, we will cover the major categories of psychiatric disorders and what is known about the sleep disturbances associated with them.

SLEEP AND DEPRESSIVE DISORDERS

Of all the psychiatric disorders, depressive disorders are the most extensively studied in the context of their relationship with sleep disturbance. Major depressive disorder (MDD), as per the DSM-5, is thought to occur when an individual has at least 5 of 9 described symptoms present consistently for at least 2 weeks, with 1 of the symptoms being either a depressed mood or loss of interest or pleasure (Box 27.1). Depression is a complex disorder that is heterogeneous in nature, with multiple neurotransmitters and neurohumoral pathways implicated, but the exact pathophysiology is still unclear.

One of the criteria for depression is sleep disturbance, classified as either insomnia or hypersomnia. The literature suggests that up to 90% of patients with depression report some type of sleep disturbance, predominately insomnia (up to 88%), and less commonly, hypersomnia (27%).[5] The relationship between sleep disturbance and depression is complex and likely bidirectional. Longitudinal

Box 27.1 Adapted DSM-5 Major Depressive Disorder Criteria

Major Depressive Disorder Diagnostic Criteria

1. Depressed mood most of the day, nearly every day, as indicated by either subjective report or observation made by others
2. Markedly diminished interest or pleasure in all, or almost all, activities most of the day, nearly every day (as indicated by either subjective account or observation)
3. Significant weight loss when not dieting or weight gain or decrease or increase in appetite nearly every day
4. Insomnia or hypersomnia nearly every day
5. Psychomotor agitation or retardation nearly every day
6. Fatigue or loss of energy nearly every day
7. Feelings of worthlessness or excessive or inappropriate guilt (which may be delusional) nearly every day
8. Diminished ability to think or concentrate, or indecisiveness, nearly every day (either by subjective account or as observed by others)
9. Recurrent thoughts of death (not just fear of dying), recurrent suicidal ideation without a specific plan, or a suicide attempt or a specific plan for committing suicide

studies have reported that insomnia significantly increases the risk of subsequent depression (relative risk 2.0–3.0).[6] Conversely, other longitudinal studies have demonstrated that insomnia is both a risk factor and a prodromal manifestation of depression.[7]

Research attempting to understand sleep disturbances in patients with depression using polysomnography (PSG) started in the 1960s. Over the next decades, studies assessing sleep architecture in depression have demonstrated alterations compared to healthy controls. The observed alterations consisted of impaired sleep efficiency (SE) and continuity, reduction in slow wave sleep (SWS), and disinhibition of rapid eye movement (REM) sleep. Specifically, REM sleep is altered, with a short initial REM sleep latency, prolongation of the first REM period, and increased REM density (increased number of rapid eye movements). It is important to note that not all studies have demonstrated these abnormalities; a meta-analysis performed subgroup analyses to exclude patients with comorbidities, and these findings were not seen, except for increased REM density.[8]

The REM sleep alterations seen in patients with depression offered a potential mechanism of antidepressant efficacy, as most classes of antidepressants suppress REM sleep. However, antidepressants such as bupropion and mirtazapine that do not suppress REM sleep are also effective in the treatment of depression, which argues against REM suppression as the primary mechanism responsible for efficacy. With initiation of pharmacological treatment of depression, there is often a lag of approximately 4 weeks before improvement of core symptoms can be seen. Unfortunately, studies have demonstrated that most patients continue to have residual sleep disturbances despite improvement in other symptoms of depression.[9] In contrast, one study suggested that patients with depression comorbid with insomnia who were treated with a combination of a selective serotonin reuptake inhibitor (SSRI), fluoxetine, and eszopiclone experienced improvement of insomnia symptoms and a quicker onset of antidepressant response.[10]

In conclusion, depression and sleep disturbance share a complex bidirectional relationship.

Clinicians need to perform a thorough evaluation of sleep complaints in patients with depression, as interventions and outcomes can differ in those with and without sleep disturbance.

SLEEP AND BIPOLAR DISORDER

This section will focus on bipolar disorder I (BD), as research investigating sleep disturbance in patients with bipolar II disorder and cyclothymic disorder is limited. BD is a chronic psychiatric illness that is characterized by recurrent (hypo)mania and depressive episodes that result in significant morbidity (Box 27.2). BD has a 12-month prevalence of 0.6%, with a male-to-female ratio of 1:1 in the United States.[11]

The relationship between sleep and BD is complex and likely bidirectional. First, there is evidence suggesting that prior to any affective episode of BD, some type of sleep disturbance

Box 27.2 Adapted DSM-5 Bipolar I Disorder Criteria

Bipolar I Disorder Diagnostic Criteria

For a diagnosis of bipolar I disorder, it is necessary to meet the following criteria for a manic episode. The manic episode may have been preceded by and may be followed by hypomanic or major depressive episodes.

A. Distinct period of abnormally and persistently elevated, expansive, or irritable mood and abnormally and persistently increased activity or energy, lasting at least 1 week and present most of the day, nearly every day (or any duration if hospitalization is necessary)

B. During the period of mood disturbance and increased energy or activity, 3 (or more) of the following symptoms (4 if the mood is only irritable) are present to a significant degree and represent a noticeable change from usual behavior:

1. Inflated self-esteem or grandiosity
2. Decreased need for sleep (e.g., feels rested after only 3 hours of sleep)
3. More talkative than usual or pressure to keep talking
4. Flight of ideas or subjective experience that thoughts are racing
5. Distractibility (i.e., attention too easily drawn to unimportant or irrelevant external stimuli), as reported or observed
6. Increase in goal-directed activity (either socially, at work or school, or sexually) or psychomotor agitation (i.e., purposeless non-goal-directed activity)
7. Excessive involvement in activities that have a high potential for painful consequences (e.g., engaging in unrestrained buying sprees, sexual indiscretions, or foolish business investments)

C. The mood disturbance is sufficiently severe to cause marked impairment in social or occupational functioning or to necessitate hospitalization to prevent harm to self or others, or there are psychotic features.

D. The episode is not attributable to the physiological effects of a substance (e.g., a drug of abuse, a medication, other treatment) or another medical condition.

(decreased need for sleep, insomnia, and/or hypersomnia) is present for greater than a year.[12] Second, the majority of patients with BD (80%) can identify sleep disturbance during the prodrome of a manic episode. Finally, induced sleep deprivation is associated with the onset of manic episodes in patients with BD.[13]

During manic episodes, the prevalence of decreased need for sleep has been reported to range from 69% to 99%.[14] Patients with BD experiencing a depressive episode suffer from hypersomnia, with estimates of 23%–78%, and/or insomnia in up to 100% of patients.[14] The majority of patients (70%) in between mood episodes (i.e. in euthymia) report ongoing sleep disturbances (longer sleep onset latency [SOL], higher pharmacological sleep aid use, and daytime dysfunction).[15] Studies evaluating chronotype and circadian rhythm in BD have observed that disruption in circadian rhythm and eveningness chronotype are more common in these patients.[16]

Objective sleep architecture studies with electroencephalography (EEG) have reported inconsistent findings, except increased SOL and increased REM density across all phases of illness.[17] Actigraphy is an exciting tool to implement for naturalistic observation; studies have demonstrated that it is a valid tool for estimating sleep length and fragmentation compared to PSG. A meta-analysis comparing actigraphy findings in patients with BD to healthy controls observed that, in general, the former are less active and tend to sleep longer.[18]

Acute treatment for BD varies by phase of illness (i.e., depression or mania), but maintenance treatment commonly consists of a mood stabilizer such as lithium or valproic acid. It is important to note that antipsychotics are often utilized as monotherapy or adjunctive therapy. Generally, antipsychotics except risperidone have more consistently been demonstrated to increase sleep duration and SE, but may vary in their effects on SWS.[19] Notably, second-generation (atypical) antipsychotics are associated with obesity and metabolic syndrome (abnormal glucose and lipid metabolism), which are risk factors for sleep-disordered breathing. Furthermore, studies have suggested that atypical antipsychotics can worsen the apnea hypopnea index (AHI) secondary to reduction in upper airway muscle tone, increasing the likelihood and severity of obstructive sleep apnea (OSA).[20] Additionally, as antipsychotics act through the dopamine system, they have been associated with sleep-related movement disorders.

Nonpharmacological interventions such as cognitive behavioral therapy for insomnia (CBT-I) have demonstrated efficacy in a variety of psychiatric and medical disorders with comorbid insomnia. Harvey and colleagues developed and studied a bipolar disorder-specific modification of CBT-I (CBTI-BP) that incorporated Interpersonal and Social Rhythm Therapy, Motivation Interviewing, and Chronotherapy and observed reduced rates of relapse along with improvement in sleep and functioning.[21]

In conclusion, the relationship between sleep and BD is complex and likely bidirectional. Sleep and circadian disturbance with eveningness chronotype are common in this patient population. Despite treatment of the underlying psychiatric disorder, sleep disturbances often persist. Evidence suggests that sleep deprivation can trigger manic episodes, highlighting the importance of targeting treatment of sleep disturbances in all phases of illness.

SLEEP AND ANXIETY DISORDERS

Anxiety disorders are common in the general population, with adult prevalence estimates of 2%–3% for generalized anxiety disorder (GAD) or panic disorder (PD).[1] In patients with anxiety disorders, sleep disturbances are frequent and are included in the diagnostic criteria. Approximately 60%–70% of patients with GAD experience "trouble sleeping," whereas in PD, prevalence ranges from 68% to 77%.[22]

Generalized Anxiety Disorder

GAD is characterized by excessive worry and anxiety that is present consistently for at least 6 months that impairs daily functioning (socially/occupationally). The cardinal feature is the preoccupation with anticipation of future threat that can result in restlessness, fatigue, difficulties concentrating, irritability, muscle tension, and sleep disturbance (Box 27.3).

In regard to disturbed sleep, the evidence is somewhat limited compared to other

Box 27.3 Adapted DSM-5 Generalized Anxiety Disorder

Generalized Anxiety Disorder Diagnostic Criteria

A. Excessive anxiety and worry (apprehensive expectation), occurring more days than not for at least 6 months, about a number of events or activities (such as work or school performance)

B. The individual finds it difficult to control the worry.

C. The anxiety and worry are associated with 3 (or more) of the following 6 symptoms (with at least some symptoms having been present for more days than not for the past 6 months):

- Restlessness or feeling keyed up or on edge
- Being easily fatigued
- Difficulty concentrating or mind going blank
- Irritability
- Muscle tension
- Sleep disturbance (difficulty falling or staying asleep, or restless, unsatisfying sleep)

D. The anxiety, worry, or physical symptoms cause clinically significant distress or impairment in social, occupational, or other important areas of functioning.

E/F. In summary, specify the need to rule out (or not better explained by) other psychiatric disorders, substance use abuse, medical conditions, or neurodevelopmental disorders.

psychiatric disorders, but studies have suggested decreased total sleep time (TST), increased stage 2 non-rapid eye movement (NREM) sleep, and increased SOL.[23,24] However, the literature on alteration in SE and REM sleep parameters is inconclusive.

Treatment of GAD is broadly divided into pharmacological (anxiolytics, antidepressants) and nonpharmacological (cognitive behavioral therapy [CBT], psychotherapy), which are generally considered equivalent in their efficacy, with some evidence suggesting that combination therapy is superior.[25] Studies have demonstrated that patients undergoing CBT for GAD experience an improvement in insomnia symptoms; however, many have residual symptoms that would meet a diagnosis of insomnia or subthreshold insomnia.[26] One small study suggested that sequential treatment of CBT for GAD followed by CBT-I is more efficacious than CBT in the reverse order.[27]

Panic Disorder

PD is characterized by recurrent unexpected panic attacks that result in multiple physical and cognitive symptoms for which no obvious cue or trigger is identified (Box 27.4). Although the criteria do not include sleep-related symptoms, sleep disturbances are estimated to occur in 68%–77% of patients.[22] Patients with PD may experience nocturnal panic attacks that awaken them from sleep, with estimates

Box 27.4 Adapted DSM-5 Panic Disorder Criteria

Panic Disorder Diagnostic Criteria

A. Recurrent unexpected panic attacks. A panic attack is an abrupt surge of intense fear or intense discomfort that reaches a peak within minutes, and during which time 4 (or more) of the following symptoms occur:

- Palpitations, pounding heart, or accelerated heart rate
- Sweating
- Trembling or shaking
- Sensations of shortness of breath or smothering
- Feelings of choking
- Chest pain or discomfort
- Nausea or abdominal distress
- Feeling dizzy, unsteady, light-headed, or faint
- Chills or heat sensations
- Paresthesias (numbness or tingling sensations)
- Derealization (feelings of unreality) or depersonalization (being detached from oneself)
- Fear of losing control or "going crazy"
- Fear of dying

B. At least one of the attacks has been followed by 1 month (or more) of one or both of the following:

1. Persistent concern or worry about additional panic attacks or their consequences (e.g., losing control, having a heart attack, "going crazy")
2. A significant maladaptive change in behavior related to the attacks (e.g., behaviors designed to avoid having panic attacks, such as avoidance of exercise or unfamiliar situations)

C/D. In summary, specify the need to rule out (or not better explained by) other psychiatric disorders, substance use abuse, medical conditions, or neurodevelopmental disorders.

of occurrence in 18%–45% of patients.[28] Those with nocturnal panic attacks report higher rates of insomnia (non-restorative sleep and frequent awakenings).

Nocturnal panic attacks typically occur in NREM sleep, during a transition from late-stage 2 to early-stage 3 NREM sleep.[29] Studies evaluating objective findings for PD have observed increased SOL, decreased SE, and decreased TST.[29] Other studies evaluating sleep architecture (e.g., percentage of time spent in the various sleep stages and REM parameters) are limited and results are conflicting.

Similar to GAD, treatment of PD consists of pharmacological (anxiolytics, antidepressants) and nonpharmacological (CBT, psychotherapy), which are generally considered equivalent in terms of efficacy, with some evidence suggesting that patients who receive CBT are less likely to experience recurrence in the following year than those treated with pharmacotherapy.[30]

SLEEP AND SCHIZOPHRENIA SPECTRUM DISORDERS

Schizophrenia is a severe chronic mental illness with disruptions in thought process, behaviors, and emotions (Box 27.5). These often present as delusions, hallucinations, difficulties with communication secondary to disorganized speech, and negative symptoms of social withdrawal. The lifetime prevalence estimates range from 0.3% to 0.7%.[31] Although the disorder does not have any sleep-specific criteria, studies have observed that approximately 30%–80% of patients with schizophrenia have some type of sleep disturbance.[32]

There have been many studies investigating sleep disturbances in schizophrenia. The literature in this area is heterogeneous, secondary to differences in the duration of illness, medication status, and decompensated versus stable psychosis. Research thus far has focused on evaluating sleep architecture abnormalities. Early findings suggested reduced SWS, increased or decreased REM duration, and reduction of initial REM sleep latency.[33] Only the reduction in initial REM sleep latency was observed in patients with schizophrenia compared to

Box 27.5 Adapted DSM-5 Schizophrenia Criteria

Schizophrenia Diagnostic Criteria

A. Two (or more) of the following, each present for a significant portion of time during a 1-month period (or less if successfully treated). At least 1 of these must be (1), (2), or (3):

1. Delusions
2. Hallucinations
3. Disorganized speech (e.g., frequent derailment or incoherence)
4. Grossly disorganized or catatonic behavior
5. Negative symptoms (i.e., diminished emotional expression or avolition)

B. For a significant portion of the time since the onset of the disturbance, level of functioning in 1 or more major areas, such as work, interpersonal relations, or self-care, is markedly below the level achieved prior to the onset.

C. Continuous signs of the disturbance persist for at least 6 months. This 6-month period must include at least 1 month of symptoms (or less if successfully treated) that meet Criterion A (i.e., active-phase symptoms) and may include periods of prodromal or residual symptoms. During these prodromal or residual periods, the signs of the disturbance may be manifested by only negative symptoms or by 2 or more symptoms listed in Criterion A present in an attenuated form

D–F: In summary, specify the need to rule out (or not better explained by) other psychiatric disorders, substance use abuse, medical conditions, or neurodevelopmental disorders.

healthy controls in a later meta-analysis; however, this finding was not observed in another study that controlled for antipsychotic-naive or antipsychotic withdrawn status.[34] Therefore, it has been debated whether these sleep architecture abnormalities are a state or trait phenomenon, or a medication effect. In recent years, there has been a shift in research focus from sleep architecture toward other parameters such as sleep EEG power and sleep-specific oscillatory rhythms (sleep spindle and slow waves). Studies have suggested deficits in sleep spindles and slow waves, but findings have been mixed.[35] Furthermore, there is evidence that this patient population suffers from disrupted circadian rhythm (phase advance, phase delay, or non-24-hour cycles) with general tendencies of wakefulness during nights and increased sleep during daytime.[36]

In treating schizophrenia, clinicians prescribe first- or second-generation antipsychotic medications that, broadly speaking, function as dopamine D2 receptor antagonists. However, these medications target a multitude of different receptors, including serotoninergic, histaminergic, and noradrenergic receptors, with varying levels of potency and affinity that result in the commonly observed adverse effects. The effects of antipsychotics on normal sleep and sleep disorders as discussed in the section on BD are also relevant here.

Multiple studies have evaluated CBT-I for patients with schizophrenia and have found improvement in various sleep parameters (TST, SE, and SOL) as well as improvement in other psychopathology.[37]

In conclusion, sleep is often disturbed in patients with schizophrenia (advanced phase, delayed phase, non-24-hour circadian rhythm, insomnia, hypersomnia). Pharmacological treatment with antipsychotics may predispose patients to sleep-disordered breathing and/or worsen its severity. Clinicians need to provide holistic care to these patients, with consideration given to both pharmacological and non-pharmacological interventions.

SLEEP AND OBSESSIVE-COMPULSIVE AND RELATED DISORDERS

Obsessive-compulsive disorder (OCD) is a debilitating illness wherein individuals have recurrent intrusive thoughts, urges, or images that cause significant distress (obsessions), and potentially repetitive behaviors or mental acts in response to their obsessions (compulsions), that are developed to reduce distress (Box 27.6). Individuals may experience obsessions, compulsions, or both to be diagnosed with the disorder. The prevalence of the disorder has been estimated to be between 1.1% and 1.8%.[1,38] Although there are no specific criteria for sleep disturbances, symptoms of OCD may interfere with sleep.

Research evaluating sleep disturbances in OCD is limited compared to other psychiatric disorders. Studies have demonstrated that patients with OCD have decreased TST and subjective sleep duration, but there is no evidence of significant deficits in sleep continuity or sleep depth.[39] Sleep architecture findings regarding REM and NREM sleep parameters in patients with OCD have been mixed, but a recent meta-analysis suggested increased REM sleep pressure.[39] Additionally, studies have demonstrated an association between delayed sleep phase and severity of OCD symptoms.[40] OCD is frequently comorbid with other psychiatric disorders, most commonly with depressive disorders, with prevalence estimates ranging from 30% to 80%.[41] Therefore, sleep disturbance may reflect the overlap between OCD and comorbid disorders.

Treatment of OCD, like other psychiatric disorders, consists of pharmacological and non-pharmacological interventions. SSRIs and clomipramine have the best evidence for treatment, with less robust evidence demonstrating the benefit of venlafaxine.[42] In contrast, CBT targeting OCD symptoms with exposure therapy and response-prevention components has been shown to have efficacy in reducing symptom burden. Studies suggest that first-line treatment with CBT is superior to pharmacotherapy.[43]

SLEEP AND EATING DISORDERS

There are various types of eating disorders; however, research related to sleep and eating disorders is quite limited. In this chapter, we will focus on anorexia nervosa and bulimia nervosa as they are more prevalent and studied. The essential features of anorexia nervosa are a persistent energy intake restriction, intense

Box 27.6 Adapted DSM-5 Obsessive-Compulsive Disorder Diagnostic Criteria

Obsessive-Compulsive Disorder

A. Presence of obsessions, compulsions, or both:

Obsessions are defined by (1) and (2):

1. Recurrent and persistent thoughts, urges, or images that are experienced, at some time during the disturbance, as intrusive and unwanted, and that in most individuals cause marked anxiety or distress.
2. The individual attempts to ignore or suppress such thoughts, urges, or images, or to neutralize them with some other thought or action (i.e., by performing a compulsion).

Compulsions are defined by (1) and (2):

1. Repetitive behaviors (e.g., hand washing, ordering, checking) or mental acts (e.g., praying, counting, repeating words silently) that the individual feels driven to perform in response to an obsession or according to rules that must be applied rigidly.
2. The behaviors or mental acts are aimed at preventing or reducing anxiety or distress, or preventing some dreaded event or situation; however, these behaviors or mental acts are not connected in a realistic way with what they are designed to neutralize or prevent, or are clearly excessive.

B. The obsessions or compulsions are time-consuming (e.g., take more than 1 hour per day) or cause clinically significant distress or impairment in social, occupational, or other important areas of functioning.

C/D. In summary, specify the need to rule out (or not better explained by) other psychiatric disorders, substance use abuse, medical conditions, or neurodevelopmental disorders.

fear of gaining weight/becoming overweight, or persistent behavior that interferes with weight gain, and a disturbance of self-perceived weight or shape. Anorexia nervosa is much more common in females than males (10:1) and estimated prevalence in young females is 0.4%.[44,45] In contrast, bulimia nervosa consists of recurrent episodes of binge eating, recurrent inappropriate compensatory behaviors to prevent weight gain, and self-evaluation that is influenced by body shape and weight. Often, these patients are normal to overweight in body mass index measurements in comparison to anorexia nervosa, where patients are more commonly underweight. The prevalence of bulimia nervosa in young females is 1%–1.5%, with a similar 10:1 female to male prevalence ratio.[46,47]

Anorexia Nervosa

Research exploring the overlap between eating disorders and sleep is scarce. Generally speaking, the prevalence of disturbed sleep in patients with eating disorders is estimated to be 50.3%, with no major differences between bulimia and anorexia.[48] Similar to other psychiatric disorders, the relationship between eating disorders and sleep is complex for several reasons. First, it is important to note that anorexia is often comorbid with depression, with estimates of up to 80%; therefore, sleep disturbances related to the mood disorder may be present. Second, patients with anorexia experience significant malnutrition that may impact sleep, with proposed theories of differing orexin-A concentrations among healthy controls and patients with anorexia, although studies have not found differences between the groups.[49] Results of sleep architecture abnormalities have been mixed, and this is an area that requires further research.[48] The literature appears to indicate that sleep disturbances in this population consist of initial insomnia (56.5%), interrupted sleep (47.8%), late insomnia/daytime hypersomnolence (21.7%), and parasomnias (39%).[48]

Bulimia Nervosa

Studies evaluating sleep architecture in patients with bulimia are limited and results are similar to studies of patients with anorexia, demonstrating initial insomnia, interrupted sleep, late insomnia/daytime hypersomnolence, and parasomnias. Studies evaluating subjective sleep complaints suggest that patients with bulimia nervosa do not experience significant sleep-related difficulties, but tend to have delayed bedtime of 1 hour secondary to evening binge-eating episodes.[50]

SLEEP AND TRAUMA- AND STRESSOR-RELATED DISORDERS

Post-traumatic stress disorder (PTSD) is a complex psychiatric disorder that is characterized by the development of symptoms secondary to experiencing a traumatic event (Box 27.7). The clinical presentation varies, ranging from predominately dysphoric mood states, fear-based re-experiencing, behavioral symptoms, dissociative symptoms, and hyperarousal, to reactive-externalizing symptoms, or any combination of these symptoms. The 12-month prevalence among adults in the United States is approximately 3.5%.[1]

Subjective sleep disturbance and recurrent nightmares are so prevalent in this population that it is included in the diagnostic criteria, with an estimated prevalence of sleep-related symptoms as high as 90%.[51,52] The relationship between sleep disturbances and PTSD is multifaceted. As with depression and anxiety disorders, studies have demonstrated that disturbed sleep prior to or after a traumatic event is a risk factor for the development of PTSD.[53] Sleep disturbances in PTSD include comorbid insomnia symptoms, recurrent nightmares, panicked awakenings, and disruptive nocturnal behaviors. This unique presentation of symptoms has been proposed as its own nosological entity, "trauma-associated sleep disorder" (TSD), a parasomnia following a traumatic incident.[54]

Objective PSG-based sleep architecture investigations and meta-analyses of these studies have found that there is a decrease in SWS; other results have been mixed but are suggestive of reduced sleep continuity (as a composite including SOL, SE, and/or number of awakenings). Both studies observed an increase in REM density, but the significance of this is unclear.[55] There is also research that suggests that REM sleep fragmentation early after trauma predicts the development of PTSD symptoms.[29] Additionally, the duration of PTSD impacts REM sleep in a linear fashion, with higher REM sleep proportion (increased REM duration and shorter REM latency) observed with increasing duration of PTSD. These changes may be part of an adaptive process, as REM sleep is implicated in emotional processing.

Treatment of PTSD consists of either trauma-based psychotherapy, psychopharmacology, or a combination, based on symptoms and patient preference. Trauma-based psychotherapy should have components of exposure, but may also include cognitive therapy or eye movement desensitization.[56] Psychopharmacology options consist of serotonin reuptake inhibitors (SSRIs and serotonin noradrenaline reuptake inhibitors) that have demonstrated efficacy in the reduction of core PTSD symptoms.[57] Prazosin was the pharmacological agent of choice in patients with recurrent nightmares and was recommended by the American Academy of Sleep Medicine (AASM), but a large randomized controlled trial (RCT) of military veterans did not demonstrate benefit and it was downgraded.[58] However, 2 more recent meta-analysis studies have demonstrated that in patients with recurrent nightmares, prazosin has demonstrated moderate efficacy.[59,60] Furthermore, imagery rehearsal therapy is a

Box 27.7 Adapted DSM-5 Post-Traumatic Stress Disorder Diagnostic Criteria

A. Exposure to actual or threatened death, serious injury, or sexual violence in 1 (or more) of the following ways:

1. Directly experiencing the traumatic event(s)
2. Witnessing, in person, the event(s) as it occurred to others
3. Learning that the traumatic event(s) occurred to a close family member or close friend. In cases of actual or threatened death of a family member or friend, the event(s) must have been violent or accidental.
4. Experiencing repeated or extreme exposure to aversive details of the traumatic event(s) (e.g., first responders collecting human remains; police officers repeatedly exposed to details of child abuse)

B. Presence of 1 (or more) of the following intrusion symptoms associated with the traumatic event(s), beginning after the traumatic event(s) occurred:

1. Recurrent, involuntary, and intrusive distressing memories of the traumatic event(s)
2. Recurrent distressing dreams in which the content and/or affect of the dream are related to the traumatic event(s)
3. Dissociative reactions (e.g., flashbacks) in which the individual feels or acts as if the traumatic event(s) were recurring. (Such reactions may occur on a continuum, with the most extreme expression being a complete loss of awareness of present surroundings.)
4. Intense or prolonged psychological distress at exposure to internal or external cues that symbolize or resemble an aspect of the traumatic event(s)
5. Marked physiological reactions to internal or external cues that symbolize or resemble an aspect of the traumatic event(s)

C. Persistent avoidance of stimuli associated with the traumatic event(s), beginning after the traumatic event(s) occurred, as evidenced by 1 or both of the following:

1. Avoidance of or efforts to avoid distressing memories, thoughts, or feelings about or closely associated with the traumatic event(s)
2. Avoidance of or efforts to avoid external reminders (people, places, conversations, activities, objects, situations) that arouse distressing memories, thoughts, or feelings about or closely associated with the traumatic event(s)

(*Continued*)

Box 27.7 Adapted DSM-5 Post-Traumatic Stress Disorder Diagnostic Criteria (cont.)

D. Negative alterations in cognitions and mood associated with the traumatic event(s), beginning or worsening after the traumatic event(s) occurred, as evidenced by 2 (or more) of the following:

1. Inability to remember an important aspect of the traumatic event(s) (typically due to dissociative amnesia and not to other factors such as head injury, alcohol, or drugs)
2. Persistent and exaggerated negative beliefs or expectations about oneself, others, or the world (e.g., "I am bad," "No one can be trusted," "The world is completely dangerous," "My whole nervous system is permanently ruined")
3. Persistent, distorted cognitions about the cause or consequences of the traumatic event(s) that lead the individual to blame himself/herself or others
4. Persistent negative emotional state (e.g., fear, horror, anger, guilt, or shame)
5. Markedly diminished interest or participation in significant activities
6. Feelings of detachment or estrangement from others
7. Persistent inability to experience positive emotions (e.g., inability to experience happiness, satisfaction, or loving feelings)

E. Marked alterations in arousal and reactivity associated with the traumatic event(s), beginning or worsening after the traumatic event(s) occurred, as evidenced by 2 (or more) of the following:

1. Irritable behavior and angry outbursts (with little or no provocation) typically expressed as verbal or physical aggression toward people or objects
2. Reckless or self-destructive behavior
3. Hypervigilance
4. Exaggerated startle response
5. Problems with concentration
6. Sleep disturbance (e.g., difficulty falling or staying asleep or restless sleep)

F. Duration of the disturbance (Criteria B, C, D, and E) is more than 1 month.

G. The disturbance causes clinically significant distress or impairment in social, occupational, or other important areas of functioning.

H. The disturbance is not attributable to the physiological effects of a substance (e.g., medication, alcohol) or another medical condition.

type of psychotherapy intervention that has been most extensively studied in the treatment of recurrent nightmares that has demonstrated benefit in nightmare frequency, sleep quality, and core PTSD symptoms.[61] Despite treatment, patients with PTSD often have residual symptoms of sleep disturbances.[62] Research has demonstrated that these patients may benefit from CBT specifically targeting sleep.[63]

SLEEP AND PERSONALITY DISORDERS

Personality disorders are prevalent in the general population, with estimates ranging from 9.1% to 15%.[64] Multiple studies have observed that this patient population suffers from some type of sleep disturbance, with prevalence rates of 50%–93%.[65,66] There are is a multitude of personality disorders; however, from a clinical perspective, borderline personality disorder (BPD) is most commonly encountered by clinicians. Patients with BPD have an estimated prevalence of 1%–6% in the adult general population and consist of 10%–20% of psychiatric inpatients.[67] BPD is described by the DSM-5 as a pervasive pattern of instability of interpersonal relationships, self-image, affects, and marked impulsivity.

Research on sleep disturbances and personality disorders has been mainly focused on BPD. As with other studies, results are mixed, but a meta-analysis suggested that in patients with BPD, after controlling for comorbid depression, there were significant differences in objective sleep measures (longer SOL, greater wake time after sleep onset, and REM density, shorter TST and REM latency, and lower SE) in comparison to healthy controls.[68] However, results of sleep architecture changes from the literature are mixed, making it difficult to draw firm conclusions. It is important to note that BPD is often comorbid with substance use and depression, which should be thoroughly evaluated as both can affect sleep.

In patients with BPD, the first-line treatment option is psychotherapy (dialectical behavior therapy, cognitive and behavioral therapies, Scheme-focused therapy, and others) that is supported by evidence.[69] Furthermore, patients with BPD are often prescribed adjunctive psychotropic medications (mood stabilizers, antipsychotics, antidepressants) to target specific symptoms of the disorder, and these can impact sleep. Studies have demonstrated that at least 50% of patients will achieve remission over a period of 10 years. However, in patients that do not achieve recovery, studies suggest ongoing disturbed sleep (increased global Pittsburgh Sleep Quality Index score, longer SOL, increased odds of using sleep medication, and daytime dysfunction) in comparison to patients who achieve recovery.[70]

SLEEP AND NEURODEVELOPMENTAL DISORDERS

Neurodevelopmental disorders are a diverse group of conditions that occur during the developmental period, with deficits that can result in significant impairment in multiple or specific domains (personal, social, academic, or occupational functioning). In this section, we will focus on the most prevalent conditions, consisting of autism spectrum disorder (ASD) and attention deficit hyperactivity disorder (ADHD). It is important to note that even within these disorders, presentation and deficits can vary significantly.

Autism Spectrum Disorder

The core features of ASD are persistent impairment in reciprocal social communication/interaction, and restricted, repetitive patterns of behavior, interests, or activities. The symptoms are present from early childhood and impact everyday functioning. As the disorder is labeled "spectrum," the presentation can vary significantly, with or without associated language impairment or intellectual impairment.[2] The prevalence of ASD in the United States is 1 in 59 in children aged 8 years old.[71]

Although there are no criteria for sleep disturbance in ASD, studies have demonstrated that approximately 50%–80% of children and adolescents suffer from some type of sleep difficulty.[72,73] This patient population experiences difficulties with initiating and maintaining sleep, intermittent nighttime awakenings, early morning waking, and irregular sleep-wake schedules.[74] Studies evaluating objective findings in ASD with PSG and/or actigraphy have demonstrated consistent findings in the pediatric population indicating shorter TST, longer

SOL, and decreased SE compared to healthy controls.[75,76] In contrast, in the adult ASD population, a recent meta-analysis observed that actigraphy measurements demonstrated shorter TST, longer SOL, and decreased SE, but this difference was not observed on PSG measurements compared to healthy controls.[77] Poor sleep in the pediatric ASD population has been associated with problematic daytime behaviors such as aggression, self-injury, anxiety, hyperactivity, and inattention.[78,79] As the sleep difficulties are so prevalent in this population, a thorough sleep evaluation should be conducted during clinical encounters. Multiple questionnaires are available (Modified Simonds, Parraga Sleep, Children's Sleep Habits, and Pediatric Sleep Clinical Global Impressions Scale) that can be implemented, along with evaluating for comorbidities such as restless legs syndrome (RLS), OSA, craniofacial abnormalities, epilepsy, and parasomnias.

Non-pharmacological treatment of insomnia in the pediatric ASD population consists of parent education in behavioral interventions (sleep hygiene, positive bedtime routines, extinction, sleep restriction, bedtime fading, etc.).[80]

There are no Food and Drug Administration (FDA)-approved medications for the treatment of insomnia in the pediatric population. Melatonin has been the most extensively studied agent and has demonstrated benefit and safety in multiple domains, including increased sleep duration, decreased sleep latency, improvement in daytime externalizing behaviors, and caregiver quality of sleep.[81-83] Additionally, patients with comorbid aggression and irritability may have FDA-approved antipsychotics prescribed, such as risperidone or aripiprazole, and dosing in the evening can utilize their sedative properties to potentially target insomnia. Furthermore, if patients have comorbid ADHD or Tourette syndrome, then alpha-agonists used to target either disorder can potentially be beneficial due to their sedative effects.

Attention Deficit Hyperactivity Disorder (ADHD)

The core feature of ADHD is a persistent pattern of inattention and/or hyperactivity-impulsivity that interferes with daily functioning or development (DSM-5). The estimated prevalence of ADHD is 5% in children and adolescents and 2.5% of the adult population worldwide.[84]

In children with ADHD, sleep disturbance has been reported in up to 70%, compared to 20%–30% in healthy controls.[85-87] Sleep disorders such as insomnia, circadian rhythm disturbances, RLS, and OSA are commonly comorbid with ADHD.[88] Furthermore, there appears to be a complicated bidirectional relationship between sleep disturbance and externalizing behaviors in ADHD.

Studies evaluating objective measures of sleep in patients with ADHD have resulted in mixed findings. A meta-analysis examining sleep measures using PSG in the pediatric ADHD population found that patients spent more time in stage 1 NREM sleep than healthy controls, suggesting increased light sleep. In contrast, multiple meta-analyses of studies evaluating sleep parameters utilizing PSG in adults with ADHD did not observe this finding.[89,90] At this time, there does not appear to be any consistent objective findings of sleep alterations on PSG in patients with ADHD.

The high prevalence of sleep disturbance prevalence in patients with ADHD should prompt clinicians to perform sleep assessments on a routine basis in these patients to evaluate for maladaptive sleep patterns or comorbid sleep disorders. If sleep disorders are identified, then appropriate intervention should be pursued. It is important to note that clinicians should be careful to distinguish between insomnia and delayed sleep-wake phase disorder (DSWPD), as the treatment for these 2 conditions varies. Evidence supports the efficacy of CBT-I in adolescents with insomnia.[91] In contrast, treatment of comorbid DSWPD could consist of light therapy, chronotherapy, CBT-I, and timed melatonin treatment.[92]

REFERENCES

1. Kessler RC, Chiu WT, Demler O, Merikangas KR, Walters EE. Prevalence, severity, and comorbidity of 12-month DSM-IV disorders in the National Comorbidity Survey Replication. *Arch Gen Psychiatry*. 2005 Jun;62(6):617–627. doi:10.1001/archpsyc.62.6.617.
2. American Psychiatric Association. *Diagnostic and Statistical Manual of Mental Disorders*. 5th ed. American Psychiatric Publishing; 2013.

3. Morin CM, Jarrin DC. Epidemiology of insomnia: Prevalence, course, risk factors, and public health burden. *Sleep Med Clin*. 2022 Jun;17(2):173–191. doi:10.1016/j.jsmc.2022.03.003.
4. Sarsour K, Morin CM, Foley K, Kalsekar A, Walsh JK. Association of insomnia severity and comorbid medical and psychiatric disorders in a health plan-based sample: Insomnia severity and comorbidities. *Sleep Med*. 2.010 Jan;11(1):69–74. doi:10.1016/j.sleep.2009.02.008
5. McCall WV, Reboussin BA, Cohen W. Subjective measurement of insomnia and quality of life in depressed inpatients. *J Sleep Res*. 2000 Mar;9(1):43–48. doi:10.1046/j.1365-2869.2000.00186.x.
6. Li L, Wu C, Gan Y, Qu X, Lu Z. Insomnia and the risk of depression: A meta-analysis of prospective cohort studies. *BMC Psychiatry*. 2016 Nov 5;16(1):375. doi:10.1186/s12888-016-1075-3.
7. Neckelmann D, Mykletun A, Dahl AA. Chronic insomnia as a risk factor for developing anxiety and depression. *Sleep*. 2007 Jul;30(7):873–880. doi:10.1093/sleep/30.7.873.
8. Baglioni C, Nanovska S, Regen W, et al. Sleep and mental disorders: A meta-analysis of polysomnographic research. *Psychol Bull*. 2016 Sep;142(9):969–990. doi:10.1037/bul0000053
9. Nierenberg AA, Husain MM, Trivedi MH, et al. Residual symptoms after remission of major depressive disorder with citalopram and risk of relapse: A STAR*D report. *Psychol Med*. 2010 Jan;40(1):41–50. doi:10.1017/s0033291709006011.
10. Fava M, McCall WV, Krystal A, et al. Eszopiclone co-administered with fluoxetine in patients with insomnia coexisting with major depressive disorder. *Biol Psychiatry*. 2006 Jun 1;59(11):1052–1060. doi:10.1016/j.biopsych.2006.01.016.
11. Merikangas KR, Akiskal HS, Angst J, et al. Lifetime and 12-month prevalence of bipolar spectrum disorder in the National Comorbidity Survey replication. *Arch Gen Psychiatry*. 2007 May;64(5):543–552. doi:10.1001/archpsyc.64.5.543.
12. Pancheri C, Verdolini N, Pacchiarotti I, et al. A systematic review on sleep alterations anticipating the onset of bipolar disorder. *Eur Psychiatry*. 2019 May;58:45–53. doi:10.1016/j.eurpsy.2019.02.003.
13. Wehr TA, Sack DA, Rosenthal NE. Sleep reduction as a final common pathway in the genesis of mania. *Am J Psychiatry*. 1987 Feb;144(2):201–204. doi:10.1176/ajp.144.2.201.
14. Harvey AG. Sleep and circadian rhythms in bipolar disorder: Seeking synchrony, harmony, and regulation. *Am J Psychiatry*. 2008 Jul;165(7):820–829. doi:10.1176/appi.ajp.2008.08010098.
15. Cretu JB, Culver JL, Goffin KC, Shah S, Ketter TA. Sleep, residual mood symptoms, and time to relapse in recovered patients with bipolar disorder. *J Affect Disord*. 2016 Jan 15;190:162–166. doi:10.1016/j.jad.2015.09.076.
16. Melo MCA, Abreu RLC, Linhares Neto VB, de Bruin PFC, de Bruin VMS. Chronotype and circadian rhythm in bipolar disorder: A systematic review. *Sleep Med Rev*. 2017 Aug;34:46–58. doi:10.1016/j.smrv.2016.06.007.
17. Zangani C, Casetta C, Saunders AS, Donati F, Maggioni E, D'Agostino A. Sleep abnormalities across different clinical stages of bipolar disorder: A review of EEG studies. *Neurosci Biobehav Rev*. 2020 Nov;118:247–257. doi:10.1016/j.neubiorev.2020.07.031.
18. Kaplan KA, Talbot LS, Gruber J, Harvey AG. Evaluating sleep in bipolar disorder: Comparison between actigraphy, polysomnography, and sleep diary. *Bipolar Disord*. 2012 Dec;14(8):870–879. doi:10.1111/bdi.12021.
19. Cohrs S. Sleep disturbances in patients with schizophrenia: Impact and effect of antipsychotics. *CNS Drugs*. 2008;22(11):939–962. doi:10.2165/00023210-200822110-00004.
20. Rishi MA, Shetty M, Wolff A, Amoateng-Adjepong Y, Manthous CA. Atypical antipsychotic medications are independently associated with severe obstructive sleep apnea. *Clin Neuropharmacol*. 2010 May;33(3):109–113. doi:10.1097/WNF.0b013e3181db8040.
21. Harvey AG, Soehner AM, Kaplan KA, et al. Treating insomnia improves mood state, sleep, and functioning in bipolar disorder: A pilot randomized controlled trial. *J Consult Clin Psychol*. 2015 Jun;83(3):564–577. doi:10.1037/a0038655.
22. Ohayon M. Epidemiological study on insomnia in the general population. *Sleep*. 1996 Apr;19(3 Suppl):S7–15. doi:10.1093/sleep/19.suppl_3.s7.
23. Alfano CA, Reynolds K, Scott N, Dahl RE, Mellman TA. Polysomnographic sleep patterns of non-depressed, non-medicated children with generalized anxiety disorder. *J Affect Disord*. 2013;147(1):379–384. doi:https://doi.org/10.1016/j.jad.2012.08.015.
24. Arriaga F, Paiva T. Clinical and EEG sleep changes in primary dysthymia and generalized anxiety: A comparison with normal controls. *Neuropsychobiology*. 1990;24(3):109–114. doi:10.1159/000119471.
25. Hofmann SG, Smits JA. Cognitive-behavioral therapy for adult anxiety disorders: A meta-analysis of randomized placebo-controlled trials. *J Clin Psychiatry*. 2008 Apr;69(4):621–632. doi:10.4088/jcp.v69n0415.
26. Cousineau H, Marchand A, Bouchard S, et al. Insomnia symptoms following treatment for comorbid panic disorder with agoraphobia and generalized anxiety disorder. *J Nerv Ment Dis*. 2016 Apr;204(4):267–273.
27. Belleville G, Ivers H, Bélanger L, Blais FC, Morin CM. Sequential treatment of comorbid insomnia and generalized anxiety disorder. *J Clin Psychol*. 2016;72(9):880–896. https://doi.org/10.1002/jclp.22300.
28. Craske MG, Barlow DH. Nocturnal panic. *J Nerv Ment Dis*. 1989 Mar;177(3):160–167. doi:10.1097/00005053-198903000-00006.
29. Mellman TA. Sleep and anxiety disorders. *Sleep Med Clin*. 2008;3(2):261–268. https://doi.org/10.1016/j.jsmc.2008.01.010.
30. Mitte K. A meta-analysis of the efficacy of psycho- and pharmacotherapy in panic disorder with and without agoraphobia. *J Affect Disord*. 2005 Sep;88(1):27–45. doi:10.1016/j.jad.2005.05.003.
31. McGrath J, Saha S, Chant D, Welham J. Schizophrenia: A concise overview of incidence, prevalence, and mortality. *Epidemiol Rev*. 2008;30:67–76. doi:10.1093/epirev/mxn001.
32. Benson KL. Sleep in schizophrenia: Impairments, correlates, and treatment. *Psychiatr Clin North Am*. 2006 Dec;29(4):1033–1045; abstract ix–x. doi:10.1016/j.psc.2006.08.002.

33. Stern M, Fram DH, Wyatt R, Grinspoon L, Tursky B. All-night sleep studies of acute schizophrenics. *Arch Gen Psychiatry*. 1969;20(4):470–477. doi:10.1001/archpsyc.1969.01740160086012.
34. Chouinard S, Poulin J, Stip E, Godbout R. Sleep in untreated patients with schizophrenia: A meta-analysis. *Schizophr Bull*. 2004;30(4):957–967. doi:10.1093/oxfordjournals.schbul.a007145.
35. Castelnovo A, Graziano B, Ferrarelli F, D'Agostino A. Sleep spindles and slow waves in schizophrenia and related disorders: Main findings, challenges and future perspectives. *Eur J Neurosci*. 2018 Oct;48(8):2738–2758. doi:10.1111/ejn.13815.
36. Hofstetter JR, Lysaker PH, Mayeda AR. Quality of sleep in patients with schizophrenia is associated with quality of life and coping. *BMC Psychiatry*. 2005;5:13. doi:10.1186/1471-244X-5-13.
37. Chiu VW, Ree M, Janca A, Iyyalol R, Dragovic M, Waters F. Sleep profiles and CBT-I response in schizophrenia and related psychoses. *Psychiatry Res*. 2018;268:279–287.
38. Ruscio AM, Stein DJ, Chiu WT, Kessler RC. The epidemiology of obsessive-compulsive disorder in the National Comorbidity Survey Replication. *Mol Psychiatry*. 2010;15(1):53–63.
39. Cox RC, Parmar AM, Olatunji BO. Sleep in obsessive-compulsive and related disorders: A selective review and synthesis. *Curr Opin Psychol*. 2020;34:23–26.
40. Coles ME, Schubert JR, Sharkey KM. Delayed bedtimes and obsessive–compulsive symptoms. *Behav Sleep Med*. 2012;10(4):258–265.
41. Kolada J, Bland R, Newman S. Obsessive-compulsive disorder. *Acta Psychiatr Scand*. 1994;89:24–35.
42. Soomro GM, Altman D, Rajagopal S, Oakley-Browne M. Selective serotonin re-uptake inhibitors (SSRIs) versus placebo for obsessive compulsive disorder (OCD). *Cochrane Database Syst Rev*. 2008 Jan 23;2008(1):CD001765.
43. Öst L-G, Havnen A, Hansen B, Kvale G. Cognitive behavioral treatments of obsessive–compulsive disorder. A systematic review and meta-analysis of studies published 1993–2014. *Clin Psychol Rev*. 2015;40:156–169.
44. Hoek HW, Bartelds AI, Bosveld JJ, et al. Impact of urbanization on detection rates of eating disorders. *Am J Psychiatry*. 1995 Sep;152(9):1272–1278. doi:10.1176/ajp.152.9.1272.
45. Götestam KG, Eriksen L, Heggestad T, Nielsen S. Prevalence of eating disorders in Norwegian general hospitals 1990–1994: Admissions per year and seasonality. *Int J Eat Disord*. 1998;23(1):57–64.
46. Hoek HW. Incidence, prevalence and mortality of anorexia nervosa and other eating disorders. *Curr Opin Psychiatry*. 2006;19(4):389–394.
47. Keski-Rahkonen A, Hoek H, Linna M, et al. Incidence and outcomes of bulimia nervosa: A nationwide population-based study. *Psychol Med*. 2009;39(5):823–831.
48. Abdou TA, Esawy HI, Mohamed GAR, et al. Sleep profile in anorexia and bulimia nervosa female patients. *Sleep Med*. 2018;48:113–116.
49. Sauchelli S, Jiménez-Murcia S, Sánchez I, et al. Orexin and sleep quality in anorexia nervosa: Clinical relevance and influence on treatment outcome. *Psychoneuroendocrinology*. 2016;65:102–108.
50. Latzer Y, Tzischinsky O, Epstein R, Klein E, Peretz L. Naturalistic sleep monitoring in women suffering from bulimia nervosa. *Int J Eat Disord*. 1999;26(3):315–321.
51. Neylan TC, Marmar CR, Metzler TJ, et al. Sleep disturbances in the Vietnam generation: Findings from a nationally representative sample of male Vietnam veterans. *Am J Psychiatry*. 1998;155(7):929–933.
52. Roszell DK, McFall ME, Malas KL. Frequency of symptoms and concurrent psychiatric disorder in Vietnam veterans with chronic PTSD. *Psychiatr Serv*. 1991;42(3):293–296.
53. Wright KM, Britt TW, Bliese PD, Adler AB, Picchioni D, Moore D. Insomnia as predictor versus outcome of PTSD and depression among Iraq combat veterans. *J Clin Psychol*. 2011;67(12):1240–1258.
54. Mysliwiec V, O'Reilly B, Polchinski J, Kwon HP, Germain A, Roth BJ. Trauma associated sleep disorder: A proposed parasomnia encompassing disruptive nocturnal behaviors, nightmares, and REM without atonia in trauma survivors. *J Clin Sleep Med*. 2014;10(10):1143–1148.
55. Kobayashi I, Boarts JM, Delahanty DL. Polysomnographically measured sleep abnormalities in PTSD: A meta-analytic review. *Psychophysiology*. 2007;44(4):660–669.
56. Bisson JI, van Gelderen M, Roberts NP, Lewis C. Non-pharmacological and non-psychological approaches to the treatment of PTSD: Results of a systematic review and meta-analyses. *Eur J Psychotraumatol*. 2020;11(1):1795361.
57. Stein DJ, Ipser J, McAnda N. Pharmacotherapy of posttraumatic stress disorder: A review of meta-analyses and treatment guidelines. *CNS Spectr*. 2009;14(Suppl 1):25–31.
58. Morgenthaler TI, Auerbach S, Casey KR, et al. Position paper for the treatment of nightmare disorder in adults: An American Academy of Sleep Medicine position paper. *J Clin Sleep Med*. 2018;14(6):1041–1055.
59. Khachatryan D, Groll D, Booij L, Sepehry AA, Schuetz CG. Prazosin for treating sleep disturbances in adults with posttraumatic stress disorder: A systematic review and meta-analysis of randomized controlled trials. *Gen Hosp Psychiatry*. 2016;39:46–52.
60. Zhang Y, Ren R, Sanford LD, et al. The effects of prazosin on sleep disturbances in post-traumatic stress disorder: A systematic review and meta-analysis. *Sleep Med*. 2020;67:225–231.
61. Casement MD, Swanson LM. A meta-analysis of imagery rehearsal for post-trauma nightmares: Effects on nightmare frequency, sleep quality, and posttraumatic stress. *Clin Psychol Rev*. 2012;32(6):566–574.
62. Belleville G, Guay S, Marchand A. Persistence of sleep disturbances following cognitive-behavior therapy for posttraumatic stress disorder. *J Psychosom Res*. 2011;70(4):318–327.
63. Ho FY-Y, Chan CS, Tang KN-S. Cognitive-behavioral therapy for sleep disturbances in treating posttraumatic stress disorder symptoms: A meta-analysis of randomized controlled trials. *Clin Psychol Rev*. 2016;43:90–102.
64. Lenzenweger MF, Lane MC, Loranger AW, Kessler RC. DSM-IV personality disorders in the National Comorbidity Survey Replication. *Biol*

Psychiatry. 2007 Sep 15;62(6):553–64. doi:10.1016/j.biopsych.2006.09.019.
65. Kamphuis J, Karsten J, de Weerd A, Lancel M. Sleep disturbances in a clinical forensic psychiatric population. *Sleep Med*. 2013;14(11):1164–1169.
66. Selby EA. Chronic sleep disturbances and borderline personality disorder symptoms. *J Consult Clin Psychol*. 2013;81(5):941.
67. Gunderson JG, Stout RL, McGlashan TH, et al. Ten-year course of borderline personality disorder: Psychopathology and function from the Collaborative Longitudinal Personality Disorders study. *Arch Gen Psychiatry*. 2011;68(8):827–837.
68. Winsper C, Tang NK, Marwaha S, et al. The sleep phenotype of borderline personality disorder: A systematic review and meta-analysis. *Neurosci Biobehav Rev*. 2017;73:48–67.
69. Cristea IA, Gentili C, Cotet CD, Palomba D, Barbui C, Cuijpers P. Efficacy of psychotherapies for borderline personality disorder: A systematic review and meta-analysis. *JAMA Psychiatry*. 2017;74(4):319–328.
70. Plante DT, Frankenburg FR, Fitzmaurice GM, Zanarini MC. Relationship between sleep disturbance and recovery in patients with borderline personality disorder. *J Psychosom Res*. 2013;74(4):278–282.
71. Baio J. Prevalence of autism spectrum disorder among children aged 8 years: autism and developmental disabilities monitoring network, 11 sites, United States, 2014. *MMWR Surveill Summ*. 2018;67:1–23.
72. Elrod MG, Nylund CM, Susi AL, et al. Prevalence of diagnosed sleep disorders and related diagnostic and surgical procedures in children with autism spectrum disorders. *J Dev Behav Pediatr*. 2016;37(5):377–384.
73. Polimeni MA, Richdale A, Francis A. A survey of sleep problems in autism, Asperger's disorder and typically developing children. *J Intell Disabil Res*. 2005;49(4):260–268.
74. Williams Buckley A, Hirtz D, Oskoui M, et al. Practice guideline: Treatment for insomnia and disrupted sleep behavior in children and adolescents with autism spectrum disorder: Report of the Guideline Development, Dissemination, and Implementation Subcommittee of the American Academy of Neurology. *Neurology*. 2020;94(9):392–404.
75. Elrod MG, Hood BS. Sleep differences among children with autism spectrum disorders and typically developing peers: A meta-analysis. *J Dev Behav Pediatr*. 2015;36(3):166–177.
76. Chen X, Liu H, Wu Y, Xuan K, Zhao T, Sun Y. Characteristics of sleep architecture in autism spectrum disorders: A meta-analysis based on polysomnographic research. *Psychiatry Res*. 2021;296:113677.
77. Lugo J, Fadeuilhe C, Gisbert L, et al. Sleep in adults with autism spectrum disorder and attention deficit/hyperactivity disorder: A systematic review and meta-analysis. *Eur Neuropsychopharmacol*. 2020;38:1–24.
78. Mazurek MO, Sohl K. Sleep and behavioral problems in children with autism spectrum disorder. *J Autism Dev Disord*. 2016;46:1906–1915.
79. Goldman SE, McGrew S, Johnson KP, Richdale AL, Clemons T, Malow BA. Sleep is associated with problem behaviors in children and adolescents with autism spectrum disorders. *Res Autism Spectr Disord*. 2011;5(3):1223–1229.
80. Keogh S, Bridle C, Siriwardena NA, et al. Effectiveness of non-pharmacological interventions for insomnia in children with Autism Spectrum Disorder: A systematic review and meta-analysis. *PloS One*. 2019;14(8):e0221428.
81. Gringras P, Nir T, Breddy J, Frydman-Marom A, Findling RL. Efficacy and safety of pediatric prolonged-release melatonin for insomnia in children with autism spectrum disorder. *J Am Acad Child Adolesc Psychiatry*. 2017;56(11):948–957.
82. Schroder CM, Malow BA, Maras A, et al. Pediatric prolonged-release melatonin for sleep in children with autism spectrum disorder: Impact on child behavior and caregiver's quality of life. *J Autism Dev Disord*. 2019;49:3218–3230.
83. Maras A, Schroder CM, Malow BA, et al. Long-term efficacy and safety of pediatric prolonged-release melatonin for insomnia in children with autism spectrum disorder. *J Child Adolesc Psychopharmacol*. 2018;28(10):699–710.
84. Polanczyk G, De Lima MS, Horta BL, Biederman J, Rohde LA. The worldwide prevalence of ADHD: A systematic review and metaregression analysis. *Am J Psychiatry*. 2007;164(6):942–948.
85. Yoon SYR, Jain U, Shapiro C. Sleep in attention-deficit/hyperactivity disorder in children and adults: Past, present, and future. *Sleep Med Rev*. 2012;16(4):371–388.
86. Sung V, Hiscock H, Sciberras E, Efron D. Sleep problems in children with attention-deficit/hyperactivity disorder: Prevalence and the effect on the child and family. *Arch Pediatr Adolesc Med*. 2008;162(4):336–342.
87. Quach JL, Nguyen CD, Williams KE, Sciberras E. Bidirectional associations between child sleep problems and internalizing and externalizing difficulties from preschool to early adolescence. *JAMA Pediatrics*. 2018;172(2):e174363.
88. Instanes JT, Klungsøyr K, Halmøy A, Fasmer OB, Haavik J. Adult ADHD and comorbid somatic disease: A systematic literature review. *J Atten Disord*. 2018;22(3):203–228.
89. Diaz-Roman A, Mitchell R, Cortese S. Sleep in adults with ADHD: Systematic review and meta-analysis of subjective and objective studies. *Neurosci Biobehav Rev*. 2018;89:61–71.
90. Baglioni C, Nanovska S, Regen W, et al. Sleep and mental disorders: A meta-analysis of polysomnographic research. *Psychol Bull*. 2016;142(9):969.
91. de Bruin EJ, Bögels SM, Oort FJ, Meijer AM. Improvements of adolescent psychopathology after insomnia treatment: Results from a randomized controlled trial over 1 year. *J Child Psychol Psychiatry*. 2018;59(5):509–522.
92. Auger RR, Burgess HJ, Emens JS, Deriy LV, Thomas SM, Sharkey KM. Clinical practice guideline for the treatment of intrinsic circadian rhythm sleep-wake disorders: advanced sleep-wake phase disorder (ASWPD), delayed sleep-wake phase disorder (DSWPD), non-24-hour sleep-wake rhythm disorder (N24SWD), and irregular sleep-wake rhythm disorder (ISWRD): An update for 2015: An American Academy of Sleep Medicine clinical practice guideline. *J Clin Sleep Med*. 2015;11(10):1199–1236.

Chapter 28

Sleep and Cardio-Pulmonary Conditions

Christopher J. Lettieri and Lee A. Surkin

INTRODUCTION

Poor sleep and chronic cardiopulmonary conditions commonly coexist and share a bi-directional causal relationship. Both insufficient sleep and sleep disorders, particularly obstructive sleep apnea (OSA), have been shown to cause or contribute to the development of cardiopulmonary disorders.[1,2] Similarly, cardiovascular and respiratory diseases, as well as their treatments, frequently disrupt sleep or impair sleep quality.[3] Understanding how normal sleep can impact cardiopulmonary function, how sleep disorders can lead to the development of chronic cardiac and respiratory disease, and how cardiopulmonary diseases can disrupt sleep is crucial for understanding this complex relationship and for improving outcomes.

CARDIAC AND RESPIRATORY PHYSIOLOGIC CHANGES DURING SLEEP

There are normal physiologic changes that occur during sleep that impact respiratory function. During sleep, mucociliary clearance and cough are diminished, there is an increase in airway resistance, and there is instability in the thresholds controlling both the hypoxic and hypercapnic respiratory drives. In addition, there is a circadian nadir in pulmonary function that occurs during the night, which is more pronounced while in a state of sleep. Simply lying in the supine position alters West zones and changes in hypoxic vasoconstriction that lead to a ventilation-perfusion mismatch. These normal physiologic changes lead to a relative hypoventilatory state during sleep with an expected increase in partial pressure of carbon dioxide (pCO_2).

Normal sleep also leads to changes in cardiac and pulmonary vascular function. Alterations in blood pressure follow a typical circadian pattern, with a nadir occurring overnight in the early morning hours. This is followed by a marked increase in pressure following awakening. Cardiac output decreases by approximately 25% during sleep, which is driven by a reduction in both heart rate and stroke volume.[4] Heart rate fluctuation varies significantly between non-rapid eye movement (NREM) and rapid eye movement (REM) sleep stages, resulting in both hemodynamic stress and relaxation that continually alternate during the night. NREM sleep is closely associated with greater stability in heart rate, arterial blood pressure, and coronary blood flow. In contrast, REM sleep results in a greater degree of hemodynamic alteration in association with activation of the central nervous system.[5] Sleep also leads to an increase in pulmonary vascular pressure with transient increases in right atrial and right ventricular pressures.

These changes in cardiac and respiratory physiology are not uniform during the night and are influenced by both circadian cycles and by the stage of sleep. The alterations in respiratory and cardiac function are normal physiologic changes that occur during sleep, and for most individuals, they are clinically meaningless and a normal effect of sleeping. However, among those with underlying cardiac and/or respiratory disease, these changes can exacerbate symptoms and contribute to poor outcomes.

SLEEP AND CARDIOVASCULAR DISEASE

There is a strong link between cardiovascular disease and chronic poor sleep. Not only is there a clear causal relationship between sleep disorders and the development of cardiovascular disease, but cardiovascular diseases and their treatments frequently disrupt sleep.[6] The increased risk of cardiac disease and dysfunction have been shown in both those with chronic sleep debt, and among those with a number of underlying sleep disorders, including OSA, insomnia, restless legs syndrome, and narcolepsy.

Chronic sleep debt increases the risk for hypertension and has been shown to be an independent risk factor for heart attack, stroke, and cardiovascular death, with odds ratios greater than those seen with diabetes and smoking.[7] Insufficient sleep creates a systemic, pro-inflammatory state and an increased autonomic tone that can lead to endothelial dysfunction and impaired fibrionolysis. And insufficient sleep can cause or contribute to weight gain and insulin resistance.[8] These factors have been shown to have an independent impact on cardiovascular health. A meta-analysis of 15 prospective, longitudinal studies found that, compared with those who obtain 7–8 hours of sleep per night, short sleepers were 48% more likely to develop or die from coronary artery disease and were 13% more likely to experience or die from a stroke.[9] In addition, another cross-sectional analysis of NHANES data from 2007 to 2008 confirmed the increased association between short sleep, defined as <6 hours, with an odds ratio of just over 2.0 for myocardial infarction and stroke, and also revealed that long sleepers, defined as >8 hours, had an increased association with coronary artery disease (CAD) and angina.[10]

While several sleep disorders have been associated with the development of cardiovascular diseases, the largest body of evidence has focused on the adverse impact of OSA. Sleep-disordered breathing has been shown to increase the risk for hypertension, pulmonary vascular disease, ischemic heart disease, cerebral vascular accidents, congestive heart failure and arrhythmias, independent of confounding or concomitant risk factors.[11–21] However, despite the growing body of evidence linking OSA to the development of cardiovascular disease, the true causal relationship remains controversial. Many risk factors for OSA are also known risk factors for cardiovascular disease, such as age, male gender, and obesity. In addition, OSA is associated with numerous conditions known to increase the risk of cardiac disease, such as diabetes mellitus, hypertension, and obesity. As such, it is difficult to prove if OSA independently causes cardiovascular disease given that it is difficult to control for the numerous associated cardiovascular comorbidities.

Episodes of sleep-disordered breathing cause pathologic vascular changes and dysfunction, which can both cause and contribute to cardiovascular disease independent of confounding factors. However, the true mechanism of cardiovascular disorders associated with OSA is complicated and not fully understood.

The adverse effects that OSA imposes on cardiovascular function are thought to arise from several overlapping mechanisms. Apneic events, intermittent hypoxia, and the resulting arousals result in increased sympathetic tone, oxidative stress, intrathoracic pressure variations, endothelial dysfunction, clotting tendency, and a pro-inflammatory state.[15,22–26] The increase in sympathetic tone and associated catecholamine surges result in increased peripheral vascular resistance with associated blood pressure increases, which ultimately results in the development of hypertension. These changes also induce electrical and structural remodeling of the cardiovascular system, which contributes to the development of cardiovascular disease. [20,21,24,26,27] When apneas occur, there is an increase in sympathetic vasoconstriction due to the lack of inhibitory input from pulmonary stretch receptors that typically signal brain stem adrenergic centers. The resultant hypoxia and hypercapnia trigger an increased sympathetic discharge, resulting in expression of norepinephrine, which exerts its deleterious effects on the cardiovascular system. Repetitive respiratory events contribute to the development of comorbid cardiovascular conditions.[27] Regardless of the underlying mechanism or pathophysiologic alterations, the presence of OSA has clearly been shown to increase cardiovascular disease, major adverse cerebrovascular and cardiovascular events (MACCEs), and mortality.[29]

Hypertension

The causal link between OSA and systemic hypertension has been clearly established. Several studies have shown that sleep apnea increases the relative risk of hypertension, independent of other confounding factors.[11–14] Approximately 50% of patients with OSA have hypertension, compared with only 30% of the general public. Likewise, comorbid OSA occurs in half of patients with hypertension and in 82% of those with resistant hypertension.[30,31] In a cross-sectional analysis of over 6000 patients, the Sleep Heart Health Study showed a linear relationship between mean systolic and diastolic blood pressures and OSA severity.[11] Likewise, the prevalence of hypertension linearly increased with the presence and severity of OSA. Because of the strength of evidence linking OSA with the development of hypertension, the seventh report of the Joint National Committee on Prevention, Detection, Evaluation, and Treatment of High Blood Pressure (JNC-VII) lists sleep apnea as a significant cause of secondary hypertension.[13]

Solidifying validation of this causal relationship, treatment of OSA with either positive airway pressure (PAP) or oral appliances (OAs) leads to a reduction in blood pressure and greater control of hypertension.[32–37] This is also true in patients with resistant HTN.[35–37] Unfortunately, most clinical trials have only shown a modest reduction of systolic and diastolic blood pressure despite otherwise successful treatment of OSA. However, even a modest reduction in blood pressure confers cardiovascular benefits.

Cardiac Arrythmias

Cardiac arrhythmias, especially tachy-brady syndrome, ventricular ectopy, and atrial fibrillation, are commonly identified in patients with OSA.[19–21] The Sleep Heart Health Study observed that patients with sleep-disordered breathing had a higher likelihood of arrhythmias compared to controls.[20] Specifically, OSA was associated with a 4-fold increase in atrial fibrillation, a 3-fold increase in non-sustained ventricular tachycardia, and a 2-fold increase in complex ventricular ectopy. CPAP therapy has been shown to reduce the rates of arrhythmias even after controlling for heart failure and other independent variables.[21]

These rhythm disturbances likely correlate with nocturnal hypoxia, sleep fragmentation, and elevated sympathetic tone. OSA also produces cardiac structural changes which can result in aberrant conduction abnormalities, including, but not limited to, left atrial enlargement. There are several pathophysiologic mechanisms that lead to the development of arrythmias in these patients. Upper airway collapsibility and transient increases in upper airway resistance lead to alterations in the transpleural and intrathoracic pressure gradients. This leads to atrial stretch, enlargement, and remodeling. The repetitive oxidative stress produced by OSA leads to catecholamine release, autonomic nervous system dysregulation, elevated sympathetic tone, and an inflammatory response. These hemodynamic and sympathetic consequences of OSA are the catalyst for developing both endothelial dysfunction and complex arrythmias.

The best-understood arrythmia among patients with OSA is atrial fibrillation (AF), and there is a clear and significant association between these two disorders. OSA occurs in 17% more patients with AF compared with controls.[38] Likewise, the majority of patient with AF are found to have underlying OSA, and the prevalence of AF directly correlates with OSA severity.[39–41] In the Sleep Heart Health Study, severe OSA was associated with a 4-fold increased risk for the development of AF.[20] Not only does OSA increase the risk of developing AF, it also decreases the likelihood of a successful cardioversion, reduces the effectiveness of anti-arrhythmic therapy, and increases recurrence following ablation.[42–44] Given this close association, and the adverse impact it has on treatment and outcomes, it is strongly recommended that all patients with AF be screened for sleep-disordered breathing.

Heart Failure

Sleep and heart failure share several important relationships. Heart failure impairs sleep. Poor sleep quality is common among those with reduced cardiac function, and medications used to treat heart failure frequently cause sleep disturbances. Likewise, sleep disturbances can cause or worsen heart failure. The normal physiologic changes that occur during sleep can add further strain on the heart and pulmonary vasculature, which can exacerbate symptoms in susceptible patients. And the association between heart failure and both central sleep apnea (CSA) and OSA is well documented and accepted.

There are several reasons why a person with heart failure, especially those with a reduced left ventricular ejection fraction (LVEF), have poor sleep quality. Orthopnea can make falling asleep difficult, can fragment sleep, and lead to nocturnal awakenings. Diuretics can also cause sleep fragmentation and nocturnal awakenings. Statins, especially lipophilic preparations, can lead to daytime somnolence. In addition, betablockers can cause daytime sleepiness and have been associated with an increased risk for increase nightmares. They also reduce melatonin production, potentially leading to insomnia and fragment sleep. Not surprisingly, nearly two-thirds of those with heart failure report poor subjective sleep quality. Objectively, a reduced ejection fraction is associated with a decrease in sleep continuity, more nocturnal arousals, and a diminished amount of both slow wave and REM sleep.[6]

Underlying sleep-disordered breathing is highly prevalent among patients with heart failure, and both central and obstructive respiratory events are common in individuals with systolic and diastolic dysfunction.[16–18] The Sleep Heart Health Study found the likelihood of having heart failure was 2.4 times greater among individuals with OSA.[45] This association was independent of other known risk factors. Similarly, a prospective study of patients with LVEF found concurrent sleep apnea in 50%.[16] The occurrence and type of respiratory event is highly correlated with the ejection fraction. As cardiac function becomes more impaired, coupled with worsening hemodynamics, the frequency of obstructive events tends to decrease and central apneas begin to emerge. The prevalence of OSA versus CSA in the heart failure patient is based on multiple factors including, but not limited to, the LVEF. It has been shown that CSA is more predominant in individuals with a greater degree of LVEF reduction compared to OSA. Other risk factors for CSA include male gender, increasing age, and a low pCO_2. In fact, a pCO_2 at or near the apnea threshold was determined to be the most likely predisposing factor for CSA in the heart failure patient.[46]

Treating sleep-disordered breathing reverses, or at least abates, the pathophysiologic effects that cause or contribute to heart failure. PAP has been shown to be beneficial in those with heart failure exacerbations.[47] Intuitively, it would seem that PAP would also provide a benefit in the chronic management of heart failure, especially among those with underlying sleep-disordered breathing. However, this finding has not been consistently observed in clinical trials. Randomized controlled trials (RCTs) have shown that treatment of OSA with CPAP is associated with significant improvements in cardiac function, sympathetic activity, and quality of life.[17,18] Similarly, in the CANPAP study, CPAP improved nocturnal oxygenation, increased left ventricular function, lowered norepinephrine levels, and improved functional capacity among patients with central sleep apnea and heart failure.[48] Ultimately, however, CPAP did not improve transplant-free survival in this trial. A post-hoc analysis parsing out those patients whose CSA responded more rapidly to CPAP did reveal both an improvement in LVEF and a transplant-free survival benefit.[49] Likewise, in the study SERVE-HF (Treatment of Sleep Disordered Breathing with Predominant Central Sleep Apnea by Adaptive Servo Ventilation in Patients with Heart Failure), treatment with CPAP or adaptive servo ventilation (ASV) failed to improve outcomes, with concerns for increased mortality, among patient with HFrEF (LVEF ≤45%) complicated by CSA associated with Hunter, Cheyne Stokes breathing.[50] However, these trials have largely been limited by problems with trial design, device settings and titrations, and PAP adherence. A meta-analysis, which included 19 RCTs, compared therapeutic outcomes for patients with CSA with HFrEF.[51] This analysis found that ASV provided improvements in sleep measures but did not lead to improvements in quality of life (QOL), cardiovascular outcomes, or mortality. Similarly, while CPAP improved short-term outcomes on sleep, cardiovascular outcomes, and QOL, no longer-term benefits on cardiovascular events or mortality were observed. Given the mixed results and limitations of prior investigations, ongoing trials exploring the potential benefits of PAP and ASV utilizing different treatment algorithms in a mixed patient population including CSA and OSA are underway.

Other treatment options for patients with heart failure and CSA exist, although with less robust evidence than PAP platforms. For example, a novel treatment utilizing phrenic nerve stimulation has been shown to provide significant benefits in suppressing CSA, increasing LVEF, and improving QOL metrics; with sustained benefits noted over a 5-year observation period.[52] Acetazolamide has also proven to be beneficial in a short-term trial.[53] In addition, the potential benefit of supplemental O_2 and high-flow oxygen delivery systems are being actively investigated.

Coronary Artery Disease and the Risk of Myocardial Infarction (MI)

Despite overlapping demographics and risk factors, there is robust evidence that OSA has a causal relationship with coronary artery disease (CAD), and several studies have suggested the prevalence of CAD is 3–5 times higher in patients with OSA compared to controlled populations.[2,15,28,32,34,54,55] This is especially true with moderate to severe OSA. More importantly, long-term observational studies found that severe OSA significantly increases the risk of both fatal and nonfatal cardiovascular events.[32,55] OSA causes or contributes to hypertension, arterial noncompliance, atherosclerosis, and glucose intolerance. Additionally, OSA produces carotid arterial wall thickness in a dose-response nature, which has been shown to be a marker of cardiovascular disease and a predictor of morbidity and mortality.[56] Similarly, among patients with known CAD, the respiratory disturbance index was the only independent predictor of mortality in a 5-year study.[57] Likewise, ablation of obstructive events with PAP has been shown to decrease the risk of cardiovascular events and prevent the development of new ischemic heart disease.[57] As such, it seems clear that OSA is an independent risk factor for CAD.

While the risk of untreated OSA is clearly linked to an increased risk of cardiovascular disease, the benefit of PAP therapy on reducing these events has not yet been definitively established in randomized controlled clinical trials. In a 4-year follow-up study by Barbe et al., CPAP failed to significantly reduce the incidence of cardiovascular events.[58] Similarly, the RICCADSA trial (Randomized Intervention with Continuous Positive Airway Pressure in CAD and OSA) revealed no difference in the incidence of revascularization, MI, stroke, or cardiovascular mortality between those treated with CPAP and controls.[59] Similarly, the SAVE Trial (Sleep Apnea Cardiovascular Endpoints) compared CPAP plus usual care versus usual care alone among 2717 mostly male adults with moderate to severe OSA and known CAD or cardiovascular disease for a mean follow-up of 3.7 years. In this trial, CPAP therapy did not confer a significant effect on cardiovascular endpoints.[60] Likewise, CPAP did not reduce the incidence of subsequent cardiovascular events among patients with prior acute coronary syndrome in the ISAAC Study (Impact of Sleep Apnea syndrome in the evolution of Acute Coronary Syndrome).[61] Interestingly, this study observed that the presence of OSA was not associated with an increase in cardiovascular events.

While these studies did not demonstrate a significant impact, they primarily enrolled a population of non-sleepy patients who had poor adherence with CPAP. Mean CPAP use was only 2.8 hours per night in the ISAAC Study and 3.3 hours per night in the SAVE Trial.[60,61] These studies are limited by insufficient use of PAP with potential confounding variables reflecting a specific phenotype of OSA, which likely minimized the impact and benefits of CPAP therapy. Not surprisingly, when evaluating the results based on CPAP adherence (>4 hours per night), the RICCADSA trial found a significant benefit of CPAP on the primary endpoints after adjustment for baseline comorbidities.[59] Similarly, benefits were noted among those using CPAP at least 4 hours per night in the SAVE trial.[60] A subsequent meta-analysis that explored the impact of CPAP adherence and the risk of cerebrovascular and cardiovascular events found that, compared with no treatment, CPAP use of at least 4 hours per night was associated with significant improvements in MACCEs, especially cerebrovascular accidents (CVAs).[62]

Cerebrovascular Accidents

Disordered sleep and cerebrovascular accidents (CVA) share a common bi-directional relationship. Sleep quality is often poor following a stroke, and preexisting sleep disorders increase the risk for stroke. The presence of either comorbid or consequential sleep abnormalities portend worse outcomes among those who sustain a CVA.

Several sleep issues commonly arise following a stroke. Approximately 50% of stroke patients will report insomnia within the first month following their CVA.[63,64] This persists in the majority of patients and may be a sign of depression. However, damage to certain regions of the brain, particularly thalamic infarcts, have a higher risk of developing insomnia. Circadian rhythm misalignment is also common, with 20%–40% of patients experiencing a shift or frank inversion of their sleep-wake cycle following a CVA. Hypersomnolence is also common following strokes and can impede recovery. Parasomnias, especially REM behavior disorder (RBD), have been reported following a CVA. One observational study found that 46% of RBD patients had prior brainstem infarctions.[65] The most commonly identified sleep disorder following a CVA is sleep-disordered breathing. While OSA is a known risk factor for stroke, strokes can also induce OSA, primarily through dystonia of the oropharyngeal structures. It is observed in over two-thirds of patients following a stroke.[66] And, when left untreated, is associated with worse neurologic outcomes and a diminished response to rehabilitation programs.[67]

While poor sleep and sleep disorders commonly develop following a stroke, there are several sleep disorders that have been shown to be independent risk factors for CVAs. Chronic insufficient sleep increases the risk for stroke. One study found that the risk of stroke was 63% greater among individuals who obtained less than 6 hours per night compared to those who slept 7–8 hours.[68] The risk for stroke was even greater among those who also had poor subjective sleep quality. While insufficient sleep increases the risk for stroke, so does excessive amounts of sleep. Studies have shown that sleeping more than 9 hours per night increases the risk of stroke even after eliminating confounding factors.[69,70] Chronic insomnia has also been shown to increase the risk of stroke, especially in younger adults. In a large national cohort, the authors found that insomnia increased the likelihood of subsequent hospitalization for stroke by 54%. Further, the incidence of stroke was 8 times higher among those adults younger than 34 years.[71]

OSA is an established risk factor for CVA events. Compared with those who do not have sleep-disordered breathing, the presence of OSA is associated with a 2- to 3-fold increased risk for stroke.[72–74] A post-hoc analyses of the SAVE trial found that the degree and duration of nocturnal hypoxia were greater predictors of cardiovascular events than the apnea hypopnea index (AHI).[75] In another post hoc analysis of the SAVE trial, Li et al. explored the risk of CVAs based on the presence of snoring among patients with OSA.[76] The study found that snorers with OSA had an increased risk of CVAs, but not cardiac events. Both the frequency and intensity of snoring increased the odds ratio for CVAs. The largest study exploring the relationship between OSA severity and the incidence of stroke was provided by the Sleep Heart Health Study.[74] In this trial, the risk of stroke increased proportionately with an increasing AHI.[74] After adjustment for age, race, body mass index (BMI), smoking status, hypertension, and diabetes, the highest AHI was associated with an almost 3-fold increased risk of incident stroke.

Pulmonary Vascular Disease

OSA results in hemodynamic derangements and dysfunction of the pulmonary vasculature and may contribute to the progression of underlying pulmonary hypertension (PH). Nocturnal desaturation, hypoxic-vasoconstriction, reperfusion injuries, ventilatory instability, impaired nitric oxide synthesis, endothelial dysfunction, and vascular remodeling resulting from repetitive obstructive respiratory events can lead to the development of pulmonary vascular disease. While OSA does cause PH, elevations in mean pulmonary pressures are often mild. OSA is unlikely to, by itself, lead to moderate or severe PH. However, OSA is highly prevalent in patients with other forms of PH and can contribute to more hypoxia and progression of disease.

An ACCP Consensus panel found that PH occurred in 17%–53% of individuals with OSA.[77] Likewise, in a study of patients with WHO Group 1 PAH, sleep-disordered breathing was found in 71%, with 56% having OSA and 44% having CSA.[78] A similar review found that 82% of patients with PH had underlying sleep-disordered breathing.[14] Given the high prevalence of OSA in patients with PH, and the potential that it contributes to disease progression, the 2019 CHEST Guideline and Expert Panel Report for PAH recommends that contributing causes of PH, such as OSA, be treated aggressively.[79]

SLEEP-DISORDERED BREATHING AND RESPIRATORY DISEASE

Comorbid OSA is common among patients with chronic respiratory disorders. In a study by Pinto et al., the investigators found that approximately 25% of those with OSA had asthma or chronic obstructive pulmonary disease (COPD).[80] While common, underlying sleep-disordered breathing frequently goes unrecognized as these disease processes share similar, often overlapping, symptoms. Both may result in fragmented sleep and frequent arousals with subsequent excessive daytime somnolence. Similarly, both may manifest with recurrent episodes of choking, coughing, and breathlessness during sleep. And both involve repetitive arousals and sleep-stage changes associated with functional limitations in airflow and increasing respiratory efforts with resulting desaturation or lability in oxygenation.

Sleep and Asthma

Poor sleep quality is common with asthma. And it is both a measure of disease severity and a goal of therapy. There are several reasons why asthmatics frequently report poor sleep. As discussed previously, normal circadian alterations in respiratory mechanics and function can have a negative impact on most asthmatics and lead to nocturnal symptoms. Common treatments for asthma, such as methylxanthines, beta-agonists, and systemic corticosteroids, frequently cause sleep fragmentation, leading to non-restorative sleep. And, asthmatics commonly have underlying gastroesophageal reflux disease (GERD) and chronic rhinitis, which can further fragment sleep. While common, nocturnal symptoms are regarded as a sign of poor asthma control and an increased risk for exacerbations.

Sleep-disordered breathing is another, often overlooked cause of poor sleep among asthmatics, and the association between asthma and OSA is well-established.[80–87] This association may be due, in part, to the high prevalence of each disorder. However, it appears that this common relationship is more likely the result of overlapping pathogenesis. There is a clear association between chronic cough/asthma, obstructive sleep apnea, rhinosinusitis and esophageal reflux disease, otherwise known as the CORE syndrome.[80] These nocturnal entities not only share common symptoms, they also share common manifestations, which may contribute to the presence and severity of the others. OSA frequently results in mouth breathing, which can dry inspired air and cause bronchoconstriction. Nasal congestion is common in patients with both OSA and asthma and can manifest as snoring. And both disorders are frequently associated with

GERD, which itself is often worse at night, especially during recumbent sleep. Gastric acid secretion exhibits a circadian rhythm, with peak levels occurring during the night. Sleep reduces esophageal peristalsis, reduces gastric emptying, and relaxes lower esophageal sphincter tone. As such, reflux events are significantly more common at night. This is more pronounced among those with OSA, where upper airway closure leads to greater changes in transthoracic pressure. Acid in the distal esophagus leads to a compensatory bronchospasm, increased respiratory resistance, and increased minute ventilation, which can lead to more nocturnal asthma. Further, nocturnal reflux can cause rhinitis and upper airway dysfunction, which can both mimic and exacerbate asthma symptoms. And rhinitis can lead to snoring, sleep fragmentation, and coughing at night. In short, each component of the CORE syndrome can mimic and/or exacerbate the other conditions and should be strongly considered when treating both asthma and OSA.

OSA is more common among asthmatics compared with the general population. In one study, 49% of difficult-to-control asthmatics had mild to moderate OSA.[81] Not only is OSA more common among asthmatics, asthma itself is a risk factor for risk for developing OSA, independent of steroid use.[82] The Wisconsin Sleep Cohort found that having a diagnosis of asthma increases the risk of developing OSA, with an adjusted relative risk of 1.4.[83] Further, having OSA can impair asthma control, and individuals with OSA are 3.6 times more likely to have uncontrolled asthma and 3.4 times more likely to experience an exacerbation compared to asthmatics without OSA.[82,84] There also appears to be a correlation between OSA severity and the likelihood and severity of asthma, where a higher AHI and lower mean nocturnal oxygenation are both associated with greater asthma severity.[85] This may reflect a unique phenotype of asthma. According to the Severe Asthma Phenotyping (SARP), this association may suggest a Cluster 3 phenotype, which is characterized by greater asthma severity, an older onset of symptoms, more obesity, less atopic, and more rhinitis.[86] Due to the strong relationship between asthma and OSA, and because of the marked increased risk for poor outcomes, the National Asthma Education and Prevention Program recommends that all patients with difficult-to-control asthma be screened for OSA.[87]

Sleep and Chronic Obstructive Pulmonary Disease

The normal physiologic changes that occur during sleep can clearly contribute to symptoms among those with COPD. Not surprisingly, sleep complaints are highly prevalent in these patients. Not only does COPD lead to poor sleep quality, medications commonly used to treat COPD may all fragment sleep. The most important association between sleep and COPD is hypoventilation and its resultant hypoxia. Normal sleep creates a state of relative hypoventilation, mediated by a decrease in CO_2 sensitivity and diminished tidal breathing during sleep. This results in a modest, and often clinically meaningless, increase in serum pCO_2. However, among those with an underlying hypoventilatory disorder such as COPD, this can lead to significant alveolar hypoventilation with resultant hypoxia and CO_2 retention. Worsening ventilation, often with associated hypoxia, is more likely among those with an FEV-1 less than 50% predicted, and is especially more common among those with an FEV-1 less than 35% predicted. This should be considered and evaluated for as it is associated with poor outcomes and is linearly associated with decreased survival.[88]

OSA shares a unique and common relationship with COPD, often described as the "overlap syndrome."[89] COPD and OSA are both highly prevalent and share common demographics. As such, their relationship may be based on chance association alone. However, different clinical COPD phenotypes influence the likelihood of having coexisting OSA, which may explain the controversies that have made establishing a true causal relationship challenging. It appears that a predominant emphysema phenotype, characterized by increased lung volumes and a low BMI, may be protective against OSA. In contrast, greater peripheral edema and an increased BMI associated with the predominant chronic bronchitis phenotype likely promote OSA. Regardless, both COPD and OSA are associated with similar physiological and molecular consequences, such as hypoxia and systemic inflammation, that contribute to cardiovascular, pulmonary, and pulmonary vascular function that can adversely impact health and survival.

CONCLUSION

It is widely accepted that sleep is a pillar of health, and yet the prevalence of sleep disorders in the United States and internationally is inconsistent with the level of urgency in enhanced screening, testing, diagnosis, and treatment. Poor quality sleep from any etiology broadly contributes to adverse health consequences.

Regardless of the ability to prove a true causal relationship, cardiovascular and pulmonary diseases are predictably common among patients with OSA and are associated with adverse outcomes. It appears that OSA likely causes, or at least potentiates, cardiovascular disease and contributes to worsening underlying pulmonary disease. While OSA clearly impacts quality of life, established and growing evidence suggests that its impacts on cardiovascular health should further compel physicians to evaluate patients with OSA for these potential consequences and at least consider underlying sleep-disordered breathing in patients with known cardiovascular diseases.

While the data presented confirm strong associations between OSA, CSA, and cardiopulmonary disorders, the impact that treating OSA has on outcomes remains controversial and overall unconvincing. Several trials that delivered appropriate treatment of the underlying sleep-disordered breathing found favorable results with regard to cardiovascular outcomes. However, clinical trials with negative results have largely been limited by a lack of long-term outcomes data, insufficiently defined treatment goals, inadequately delivered therapy, poor adherence with that therapy, and inclusion of skewed patient populations, resulting in skepticism among experts. New and recently launched trials are prioritizing a phenotypic approach to subject selection and a greater degree of sophistication in study design with the hope and expectation that results will establish evidence of causality and improved outcomes.

In this chapter, we have reviewed the broad topic of sleep and cardio-pulmonary conditions. Heart disease has consistently been the most common cause of mortality in men and women for decades, and undiagnosed obstructive sleep apnea may affect as many as 40 million people in the United States and one billion worldwide. Given the tremendous prevalence of cardio-pulmonary diseases and sleep disorders, the common association of both, and considering how, when present, this association markedly worsens outcomes, healthcare systems in both the United States and globally face a growing epidemic that has and will continue to affect a significant portion of the world's population. The personal and financial consequences of sleep and cardio-pulmonary diseases are staggering and require wide adoption of public education, enhanced prevention measures, mass screening, early treatment, and enhanced support of large, well-designed trials to establish practice guidelines.

REFERENCES

1. Cappuccio FP, Cooper D, D'Elia L, et al. Sleep duration predicts cardiovascular outcomes: A systematic review and meta-analysis of prospective studies. *Eur Heart J.* 2011; 32:1484–1492.
2. Wang X, Fan JY, Zhang Y, Nie SP, et al. Association of obstructive sleep apnea with cardiovascular outcomes after percutaneous coronary intervention: A systematic review and meta-analysis. *Medicine (Baltimore).* 2018; 97:e0621.
3. Yin J, Jin X, Shan Z, et al. Relationship of sleep duration with all-cause mortality and cardiovascular events: A systematic review and dose-response meta-analysis of prospective cohort studies. *J Am Heart Assoc.* 2017; 6:e005947.
4. Miller JC, Horvath SM. Cardiac output during human sleep. *Aviat Space Environ Med.* 1976 Oct;47(10):1046–1051.
5. Somers VK, Dyken ME, Mark AL, Abboud FM. Sympathetic-nerve activity during sleep in normal subjects. *N Engl J Med.* 1993;328:303–307.
6. Floras J. Sleep apnea and cardiovascular disease. *Circ Res.* 2018;122:1741–1764.
7. Hsieh C, Maertin J. Short sleep, insomnia and cardiovascular disease. *Curr Sleep Med Rep.* 2019;5:234–242.
8. Mesarwi O, Polak J, Jun J, et al. Sleep disorders and the development of insulin resistance and obesity. *Endocrinol Metab Clin North Am.* 2013 Sep;42(3):617–634.

9. Cappuccio FP, Cooper D, D'Elia L, et al. Sleep duration predicts cardiovascular outcomes: A systematic review and meta-analysis of prospective studies. *Eur Heart J*. 2011;32:1484–1492.
10. Aggarwal S, Loomba RS, Arora RR, et al. Associations between sleep duration and prevalence of cardiovascular events. *Clin Cardiol*. 2013;36(11):671–676.
11. Nieto FJ, Young TB, Lind BK, et al. Association of sleep-disordered breathing, sleep apnea, and hypertension in a large community-based study: Sleep Heart Health Study. *JAMA*. 2000 Apr 12;283(14):1829–1836.
12. Lavie P, Herer P, Hoffstein V, et al. Obstructive sleep apnoea syndrome as a risk factor for hypertension: Population study. *BMJ*. 2000;320:479–482.
13. The National Heart, Lung, and Blood Institute. The Seventh Report of the Joint National Committee on Prevention, Detection, Evaluation, and Treatment of High Blood Pressure. NIH; 2003.
14. Krishnan V, Hassaun P, Hummers L, Collop NA. Sleep disordered breathing and pulmonary hypertension. *Sleep*. 2005;20:A300.
15. Peker Y, Kraiczi H, Hedner J, et al. An independent association between obstructive sleep apnoea and coronary artery disease. *Eur Respir J*. 1999;14:179–184.
16. Javaheri S. Sleep disorders in systolic heart failure: a prospective study of 100 male patients. *Int J Cardiol*. 2006;106:21–28.
17. Mansfield DR, Gollogly NC, Kaye DM, et al. Controlled trial of continuous positive airway pressure in obstructive sleep apnea and heart failure. *Am J Respir Crit Care Med*. 2004;169:361–366.
18. Cloward TV, Walker JM, Farney RJ, Anderson JL. Left ventricular hypertrophy is a common echocardiographic abnormality in severe obstructive sleep apnea and reverses with nasal continuous positive airway pressure. *Chest*. 2003;124:594–601.
19. Guilleminault C, Connolly SJ, Winkle RA. Cardiac arrhythmia and conduction disturbances during sleep in patients with sleep apnea syndrome. *Am J Cardiol*. 1983;52:490–494.
20. Mehra R, Benjamin EJ, Shahar E, et al. Association of nocturnal arrhythmias with sleep-disordered breathing: The Sleep Heart Health Study. *Am J Respir Crit Care Med*. 2006;173:910–916.
21. Harbison J, O'Reilly P, McNicholas WT. Cardiac rhythm disturbances in the obstructive sleep apnea syndrome, effects of nasal continuous positive airway pressure therapy. *Chest*. 2000;118:591–595.
22. Narkiewicz K, Somers VK. Sympathetic nerve activity in obstructive sleep apnoea. *Acta Physiol Scand*. 2003;177:385–390.
23. Mooe T, Franklin KA, Holmstrom K, et al. Sleep-disordered breathing and coronary artery disease: Long-term prognosis. *Am J Respir Crit Care Med*. 2001;164:1910–1913.
24. Chan KH, Wilcox I. Obstructive sleep apnea: Novel trigger and potential therapeutic target for cardiac arrhythmias. *Expert Rev Cardiovasc Ther*. 2010 Jul;8(7):981–994.
25. Vanninen E, Tuunainen A, Kansanen M, et al. Cardiac sympathovagal balance during sleep apnea episodes. *Clin Physiol Oxf Engl*. 1996 May;16(3):209–216.
26. Chan KH, Wilcox I. Obstructive sleep apnea: Novel trigger and potential therapeutic target for cardiac arrhythmias. *Expert Rev Cardiovasc Ther*. 2010 Jul;8(7):981–994.
27. Camen G, Clarenbach CF, Stöwhas A-C, et al. The effects of simulated obstructive apnea and hypopnea on arrhythmic potential in healthy subjects. *Eur J Appl Physiol*. 2013 Feb;113(2):489–496.
28. Bradley TD, Floras JS. Obstructive sleep apnoea and its cardiovascular consequences. *Lancet*. 2009;373:82–93.
29. Javaheri S, Barbe F, Campos-Rodriquez F, et al. Sleep apnea: Types, mechanisms, and clinical cardiovascular consequences. *J Am Coll Cardiol*. 2017 Feb 21;69(7):841–858.
30. Chahal A, Somers V. Secondary hypertension and obstructive sleep apnea. *J Am Soc Hypertens*. 2015 Mar;9(3):244–247.
31. Muxfelt ES, Margallo V, Guimaraes G, et al. Prevalence and associated factors of obstructive sleep apnea in patients with resistant hypertension. *Am J Hypertens*. 2014;27:1069–1078.
32. Marin JM, Carrizo SJ, Vicente E, Agusti AG. Long-term cardiovascular outcomes in men with obstructive sleep apnoea-hypopnoea with or without treatment with continuous positive airway pressure: An observational study. *Lancet*. 2005;365:1046–1053.
33. Van Haesendonck G, Dieltjen M, Kastoer C, et al. Cardiovascular benefits of oral appliance therapy in obstructive sleep apnea: A systematic review. *J Dent Sleep Med*. 2015;2(1):9–14.
34. Marin JM, Carrizo SJ, Vicente E, Agusti AGN. Long-term cardiovascular outcomes in men with obstructive sleep apnoea-hypopnoea with or without treatment with continuous positive airway pressure: An observational study. *Lancet Lond Engl*. 2005 Mar 19;365(9464):1046–1053.
35. Liu L, Cao Q, Guo Z, Dai Q. Continuous positive airway pressure in patients with obstructive sleep apnea and resistant hypertension: A meta-analysis of randomized controlled trials. *J Clin Hypertens Greenwich Conn*. 2016 Feb;18(2):153–158.
36. Martínez-García M-A, Capote F, Campos-Rodríguez F, et al. Effect of CPAP on blood pressure in patients with obstructive sleep apnea and resistant hypertension: The HIPARCO randomized clinical trial. *JAMA*. 2013 Dec 11;310(22):2407–2415.
37. Lozano L, Tovar JL, Sampol G, et al. Continuous positive airway pressure treatment in sleep apnea patients with resistant hypertension: A randomized, controlled trial. *J Hypertens*. 2010 Oct;28(10):2161–2168.
38. Gami A, Pressman G, Caples S, et al. Association of atrial fibrillation and obstructive sleep apnea. *Circulation*. 2004 Jul 27;110(4):364–367.
39. Braga B, Poyares D, Cintra F, et al. Sleep-disordered breathing and chronic atrial fibrillation. *Sleep Med*. 2009;10:212–216.
40. Bitter T, Langer C, Vogt J, et al. Sleep-disordered breathing in patients with atrial fibrillation and normal systolic left ventricular function. *Dtsch Arztebl Int*. 2009;106(10):164–170.
41. Digby G, Baranchuk A. Sleep apnea and atrial fibrillation; 2012 update. *Curr Cardio Rev*. 2012 Nov;8(4):265–272.
42. Vanderveken O, Boudewyns A, Quan N, et al. Cardiovascular implications in the treatment of

obstructive sleep apnea. *J Cardiovasc Trans Res.* 2011;4:53–60.

43. Monahan K, Brewster J, Wang L, et al. Relation of the severity of obstructive sleep apnea in response to anti-arrhythmic drugs in patients with atrial fibrillation or atrial flutter. *Am J Cardiol.* 2012;110(3):369–372.
44. Neilan T, Farhad H, Dodson J, et al. Effect of sleep apnea and continuous positive airway pressure on cardiac structure and recurrence of atrial fibrillation. *J Am Heart Assoc.* 2013;2(6)e000421.
45. Shahar E, Whitney CW, Redline S, et al. Sleep-disordered breathing and cardiovascular disease: Cross-sectional results of the Sleep Heart Health Study. *Am J Respir Crit Care Med.* 2001;163:19–25.
46. Sin D, Fitzgerald F, Parker J, et al. Risk factors for central and obstructive sleep apnea in 450 men and women with congestive heart failure. *AJRCCM.* 1999;160:1101–1106.
47. Bendjelid K, Schutz N, Suter P, et al. Does continuous positive airway pressure by face mask improve patients with acute cardiogenic pulmonary edema due to left ventricular diastolic dysfunction? *Chest.* 2005 Mar;127(3):1053–1058.
48. Bradley TD, Logan AG, Kimoff, RJ. Continuous positive airway pressure for central sleep apnea and heart failure. *N Eng J Med.* 2005;353:2025–2033.
49. Arzt M, Floras J, Logan A, et al. Suppression of central sleep apnea by continuous positive airway pressure and transplant–free survival in heart failure: A post hoc analysis of the Canadian Continuous Positive Airway Pressure for Patients with Central Sleep Apnea and Heart Failure Trial (CANPAP). *Circulation.* 2007;115:3173–3180.
50. Cowie M, Woehrle H, Wegscheider K, et al. Adaptive servo-ventilation for central sleep apnea in systolic heart failure. *N Engl J Med.* 2015;373:1095–1105.
51. Javaheri S, Brown L, Khayat R. Update on apneas of heart failure with reduced ejection fraction: Emphasis on the physiology of treatment: Part 2: Central sleep apnea. *Chest.* 2020 Jun;157(6):1637–1646.
52. Costanzo MR, Javaher S, Ponikowski P, et al. Transvenous phrenic nerve stimulation for treatment of central sleep apnea: Five-year safety and efficacy outcomes. *Nat Sci Sleep.* 2021;13:515–526.
53. Schmickl C, Landry S, Orr J, et al. Acetazolamide for OSA and central sleep apnea: A comprehensive systematic review and meta-analysis. *Chest.* 2020 Dec;158(6):2632–2645.
54. Peker Y, Hedner J, Kraiczi H, et al. Respiratory disturbance index: An independent predictor of mortality in coronary artery disease. *Am J Respir Crit Care Med.* 2000;162:81–86.
55. Mooe T, Franklin KA, Holmstrom K, et al. Sleep-disordered breathing and coronary artery disease: Long-term prognosis. *Am J Respir Crit Care Med.* 2001;164:1910–1913.
56. Unruh ML, Enright PL, Polak JF, et al. The relationship of sleep apnea to carotid wall thickness among a large cohort of older adults. *Sleep.* 2005;20:A112.
57. Doherty LS, Kiely JL, Swan V, McNicholas WT. Long-term effects of nasal continuous positive airway pressure therapy on cardiovascular outcomes in sleep apnea syndrome. *Chest.* 2005;127:2076–2084.
58. Barbe F, Duran-Cantolla J, Sanchez-de-la-Torre M, et al. Effect of continuous positive airway pressure on the incidence of hypertension and cardiovascular events in non-sleepy patients with obstructive sleep apnea: A randomized controlled trial. *JAMA.* 2012 May 23;307(20):2161–2168.
59. Peker, Y, Giantz H, Eulenburg C, et al. Effect of positive airway pressure on cardiovascular outcomes in coronary artery disease patients with non-sleepy obstructive sleep apnea: The RICCADSA randomized controlled trial. *Am J Respir Crit Care Med.* 2016 Sep 1;194(5):613–620.
60. McEvoy RD, Antic N, Heeley E, et al. CPAP for prevention of cardiovascular events in obstructive sleep apnea. *N Engl J Med.* 2016;375:919–931.
61. Sanchez-de-la-Torre M, Sanchez-de-la-Torre A, Bertran S, et al. Effect of obstructive sleep apnea and its treatment with continuous positive airway pressure on the prevalence of cardiovascular events in patients with acute coronary syndrome (ISAACC study): A randomized controlled trial. *Lancet Respir Med.* 2020 Apr;8(4):359–367.
62. Javaheri S, Martinez-Garcia M, Campos-Rodriguez F, et al. Continuous positive airway pressure adherence for prevention of major adverse cerebrovascular and cardiovascular events in obstructive sleep apnea. *Am J Respir Crit Care Med.* 2019;199:A7350.
63. Hermann DM, Bassetti CL. Sleep-related breathing and sleep-wake disturbances in ischemic stroke. *Neurology.* 2009;73:1313–1322.
64. Sterr A, Kuhn M, Nissen C, et al. Post-stroke insomnia in community-dwelling patients with chronic motor stroke: Physiological evidence and implications for stroke care. *Sci Rep.* 2018;8:8409.
65. Tang WK, Hermann DM, Chen YK, et al. Brainstem infarcts predict REM sleep behavior disorder in acute ischemic stroke. *BMC Neurol.* 2014;14:88.
66. Khot SP, Morgenstern LB. Sleep and stoke. *Stroke.* 2019;50:1612–1617.
67. Mansukhani MP, Bellolio MF, Kolla BP, Enduri S, Somers VK, Stead LG. Worse outcome after stroke in patients with obstructive sleep apnea: An observational cohort study. *J Stroke Cerebrovasc Dis.* 2011;20:401–405.
68. Ji A, Lou H, Lou P, et al. Interactive effect of sleep duration and sleep quality on risk of stroke: An 8-year follow-up study in China. *Sci Rep.* 2020;10:86–90.
69. Leng Y, Cappuccio FP, Wainwright NW, et al. Sleep duration and risk of fatal and nonfatal stroke: a prospective study and meta-analysis. *Neurology.* 2015;84:1072–1079.
70. Titova OE, Michaëlsson K, Larsson SC. Sleep duration and stroke: Prospective cohort study and Mendelian randomization analysis. *Stroke.* 2020 Nov;51(11):3279–3285.
71. Wu M-P, et al. Insomnia subtypes and the subsequent risks of stroke. *Stroke.* 2014;45:1349–1354.
72. Yaggi HK, Concato J, Kernan WN, Lichtman JH, Brass LM, Mohsenin V. Obstructive sleep apnea as a risk factor for stroke and death. *N Engl J Med.* 2005;353:2034–2041.
73. Xie W, Zheng F, Song X. Obstructive sleep apnea and serious adverse outcomes in patients with cardiovascular or cerebrovascular disease: A PRISMA-compliant

systematic review and meta-analysis. *Medicine (Baltimore)*. 2014 Dec;93(29):e336.
74. Redline S, Yenokyan G, Gottlieb DJ, et al. Obstructive sleep apnea-hypopnea and incident stroke: The Sleep Heart Health Study. *Am J Resp Crit Care Med*. 2010;182:269–77.
75. Linz D, Loffler K, Sanders P, et al. Prognostic value of novel nocturnal metrics in patients with OSA and high cardiovascular event risk: Post hoc analyses of the SAVE study. *Chest*. 2020;158:2621–2631.
76. Li J, Zheng D, Loffler KA, et al.; SAVE Investigators. Sleep duration and risk of cardiovascular events: The SAVE study. *Int J Stroke*. 2020;15(8):858–865.
77. Rubin LJ; American College of Chest Physicians. Diagnosis and management of pulmonary arterial hypertension: ACCP evidence-based clinical practice guidelines. *Chest*. 2004;126(Suppl 1):7S–10S.
78. Minic M, Granton JT, Ryan CM. Sleep disordered breathing in group 1 pulmonary arterial hypertension. *J Clin Sleep Med*. 2014;10(3):277–283.
79. Klinger JR, Elliott CG, Levine DJ, et al. Therapy for pulmonary arterial hypertension in adults: Update of the CHEST guideline and expert panel report. *Chest*. 2019 Mar;155(3):565–586.
80. Kasasbeh A, Kasabeh E, Krishnaswamy G. Potential mechanisms connecting asthma, esophageal reflux, and obesity/sleep apnea complex: A hypothetical review. *Sleep Med Rev*. 2007 Feb;11(1):47–58.
81. Taillé C, Rouvel-Tallec A, Stoica M, et al. Obstructive sleep apnoea modulates airway inflammation and remodelling in severe asthma. *PLoS One*. 2016;11(3):e0150042.
82. Teodorescu M, Consens F, Bria W, et al. Predictors of habitual snoring and obstructive sleep apnea risk in patients with asthma. *Chest*. 2009 May;135(5):1125–1132.
83. Theodorescu M, Barnet J, Hagen E, et al. Association between asthma and risk of developing obstructive sleep apnea. *JAMA*. 2015 Jan 13;313(2):156–164.
84. Brink AT, Sterk P, Masclee A, et al. Risk factors of frequent exacerbations in difficult-to-treat asthma. *Eur Respir J*. 2005 Nov;26(5):812–818.
85. Julien JY, Martin J, Ernst P, et al. Prevalence of obstructive sleep apnea-hypopnea in severe versus moderate asthma. *J Allergy Clin Immunol*. 2009 Aug;124(2):371–376.
86. Teague WG, Phillips BR, Fahy JV, et al. Baseline features of the Severe Asthma Research Program (SARP III) cohort: Differences with age. *J Allergy Clin Immunol Pract*. 2018 Mar–Apr;6(2):545–554.
87. Expert Panel Report 3 (EPR-3). Guidelines for the diagnosis and management of asthma: Summary report 2007. *J Allergy Clin Immunol*. 2007;120(Suppl 5):S94–S138.
88. Kent BD, Mithcell P, McNicholas W. Hypoxemia in patients with COPD: Cause, effects, and disease progression. *Int J Chron Obstruct Pulmon Dis*. 2011;6:199–208.
89. McNichols W. COPD-OSA overlap syndrome: Evolving evidence regarding epidemiology, clinical consequences, and management. *Chest*. 2017 Dec;152(6):1318–1326.

Chapter 29

Sleep-Disordered Breathing in Pediatrics

Fauziya Hassan, Chandra M. Cherukuri, and Neeraj Kaplish

PEDIATRIC OBSTRUCTIVE SLEEP APNEA

Sleep-disordered breathing (SDB) refers to a wide spectrum consisting of habitual snoring (3 nights of the week or more) to obstructive sleep apnea (OSA) characterized by recurrent episodes of partial and/or complete upper airway obstruction (hypopneas or obstructive apneas) with associated arousals, awakenings or oxyhemoglobin desaturations. It may be associated with disruption in ventilation and sleep architecture.[1–3] Prevalence of primary snoring is 10%–12% of children within the United States, and prevalence of OSA is 1%–4%.[4–6] OSA has certain genetic influences, such as skeletal and soft tissue characteristics, body habitus, and respiratory control differences. In addition, certain environmental influences, such as cigarette smoking and allergies, may have an impact. There are predisposing factors that place children at higher risk of OSA, such as adenotonsillar hypertrophy, prematurity, and twin gestation. Neuromuscular disorders with hypotonia have upper airway muscle weakness and are predisposed to airway collapse. Studies of children with neurodevelopmental disorders (NDDs) such as Down syndrome (DS) and Prader Willi syndrome (PWS) have found that there is a high prevalence of OSA (>50%) due to obstruction at multiple sites of the upper airway. Children with craniofacial syndromes such as Goldenhaar, Apert, Crouzon, and Pierre Robin syndrome are at high risk for OSA due to retrognathia or micrognathia and midface hypoplasia.[7] However, authors of these studies also note that the prevalence of OSA is likely underestimated because of inconsistent evaluation and screening of affected children.

Untreated OSA syndrome (OSAS) includes consequences of OSA; the most prominent consequences among children are neurocognitive effects.[8–10] Children with OSAS are also at an increased risk of psychosocial problems, including poor socialization, poor school performance, and aggressive behavior.[11] Systemic side effects, such as metabolic dysfunction, insulin resistance, increase in inflammatory markers, systemic and pulmonary hypertension deficits, have also been associated with pediatric OSAS.[12–13] The consequences of pediatric hypertension in particular may be long lasting, with elevated blood pressure and metabolic syndrome into adulthood.[14]

Clinical History

The American Academy of Pediatrics (AAP) guidelines recommend universal screening for snoring in all children. Parents or caregivers may report disturbed or restless sleep, gasping, and witnessed apneas.[3] A comprehensive evaluation by a sleep medicine physician would be helpful to identify patients with SDB with a detailed sleep history, focusing on characteristics of snoring, witnessed apneic events, gasping arousals, labored, paradoxical breathing, or obstructed breathing during sleep.[15] There may be under-reporting of snoring by parents; sensitivity and specificity of history and physical examination can be poor.[16] The absence of witnessed apneas does not preclude a diagnosis of SDB. Infants as well as children with neuromuscular disorders (NMD) or syndrome may not have a clear-cut history of snoring, witnessed apneas, desaturations, or abnormal breathing.[17]

Details of sleep duration and schedule should be evaluated, including latency to sleep onset, bed and wake-up times. They should also be queried about non-rapid eye movement (NREM) parasomnias such as sleep talking, confusional arousals, night terrors, and sleepwalking, and rapid eye movement (REM) parasomnias such as nightmares. Night time enuresis, particularly secondary enuresis, in particular, has been strongly linked to OSA.[18] OSAS may result in significant neurocognitive consequences among children, including hyperactivity, inattention, behavioral issues, learning problems, and sleepiness, even early on with improvement in school performance after adeno-tonsillectomy (T&A).[8–10,19] Overall, daytime sleepiness is less common in children than in adults; however, excessive sleepiness is frequently reported in children with PWS, cerebral palsy (CP), and DS. Presence of excessive daytime sleepiness in a child should alert a clinician to consider additional alternative etiologies such as sleep deprivation, medications or drug effect in a child with OSA.

Standardized Questionnaires

Multiple sleep questionnaires were developed to characterize the signs and symptoms of SDBs; however, these questionnaires are limited in sensitivity or specificity and are designed for certain patient populations. The Pediatric Sleep Questionnaire (PSQ) is validated to screen for OSA with a high sensitivity (83%) and specificity (87%); however, it has only been validated among healthy children age 2–18 years.[15] Among children with craniofacial deformities, use of PSQ is less likely to predict OSA prevalence, given that some of the questions may not accurately pertain to this patient population.[20] Other questionnaires, like the Children's Sleep Habits Questionnaire (CSHQ), have been shown to have a sensitivity and specificity of >70% for SDB in otherwise healthy elementary school-age children.[21] The OSA-18 has been developed to measure SDB quality of life and was validated in otherwise healthy children, and was subsequently validated in children with syndromic craniosynostosis.[22–23]

It is, however, important to acknowledge the limitations of sleep questionnaires. Few surveys have been used specifically for the evaluation of children with NDDs. Further studies would be required to validate these questionnaires prior to widespread implementation and also to consider the relevant patient population.

Physical Examination

Physical evaluation should involve a general assessment of behavior and sleepiness. Children with severe OSA may appear somnolent or have a history of daytime hypersomnolence. Body mass index (BMI) is important, as children with obesity are 4–6 times more likely to have OSA than non-obese children.[24] In children with DS, BMI is associated with an increased risk of OSA, even after adjusting for age and sex.[25] However, the association between obesity and sleep-related breathing disorders (SRBDs) may not always be as straightforward.

Nasal exam should include evaluation for turbinate hypertrophy, polyps, nasal septum deviation, and hypoplasia of nares, either unilateral or bilateral. Signs of nasal adenoid facies, which are elongated facial features with

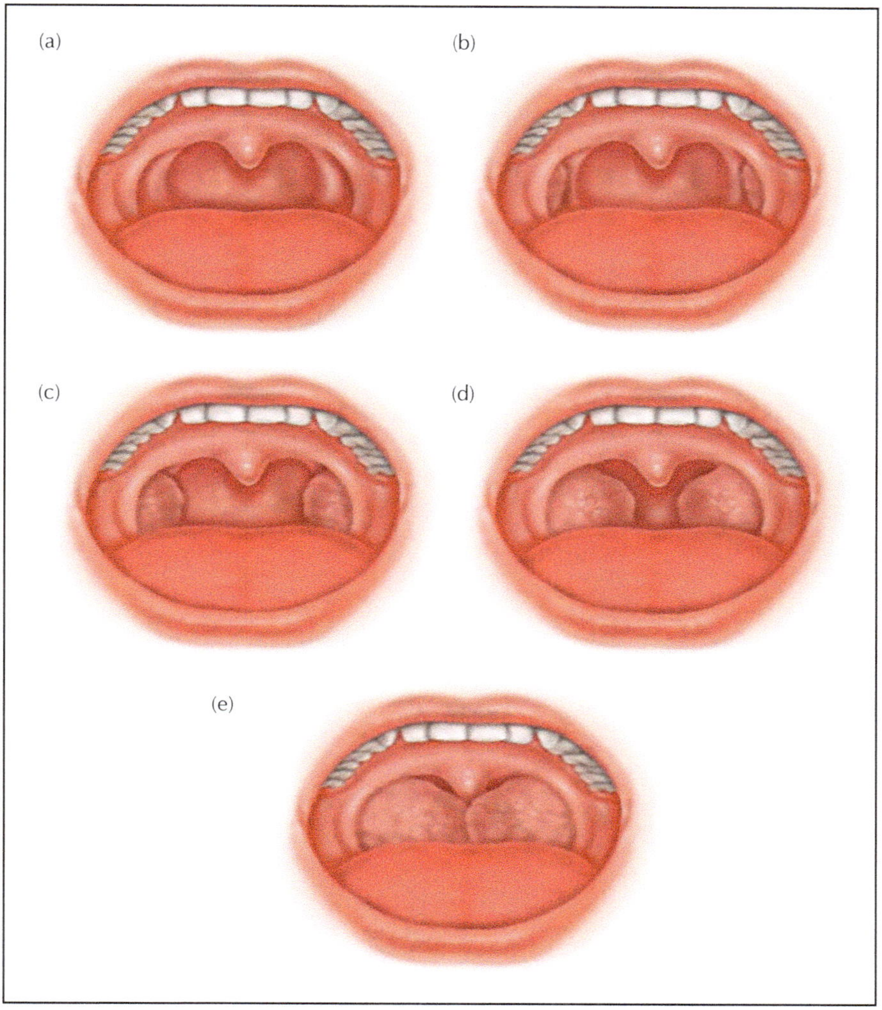

Figure 29.1. Grading of palatine tonsil size from 0 to IV.

Friedman tonsil size grading: (a) Grade 0: tonsils surgically absent; (b) Grade I: located within the tonsillar pillars; (c) Grade II: extend just beyond the tonsillar pillars; (d) Grade III: extend >50% toward the midline; and (e) Grade IV: make contact at the midline.[28]

mouth breathing associated with adenoidal hypertrophy, may also be noted among children with OSA. A systematic review reported a significant association between allergic rhinitis and SDB.[26] Anterior rhinoscopy may also demonstrate other causes of obstruction, such as inferior turbinate hypertrophy, septal deviation, or nasal polyps.

Oral exam should include evaluation of dentition, tongue, palate and tonsillar size, and visualization of the posterior oropharynx. A 4-point grading system with regard to tonsillar size (Figure 29.1) has been shown to have both acceptable inter-observer and intra-observer reproducibility.[27]

In addition, examination of oropharyngeal crowding helps predict risk of OSA and this is done with the help of scoring with the tongue protrusion without phonation (Mallampati score), though Friedman scoring system can be more appropriate done with the tongue not in protrusion and no phonation (Figure 29.2).

The presence of retrognathia and/or micrognathia should be assessed, particularly among

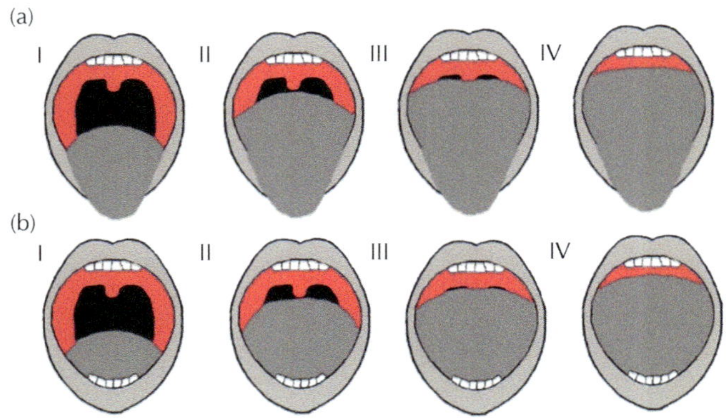

Figure 29.2. Top row (A) showing Mallampati score with tongue protruded. Bottom row (B) showing Friedman score with tongue not in protrusion position. Mallampati tongue/palate position grading (A). Grade I: entire uvula, palate, and tonsillar pillars visible; Grade II: uvula and palate visible; Grade III: palate and base of uvula visible; Grade IV: only hard palate visible.

Friedman tongue/palate position grading (B). Grade I: entire uvula, palate, tonsils/pillars visible; Grade II: base of uvula, palate visible, but tonsils/pillars not visible; Grade III: only soft and hard palate visible; Grade IV: pnly hard palate visible.[29]

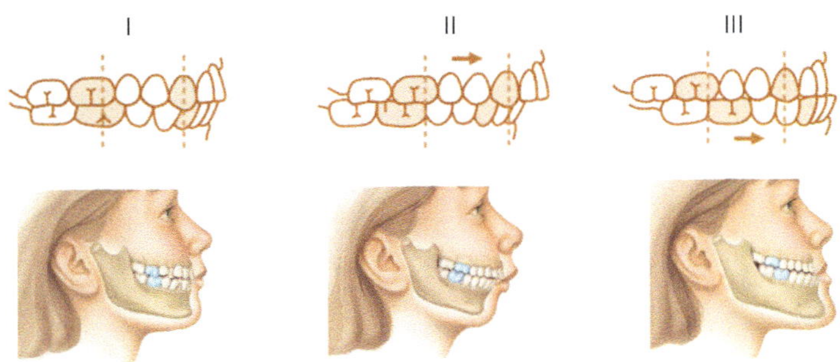

Figure 29.3. Angle's classification of malocclusion. Class I: maxillary second molar cusp occludes with the groove of the mandibular second molar. Class II: maxillary second molar cusp occludes with the interdental space between primary mandibular first and second molar. Can cause overbite or overjet. Class III: maxillary second molar cusp occludes with the distal surface of the primary mandibular second molar.[92,93]

children with other craniofacial disorders such as Pierre Robin sequence, which would predispose to upper airway obstruction particularly due to obstruction at the base of the tongue.[30] Midface and maxillary hypoplasia are features of children with Down syndrome, Crouzon syndrome, and Angelman syndrome.

Relative macroglossia is a condition in which a patient has a normal-sized tongue in a small oral cavity. This is found in DS or among children born prematurely or a product of twin pregnancy. The palate should also be evaluated for any evidence of midline defects, including overt clefts of the hard and soft palate, soft palate sub-mucosal cleft, and the presence of a bifid uvula. Also, dental occlusion should be evaluated using Angle's classification of malocclusion (Figure 29.3): class I (normal), class II (overbite or overjet), and class III (underbite); class II and III malocclusion are significantly correlated with OSA.[31]

Nasal endoscopy and flexible laryngoscopy are methods primarily used in otolaryngology clinics to visualize the upper airway, including nasal cavity, adenoids, oropharynx, pharyngeal walls, base of tongue, lingual tonsils, hypopharynx, supraglottis, and glottis. The upper airway scope is limited by visualization in an upright position, which may vary during sleep and in the supine position.

Laboratory Evaluation

Laboratory studies are generally not required in the workup of OSA. Thyroid function studies are suggested among children with OSA who are overweight or obese and may have prominent or scalloped tongue. Complete blood count is recommended to identify polycythemia which could be noted in severe OSA with intermittent severe hypoxemia. Gas exchange abnormalities during sleep can occur in OSA, which is elevated CO_2; however, utilization of blood gas as a diagnostic tool for sleep-related hypoventilation would not be accurate, nor would basic chemistry for assessment of bicarbonate values, as both may be within normal limits.

Imaging

Among children with OSA, lateral neck x-rays have been utilized to evaluate adenoid size in a systematic review; however, given the risk of radiation exposure, it is currently recommended that lateral neck films be reserved for children who cannot tolerate flexible nasal endoscopy, which is the current standard of care.[32–33] Among infants in whom pyriform aperture stenosis or choanal atresia is suspected, computed tomography (CT) imaging without contrast is utilized to evaluate the upper airways to delineate the site of obstruction.

Drug-Induced Sleep Endoscopy (DISE) and Cine Magnetic Resonance Imaging (MRI)

Drug induced sleep endoscopy (DISE) has been used to identify areas of airway obstruction, among children with OSA, when tonsils and adenoids are small and considered nonobstructive. DISE allows for dynamic examination of the upper airway under sedation from the nares to the supraglottis (adenoids, velum, lateral pharyngeal wall/tonsils, tongue base, supraglottis) using an ordinal scale; 0 = no obstruction; 1 = 0%–50% obstruction; 2 = 50%–99% obstruction; 3 = complete obstruction. DISE has been shown to be valid and reliable in both adults and children.[34–35] This procedure is particularly useful for children who can have obstruction at multiple sites and have a high likelihood of persistent OSA after T&A, such as those with obesity or Down syndrome.[36–37] DISE would help quantify sites of obstruction of the upper airway either due to syndromic pathogenesis, NMDs, or anatomic abnormalities associated with other NDDs who are likely to have persistent OSA after surgical intervention.[38]

Sleep cine magnetic resonance imaging (cMRI) is a useful imaging technique to evaluate children with OSA after T&A. cMRI allows for high-resolution examination of the upper airway with and without sedation and without radiation, while spontaneously breathing. Images are collected with the patient in a supine position from the superior-most aspect of the nasopharynx to the level of the lower cervical trachea in a 1–2-minute period and combined to create real-time images demonstrating upper airway dynamic motion. Evaluation is done at 3 main anatomic sites: nasopharynx, oropharynx, and hypopharynx. cMRI can be used as an alternative to DISE among patients who have persistent OSA following T&A. cMRI allows multiple overlapping areas of obstruction to be evaluated simultaneously.[39–40] cMRI has limitations; it does not identify obstruction well in the nasal passages or the larynx, and availability is limited to a few tertiary care centers.[41]

Polysomnography (PSG)

Attended in-laboratory PSG is the gold standard and the only recommended test to diagnose OSA in children. The American Academy of Sleep Medicine (AASM) and the American Academy of Pediatrics (AAP) recommend that PSG should be performed among children and adolescents with snoring and symptoms and signs of OSAS prior to T&A, as tonsillar size does not predict OSA.[3,42] The American Academy of Otolaryngology–Head and Neck Surgery (AAO-HNS) recommends PSG prior to operative intervention in high-risk patients such as children with obesity, DS, PWS, craniofacial abnormalities, and neuromuscular disease.[43] These guidelines also emphasize the need for repeat postoperative evaluation and PSG with high risk for persistent SRBDs after treatment among children with obesity, neuromuscular disorders, syndromes, and craniofacial abnormalities.

PSG involves simultaneous monitoring and recording of multiple physiologic parameters, including but not limited to airflow, respiratory effort, pulse oximetry, capnography, electroencephalography, electrooculography, and electromyography (EMG).[44] Airflow is monitored via nasal pressure transducer, oronasal thermal airflow. Respiratory inductance plethysmography (RIP) sum and RIP flow both calibrated and uncalibrated, polyvinylidene film based sensor (PVDF) sum belts are acceptable for recording respiratory effort. In addition, end-tidal capnography ($EtCO_2$) monitoring can be used as an alternative for scoring apneas.[45] $EtCO_2$ monitoring is used as a standard on baseline PSG among children as gas exchange abnormalities can occur with OSA along with snoring and flow limitation. Transcutaneous CO_2 (TCO_2) monitoring can be used as a surrogate. Additional monitoring sensors include pulse oximetry, electrocardiography, and surface limb EMG monitoring.[44] Thoracic and abdominal belts are used to detect respiratory effort, allowing for the differentiation between central and obstructive apneas. Dual thoracoabdominal PVDF belts are considered acceptable for recording respiratory effort events.[45] Based on the review of available literature, home sleep apnea testing has not been recommended for diagnosis of OSA among children <18 years.[46]

PSG scoring guidelines differ from adults ≥18 years versus children <18 years, with the most significant difference being respiratory events are 2 breaths in duration, based on the duration of previous breaths. Respiratory events must last 10 seconds to be scored in an adult. Obstructive hypopneas among adults and children require (1) presence of snoring during the event, (2) increased inspiratory flattening of nasal pressure or equivalent during the event, or (3) associated thoraco-abdominal paradox during the event. The absence of these findings signifies that the event is a central hypopnea with a lack of thoracic and abdominal belt effort. Other key differences are also in the scoring of mixed apneas; among adults there is absent inspiratory effort during the initial portion of the event with resumption of inspiratory effort during the second half. In children <18 years of age, mixed apnea is for a duration of at least 2 breaths, in the absence of inspiratory effort in 1 breath and present in the other.[44] Adult scoring guidelines can be used in children ≥13 years of age, which includes scoring of respiratory effort related arousals (RERAs) and calculation of respiratory disturbance index (RDI) as opposed to apnea hypopnea index (AHI) for diagnosis of OSA (Table 29.1; Figures 29.4, 29.5, 29.6).

Pediatric OSA is defined as an obstructive AHI of ≥1/hr or obstructive hypoventilation (25% of total sleep time (TST with $PaCO_2$ >50 mm Hg or surrogate - EtCO2 or TCO2 values > 50 mm Hg for 25% of TST) with associated snoring, flattening of inspiratory nasal pressure waveform or paradoxical thoraco-abdominal motion.[1]

Treatment Options

WATCHFUL WAITING

A multicenter Childhood Adenotonsillectomy Trial (CHAT) for pediatric OSA, lasting 7 months, evaluated early adeno-tonsillectomy (eAT) versus watchful waiting (WW). Among those assigned to WW, the majority of whom had mild OSA, a significant proportion (46%) exhibited normalization of their respiratory disturbances during sleep in follow-up PSG.[47] In a randomized controlled trial (RCT) among 60 children age 2–4 years with mild to moderate OSA and repeat PSG after 9 months, findings suggested that WW could be an alternative for mild OSA (AHI <5) with repeat PSG, as there was a reduction in AHI by −1.9 in the WW group, though the improvement was more pronounced in eAT group with reduction in AHI by −2.9 and more significant improvement in OSA scores, reduction by −18.[48]

ADENO-TONSILLECTOMY

T&A is first-line therapy for children with OSA. The CHAT study demonstrated T&A to be 79% effective in normalization of PSG findings of OSA among children 5–9 years of age. Nearly half of the patients in this study were overweight or obese (BMI z score <3). Normalization of PSG findings was higher among those who were not Black versus Black race, non-obese versus obese. There was also a greater chance of normalization of PSG if the AHI was at or below the median AHI (WW AHI: 4.5 vs. eAT AHI: 4.8).[47] Among children who were obese, OSA was noted to be more severe with higher AHI, and though there is

Table 29.1 **Rules for Scoring Respiratory Events Among Children (<18 Years)**

Obstructive Apnea	Event: Drop in peak signal excursion by >90% of pre-event baseline using oro-nasal thermal sensor or equivalent (Need both a + b) a. Event duration of at least 2 breaths AND b. Associated with ongoing respiratory effort through the period of apnea.
Central Apnea	(Either a or b or c) a. Event duration lasts >20 seconds OR b. Event duration of at least 2 breaths + >3% oxygen desaturation (or) cortical arousal OR c. Event duration of at least 2 breaths + Among infants <1 yr: decrease in heart rate (HR) to <50 bpm for >5 seconds (or) HR <60 bpm for >15 seconds
Mixed Apnea	(Need both a + b) a. Event duration of at least 2 breaths AND b. Absence of inspiratory effort in one breath and present in the other
Hypopnea	(Need a + b + c) a. Event: Drop in peak signal excursion by >30% of pre-event baseline using nasal pressure sensor or equivalent b. Duration of event at least 2 breaths c. Event is associated ≥3% oxygen desaturation or a cortical arousal If ANY of the below are present, then it is an Obstructive Hypopnea If NONE of the below are present, then it is a Central Hypopnea · Snoring during the event · Increased inspiratory flattening of nasal pressure or equivalent during event · Associated thoraco-abdominal paradox during event

Pediatric OSA is defined as an obstructive AHI of ≥1/hr or obstructive hypoventilation (25% of total sleep time) (TST with $PaCO_2$ >50 mm Hg or surrogate – EtCO2 or TCO2 values >50 mm Hg for 25% of TST) with associated snoring, flattening of inspiratory nasal pressure waveform, or paradoxical thoraco-abdominal motion.[1,44]

improvement after T&A, complete resolution of OSA is less likely.[49–50] Per the revised pediatric otolaryngology guidelines, overnight inpatient monitoring is recommended after T&A for children <3 years of age, or who have severe OSA (obstructive AHI ≥10 events per hour or oxygen saturation nadir <80% or both) due to higher risk of respiratory compromise after surgery. There should also be a low threshold to monitor children in an inpatient setting after T&A, if the children have complicated comorbid diagnosis such as cardiac complications of OSA, DS, neuromuscular disorders, failure to thrive, craniofacial anomalies, recent or current respiratory infection, obese children (BMI >95th percentile without PSG to characterize severity), and children with behavioral issues that would predict poor oral intake or pain management.[43]

Incomplete resolution of OSA is more common in children with NDD, especially for those with DS, PWS, neuromuscular disorders, and craniofacial abnormalities. AAP and AAO-HN recommend that children at high risk for having persistent OSA or who have persistent symptoms undergo repeat PSG to evaluate for residual OSA after T&A.[3,43] For children with persistent or recurrent OSA after T&A, there are other surgical and non-surgical options, though these are second-line treatment and the efficacy is still uncertain and dependent on the assessment of the site of obstruction.

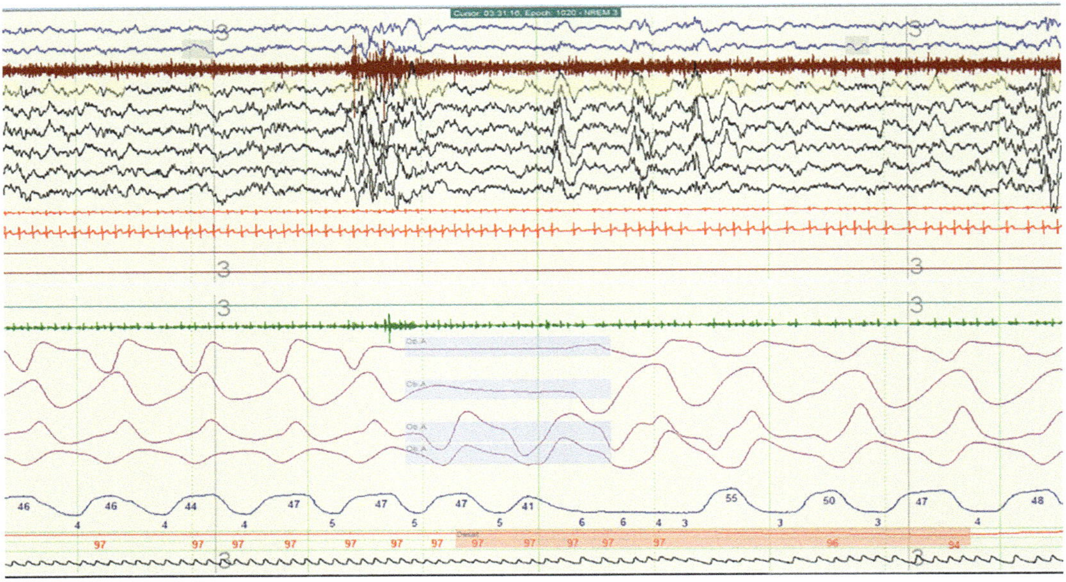

Figure 29.4. Pediatric obstructive apnea as noted on polysomnogram. A 60-second epoch demonstrating obstructive apnea. Note the drop in peak signal excursion by >90% of pre-event baseline using oro-nasal thermal sensor or equivalent with retained respiratory effort as seen in the chest and abdominal inductance plethysmography belts. The event lasts at least the duration of 2 breaths.

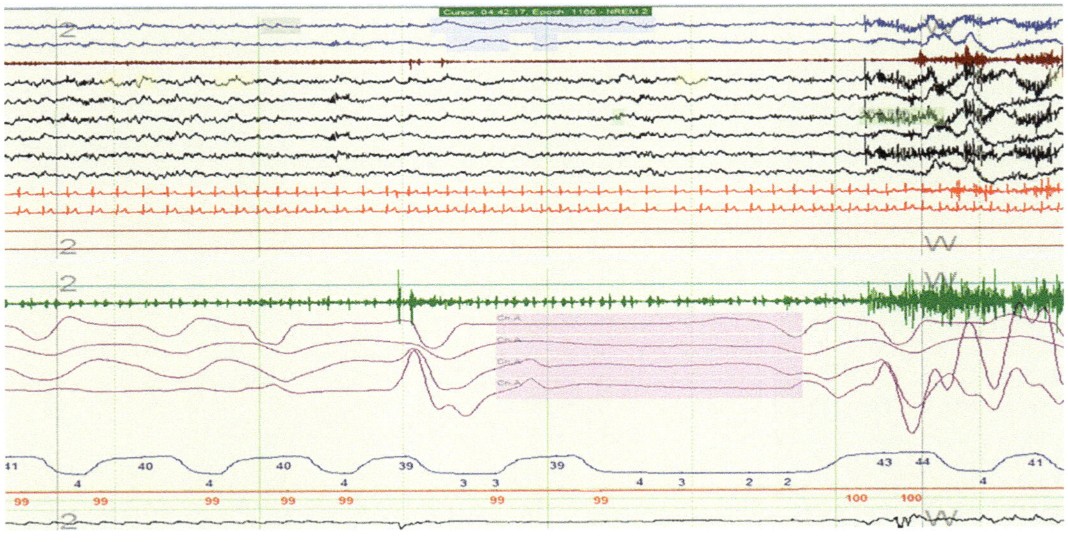

Figure 29.5. Pediatric central apnea as noted on polysomnogram. A 60-second epoch demonstrating obstructive apnea. Note the drop in peak signal excursion by >90% of pre-event baseline using oro-nasal thermal sensor or equivalent without respiratory effort as seen in the chest and abdominal inductance plethysmography belts. The event lasts at least the duration of 2 breaths.

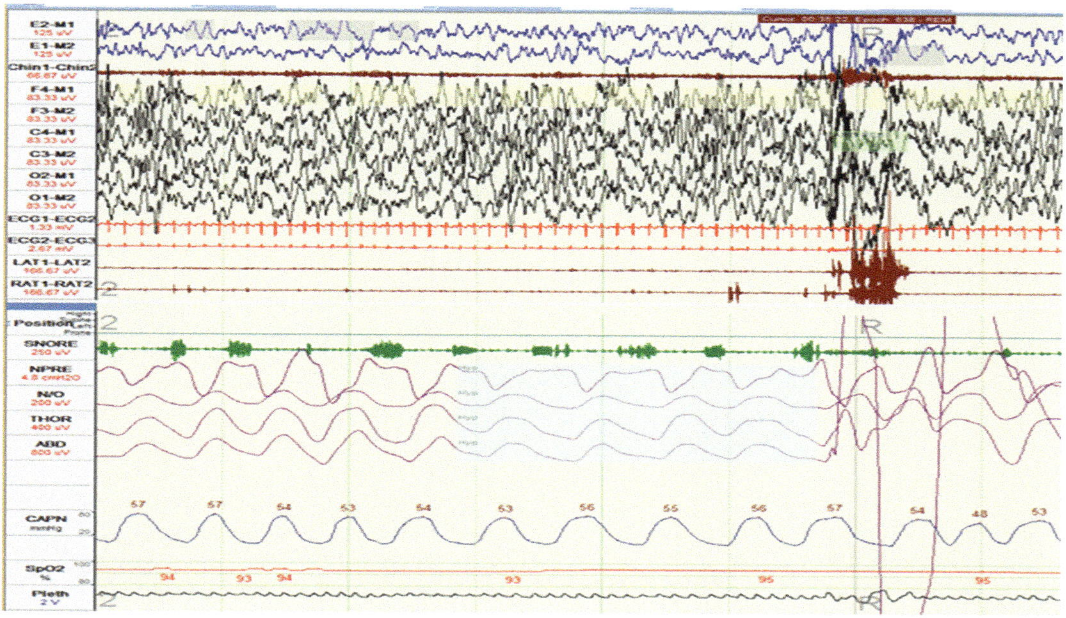

Figure 29.6. Pediatric hypopnea as noted on polysomnogram. A 60-second epoch demonstrating obstructive hypopnea. Note the drop in peak signal excursion by >30% of pre-event baseline using oro-nasal thermal sensor or equivalent with retained effort seen in the chest (THOR) and abdominal (ABD) inductance plethysmography belts. The event lasts at least the duration of 2 breaths.

POSITIVE AIRWAY PRESSURE (PAP) THERAPY

Positive airway pressure (PAP) therapy typically consists of 2 modalities: continuous positive airway pressure (CPAP), or bilevel positive airway pressure therapy (BPAP) which is a standard therapy for treatment of pediatric OSA. This therapy can be highly effective; however, finding an appropriately sized and fitted mask can often be a challenge among children, particularly those with craniofacial issues or younger children. The recommendations for increase in settings during the CPAP titration studies vary from adults to pediatrics. Among children <12 years of age, settings can be increased by 1 cm of water for 1 obstructive apnea, 1 hypopnea, 3 respiratory effort-related arousals (RERAs), or 1 minute of loud or unambiguous snoring or flow limitation, in contrast to those ≥12 years of age, where the recommendation is to increase the pressure by 1 cm of water for any one of the following: 2 obstructive apneas, 3 hypopneas, 5 RERAs, or 3 minutes of loud or unambiguous snoring. The maximum CPAP pressure for children <12 years of age is 15 cm of water after which they should be transitioned to BPAP, and it is 20 cm of water for those ≥12 years of age.[51] Increase of IPAP and EPAP is recommended for obstructive apneas, and increase in IPAP is recommended for hypopneas, RERAs, and snoring to a maximum IPAP of 20 cm of water for BPAP <12 years of age and 30 cm of water for ≥12 years of age.

Auto-PAP devices are not indicated for the treatment of pediatric OSA. The duration of the apneas and hypopneas is defined as reduction in ventilation for at least 10 seconds; ResMed™ devices indicate a reduction in flow by 50% from the baseline for hypopneas.[52] In addition, close attention should be paid to current FDA approvals for weight requirements, which are 66 pounds for CPAP and BPAP and 35 pounds for BPAP with backup rate for both ResMed™ and Respironics™ devices. These weight approvals can change over time.

PAP therapy for the management of OSA has been associated with decreased insulin resistance and systolic pressure load and other inflammatory markers which did not show a statistically significant response in this small patient population of 27 children aged 8–16 years with moderate to severe OSA.[53] There was improvement in neurobehavioral abnormalities and daytime sleepiness at 3 months, which was also dependent on adherence.[54] Research indicates, however, that CPAP adherence is often suboptimal, with one multicenter study reporting that among the 29 children studied, one-third dropped out prior to the 6-month mark. Among the 21 remaining children, 6-month objective adherence data was only 5.3 ± 2.5 hours per evening with an overestimation by parental estimates.[55]

The literature varies on the adverse effects of long-term PAP therapy. A study utilizing cephalometric variables in about 50 children who were compliant with nasal PAP therapy (mean age 10.42 years) for an average of 2.57 years, compared to 50 noncompliant subjects (mean age 8.53 years). Compliant patients demonstrated midface retrusion and upper incisor flaring compared to noncompliant subjects.[56] In contrast, a study with smaller population of 12 children compliant on CPAP therapy with nasal mask (6 hours of nightly use for mean duration of 35.8 ± 25.8 months) versus 11 age-matched controls did not demonstrate association between duration of PAP therapy and cephalometric variables impacting midface growth.[57]

MEDICATIONS

Nasal steroids have been used for the treatment of OSA and may be effective in children with mild to moderate disease. A 6-week course of fluticasone nasal spray among children with adeno-tonsillar hypertrophy and OSA (AHI 10.7 ± 2.6) versus placebo has been shown to reduce AHI (6.3 ± 1.2).[58] Similarly, a double-blind randomized crossover trial of intranasal budesonide for 6 weeks or placebo, followed by an alternative treatment for 6 weeks and a 2-week washout, demonstrated similar results. There was an improvement of mild OSA with resolution of OSA among 54% of patients.[59] A prospective randomized double-blind trial of oral montelukast 4 and 5 mg for 12 weeks versus placebo of a small number of patients had modest benefit in the treatment of mild to moderate OSA (reduction of AHI by 50% in 65% of patients), and it proved to be effective in reducing adenoid hypertrophy and improving OSA symptoms.[60] A group of children who were post T&A with mild OSA (AHI >1 but <5/hr): 22 children were treated with combined intranasal budesonide and oral montelukast for 12 weeks versus 14 children in the control arm. There was a small improvement in AHI from the post T&A pretreatment study (AHI 3.9 ± 1.2 vs. control group AHI 3.6 ± 1.4) by AHI of 0.3 ± 0.3 in the treatment group with slightly better improvement in baseline oxygen saturation 92.5% ± 3.0%, and no statistically significant results were found in the control group.[61]

WEIGHT LOSS

There are various factors that contribute to upper airway obstruction in obese individuals which may be a combination of positive airway critical closing pressure causing airway collapse during sleep with mild negative inspiratory pressure and altered neuromuscular tone. Weight loss should be strongly advocated for overweight and obese children, as the surgical outcomes are worse among obese children, such as T&A.[49] Weight loss continues to be considered as an adjunctive therapy in treatment of OSA. Weight loss surgery is being performed in adolescents with severe OSA although outcomes in children are unclear. Bariatric surgery has been shown to result in significant improvement in OSA severity in adults.[62]

MAXILLARY EXPANSION

Recent literature has supported the use of rapid maxillary expansion as a non-surgical option in the treatment of mild to moderate OSA. A study of 14 non-overweight children age 6.9 ± 2.2 years demonstrated statistically significant improvement in OSA from baseline PSG versus 12 months PSG (AHI: 5.8 ± 6.8 vs. 1.5 ± 1.6; $p = 0.005$).[63] Even among a smaller cohort of 9 children with higher AHI (mean AHI 17.4) there was an improvement in severity of OSA, though not complete resolution with a PSG at 12 months (mean AHI 5.4).[64]

MANDIBULAR ADVANCEMENT DEVICES

The intraoral protrusion devices result in forward and downward position of the lower jaw during sleep and improves airway patency. It is more effective for mild to moderate OSA that is more prominent during supine sleep. Higher treatment success has been noted among less obese patients and female patients. Very limited data are available among children, especially younger than 16 years of age, as it has an impact on dental occlusion and bite. Systematic review of 4 prospective studies among children 18 years of age demonstrated improvement in AHI, though not complete resolution of OSA.[65]

OTHER OPTIONS

There are other, less often used options that deserve a brief mention. Use of nasopharyngeal airway (NPA) has been utilized in treatment of OSA and there are clinical trials underway regarding use of 3D printed NPA. Use of positional therapy that would result in avoidance of supine sleep when OSA occurs exclusively during supine sleep, such as T-shirts with tennis balls or other devices, can be used, though long-term compliance has been noted to be low and these could be considered adjunctive therapy at best.

SURGICAL OPTIONS

There are surgical options as possible treatment options for OSA that may be considered for children with persistent OSA following T&A, especially if they are not optimal candidates for PAP therapy due to seizures disorder, particularly nocturnal seizures, sialorrhea, or other contraindications. Typical sites of obstruction are at the base of the tongue, the palate, or both, and often require cine MRI or DISE to delineate. Lingual tonsillectomy has been a surgical option in the improvement of OSA with a success rate of 17% in resolution of OSA (AHI <1) and 51% success in reduction of AHI to < 5.[66] In this systemic review, patient populations were small and included patients who were obese, or may have had other comorbid diagnoses like DS, muco-polysaccharidosis, or Noonans syndrome. For infants with laryngomalacia or older children with sleep-state-dependent laryngomalacia, supraglottoplasty can be considered. Studies examining supraglottoplasty are limited by small sample size, but the consensus is that there seems to be an improvement in AHI but not complete resolution. A systematic review evaluated supraglottoplasty outcomes in infants and children (≥12 months) with NDDs or syndromes and found that resolution of OSA after surgery is low and additional surgeries were required after supraglottoplasty.[67] Modified uvulopalatopharyngoplasty (UPPP) is resection of the soft palate with uvulectomy and preservation of the soft palate musculature. Data are limited on the efficacy of this surgical option among children. A study of 15 children, 12 with neurologic impairment who had OSA (utilizing PSG data) underwent UPPP and T&A; the AHI improved from a preoperative mean AHI of 19 to a postoperative mean AHI of 2.5.[68]

Maxillary mandibular advancement (MMA) is a surgical option with improved outcomes data among adults. Among the pediatric population outcomes, data are sparse, but it could be a viable option for treatment of severe OSA. In a retrospective analysis of 15 adolescents and young adults (14–20 years of age) MMA done for malocclusion also demonstrated improvement of OSA with a reduction of AHI from preoperative AHI of 28.9 ± 16.0 to postoperative AHI of 5.7 ± 4.6, reflecting an 80% reduction in AHI.[69]

Other surgical options that are performed typically by oral-maxillofacial surgeons are hyoid suspension, a procedure where the free-floating hyoid bone is pulled forward, in effect pulling the tongue base forward to the lower jaw as the tongue muscle is attached to the hyoid bone. Genioglossus advancement pulls the tongue base forward by advancing the part of the lower jaw bone to which the tongue base is attached. Otolaryngologists perform other surgeries like epiglottopexy, a surgical technique that pulls the epiglottis away from the back wall of the throat by suturing it forward to the tongue base, and posterior or midline glossectomy among patients with a large or prominent tongue, which involves removal of the central portion of the muscle from the base of the tongue. Prior to selection of these surgical options, a multidisciplinary team approach is important to assess sites of maximal obstruction of the upper airway which could involve DISE and cephalometric imaging or cone beam CT.

Hypoglossal nerve stimulator (HGNS) for DS children age 10–18 years with moderate to severe OSA (AHI 10–50 events/hr) is under clinical trials at certain select pediatric children's hospitals. The exclusionary criteria is obesity (BMI >97th percentile) using the DS growth chart, which would exclude a significant proportion of patients. There should also not be concentric collapse of the upper airway, which is an exclusionary criterion for the placement of HGNS among adults as well. It is FDA approved for use above 18 years of age with certain caveats. It is approved for use among patients who are non-adherent or intolerant of positive airway pressure therapy, with moderate to severe OSA, and a BMI of ≤32 kg/m^2. Some of the insurance providers have relaxed BMI guidelines to allow implantation in patients with a BMI of <35 kg/m^2.[70]

CENTRAL SLEEP APNEA

Central sleep apnea (CSA) is divided primarily into 3 diagnostic categories among children, based on the age at the time of diagnosis: primary central sleep apnea, primary sleep apnea of infancy, primary sleep apnea of prematurity.[1] The diagnosis of central sleep apnea is dependent on exclusion of other underlying medical or neurological diagnosis.

Primary Central Sleep Apnea

Primary CSA is considered to be a diagnosis when the central apneas are of unknown etiology. Symptoms are typically daytime sleepiness or insomnia, difficulty initiating or maintaining sleep, with frequent nighttime awakenings and disruption in sleep quality. There may be possible reports of snoring, witnessed apneas, or awakening feeling short of breath. The daytime effects of CSA may not always be evident. The diagnostic criteria for CSA are 5 or more central apneas and/or central hypopneas per hour of sleep as determined by PSG.[1] There should be no evidence of sleep-related or daytime hypoventilation. Scoring criteria for central apneas and hypopneas among children <18 years is discussed earlier in this chapter. Primary central sleep apnea is relatively rare among children, with a retrospective study demonstrating only 5.4% of children had a diagnosis of CSA, and among those, 24% had associated sleep-related hypoventilation, which would exclude the diagnosis of primary CSA.[71]

Testing

Diagnosis of primary CSA is done by PSG and excluding OSA and hypoventilation as the primary diagnosis. Pediatric PSG is done with CO_2 monitoring, and the predisposing factor for primary CSA appears to be drop in arterial PCO_2 ($PaCO_2$) below the hypocapnic apnea threshold (HAT), so a determination of blood gas would reveal normal to low $PaCO_2$. The HAT is typically close in values to the awake $PaCO_2$.[1] PSG criteria for scoring hypopneas and central apneas are mentioned in Table 29.1.[44–45] Children with idiopathic CSA should undergo imaging of the brain, preferably a brain MRI, to rule out a CNS pathology as a cause for CSA, as the diagnostic yield of MRIs exceeds 50%.[2]

Differential Diagnosis

Primary CSA is typically a diagnosis of exclusion, and children with OSA as the primary diagnosis can have central apneas during the diagnostic studies or treatment-emergent central apneas during the titration studies. The central apneas do tend to improve over time on PAP therapy. Central apneas can occur secondary to neurological disorders like Chiari malformation and achondroplasia, cardiac disorders, and medications like narcotics.[71] Sleep-related hypoventilation can be associated with central apneas among disorders such as abnormalities of ventilatory control like central congenital hypoventilation syndrome (CCHS), rapid onset obesity, hypothalamic dysregulation, hypoventilation and autonomic dysfunction (ROHHAD), and neuromuscular disorders which can present initially with central apneas without hypoventilation in a small subset, restrictive chest wall disorders, and parenchymal lung disease.[72–73] Among patients with CCHS, SDB improves during REM sleep, unlike neuromuscular and restrictive chest wall disorders, which are worse during REM sleep.

Treatment Options

Acetazolamide has been reported to help with the treatment of CSA, though the studies have been among adults.[74] There are case reports of success utilizing acetazolamide for the treatment of CSA among children. Treatment options among pediatric CSA are not well studied, and data are often extrapolated from adult population and include supplemental oxygen, PAP therapy including CPAP, and noninvasive ventilation, which is use of BPAP with backup rate.[75]

Primary Central Sleep Apnea of Infancy

Primary central sleep apnea of infancy (CSAI) is the occurrence of central apneas among infants ≥37 weeks post-conceptual age (PCA). It occurs in the first 6 months of life and typically in the first few months of life.[1] Immaturity of the respiratory control system is considered to be the underlying etiology, along with lower functional residual capacity and compliant chest wall. Symptomatic CSA occurs in 0.5% of infants, and 2% of healthy asymptomatic full-term infants will have at least 1 observed central event. The scoring criteria among infants are discussed in the prior portion of the chapter, and a significant difference is decline in heart rate used to score central apneas, as well as possible need for intervention like stimulation or resuscitation (Table 29.2).

In 2016, the American Academy of Pediatrics (AAP) outlined clinical practice guidelines for the evaluation of infants who suffered an apparent life-threatening event (ALTE). This guideline accomplishes 3 objectives. First, the term ALTE was relabeled with a new, more specifically defined term: brief resolved unexplained event (BRUE). Second, there was a need to stratify infants into low or high risk based on the likelihood of a serious underlying condition. Lastly, there was a need to provide evidence-based management recommendations and key action statements for lower-risk infants. BRUE is defined as a sudden, brief (<1 min), resolved event occurring in an infant less than 12 months of age, witnessed by an observer, characterized by ≥1 of the following: cyanosis or pallor, absent/decreased/irregular breathing, marked change in tone, and an altered level of responsiveness.[76]

Testing

PSG has a role in quantifying SDB. The normative data are limited on infant PSG, and AHI is variable, with improvement in AHI with increase in PCA, and extent of oxygen desaturation may be more of clinical consequence.[77] This review is limited by the studies utilizing variable methods for determining SDB from infant PSG or pulse oximetry and different channels, as well as different configurations and scoring criteria used during PSG. Prior studies using unattended polygraphy have indicated higher central apnea index (CAI) among infants (1–3 months of age) and higher obstructive apnea index (OAI) (<8 weeks of age).[78–79] In a more recent study with 38 healthy newborns (<1 month of age), 7 did not show SDB and 31 underwent PSG with $EtCO_2$ monitoring using AASM criteria for scoring. Mean AHI was 14.9/hr with hypopneas the most common scored events. Periodic breathing was noted in 40% of newborns and median oxygen saturation was 98% with an oxygen nadir of 85%.[80] Typically SDB is worse during REM sleep.

Differential Diagnosis

Infant sleep apnea can be result from underlying comorbid conditions like gastroesophageal reflux (GERD), neurological conditions such as Chiari malformation, brainstem malformation, metabolic disease, and syndromes such as

Table 29.2 **Diagnostic Criteria of Central Sleep Apnea of Infancy**

AASM Diagnostic Criteria: should satisfy A + B + C + D*

A	B	C	D
Apnea or cyanosis noted by observer or central apnea or desaturation detected by monitoring	Infant has post-conceptual age of ≥37 wks	PSG or alternative monitoring in hospital/ home apnea monitor Recurrent prolonged (>20 sec) central apneas Periodic breathing for ≥5% of total sleep time (TST)	Not explained by another sleep disorder or medical, neurological disorder, or medication

* *International Classification of Sleep Disorders* (ICSD-3)

Pierre Robin, Trisomy 21, 18, and 13, central congenital hypoventilation syndrome (CCHS), and Prader Willi syndrome (PWS), as well as cyanotic heart diseases. Some of these comorbid conditions, such as myelo-meningocele, may present as SDB with higher proportion of hypopneas that are difficult to differentiate into central versus obstructive pathology with higher AHI compared to their age-matched controls.[81] Lower gestational age and structural abnormalities seem to be correlated with higher obstructive apnea index and does not seem to improve with increase in gestational age.[82] Impaired oxygen and infections, particularly certain viral infections, can cause apneas such as RSV and pertussis.

Primary Central Sleep Apnea of Prematurity

Primary CSA of prematurity is defined as central apneas demonstrated on PSG among infants <37 weeks PCA when symptoms are first noted, not explained by associated sleep, medical, or neurologic conditions. It is diagnosed in nearly all infants born at <29 weeks or with a birth weight of <1000 g, 54% of infants born at 30–31 weeks, 15% of infants born at 32–33 weeks, and 7% of infants born at 34–35 weeks.[83] This condition typically resolves by 36–40 weeks conceptional age.[1] The diagnostic criteria for primary CSA of prematurity are described in Table 29.3. The underlying etiology is considered to be immaturity of control of breathing with nerve conduction delays and pulmonary physiology, which is a compliant chest wall and reduced functional residual capacity.[84–85] Infants with chronic lung disease, neurological abnormalities, metabolic disturbances, or GERD may have slower rates of improvement of CSA.

Testing

The diagnosis of CSA of prematurity is done by cardiorespiratory monitoring in the neonatal intensive care unit (NICU). PSG can be done on some occasions. The normative data on AHI are unclear as is the number of central apneas per hours of sleep. The oxygen desaturations associated with brief central apneas can be due to decreased pulmonary reserve, which would improve over time. Obstructive and mixed apneas as well as hypopneas may also occur at a higher frequency particularly during REM sleep. There can be a higher preponderance of mixed and obstructive apneas among premature infants.[86] CSA of prematurity should improve by 43 weeks PCA.

Management

Full-term and premature infants with CSA are generally managed with supportive therapy. Depending on the severity of disease, interventions include observation, oxygen supplementation, and pharmacologic therapy. Observation may be employed when children have mild CSA and are in a monitored setting. Oxygen therapy may be utilized to support infants until CSA resolves. Both caffeine and theophylline have been used as central nervous system stimulators in children with CSA. Currently, caffeine is preferred because of its longer lasting effect and safety profile.[83]

Table 29.3 **Diagnostic Criteria for Primary Sleep Apnea of Prematurity**

AASM Diagnostic Criteria- should satisfy A + B + C + D*

A	B	C	D
Apnea or cyanosis noted by observer or central apnea is noted during sleep or oxygen desaturation or bradycardia detected by hospital monitoring	Gestational age of <37 wks	PSG or home apnea device or hospital monitoring shows Recurrent, prolonged (>20 sec) central apnea or Periodic breathing for ≥5% of TST	Not explained by another sleep disorder or medical or neurological disorder, or medication

* *International Classification of Sleep Disorders* (ICSD-3)

It has been shown that earlier initiation of caffeine has been associated with shorter duration of mechanical ventilation and lower incidence of bronchopulmonary dysplasia (BPD).[87] Profound CSA at times requires treatment with CPAP or noninvasive or invasive positive pressure ventilation. Preterm infants appear to have an exaggerated laryngeal chemoreflex response, and there have been studies conducted to demonstrate the association between GERD and apneas, though temporal association has not been proven.[87]

HYPOVENTILATION

Elevation in carbon dioxide (CO_2) values can be present during daytime with blood gas or surrogate CO_2 values, either $EtCO_2$ or TCO_2 values, >45 mmHg. Hypoventilation can be either central in etiology due to impact on central chemoreceptors located in the medullary respiratory control center or from weakness of the respiratory muscles or restriction of the chest wall. Scoring guidelines in sleep-related hypoventilation differ from adult to pediatrics in that in children <18 years of age, arterial PCO_2 ($PaCO_2$) level or surrogate value should be >50 mmHg for >25% of total sleep time (TST).[1] Among neuromuscular disorders such as Duchenne muscular dystrophy, the scoring criteria for hypoventilation have changed and an elevation in CO_2 values for 2% of sleep time is considered diagnostic of sleep-related hypoventilation.[88]

Central hypoventilation is from the inability to maintain adequate respiratory drive, which is impacted from the dorsal respiratory group of neurons associated with inspiration, and the pre-Botzinger complex, which is essential for generating the rhythm of respiration.[89] Central hypoventilation has variable presentation from mild hypoventilation during sleep to life-threatening inability to maintain spontaneous ventilation. Hypoventilation in children can be congenital or acquired. Congenital disorders include CCHS, ROHHAD (rapid-onset obesity, hypothalamic dysfunction, hypoventilation, and autonomic dysregulation) syndrome, Chiari malformations/myelomeningocele, achondroplasia, Prader-Willi syndrome (PWS), Leigh syndrome, Joubert syndrome, and familial dysautonomia, secondary to CNS injury during birth. Acquired etiologies of central hypoventilation include brain tumors, infection, infarction, or after neurologic surgery, and metabolic diseases.

Prader-Willi syndrome (PWS) is a syndrome that deserves special mention as it has variable presentation depending on the age of symptom recognition. It is a rare neurodevelopmental genetic disorder caused by deletion in the paternally derived chromosome 15(15q11-q13).[90,91] There is developmental delay, hypotonia, hypogonadism, hyperphagia, obesity, intellectual disability, and behavioral abnormalities. Hypotonia is prominent in the neonatal period, presenting initially as failure to thrive (FTT) due to poor sucking reflex, decreased arousal, and generalized weakness, but slight improvement in tone is noted. Hypotonia gradually improves and becomes milder in severity but persists throughout life. Though the initial presentation is FTT during infancy, they eventually develop significant hyperphagia and morbid obesity, which is the most recognizable hallmark feature of PWS. Children with PWS can have the entire spectrum of SDB, from central apneas during infancy and hypoventilation to OSA due to obesity and hypotonia, as well as hypoventilation.

Hypoventilation can occur when muscles of respiration such as the diaphragm, intercostal muscles, abdominal muscles, and accessory muscles are impacted, or there is restriction to the chest wall.[88] Neuromuscular disorders such as Duchenne muscular dystrophy and spinal muscular atrophy are associated with muscle weakness, and other skeletal abnormalities, such as Jeune syndrome and neuromuscular scoliosis, demonstrate restriction to the chest wall.[73,88]

For differentiation of disorders of hypoventilation as well as use of PSG and treatment options, please refer to Chapter 10 on hypoventilation. Children should undergo arterial blood gas (ABG) or blood gas analysis to confirm daytime hypercapnia or surrogate such as TCO_2 or $EtCO_2$ monitoring. Blood gas may also demonstrate compensatory respiratory acidosis, and ABG or pulse oximetry can help if there is hypoxemia associated with hypoventilation. Chemistry with estimation of bicarbonate values can help with estimation of renal compensation; sleep-related hypoventilation is profound, with resultant daytime hypoventilation. They should also undergo a complete blood count (CBC) to identify possible polycythemia associated with chronic hypoxemia.

Noninvasive ventilation and invasive ventilation are considered to be standard of care depending on the severity and age of presentation as well as hours of ventilatory support required.

SLEEP-RELATED HYPOXEMIA

It is diagnosed when PSG or nocturnal oximetry demonstrates arterial oxygen saturation <90% for ≥5 minutes in the absence of sleep-related hypoventilation.[1] Hypoxemia is worse during REM sleep, which is due to muscle weakness. When hypoxemia demonstrates worsening, there is daytime hypoxemia. Hypoxemia can be noted with worsening hypoventilation, such as central disorders of hypoventilation and neuromuscular syndromes. OSA or CSA should not be considered as the underlying cause of hypoxemia as the respiratory events related to SDB should not result in low baseline oxygen saturations. There may be underlying causes of sleep-related hypoxemia (SRH) such as shunt, ventilation perfusion mismatch, diffusion impairment, or high altitude.[89] Cyanotic congenital heart diseases are associated with daytime hypoxemia, which are ameliorated after surgical interventions that are often staged, though SRH may persist. There can be worsening of SRH with exacerbation of respiratory disorders.

There are comorbidities associated with SRH which are pulmonary artery hypertension, cor pulmonale, polycythemia, and impact on neurocognitive functioning. Oxygen supplementation is typically the treatment option for SRH. This should be considered if there is no associated hypoventilation. Noninvasive and invasive ventilation can be considered for profound hypoxemia.

REFERENCES

1. American Academy of Sleep Medicine. *International Classification of Sleep Disorders*. 3rd ed. American Academy of Sleep Medicine; 2014.
2. Beck SE, Marcus CL. Pediatric polysomonography. *Sleep Med Clin*. 2009;4(3):393–406.
3. Marcus CL, Brooks LJ, Draper KA, et al. Diagnosis and management of childhood obstructive sleep apnea syndrome. *Pediatrics*. 2012;130(3):e714–e755.
4. Ali NJ, Pitson DJ, Stradling JR. Snoring, sleep disturbance, and behavior in 4-5 year olds. *Arch Dis Child*. 1993;68(3):360–366.
5. Tarasiuk A, Greenberg-Dotan S, Simon-Tuval T, et al. Elevated morbidity and health care use in children with obstructive sleep apnea syndrome. *Am J Respir Crit Care Med*. 2007;175(1):55–61.
6. Schwengel DA, Sterni LM, Tunkel DE, Heitmiller ES. Perioperative management of children with obstructive sleep apnea. *Anesth Analg*. 2009;109(1):60–75.
7. Hoeve LJ, Pijpers M, Joosten KF. OSAS in craniofacial syndromes: An unsolved problem. *Int J Pediatr Otorhinolaryngol*. 2003;67(Suppl 1):S111–S113.
8. Gozal D. Sleep-disordered breathing and school performance in children. *Pediatrics*. 1998 Sep;102(3):616–620.
9. Chervin RD, Archbold KH, Dillon JE, et al. Inattention, hyperactivity, and symptoms of sleep-disordered breathing. *Pediatrics*. 2002 Mar;109(3):449–456.
10. O'Brien LM, Holbrook CR, Mervis CB, et al. Sleep and neurobehavioral characteristics of 5- to 7-year-old children with parentally reported symptoms of attention-deficit/hyperactivity disorder. *Pediatrics*. 2003;111(3):554–563.
11. Mitchell RB. Sleep-disordered breathing in children: Are we underestimating the problem? *Eur Respir J*. 2005;25(2):216–217.
12. Gozal D, Capdevila OS, Kheirandish-Gozal L. Metabolic alterations and systemic inflammation in obstructive sleep apnea among nonobese and obese prepubertal children. *Am J Respir Crit Care Med*. 2008;177(10):1142–1149.
13. Ng DK, Wong JC, Chan CH, Leung LCK, Leung S. Ambulatory blood pressure before and after adenotonsillectomy in children with obstructive sleep apnea. *Sleep Med*. 2010;11(7):721–725.
14. Sun SS, Grave GD, Siervogel RM, Pickoff AA, Arslanian SS, Daniels SR. Systolic blood pressure in childhood predicts hypertension and metabolic syndrome later in life. *Pediatrics*. 2007;119(2):237–246.
15. Chervin RD, Hedger K, Dillon JE, Pituch KJ. Pediatric Sleep Questionnaire (PSQ): Validity and reliability of scales for sleep disordered breathing, snoring, sleepiness, and behavioral problems. *Sleep Med*. 2000;1(1):21–32.
16. Blunden S, Lushington K, Lorenzen B, Wong J, Balendran R, Kennedy D. Symptoms of sleep breathing disorders in children are underreported by parents at general practice visits. *Sleep Breath*. 2003;7(4):167–176.
17. American Thoracic Society. Standards and indications for cardiopulmonary sleep studies in children. *Am J Respir Crit Care Med*. 1996;153(2):866–878.
18. Brooks LJ, Topol HI. Enuresis in children with sleep apnea. *J Pediatr*. 2003;142(5):515–518.
19. Bonuck K, Freeman K, Chervin RD, Xu L. Sleep-disordered breathing in a population-based cohort: Behavioral outcomes at 4 and 7 years. *Pediatrics*. 2012;129(4):e857–e865.
20. Paliga JT, Tahiri YT, Silvestry J, Taylor JA. Screening for obstructive sleep apnea in children treated at a major craniofacial center. *J Craniofac Surg*. 2014;25:1762–1765.
21. Owens A, Spirito A, McGiunn M, Nobile C. Sleep habits and sleep disturbance in elementary school-aged children. *J Dev Behav Pediatr*. 2000;21(1):27–36.
22. Borgström A, Nerfeldt P, Friberg D. Questionnaire OSA-18 has poor validity

compared to polysomnography in pediatric obstructive sleep apnea. *Int J Pediatr Otorhinolaryngol.* 2013;77(11):1864–1868.

23. Bannink N, Maliepaard M, Raat H, Joosten KF, Mathijssen IM. Reliability and validity of the obstructive sleep apnea-18 survey in healthy children and children with syndromic craniosynostosis. *J Dev Behav Pediatr*. 2011;32(1):27–33.
24. Speiser PW, Rudolf MC, Anhalt H, et al. Childhood obesity. *J Clin Endocrinol Metab.* 2005;90(3):1871–1887.
25. Shires CB, Anold SL, Schoumacher RA, Dehoff GW, Donepudi SK, Stocks RM. Body mass index as an indicator of obstructive sleep apnea in pediatric Down syndrome. *Int J Pediatr Otorhinolaryngol.* 2010;74(7):768–772.
26. Lin SY, Melvin TA, Boss EF, Ishman SL. The association between allergic rhinitis and sleep-disordered breathing in children: A systematic review. *Int Forum Allergy Rhinol.* 2013;3(6):504–509.
27. Ng SK, Lee DL, Li AM, Wing YK, Tong MC. Reproducibility of clinical grading of tonsillar size. *Arch Otolaryngol Head Neck Surg.* 2010;136(2):159–162.
28. Friedman M, Salapatas AM, Bonzelaar LB. Updated Friedman staging system for obstructive sleep apnea. *Adv Otorhinolaryngol.* 2017;80:41–48.
29. Yu JL, Rosen I. Utility of the modified Mallampati grade and Friedman tongue position in the assessment of obstructive sleep apnea. *J Clin Sleep Med.* 2020;16(2):303–308.
30. Anderson IC, Sedaghat AR, McGinley BM, Redett RJ, Boss EF, Ishman SL. Prevalence and severity of obstructive sleep apnea and snoring in infants with Pierre Robin sequence. *Cleft Palate Craniofac J.* 2011;48(5):614–618.
31. Anselmo M, de Siqueira J, Dal'Fabbro C, Tufik S. Type of dental occlusion in children and adolescents presenting sleep disorders. *Sleep Sci.* 2008;1:46–48.
32. Feres MFN, Hermann JS, Cappellette M, et al. Lateral X-ray view of the skull for the diagnosis of adenoid hypertrophy: A systematic review. *Int J Pediatr Otorhinolaryngol.* 2011;75:1–11.
33. Baldassari CM, Choi S. Assessing adenoid hypertrophy in children: X-ray or nasal endoscopy? *Laryngoscope.* 2014;124(7):1509–1510.
34. Chan DK, Liming BJ, Horn DL, Parikh SR. A new scoring system for upper airway pediatric sleep endoscopy. *JAMA Otolaryngol Head Neck Surg.* 2014;140(7):595–602.
35. Fishman G, Zemel M, DeRowe A, Sadot E, Sivan Y, Koltai PJ. Fiber-optic sleep endoscopy in children with persistent obstructive sleep apnea: Inter-observer correlation and comparison with awake endoscopy. *Int J Pediatr Otorhinolaryngol.* 2013;77(5):752–755.
36. Hyzer JM, Milczuk HA, Macarthur CJ, King EF, Quintanilla-Dieck L, Lam DJ. Drug-induced sleep endoscopy findings in children with obstructive sleep apnea with vs without obesity or Down syndrome. *JAMA Otolaryngol Head Neck Surg.* 2021;147(2):175–181.
37. Donnelly LF, Shott SR, LaRose CR, Chini BA, Amin RS. Causes of persistent obstructive sleep apnea despite previous tonsillectomy and adenoidectomy in children with Down syndrome as depicted on static and dynamic cine MRI. *AJR.* 2004;183:175–181.
38. Park JS, Chan DK, Parikh SR, Meyer AK, Rosbe KW. Surgical outcomes and sleep endoscopy for children with sleep-disordered breathing and hypotonia. *Int J Pediatr Otorhinolaryngol.* 2016;90:99–106.
39. Shott SR. Sleep cine magnetic resonance imaging: A dynamic evaluation of the airway. *Oper Tech Otolaryngol.* 2012;23:19–24.
40. Brietzke SE, Gallagher D. The effectiveness of tonsillectomy and adenoidectomy in the treatment of pediatric obstructive sleep apnea/hypopnea syndrome: A meta-analysis. *Otolaryngol Head Neck Surg.* 2006;134(6):979–984.
41. Isaiah A, Kiss E, Olomu P, Koral K, Mitchell RB. Characterization of upper airway obstruction using cine MRI in children with residual obstructive sleep apnea after adenotonsillectomy. *Sleep Med.* 2018;50:79–86.
42. Aurora RN, Zak RS, Karippot A, et al. Practice parameters for the respiratory indications for polysomnography in children. *Sleep.* 2011;34(3):379–388.
43. Mitchell RB, Archer SM, Ishman SL, et al. Clinical practice guideline: Tonsillectomy in children (update). *Otolaryngol Head Neck Surg.* 2019;160(Suppl 1):S1–S42.
44. American Academy of Sleep Medicine. *AASM Manual for the Scoring of Sleep and Associated Events.* Version 2.5.0. American Academy of Sleep Medicine; 2018.
45. American Academy of Sleep Medicine. *Summary of Updates for the Manual for Scoring Sleep and Associated Events.* Version 2.6. American Academy of Sleep Medicine; Jan 2020.
46. Kirk V, Baughn J, D'Andrea L, et al. American Academy of Sleep Medicine position paper for the use of a home sleep apnea test for the diagnosis of OSA in children. *J Clin Sleep Med.* 2017;13(10):1199–1203.
47. Marcus CL, Moore RH, Rosen CL, et al. A randomized trial of adenotonsillectomy for childhood sleep apnea. *N Engl J Med.* 2013;368(25):2366–2376. doi:10.1056/NEJMoa1215881.
48. Fehrm J, Nerfeldt P, Browaldh N, Friberg, D. Effectiveness of adenotonsillectomy vs watchful waiting in young children with mild to moderate obstructive sleep apnea: A randomized clinical trial. *JAMA Otolaryngol Head Neck* Surg. 2020;146(7):647–654.
49. Ye J, Liu H, Zhang G, et al. Outcome of adenotonsillectomy for obstructive sleep apnea syndrome in children. *Ann Otol Rhinol Laryngol.* 2010;119(8):506–513.
50. Mitchell RB, Kelly J. Adenotonsillectomy for obstructive sleep apnea in obese children. *Otolaryngol Head Neck Surg.* 2004;131(1):104–108.
51. Kushida CA, Chediak A, Berry RB, et al.; Positive Airway Pressure Titration Task Force of the American Academy of Sleep Medicine. Clinical guidelines for the manual titration of positive airway pressure in patients with obstructive sleep apnea. *J Clin Sleep Med.* 2008;4(2):157–171.
52. Johnson KG, Johnson DC. Treatment of sleep-disordered breathing with positive airway pressure devices: Technology update. *Med Devices (Auckl).* 2015;8:425–437.
53. Katz SL, MacLean JE, Hoey L et al. Insulin Resistance and Hypertension in Obese Youth With Sleep-Disordered Breathing Treated With Positive Airway Pressure: A Prospective Multicenter Study. *J Clin Sleep Med.* 2017 Sep 15;13(9):1039–1047.

54. Marcus CL, Radcliffe J, Konstantinopoulou S, et al. Effects of positive airway pressure therapy on neurobehavioral outcomes in children with obstructive sleep apnea. *Am J Respir Crit Care Med*. 2012;185(9):998–1003.
55. Marcus CL, Rosen G, Ward SL, et al. Adherence to and effectiveness of positive airway pressure therapy in children with obstructive sleep apnea. *Pediatrics*. 2006;117(3):e442–e451.
56. Roberts SD, Kapadia H, Greenlee G, Chen ML. Midfacial and dental changes associated with nasal positive airway pressure in children with obstructive sleep apnea and craniofacial conditions. *J Clin Sleep Med*. 2016;12(4):469–475.
57. Korayem MM, Witmans M, MacLean J. Craniofacial morphology in pediatric patients with peristent obstructive sleep apnea with or without positive airway pressure therapy: A cross sectional cephalometric comparison with controls. *Am J Orthod Dentofacial Orthop*. 2013;144:78–85.
58. Brouillette RT, Manoukian JJ, Ducharme FM, et al. Efficacy of fluticasone nasal spray for pediatric obstructive sleep apnea. *J Pediatr*. 2001 Jun;138(6):838–844. doi:10.1067/mpd.2001.114474. PMID: 11391326.
59. Kheirandish-Gozal L, Gozal D. Intranasal budesonide treatment for children with mild obstructive sleep apnea syndrome. *Pediatrics*. 2008 Jul;122(1):e149–e155.
60. Goldbart AD, Greenberg-Dotan S, Tal A. Montelukast for children with obstructive sleep apnea: A double-blind, placebo-controlled study. *Pediatrics*. 2012 Sep;130(3):e575–e580.
61. Kheirandish L, Goldbart AD, Gozal D. Intranasal steroids and oral leukotriene modifier therapy in residual sleep-disordered breathing after tonsillectomy and adenoidectomy in children. *Pediatrics*. 2006;117(1):e61–e66.
62. Quintas-Neves M, Preto J, Drummond M. Assessment of bariatric surgery efficacy on obstructive sleep apnea (OSA). *Rev Port Pneumol*. (2006). 2016;22(6):331–336.
63. Villa MP, Malagola C, Pagani J, et al. Rapid maxillary expansion in children with obstructive sleep apnea syndrome: 12-month follow-up. *Sleep Med*. 2007;8:128–134.
64. Miano S, Rizzoli A, Evangelisti M, et al. NREM sleep instability changes following rapid maxillary expansion in children with obstructive apnea sleep syndrome. *Sleep Med*. 2009;10:471–478.
65. Al-Jewair TS, Gaffar BO, Flores-Mir C. Quality assessment of systematic reviews on the efficacy of oral appliance therapy for adult and pediatric sleep-disordered breathing. *J Clin Sleep Med* 2016;12(8):1175–1183.
66. Kang KT, Koltai PJ, Lee CH, Lin MT, Hsu WC. lingual tonsillectomy for treatment of pediatric obstructive sleep apnea: A meta-analysis. *JAMA Otolaryngol Head Neck Surg*. 2017;143(6):561–568. doi:10.1001/jamaoto.2016.4274.
67. Durvasula VS, Lawson BR, Bower CM, Richter GT. Supraglottoplasty outcomes in neurologically affected and syndromic children. *JAMA Otolaryngol Head Neck* Surg. 2014 Aug;140(8):704–711.
68. Kosko JR, Derkay CS. Uvulopalatopharyngoplasty: Treatment of obstructive sleep apnea in neurologically impaired pediatric patients. *J Pediatr Otorhinolaryngol*. 1995;32:241–246.
69. Best DL, Chadha S, Harriman E, Wang CS, Troost JP, Aronovich S. Maxillomandibular advancement effectively treats obstructive sleep apnea in adolescents at short-term follow-up. *Oral Surg Oral Med Oral Pathol Oral Radiol*. 2021;132(4):386–392.
70. Hassan F, Kaplish N. A Novel Treatment Approach for OSA - Overview of Treatment, Including Diagnostic and Patient Criteria and Procedural Terminology Codes. *Chest*. 2021;160(4):1406–1412.
71. Kritzinger FE, Al-Saleh S, Narang I. Descriptive analysis of central sleep apnea in childhood at a single center. *Pediatr Pulmonol*. 2011 Oct;46(10):1023–1030.
72. Weese-Mayer DE, Berry-Kravis EM, Ceccherini I, Keens TG, Loghmanee DA, Ha Trang DE. An official ATS clinical policy statement: Congenital central hypoventilation syndrome. *Am J Respir Crit Care Med*. 2010;181:626–644.
73. Finkel RS, Mercuri E, Meyer OH, et al. Diagnosis and management of spinal muscular atrophy: Part 2: Pulmonary and acute care; medications, supplements and immunizations; other organ systems; and ethics. *Neuromusc Disord*. 2018;28(3);197–207.
74. Schmickl CN, Landry SA, Orr JE, et al. Acetazolamide for obstructive and central sleep apnea: A comprehensive systematic review and meta-analysis. *Chest*. 2020;158(6):2632–2645.
75. Felix O, Amaddeo A, Arroyo JO, et al. Central sleep apnea in children: Experience at a single center. *Sleep Med*. 2016;25:24–28.
76. Tieder JS, Bonkowsky JL, Etzel RA, et al.; Subcommittee on Apparent Life Threatening Events. Brief resolved unexplained events (formerly apparent life-threatening events) and evaluation of lower-risk infants. *Pediatrics*. 2016 May;137(5):e20160590.
77. Ng DK, Chan CH. A review of normal values of infant sleep polysomnography. *Pediatr Neonatol*. 2013 Apr;54(2):82–87.
78. Brockman PE, Poets A, Poets CF. Reference values for respiratory events in overnight polygraphy from infants aged 1 and 3 months. *Sleep Med*. 2013;14:1323–1327.
79. Kato I, Franco P, Groswasser J, Kelmanson I, Togari H, Kahn A. Frequency of obstructive and mixed sleep apneas in 1,023 infants. *Sleep*. 2000;23(4):487–492.
80. Daftarya AS, Jaloua HE, Shivelya L, Slavenb JE, Davis SD. Polysomnography reference values in healthy newborns. *J Clin Sleep Med*. 2019;15(3):437–443.
81. Shellhaas RA, Kenia PV, Hassan F, Barks JD, Kaciroti N, Chervin RD. Sleep-disordered breathing is ubiquitous among newborns with myelomeningocele. *J Pediatrics*. 2018;194:244–247.
82. Matlen LB, Hassan F, Shellhaas RA. Associations between age and sleep apnea risk among newborn infants. *Pediatr Pulmonol*. 2019 Aug;54(8):1297–1303.
83. Zhao J, Gonzalez F, Mu, D. Apnea of prematurity: From cause to treatment. *Eur J Pediatr*. 2011;170:1097–1105.
84. lvaro RE. Control of breathing and apnea of prematurity. *Neo Rev*. 2018;19(4)227.

85. Henderson-Smart DJ, Pettigrew AG, Campbell DJ. Clinical apnea and brain-stem neural function in preterm infants. *N Engl J Med.* 1983 Feb 17;308(7):353–357.
86. Davis RP, Mychaliska GB. Neonatal pulmonary physiology. *Semin Pediatr Surg.* 2013 Nov;22(4):179–184.
87. Eichenwald EC, Committee on Fetus and Newborn, Watterberg KL, et al. Apnea of rematurity. *Pediatrics.* 2016;137(1):e20153757.
88. Birnkrant DJ, Bushby K, Bann CM, et al.; DMD Care Considerations Working Group. Diagnosis and management of Duchenne muscular dystrophy: Part 2: Respiratory, cardiac, bone health, and orthopaedic management. *Lancet Neurol.* 2018 Apr;17(4):347–361.
89. West JB, Luks A. *Respiratory Physiology: The Essentials.* 9th ed. Williams and Wilkins; 2012.
90. Vogels A, Van Den Ende J, Keymolen K, et al. Minimum prevalence, birth incidence and cause of death for Prader–Willi syndrome in Flanders. *Eur J Hum Genet.* 2004;12(3):238–240.
91. Kaplan J, Fredrickson PA, Richardson JW. Sleep and breathing in patients with the Prader-Willi syndrome. *Mayo Clin Proc.* 1991;66:1124–1126.

Chapter 30

Sleep and the Workplace

Salma Batool-Anwar and Lawrence J. Epstein

NECESSITY OF SLEEP

Sleep is an essential behavior for both physical and mental well-being. Although we spend almost one-third of our lives in sleep, there is a lack of understanding about the importance of getting an adequate amount of sleep. Sleep serves many functions, playing a role in development, energy conservation, brain waste clearance, modulation of immune responses, cognition, performance, vigilance, disease, and psychological state.[1] Getting insufficient sleep, whether through not getting enough, or due to a sleep disorder that interferes with sleep continuity, increases the likelihood of negative health consequences, poor performance, impaired work productivity, and accidents.

Appropriate sleep requirements vary across the lifespan, declining from childhood to adulthood among healthy individuals.[2] Recommendations from the American Academy of Sleep Medicine and Sleep Research Society for sufficient sleep range from 12–16[3] hours for newborns to 7 or more[4] hours for adults. However, it is estimated that about a third of U.S. adults sleep less than the recommended amount.[5] Sleep deprivation is prevalent among adolescents, with 72.7% of students reporting an average of <8 hours of sleep on school nights.[6] Moreover, only 65.2% of respondents reported a healthy sleep duration to the 2014 Behavioral Risk Factor Surveillance System (BRFSS) survey.[7]

Sleep disturbances and sleep deprivation are detrimental to population health and have a negative impact on the economic health of society. Over the past few decades, several studies have demonstrated an association between short sleep duration and poor health outcomes. A sleep duration of less than 6 hours has been shown to increase the risk of developing diabetes and impaired glucose tolerance.[8] In addition, poor sleep quality and short sleep duration have been found to be independently associated with the risk of developing coronary heart disease.[9] Moreover, both short and long sleep durations have been linked with increased mortality. A meta-analysis of prospective studies demonstrated that short sleepers (<5–7 hr per night) have a 12% greater risk, and long sleepers (>8 or 9 hr per night) a 30% greater risk, of dying than those sleeping 7–8 hours per night.[10] Sleep disturbances have also been found in psychiatric disorders, and researchers have found an association between sleep disturbance and cognitive impairment.[11]

In addition to these negative health outcomes, chronic sleep loss has serious consequences for performance and safety.[12] Insufficient sleep can impair cognitive performance, increasing the risk of motor vehicle crashes, work-related accidents, industrial and medical errors, and loss of work productivity.[7]

Healthy People 2030 is a Department of Health and Human Services initiative to improve the health and well-being of the American public. One of the objectives of Healthy People 2030 is to increase the proportion of adults who get enough sleep.[13] Therefore, identifying people at risk of insufficient sleep and improving the quality of sleep are vital if we are to achieve this objective.

FACTORS AFFECTING SLEEP DURATION

Sleep duration is influenced by multiple factors, including demographic characteristics such as gender and race/ethnicity, as well as environmental and societal determinants.

Demographic Factors

Several studies have suggested differences in sleep duration between ethnic and racial groups. Additionally, sleep duration is socially driven and subject to environmental and societal factors. Sleep disorders can result in insufficient sleep, and the same factors influencing sleep duration can affect the prevalence of sleep disorders. The work environment, work schedule, and type of work also have a large influence on sleep duration.

Chen et al. reported short sleep duration among Blacks, Hispanics, and Chinese as compared to whites.[14] Cross-sectional data from U.S.-born and foreign-born adults demonstrated that, compared to whites, Blacks and Asians had a higher likelihood of short sleep regardless of their place of birth. In contrast, U.S. born Hispanics but not foreign-born Hispanics had a higher likelihood of short sleep.[15] In another study, the rate of very short sleep (≤4 hours) among Blacks, African Americans, and Asians was at least 2.5 times those of non-Hispanic whites.[16]

Socioeconomic status is thought to play a vital role, as immigrants and racially diverse people may be employed in low-skilled jobs requiring them to work odd shifts.[17] Racial discrimination has also been shown to negatively impact sleep, and the sleep disturbances seen were independent of the effect of race, sociodemographic factors, and mood.[18]

Gender differences in sleep have also been described, with women reporting shorter sleep and increased rates of insomnia.[16,19] In contrast, some sleep disorders are more common among men. Obstructive sleep apnea (OSA) is more prevalent among men and results in increased mortality related to its complications,[20,21] and REM behavior disorder also affects more men than women.

Insufficient sleep is becoming a global public health problem. Studies have suggested that sleep disturbances and sleep deprivation are common among modern societies and there has been a steady decline in sleep duration in industrialized countries.[22] One of the major disruptive changes to sleep is the adoption of 24/7 lifestyles with long and extended work hours. Because of globalization, increased social and commercial interactions, as well as work responsibilities outside of routine work hours, negatively affect sleep duration. People working multiple jobs have also been shown to be at risk for short sleep duration. While work schedule influences sleep duration, the stress of not working can also alter sleep time. In one study, employed individuals reported lower rates of self-reported sleep disturbance compared to the unemployed individuals.[23]

Occupation and Work Schedule Factors

Occupational characteristics, such as industry type and work schedule, also significantly impact sleep duration.

OCCUPATION TYPE

The likelihood of getting insufficient sleep is related to occupation type. A CDC survey[24] ranked occupations by the percentage of workers getting <7 hours of sleep per night and found that the 5 major occupation groups of the Standard Occupational Classification System with the highest prevalence of short sleep duration were production, healthcare support, healthcare practitioners and technicians, food preparation and serving-related, and protective services. Multiple industries, such as the airlines, long-haul trucking, and shift-work manufacturing, have recognized the detrimental effects of sustained sleep disturbance on health[25] and performance. In addition, disturbed sleep has been reported among manual workers as opposed to the managing directors.[26] In a retrospective study, white-collar workers above the age of 75 reported better sleep than blue-collar workers.[27]

SHIFT WORK

Shift work has traditionally been defined as when a portion of the shift occurs between 7 PM and 6 AM.[28] The exact prevalence of shift work is difficult to determine; however, it is estimated that about 20% of the U.S. workforce meets this definition.[29] In addition, about 2.7%–4.3% of U.S. workers have rotating shifts, with their schedule changing every week.[30]

Shift work is more common among service industry workers, that is, law enforcement, food service, fire safety, transportation (both ground and air), and healthcare. Based upon data from U.S. Department of Labor, shift work is classified as: night shift workers, early morning shift workers, evening/afternoon shift workers, rotating shift workers, irregular, and split shift.[31]

The difficulty posed by shift work is due to circadian misalignment. Internal circadian clocks control the timing of human physiology, including when we sleep. Sleep is promoted at night when the levels of melatonin are high. In contrast, wakefulness is promoted during the day when melatonin levels are low.[32] The internal circadian clock is slightly longer than 24 hours in humans[33] but gets reset (termed *entrainment*) to the 24-hour day of the person's environment. Light is the dominant environmental cue that entrains human circadian clocks to the light-dark cycle and 24-hour day. Circadian misalignment occurs when the person tries to do activities counter to their circadian phase. For example, shift workers work during their circadian sleep phase, and sleep during their awake period.

Because shift workers are functioning against their circadian clocks, they are in constant conflict with their endogenous sleep rhythm, resulting in sleep impairments and difficulty with wakefulness. Sleepiness and insomnia are commonly encountered among shift workers. Night shift workers' daytime sleep is approximately 2 hours shorter than when they sleep[34] at night, and they are prone to unintentional sleep while at work. It has been reported that 7% of shift workers fall asleep at work several times per month, increasing the risk of work-related accidents. This is of great concern for safety-sensitive occupations.[35,36] Several epidemiologic studies have established a link between shift work and accidents, with one reporting a 50% increase in road accidents among night shift workers.[37] Similarly, in a large sample of night shift nurses, 79.5% reported at least 1 drowsy driving incident.[38] Studies have also indicated that cardiometabolic stress and cognitive impairments are increased among shift workers.[39] In 2019, the International Agency for Research on Cancer[40] reported that there was sufficient evidence to conclude that night shift work is carcinogenic due to disturbed chronobiology.

IMPACT OF INSUFFICIENT SLEEP ON WORK

Insufficient sleep has been linked to impaired decision-making, and decreased productivity in the workplace. In addition, sleep deprivation imposes substantial economic costs through lost workdays, decreased efficiency, and increased healthcare utilization."

Economics

Sleep-deprived workers have reduced productivity, higher numbers of lost workdays, and increased healthcare costs. A recent study by the Rand Corporation estimated that a worker sleeping 6 hours or less per night loses 6 working days more per year due to absenteeism or presenteeism than a worker sleeping 7–9 hours. This results in a 2.4% higher productivity loss than workers getting sufficient sleep. U.S. companies lose about 1.23 million working days due to insufficient sleep, resulting in an economic loss between $280 billion and $411 billion annually. Another study examining sleep disturbances in >4000 employees demonstrated lower at-work productivity, impaired performance, and poor safety outcomes. While fatigue-related productivity losses for those with insufficient sleep was double the losses for those with good sleep, the greatest economic impact was seen among people with insomnia, with a work productivity loss of $ 3156/year.[41] Increased employer costs of over $3000 for those with insomnia compared to less than $1300 for well-rested employees has also been reported.[41] Additional healthcare costs of $3600–$5200 per person per year have been reported for those with difficulty sleeping.[42] An American Academy of Sleep Medicine report attributed $6.5 billion in workplace accidents, $26.2 billion in motor vehicle crashes, and $86.9 billion to lost productivity among patients with undiagnosed OSA, along with an estimated $30 billion in costs from OSA-related comorbid diseases. In addition to the loss of life and decreased quality of life, occupational injuries negatively impact the health and productivity of a country.[43] The economic burden of work-related injuries has been estimated to account for 3%–10% of gross domestic product (GDP).[43]

Performance and Safety

Lack of adequate sleep has been linked to reduced cognitive performance and chronic sleep deprivation can increase the risk of occupational accidents and errors, particularly in safety-sensitive industries.

PERFORMANCE

The negative impact of sleep deprivation on cognitive function and task performance is well established. Van Dongen et al.[44] found that errors on the Psychomotor Vigilance Test increased linearly with chronic sleep deprivation, with the decrease in performance after 14 days of 6 hours/night of sleep the same as seen after 24 hours of acute sleep deprivation. Subjects displayed increased errors, decreased cognitive accuracy, and reduced speed of response. Sleep deprivation interferes with visual learning and memory consolidation.[45,46] Multiple studies have shown decreases in performance on a variety of work-related tasks, including errors in detection of cardiac arrhythmias on electrocardiograms,[47] reduction in surgical simulator speed,[48] increased medical errors,[49] and impaired performance on driving simulators.[50]

WORKPLACE ACCIDENTS

Sleep plays a vital role among safety-sensitive occupations, and adequate sleep is required for optimal performance. Globally, 250 million occupational injuries and 350,000 fatalities have been reported as work related.[51] Sleep problems have been linked with 13% of work injuries, and studies demonstrate a 1.62 times higher risk of injuries among people with sleep disorders.[52] Researchers have attributed the catastrophes at the nuclear power plants at Three Mile Island in Pennsylvania in 1979 and Chernobyl in the Ukraine in 1986, as well as the Exxon Oil spill in Alaska in 1989, to sleep deprivation.[53,54] Other examples of sleep-related work accidents include: an oil tanker that ran aground off the coast of Rhode Island while under the command of a sleep-deprived shipmaster who had been up for 36 hours; a medical resident in Los Angeles who prescribed a wrong medication that caused a patient to go into coma after working 120 hours per week; and a train crash in Wyoming where the engine of a freight train plowed into the rear of anther train[54] after the engineer and brakeman fell asleep at the controls. According to the U.S. Bureau of Labor Statistics, 2122 deaths in the United States were attributed to transportation-related occupational injuries.[55]

SLEEP AND DRIVING

Transportation accidents are among the most frequent preventable injuries. Motor vehicle injury causes an enormous burden on society and has been found to be one of the leading causes of death and disability globally.[56,57] In 2018, the World Health Organization reported that 1.35 million people die every year from road traffic accidents.[58]

There has been a steady decline in total sleep duration in industrialized countries, with about 20%–35% of adults sleeping <6 hours per 24 hours,[59] thereby increasing the risk of sleepiness while driving. The prevalence of motor vehicle crashes from sleepiness varies between countries. In the United States, the National Transportation Safety Board (NTSB) reported that approximately 42,000 drivers die yearly in traffic-related accidents.[60] Additionally, the National Sleep Foundation (NSF) Poll reported that 51% of adult drivers admitted to driving drowsy, and 17% reported falling asleep at the wheel in the previous year.[61] In a large population-based study conducted in 19 European countries, the prevalence of falling asleep at the wheel was 17%.[62] Similarly, a study of French drivers found that 5.2% of drivers reported a sleep-related accident and 28% reported an episode of severe sleepiness[63] requiring them to stop driving. In a survey of over 4600 male drivers in the United Kingdom, 29% of participants reported feeling sleepy or falling asleep at the wheel at least once in the previous year.[64] The most frequent cause of sleepiness is related to insufficient sleep, either from reduced or fragmented sleep or in the setting of circadian variations in alertness.[65]

In addition to the insufficient sleep, sleep disorders, particularly OSA, have been shown to increase the risk of motor vehicle crashes and work-related accidents. In a study done in Lausanne, Switzerland. Moderate or severe OSA was found to be highly prevalent affecting 20%–30% of men and 10%–15% of women.[66]

A French cohort of OSA patients was investigated between 2007 and 2017; it was found that 35% of the participants reported sleepiness at the wheel, and 20% were involved in a car crash or near-miss accident in the preceding year.[67] Studies have also demonstrated that young drivers not only are at increased risk of serious injuries requiring hospitalization but are over-represented in fatal crashes.[68] Substantial economic cost has also been reported in young drivers' crashes.[69]

Some of the most common signs of sleepy driving are single or repetitive head drops (called microsleeps = lapses of ≥500 ms), heavy eyelids with frequent eye closures, and yawning. These signs are often ignored by the driver, and it has been reported that subjects who fell asleep while driving usually were aware of these signs and had experienced sleepiness while driving prior to the crash.[70]

While there is no paucity of literature on the hazards of drowsy driving, there remains a wide gap between the scientific data and public understanding. A good example of the system's failure is the death of 20-year-old student Maggie McDonald in 1997, who was killed after her car was hit head-on by a man who fell asleep at the wheel after 30 hours without sleep. It was only after the family's intense lobbying and persistence in obtaining justice that the New Jersey legislature enacted "Maggie's Law." This first of its kind legislation authorizes criminal penalties for drowsy drivers who are involved in deadly automobile accidents.

Sleepiness is considered a greater traffic hazard than alcohol. Compared to the level of impairment from alcohol intoxication, it has been shown that decline in cognitive functioning from modest sleep deprivation (20 hr of wakefulness) approaches the level of impairment caused by blood alcohol levels of 0.1%.[71]

This level of impairment has been replicated by other researchers. In one study, cognitive psychomotor performance after 17 hours of wakefulness decreased to a level equivalent to that observed at blood alcohol concentration of 0.05%. Further increasing the sleep deprivation to 24 hours of sustained wakefulness decreased the psychomotor performance to a level equivalent to that observed at blood alcohol concentration of 0.10%.[72] Similar levels of impairment have also been noted in other driving simulation studies.[73]

Impact of Sleep Disorders

Obstructive sleep apnea, a common and yet under-recognized disorder, has been shown to increase morbidity[74] and mortality and increase the number of lost workdays. In a study of public-sector employees, the rate of lost workdays was found to be 1.6 times greater for men and 1.8 times greater for women during the 5 years period preceding the diagnosis of OSA.[75] Similarly, a relationship between excessive daytime sleepiness from untreated sleep apnea and limitation in work performance has been described using a validated measure[76] of sleepiness. In this study, every 1-point increase on the Epworth Sleepiness Scale reported by patients with OSA was associated with an additional 1% of time spent at suboptimal work performance. In addition to excessive daytime sleepiness, other traits of OSA, such as decreased vigilance, difficulty in concentration, and impairment in memory and executive functions, are thought to contribute to work-related injuries.[77] In a meta-analysis, researchers reported a 2-fold increased risk (OR: 2.18; 95% CI: 1.53–3.10; p <0.0001) of occupational injuries among individuals with OSA.[78] Another recent meta-analysis[79] showed that individuals with OSA have a 1.64-fold increased risk of work-related injuries.

Similar impact on job performance, productivity, and workplace accidents has been found for other sleep disorders. Insomnia has been associated with increased lost workdays,[80] lost work performance due to presenteeism,[81] higher rates of workplace accidents[82] and errors, and increased healthcare costs.[83] Narcolepsy patients report greater percentages of absenteeism, presenteeism, overall work impairment, activity impairment, and long-term disability.[84]

JOB-SPECIFIC IMPACT

sleep deprivation can significantly compromise safety, productivity, decision-making, and emotional stability. Here's a breakdown of impairments by job type:

Transportation Industry

Given the impact of insufficient sleep on driving performance, safety in the commercial driving industry is of great concern. The Federal Motor Carrier Safety Administration (FMCSA) and the National Highway Traffic Safety Administration (NHTSA) conducted a multi-year, nationwide study of factors that contribute to truck crashes and found that driver fatigue was a prominent factor. When the driver was at fault in a large truck accident, fatigue was listed as a cause in 13% of the cases.[85]

There are multiple potential contributors to sleepiness in drivers. These include acute sleep deprivation from a prolonged wake period, chronic sleep deprivation from a regularly shortened sleep period, time of day driving, and presence of sleep disorders. The impact of sleep deprivation on performance has been described previously. The impact of time of driving is related to circadian dyssynchrony. Driving at night, during the circadian sleep phase, increases the risk of drowsy driving and accidents. Several studies have shown that the highest number of fatigue-related crashes[86] and fatigue-related single-vehicle truck accidents[87] occur in the early morning hours, even though there are the fewest number of vehicles on the road at that time.

Recently, much interest has focused on screening commercial motor vehicle (CMV) drivers for sleep disorders, particularly OSA. In a survey of >2500 Australian CMV drivers,[88] 24% reported chronic sleepiness and 16% were diagnosed with OSA syndrome, with similar rates found in other countries. Multiple studies have found OSA prevalent among professional drivers (28%–78%)[89–91] and, unfortunately, professional drivers also are at increased risk for OSA due to obesity related to a sedentary lifestyle, as well as a higher proportion of male gender.[92–94]

Treatment of OSA reduces the risk of motor vehicle crashes. A meta-analysis commissioned by the FMCSA[95] found the odds that a driver with untreated OSA will have a crash is 243% higher than a driver without OSA, but treatment of OSA with continuous positive airway pressure (CPAP) lowers crash risk to the same level as seen in individuals without OSA. Although the available data on crash risk among CMV drivers with OSA are limited, the data suggest that OSA treatment reduces crash risk. A large commercial company, Schneider Trucking, instituted a mandatory screening program and offered PAP therapy to drivers confirmed to have OSA. They monitored objective PAP adherence rates and crash rates. Those who were non-adherent to PAP had a crash rate that was 5-fold higher than adherent drivers, whose rates were equivalent to those without OSA.[96]

Programs to screen and treat CMV drivers for OSA have also been shown to be cost effective. One study[97] estimated that not screening or treating commercial drivers costs the trucking industry about $2.4 billion/year, or $689/driver, due to vehicular accidents alone. In a study[98] of commercial drivers undergoing a company-instituted OSA detection and treatment program, CPAP treatment resulted in a reduction of $153,042/100 drivers in healthcare spending for an average savings of $441 per driver per month.

However, implementing screening and treatment programs remains controversial. CMV drivers undergo biannual commercial license examinations by Department of

Transportation–certified medical examiners. The purpose of the examination is to determine if the CMV driver meets the physical qualification standards to operate a CMV. OSA[99] was listed in the *Medical Examiner Handbook* as a respiratory condition that interferes with oxygen exchange and may result in gradual or sudden incapacitation until 2015. In 2011 the FMCSA tasked the Motor Carrier Safety Advisory Committee (MCSAC) and the Medical Review Board (MRB) to develop regulatory guidance about how to address drivers with OSA. In 2012 the MCSAC and MRB found that untreated OSA should preclude unconditional certification. They proposed[100] that CMV drivers be screened for OSA, those with moderate to severe OSA should be treated before being granted a license, and compliance to therapy should be demonstrated at yearly evaluations. The FMCSA proposed regulations in the Federal Register[101] in 2013 but implementation has been blocked.[102] Guidelines for screening and testing for OSA were included in the 2020 edition of the *Medical Examiner Handbook*[103] but this document remains in draft form only. Currently, evaluation, testing, and treatment for OSA are left to the discretion of the medical examiner.

Aviation

Military and civil aviation fatigue has been a topic of discussion for safety issues. Comparable to other shift workers, aviation personnel suffer from chronic fatigue related to unpredictable schedules, work periods requiring night-time alertness, and layovers in different time zones,[104] causing circadian misalignment. Circadian disruptions are also known to have a negative impact on body weight and to increase the risk of metabolic syndrome among pilots. Fatigue has been identified as the probable cause of 21%–23% of major aviation accidents investigations.[104,105] Despite these statistics, United States Air Force aviators averaged only 6.6 (SD 1.8) hours of sleep per night,[106] and 68.3% of commercial airline pilots reported severe fatigue on the Fatigue Severity Scale.[107]

The Federal Aviation Administration (FAA) considers OSA a potentially disqualifying[108] condition for pilots unless treated. Pilots undergo qualifying examinations every 2 years from a certified aviation medical examiner (AME). The AME is tasked with identifying pilots at risk for OSA, according to the Clinical Guidelines[109] of the American Academy of Sleep Medicine (AASM). Ongoing certification[110] is dependent on demonstrating compliance to therapy for OSA.

Law Enforcement

Several studies have shown that sleep disturbances are common among police officers, particularly sleep apnea, insomnia, and shift work disorder. In one study, police officers with increased risk of sleep disorders were found to be more at risk for falling asleep at work and using unnecessary violence against citizens.[111,112]

In a cross-sectional survey of police officers, 40.4% of participants reported at least 1 sleep disorder, and 28.5% reported excessive sleepiness.[112] In another study examining shift work–induced fatigue and critical operational performance using a driving simulator, lane deviation, lapses in attention, and subjective sleepiness were worse after night shift work,[113] indicating that active-duty police officers are susceptible to performance degradation as a consequence of working nights. The Buffalo Cardio-Metabolic Occupational Police Stress study revealed that midnight shift workers had significantly higher risk of injury compared to those who predominantly worked day or afternoon shift.[114] Moreover, officers working extended hours have experienced significant decrease in sleep duration and sleep quality, as well as suffering from impaired cognitive function and poor quality of life.[115] There is an increase in the rates of police vehicle collisions[116] between the hours of 12:00 AM and 3:00 AM, coinciding with lowered circadian alertness levels. Like other professionals, many police officers work second jobs or overtime to supplement their income at the expense of their sleep.

Healthcare

Healthcare workers suffer from fatigue related to poor sleep quality, which contributes to poor outcomes.[117] An astonishing number of patients are annually affected by medical errors, impacting clinical outcomes and increasing healthcare costs.[118]

RESIDENTS' WORK HOURS

Due to the nature of healthcare delivery, healthcare workers' schedules include rotating shifts. Medical residents have chronic and acute sleep deprivation due to extended training hours, and there is evidence that sleep deprivation negatively impacts the performance of medical residents. The loss of sleep among residents is cumulative and results in chronic sleep deprivation. In addition, interruptions during night call result in sleep inertia, which can impair performance for up to 30 minutes after waking.[119] Studies have suggested that sleep-deprived residents make errors and can compromise patient safety. In a randomized controlled trial, residents working frequent 24-hour shifts were found to make 36% more serious errors compared to those working less than 16 hours.[120]

In 2003, work-hour regulations were implemented by the Accreditation Council for Graduate Medical Education (ACGME).[121] Work-hour limits have been shown to decrease patients' intensive care unit (ICU) stay, improve discharge from the hospital, and decrease pharmacy intervention to prevent errors.[122] These improved patient outcomes were thought to be from reduced fatigue among the house staff. Similarly, the implementation of work-hour regulations have decreased short-term mortality among high-risk medical patients.[123]

NURSES

Nurses constitute the largest group of healthcare workers and are responsible for the majority of patient care. The risk for making critical safety mistakes in medication administration, clinical judgment, or failing to intercept errors by other healthcare teams is high among fatigued nurses.[124] Several studies have reported that nurses often sleep less than the recommended amounts, interfering with their health and performance at work.[125,126] High levels of sleepiness on at least 1 of 3 consecutive 12-hour shifts were reported among 45% of hospital nurses.[127] In one study, 65% of the participating nurses endorsed exhaustion at work, and 20% admitted to falling asleep during the shift.[128] In another cross-sectional study, rotating night-shift nurses reported lower scores in sleep quality and quantity compared to day-shift nurses and particularly suffered from sleepiness during morning shift (p <0.001).[129] Similarly, another study suggested that nurses struggling to stay awake at work are more likely to report an error (OR: 2.4; 95% CI: 1.17, 4.91).[130]

In line with the effect of residents' work hours on performance, nurses have also shown lower scores on intellectual ability, mental speed, and reaction times after performing a night shift.[131] These effects were thought to be due to alterations in sleep-wake rhythm affecting the executive functions. Although work hours are regulated for truck drivers, locomotive engineers, pilots, and medical residents to protect the public from fatigue-related errors, there are currently no limitations on work hours for nurses[132] or attending physicians.

First Responders

Sleep deprivation significantly impairs the performance of first responders, affecting reaction time, decision-making, and situational awareness. Chronic sleep loss in this population has also been associated with increased risk of burnout, mental health issues, and reduced operational effectiveness.

EMERGENCY MEDICAL SERVICES (EMS)

EMS workers provide medical care and emergency transportation 24 hours a day. As their work involves operating ambulances at high speeds and stabilizing patients under uncontrolled settings, EMS workers are at increased risk of workplace injury.[133] Mental and physical fatigue among EMS workers has been linked to personal injury, patient care errors, and adverse events.[134] Consistent with other shift-work groups, EMS personnel have disrupted sleep and circadian rhythm patterns contributing to fatigue.[135] As a result, EMS workers suffer from work-related fatigue and generally have poor sleep quality.[136]

FIREFIGHTERS

Similar to the EMS work schedules, the firefighters also do not get adequate amounts of sleep during their shift work.[137] Poor sleep among firefighters affects their psychological well-being and is a contributor to work stress.[138] Firefighters[139] demonstrate a significant decrease in alertness and increase in reaction times over a 24-hour shift. Additionally, firefighters working a 48/96 schedule (a 6-day rotation in which they work 48 hours consecutively, followed by 96 hours off)[140] demonstrate increases in disciplinary measures, use of sick leave, and traffic collisions.

IMPACT OF COVID-19 PANDEMIC ON SLEEP AND WORK

The COVID-19 pandemic not only has affected physical health but also has contributed to the development of mental health problems and sleep disturbances that interfere with work. Several studies have reported a major impact on daily functioning and nighttime sleep.[141,142] Sleep disorders such as insomnia, circadian rhythm sleep disorders, and sleep fragmentation have been seen at higher rates during the COVID-19 pandemic. Sleep disturbances can potentially be a *direct* consequence of SARS-CoV-2 infection, or an *indirect* consequence of the mitigation measures to prevent the spread of SARS-CoV-2 infection. The isolation and quarantine used to combat the spread of the virus resulted in disturbed sleep quality during the pandemic. Other factors affecting sleep during the pandemic include excessive time in bed, stress from work, health concern, lack of preparedness for sudden lockdowns, and uncertainly about the future.

Although the risk of COVID-19 exposure varies, nearly all occupations are affected. Increasing job strain from high psychological demands or low decision latitudes negatively impact sleep.[143] Healthcare workers are among the highest risk category for developing psychological distress.[144] Workers from other occupations have also been affected, either from job loss or increased risk of viral infection. Sudden loss of job has been shown to be traumatic for many individuals and leads to negative emotions.[145,146]

First responders are particularly vulnerable to psychological distress during pandemics, which can elicit post-traumatic stress disorder under exceptionally stressful events.[147] Several cross-sectional studies have documented the psychological impact of the COVID-19 pandemic on front-line health workers.[148] A systematic meta-analysis of 13 cross-sectional studies has demonstrated sleep disturbances in 38.9% of female nurses compared to male nurses and physicians.[149] In another study, healthcare workers were more likely to experience poor sleep quality and develop psychological issues compared to the general population.[150] Furthermore, 6–12 months after recovering from COVID-19, healthcare workers continue to show disturbed sleep.[151–153] Healthcare workers had a prevalence of insomnia of 36% during the pandemic using the Insomnia Severity Index. Similarly, increased insomnia levels of 60% have been demonstrated among EMS workers.[154]

Nurses in particular are at increased risk of suffering from insomnia due to the nature of their job: increased responsibility, heavy workload, and need to work in shifts.[155] During the pandemic an incidence of insomnia as high as 64.1% has been reported among front-line nurses. Increased fatigue, stress, and the fear of COVID-19 were thought to be the predicting factors of insomnia in this study.

The change in work timing, reduction in travel time as a result of pandemic-related quarantines, and shift to working at home benefited a segment of the population. A study[156] using smartphone data found that average estimated sleep duration increased in the months after the onset of the COVID-19 pandemic. Another study found that during the COVID-19 lockdown people went to bed and woke up later, which could specifically benefit those with circadian rhythm disorders such as delayed sleep wake phase disorder.[157]

Fatigue Management

While there is no substitute for getting an adequate amount of sleep, there are strategies that can be implemented to reduce the impact of unavoidable sleep deprivation due to work schedules. Multiple industries[158] have implemented fatigue risk management systems to try to reduce injuries, accidents, and decrements in performance, including the mining, healthcare, pipeline and hazardous materials, and petrochemical and refining industries.

Box 30.1 Elements of a Fatigue Management Program (FMP)

- Fatigue and risk assessment
- Detailed management plan
- Commitment of appropriate resources
- Educate work personnel
- Implement FMP
  - Schedule optimization
  - Countermeasures
  - Sleep disorders management
- Monitor
- Review and revise

The elements of a fatigue management program (FMP) are listed in Box 30.1. It should start with a fatigue and risk assessment. Review work schedules, number and timing of shift changes, and how the work environment contributes to fatigue and accident risk. Identify past patterns of accidents and injuries to look for contributing factors and ongoing risk. Once the problems have been identified, develop a comprehensive management plan that addresses as many of the issues as possible. The American College of Occupational and Environmental Medicine has published[158] a detailed methodology for conducting such a review and planning program. Once the plan is developed, ensure that appropriate resources are committed to allow completion of the program. Before initiating the FMP, educate workers and management on the rationale, processes, and expectations for the program. Implementation should be accompanied by a reporting system to identify problems and allow auditing of the impact of the changes. Finally, review and reassessment should be done at regular intervals to see what has worked and what part of the plan needs modification.

A number of fatigue countermeasures can be implemented. First, optimization of worker staffing levels and length and direction of shift schedules can improve fatigue-related outcomes. An assessment of staffing needs may reveal understaffing that can lead to longer shifts and more overtime that result in increased fatigue[159] and decreased performance. Reducing shift length improves worker safety. A review[160] that evaluated different durations of shift work found a significant reduction in negative outcomes for shifts <24 hours compared to those >24 hours. Further comparison of 8-hour versus 12-hour shifts identified no convincing pattern of evidence in favor of specific shift durations. The direction of rotating shifts also affects sleep deprivation and fatigue. A study[161] comparing nurses working different schedules found that fast forward-rotating shifts (i.e., morning to afternoon to night) were associated with lower levels of tiredness and sleepiness and higher levels of sustained attention compared with backward-rotating shifts (i.e., afternoon to morning to night), though both shift-rotation models were negatively associated with health and cognitive performance.

Specific countermeasures can also be used during shifts to combat decreased alertness. Bright[162] light exposure can reduce the likelihood of falling asleep during a night shift and reduce awakenings during daytime sleep. In-shift naps[163] shorter than 1 hour improve alertness during night shifts but can produce sleep inertia upon awakening. Caffeine is a stimulant[164] that suppresses adenosine-mediated sleep drive and improves mood and performance, increases alertness, and reduces fatigue. A study[165] comparing caffeine and napping found that 200 mg of caffeine and a 30-minute nap produced similar improvements in middle of the night driving simulator performance compared to placebo. To evaluate a combined intervention, one group[166] compared nighttime cognitive performance in subjects who had a pre-work nap, 4 mg/kg of caffeine, both caffeine and a nap, or a placebo, and found the combination resulted in improved performance compared to either napping or caffeine alone, both of which were better than placebo. Pharmacotherapy to maintain alertness during night shifts or improve post-shift sleep has not been extensively studied. A Cochrane review[167] concluded that, based on limited data, both modafinil and armodafinil increase alertness and reduce sleepiness in employees who suffer from shift-work sleep disorder, but they can be associated with adverse events, predominantly headache and blood pressure increases. In a single trial, hypnotic medication did not result in significantly longer daytime sleep length compared to placebo.

Because of the known negative impact of sleep disorders on performance and safety, a screening program for sleep disorders should be included in an FMP. Screening can be done through questionnaires, sleep wellness programs, or during certification examinations. When selecting a screening program, it is important to understand the dynamics and concerns of the employees. Concern over impact on employment can lead to underreporting, a worrisome problem when alertness is critical to the mission. For example, one study[168] of truck drivers undergoing certification examinations found that none responded positively to questions about OSA symptoms on their certification questionnaire, but 13% were found to have OSA by sleep testing that was triggered by a screening evaluation[169] based on objective findings such as body mass index (BMI) and hypertension.

CONCLUSION

Obtaining an adequate amount of sleep is necessary for optimal alertness, performance, and safety. Inability to get sufficient sleep can be due to work type or schedule, socioeconomic factors, timing of the sleep period, or the presence of sleep disorders. Insufficient sleep contributes to decreased performance, increased accidents, decreased productivity, and higher healthcare costs. Implementation of an FMP can improve productivity and safety. Including a sleep disorders screening program can further maximize the benefits of an FMP.

REFERENCES

1. Zielinski MR, McKenna JT, McCarley RW. Functions and mechanisms of sleep. *AIMS Neurosci*. 2016;3:67.
2. Ohayon MM, Carskadon MA, Guilleminault C, Vitiello MV. Meta-analysis of quantitative sleep parameters from childhood to old age in healthy individuals: Developing normative sleep values across the human lifespan. *Sleep*. 2004;27:1255–1273.
3. Paruthi S, Brooks LJ, D'Ambrosio C, et al. Recommended amount of sleep for pediatric populations: A consensus statement of the American Academy of Sleep Medicine. *J Clin Sleep Med*. 2016;12:785–786.
4. Panel CC, Watson NF, Badr MS, et al. Recommended amount of sleep for a healthy adult: A joint consensus statement of the American Academy of Sleep Medicine and Sleep Research Society. *J Clin Sleep Med*. 2015;11:591–592.
5. Institute of Medicine (U.S.) Committee on Sleep Medicine and Research; Colten HR, Altevogt BM, eds. *Sleep Disorders and Sleep Deprivation: An Unmet Public Health Problem*. National Academies Press; 2006. https://www.ncbi.nlm.nih.gov/books/NBK19961. Accessed April 11, 2022.
6. Wheaton AG, Jones SE, Cooper AC, Croft JB. Short sleep duration among middle school and high school students—United States, 2015. *MMWR*. 2018;67:85.
7. Liu Y, Wheaton AG, Chapman DP, Cunningham TJ, Lu H, Croft JB. Prevalence of healthy sleep duration among adults—United States, 2014. *MMWR*. 2016;65:137–141.
8. Gottlieb DJ, Punjabi NM, Newman AB, et al. Association of sleep time with diabetes mellitus and impaired glucose tolerance. *Arch Intern Med*. 2005;165:863–867.
9. Lao XQ, Liu X, Deng H-B, et al. Sleep quality, sleep duration, and the risk of coronary heart disease: A prospective cohort study with 60,586 adults. *J Clin Sleep Med*. 2018;14:109–117.
10. Cappuccio FP, D'Elia L, Strazzullo P, Miller MA. Sleep duration and all-cause mortality: A systematic review and meta-analysis of prospective studies. *Sleep*. 2010;33:585–592.
11. Vitiello MV, Borson S. Sleep disturbances in patients with Alzheimer's disease. CNS Drugs. 2001;15:777–796.
12. Institute of Medicine (U.S.) Committee on Sleep Medicine and Research; Colten HR, Altevogt BM, eds. *Sleep Disorders and Sleep Deprivation: An Unmet Public Health Problem*. National Academies Press; 2006:3, Extent and health consequences of chronic sleep loss and sleep disorders. https://www.

ncbi.nlm.nih.gov/books/NBK19961. Accessed April 10, 2022.
13. https://health.gov/healthypeople/objectives-and-data/browse-objectives/sleep/increase-proportion-adults-who-get-enough-sleep-sh-03. Accessed January 17, 2022.
14. Chen X, Wang R, Zee P, et al. Racial/ethnic differences in sleep disturbances: The Multi-Ethnic Study of Atherosclerosis (MESA). *Sleep*. 2015;38:877–888.
15. Cunningham TJ, Wheaton AG, Ford ES, Croft JB. Racial/ethnic disparities in self-reported short sleep duration among US-born and foreign-born adults. *Ethn Health*. 2016;21:628–638.
16. Whinnery J, Jackson N, Rattanaumpawan P, Grandner MA. Short and long sleep duration associated with race/ethnicity, sociodemographics, and socioeconomic position. *Sleep*. 2014;37:601–611.
17. Chung-Bridges K, Muntaner C, Fleming LE, et al. Occupational segregation as a determinant of US worker health. *Am J Ind Med*. 2008;51:555–567.
18. Grandner MA, Hale L, Jackson N, Patel NP, Gooneratne NS, Troxel WM. Perceived racial discrimination as an independent predictor of sleep disturbance and daytime fatigue. *Behav Sleep Med*. 2012;10:235–249.
19. Green MJ, Espie CA, Hunt K, Benzeval M. The longitudinal course of insomnia symptoms: Inequalities by sex and occupational class among two different age cohorts followed for 20 years in the west of Scotland. *Sleep*. 2012;35:815–823.
20. Peppard PE, Young T, Barnet JH, Palta M, Hagen EW, Hla KM. Increased prevalence of sleep-disordered breathing in adults. *Am J Epidemiol*. 2013;177:1006–1014.
21. Punjabi NM, Caffo BS, Goodwin JL, et al. Sleep-disordered breathing and mortality: A prospective cohort study. *PLoS Med*. 2009;6:e1000132.
22. Ford ES, Cunningham TJ, Croft JB. Trends in self-reported sleep duration among US adults from 1985 to 2012. *Sleep*. 2015;38:829–832.
23. Grandner MA, Patel NP, Gehrman PR, et al. Who gets the best sleep? Ethnic and socioeconomic factors related to sleep complaints. *Sleep Med*. 2010;11:470–478.
24. Shockey TM, Wheaton AG. Short sleep duration by occupation group—29 states, 2013–2014. *MMWR*. 2017;66:207.
25. Cappuccio F, Miller MA, Lockley SW. *Sleep, Health, and Society: From Aetiology to Public Health*. Oxford University Press; 2010.
26. Partinen M, Eskelinen L, Tuomi K. Complaints of insomnia in different occupations. *Scand J Work Environ Health*. 1984:467–469.
27. Geroldi C, Frisoni GB, Rozzini R, De Leo D, Trabucchi M. Principal lifetime occupation and sleep quality in the elderly. *Gerontology*. 1996;42:163–169.
28. Caruso CC. Negative impacts of shiftwork and long work hours. *Rehabil Nurs*. 2014;39:16–25.
29. McMenamin TM. A time to work: Recent trends in shift work and flexible schedules. *Monthly Lab Rev*. 2007;130:3.
30. U.S. Congress. *Biological Rhythms: Implications for the Worker: New Developments in Neuroscience*. U.S. Government Printing Office; 2005.
31. https://www.bls.gov/news.release/flex2.t07.htm. Accessed April 29, 2022.
32. Dijk D-J, Edgar DM. Circadian and homeostatic control of wakefulness and sleep. *Lung Biol Health Dis*. 1999;133:111–147.
33. Czeisler CA, Duffy JF, Shanahan TL, et al. Stability, precision, and near-24-hour period of the human circadian pacemaker. *Science*. 1999;284:2177–2181.
34. Tilley AJ, Wilkinson R, Warren P, Watson B, Drud M. The sleep and performance of shift workers. *Hum Factors*. 1982;24:629–641.
35. Åkerstedt T. Shift work and disturbed sleep/wakefulness. *Occup Med*. 2003;53:89–94.
36. Ohayon MM, Smolensky MH, Roth T. Consequences of shiftworking on sleep duration, sleepiness, and sleep attacks. *Chronobiol Int*. 2010;27:575–589.
37. Smith L, Folkard S, Poole C. Increased injuries on night shift. *Lancet*. 1994;344:1137–1139.
38. Scott LD, Hwang W-T, Rogers AE, Nysse T, Dean GE, Dinges DF. The relationship between nurse work schedules, sleep duration, and drowsy driving. *Sleep*. 2007;30:1801–1807.
39. Kecklund G, Axelsson J. Health consequences of shift work and insufficient sleep. *BMJ*. 2016;355.
40. Ward EM, Germolec D, Kogevinas M, et al. Carcinogenicity of night shift work. *Lancet Oncol*. 2019;20:1058–1059.
41. Rosekind MR, Gregory KB, Mallis MM, Brandt SL, Seal B, Lerner D. The cost of poor sleep: workplace productivity loss and associated costs. *J Occup Environ Med*. 2010 Jan;52(1):91–98.
42. Hui S-KA, Grandner MA. Associations between poor sleep quality and stages of change of multiple health behaviors among participants of employee wellness program. *Prev Med Rep*. 2015;2:292–299.
43. Tompa E, Mofidi A, van den Heuvel S, et al. Economic burden of work injuries and diseases: A framework and application in five European Union countries. *BMC Public Health*. 2021;21:1–10.
44. Van Dongen H, Maislin G, Mullington JM, Dinges DF. The cumulative cost of additional wakefulness: Dose-response effects on neurobehavioral functions and sleep physiology from chronic sleep restriction and total sleep deprivation. Sleep. 2003;26:117–126.
45. Stickgold R, James L, Hobson JA. Visual discrimination learning requires sleep after training. *Nat Neurosci*. 2000;3:1237–1238.
46. Walker MP, Stickgold R. Sleep-dependent learning and memory consolidation. *Neuron*. 2004;44:121–133.
47. Friedman RC, Bigger JT, Kornfeld DS. The intern and sleep loss. *N Engl J Med*. 1971 Jul 22;285(4):201–203.
48. Grantcharov TP, Bardram L, Peter F-J, Rosenberg J. Laparoscopic performance after one night on call in a surgical department: Prospective study. *BMJ*. 2001;323:1222–1223.
49. Barger LK, Ayas NT, Cade BE, et al. 2006. Impact of extended-duration shifts on medical errors, adverse events, and attentional failures. *PLoS Med*. 2006 Dec;3:e487.
50. Jackson ML, Croft RJ, Kennedy G, Owens K, Howard ME. Cognitive components of simulated driving performance: Sleep loss effects and predictors. *Accid Anal Prev*. 2013;50:438–444.
51. Hämäläinen P, Takala J, Saarela KL. Global estimates of occupational accidents. *Safety Sci*. 2006;44:137–156.
52. Uehli K, Mehta AJ, Miedinger D, et al. Sleep problems and work injuries: A systematic review and meta-analysis. *Sleep Med Rev*. 2014;18:61–73.

53. Lamberg L. Sleep deprivation recognized as public-safety issue. *Psychiatr News*. 2005;40(12):22–22.
54. Vila B, Morrison GB, Kenney DJ. Improving shift schedule and work-hour policies and practices to increase police officer performance, health, and safety. *Police Q*. 2002;5:4–24.
55. U.S. Bureau of Labor Statistics. Census of fatal occupational injuries. 2020. https://www.bls.gov/iif/oshcfoi1.htm. Accessed January 17, 2022.
56. Murray CJ, Lopez AD. Alternative projections of mortality and disability by cause 1990–2020: Global Burden of Disease Study. *Lancet*. 1997;349:1498–1504.
57. Connor J, Whitlock G, Norton R, Jackson R. The role of driver sleepiness in car crashes: a systematic review of epidemiological studies. *Accid Anal Prev*. 2001;33:31–41.
58. World Health Organization. *Global Status Report on Road Safety 2018: Summary*. World Health Organization; 2018.
59. Léger D, Pepin E, Caetano G. The economic burden of sleepy driving. *Sleep Med Clin*. 2019;14:423–429.
60. Powell NB, Chau JK. Sleepy driving. *Med Clin North Am*. 2010;94:531–540.
61. Drobnich D. A National Sleep Foundation's Conference summary: The National Summit to Prevent Drowsy Driving and a new call to action. *Ind Health*. 2005;43:197–200.
62. Gonçalves M, Amici R, Lucas R, et al. Sleepiness at the wheel across Europe: A survey of 19 countries. *J Sleep Res*. 2015;24:242–253.
63. Sagaspe P, Taillard J, Bayon V, et al. Sleepiness, near-misses and driving accidents among a representative population of French drivers. *J Sleep Res*. 2010;19:578–584.
64. Maycock G. Sleepiness and driving: The experience of UK car drivers. *Accid Anal Prev*. 1997;29:453–462.
65. Drake C, Roehrs T, Breslau N, et al. The 10-year risk of verifed motor vehicle crashes in relation to physiologic sleepiness. *Sleep*. 2010;33:745–752.
66. Heinzer R, Vat S, Marques-Vidal P, et al. Prevalence of sleep-disordered breathing in the general population: The HypnoLaus study. *Lancet Respir Med*. 2015;3:310–318.
67. Sabil A, Bignard R, Gervès-Pinquié C, et al. Risk factors for sleepiness at the wheel and sleep-related car accidents among patients with obstructive sleep apnea: Data from the French Pays de la Loire Sleep Cohort. Nature Sci Sleep. 2021;13:1737.
68. Williams AF. Teenage drivers: patterns of risk. *J Safety Res*. 2003;34:5–15.
69. Watling CN. Young drivers who continue to drive while sleepy: What are the associated sleep- and driving-related factors? *J Sleep Res*. 2020;29:e12900.
70. Reyner L, Horne JA. Falling asleep whilst driving: Are drivers aware of prior sleepiness? *Int J Legal Med*. 1998;111:120–123.
71. Williamson AM, Feyer A-M, Mattick RP, Friswell R, Finlay-Brown S. Developing measures of fatigue using an alcohol comparison to validate the effects of fatigue on performance. *Accid Anal Prev*. 2001;33:313–326.
72. Dawson D, Reid K. Fatigue, alcohol and performance impairment. *Nature*. 1997;388:235–235.
73. Powell NB, Schechtman KB, Riley RW, Li K, Troell R, Guilleminault C. The road to danger: The comparative risks of driving while sleepy. *Laryngoscope*. 2001;111:887–893.
74. Yaggi HK, Concato J, Kernan WN, Lichtman JH, Brass LM, Mohsenin V. Obstructive sleep apnea as a risk factor for stroke and death. *N Engl J Med*. 2005;353:2034–2041.
75. Sjösten N, Vahtera J, Salo P, et al. Increased risk of lost workdays prior to the diagnosis of sleep apnea. *Chest*. 2009;136:130–136.
76. Mulgrew A, Ryan C, Fleetham J, et al. The impact of obstructive sleep apnea and daytime sleepiness on work limitation. *Sleep Med*. 2007;9:42–53.
77. Day R, Gerhardstein R, Lumley A, Roth T, Rosenthal L. The behavioral morbidity of obstructive sleep apnea. *Prog Cardiovasc Dis*. 1999;41:341–354.
78. Garbarino S, Guglielmi O, Campus C, et al. Screening, diagnosis, and management of obstructive sleep apnea in dangerous-goods truck drivers: To be aware or not? *Sleep Med*. 2016;25:98–104.
79. Chou KT, Tsai YL, Yeh WY, Chen YM, Huang N, Cheng HM. Risk of work-related injury in workers with obstructive sleep apnea: A systematic review and meta-analysis. *J Sleep Res*. 2022;31:e13446.
80. Ozminkowski RJ, Wang S, Walsh JK. The direct and indirect costs of untreated insomnia in adults in the United States. *Sleep*. 2007;30:263–273.
81. Kessler RC, Berglund PA, Coulouvrat C, et al. Insomnia and the performance of US workers: Results from the America insomnia survey. *Sleep*. 2011;34:1161–1171.
82. Shahly V, Berglund PA, Coulouvrat C, et al. The associations of insomnia with costly workplace accidents and errors: Results from the America Insomnia Survey. *Arch Gen Psychiatry*. 2012;69:1054–1063.
83. Wickwire EM, Tom SE, Scharf SM, Vadlamani A, Bulatao IG, Albrecht JS. Untreated insomnia increases all-cause health care utilization and costs among Medicare beneficiaries. *Sleep*. 2019;42:zsz007.
84. Flores NM, Villa KF, Black J, Chervin RD, Witt EA. The humanistic and economic burden of narcolepsy. *J Clin Sleep Med*. 2016;12:401–407.
85. U.S. Department of Transportation and Federal Motor Carrier Safety Administration. *Report to Congress on the Large Truck Causation Crash Study*. MC-R/MC-RIA; 2006. https://www.fmcsa.dot.gov/safety/research-and-analysis/report-congress-large-truck-crash-causation-study. Accessed April 25, 2022.
86. Pack AI, Pack AM, Rodgman E, Cucchiara A, Dinges DF, Schwab CW. Characteristics of crashes attributed to the driver having fallen asleep. *Accid Anal Prev*. 1995;27:769–775.
87. National Transportation Safety Board. *Safety Study: Factors That Affect Fatigue in Heavy Truck Accidents*. Vol 1: *Analysis* (SS-1995/01). NTSB; 1995. https://www.ntsb.gov/safety/safety-studies/Documents/SS9501.pdf. Accessed April 25, 2022.
88. Howard ME, Desai AV, Grunstein RR, et al. Sleepiness, sleep-disordered breathing, and accident risk factors in commercial vehicle drivers. *Am J Respir Crit Care Med*. 2004;170:1014–1021.
89. Kales SN, Straubel M. Obstructive sleep apnea in North American commercial drivers. *Ind Health*. 2014;52(1):13–24.
90. Pack AI, Dinges D, Maislin G. A study of prevalence of sleep apnea among commercial truck drivers: United States. Federal Motor Carrier Safety Administration; 2002.

91. Stoohs RA, Itoi A, Guilleminault C, Dement WC. Sleep and sleep-disordered breathing in commercial long-haul truck drivers. *Chest*. 1995;107:1275–1282.
92. Mohebbi I, Saadat S, Aghassi M, Shekari M, Matinkhah M, Sehat S. Prevalence of metabolic syndrome in Iranian professional drivers: Results from a population based study of 12,138 men. *PLoS One*. 2012;7:e31790.
93. Wong CK, Fung CS, Siu S-C, et al. The impact of work nature, lifestyle, and obesity on health-related quality of life in Chinese professional drivers. *J Occup Environ Med*. 2012;54(8):989–994.
94. Xie W, Chakrabarty S, Levine R, Johnson R, Talmage JB. Factors associated with obstructive sleep apnea among commercial motor vehicle drivers. *J Occup Environ Med*. 2011;53(2):169–173.
95. Tregear S, Reston J, Schoelles K, Phillips B. Continuous positive airway pressure reduces risk of motor vehicle crash among drivers with obstructive sleep apnea: Systematic review and meta-analysis. *Sleep*. 2010;33:1373–1380.
96. Burks SV, Anderson JE, Bombyk M, et al. Nonadherence with employer-mandated sleep apnea treatment and increased risk of serious truck crashes. *Sleep*. 2016;39:967–975.
97. Gurubhagavatula I, Nkwuo JE, Maislin G, Pack AI. Estimated cost of crashes in commercial drivers supports screening and treatment of obstructive sleep apnea. *Accid Anal Prev*. 2008;40:104–115.
98. Burks SV, Anderson JE, Panda B, et al. Employer-mandated obstructive sleep apnea treatment and healthcare cost savings among truckers. *Sleep*. 2020;43(4):1–15. doi:10.1093/sleep/zsz262.
99. National Registry of Certified Medical Examiners. *Medical* Examiner Handbook. Federal Motor Carrier Safety Administration (FMCSA); 2015. https://www.fmcsa.dot.gov/sites/fmcsa.dot.gov/files/docs/mission/advisory-committees/mrb/83401/fmcsamedicalexaminerhandbook_0.pdf. Accessed April 27, 2022.
100. Federal Motor Carrier Safety Administration. February 6, 2012 MCSAC and MRB Task 11-05-Final Report on Obstructive Sleep Apnea (OSA). 2012. https://www.fmcsa.dot.gov/february-6-2012-mcsac-and-mrb-task-11-05-final-report-obstructive-sleep-apnea-osa. Accessed April 27, 2022.
101. Federal Motor Carrier Safety Administration. Proposed recommendations on obstructive sleep apnea. *Federal Register*. 2012 Apr 20;77(77). https://www.federalregister.gov/documents/2012/04/20/2012-9555/proposed-recommendations-on-obstructive-sleep-apnea. Accessed April 29, 2022.
102. Federal Motor Carrier Safety Administration. Proposed recommendations on obstructive sleep apnea [FMCSA–2012–0102]. *Federal Register*. 2012;77(82):25226–25227. https://www.federalregister.gov/documents/2012/04/27/2012-10176/proposed-recommendations-on-obstructive-sleep-apnea. Accessed April 23, 2022.
103. Federal Motor Carrier Safety Administration (FMCSA), National Registry of Certified Medical Examiners Program. *Medical Examiner Handbook*. 2020 edition. https://www.fmcsa.dot.gov/advisory-committees/mrb/draft-fmcsa-medical-examiner-handbook-4-23-2020. Accessed April 27, 2022.
104. Caldwell JA. Crew schedules, sleep deprivation, and aviation performance. *Curr Dir Psychol Sci*. 2012;21:85–89.
105. Marcus JH, Rosekind MR. Fatigue in transportation: NTSB investigations and safety recommendations. *Injury Prev*. 2017;23:232–238.
106. Tvaryanas AP, Thompson WT. Fatigue in military aviation shift workers: Survey results for selected occupational groups. *Aviat Space Environ Med*. 2006;77:1166–1170.
107. Aljurf TM, Olaish AH, BaHammam AS. Assessment of sleepiness, fatigue, and depression among Gulf Cooperation Council commercial airline pilots. *Sleep Breath*. 2018;22:411–419.
108. Federal Aviation Administration. *Guide for Aviation Medical Examiners*. Oct 2023. https://www.faa.gov/about/office_org/headquarters_offices/avs/offices/aam/ame/guide/special_iss/all_classes/. Accessed May 19, 2025.
109. Epstein LJ, Kristo D, Strollo PJ Jr, et al. Clinical guideline for the evaluation, management and long-term care of obstructive sleep apnea in adults. *J Clin Sleep Med*. 2009;5:263–276.
110. Federal Aviation Administration. *Decision Considerations Disease Protocols: Obstructive Sleep Apnea (OSA)*. Oct 2023. https://www.faa.gov/about/office_org/headquarters_offices/avs/offices/aam/ame/guide/dec_cons/disease_prot/osa/. Accessed May 19, 2025.
111. Grandner MA, Pack AI. Sleep disorders, public health, and public safety. *JAMA*. 2011;306.23 (2011):2616–2617.
112. Rajaratnam SM, Barger LK, Lockley SW, et al. Sleep disorders, health, and safety in police officers. *JAMA*. 2011;306:2567–2578.
113. Waggoner LB, Grant DA, Van Dongen HP, Belenky G, Vila B. A combined field and laboratory design for assessing the impact of night shift work on police officer operational performance. *Sleep*. 2012;35:1575–1577.
114. Violanti JM, Fekedulegn D, Andrew ME, et al. Shift work and the incidence of injury among police officers. *Am J Ind Med*. 2012;55:217–27.
115. Bell LB, Virden TB, Lewis DJ, Cassidy BA. Effects of 13-hour 20-minute work shifts on law enforcement officers' sleep, cognitive abilities, health, quality of life, and work performance: The Phoenix Study. *Police Q*. 2015;18:293–337.
116. Horne JA, Reyner LA. Sleep related vehicle accidents. *BMJ*. 1995;310:565–567.
117. West CP, Tan AD, Habermann TM, Sloan JA, Shanafelt TD. Association of resident fatigue and distress with perceived medical errors. *JAMA*. 2009;302:1294–300.
118. Kohn LT, Corrigan JM, Donaldson MS. *To Err Is Humain: Building a Safer Health Care System*. National Academy Press; 2000.
119. Bruck D, Pisani DL. The effects of sleep inertia on decision-making performance. *J Sleep Res*. 1999;8:95–103.
120. Landrigan CP, Rothschild JM, Cronin JW, et al. Effect of reducing interns' work hours on serious medical errors in intensive care units. *N Engl J Med*. 2004;351:1838–1848.

121. Accreditation Council for Graduate Medical Education. *Common Program Requirements, Section VF*. 2004 Feb. www.acgme.org/acWebsite/dutyHours/dh_Lang703.pdf. Accessed January 20, 2007.
122. Horwitz LI, Kosiborod M, Lin Z, Krumholz HM. Changes in outcomes for internal medicine inpatients after work-hour regulations. *Ann Intern Med*. 2007;147:97–103.
123. Shetty KD, Bhattacharya J. Changes in hospital mortality associated with residency work-hour regulations. *Ann Intern Med*. 2007;147:73–80.
124. Dorrian J, Lamond N, van den Heuvel C, Pincombe J, Rogers AE, Dawson D. A pilot study of the safety implications of Australian nurses' sleep and work hours. *Chronobiol Int*. 2006;23:1149–1163.
125. Garde AH, Hansen ÅM, Hansen J. Sleep length and quality, sleepiness and urinary melatonin among healthy Danish nurses with shift work during work and leisure time. *Int Arch Occup Environ Health*. 2009;82:1219–1228.
126. Waage S, Pallesen S, Moen BE, et al. Predictors of shift work disorder among nurses: A longitudinal study. *Sleep Med*. 2014;15:1449–1455.
127. Geiger-Brown J, Rogers VE, Trinkoff AM, Kane RL, Bausell RB, Scharf SM. Sleep, sleepiness, fatigue, and performance of 12-hour-shift nurses. *Chronobiol Int*. 2012;29:211–219.
128. Rogers AE, Hwang W-T, Scott LD, Aiken LH, Dinges DF. The working hours of hospital staff nurses and patient safety. *Health Aff*. 2004;23:202–212.
129. Ferri P, Guadi M, Marcheselli L, Balduzzi S, Magnani D, Di Lorenzo R. The impact of shift work on the psychological and physical health of nurses in a general hospital: A comparison between rotating night shifts and day shifts. *Risk Manage Healthc Policy*. 2016;9:203.
130. Stimpfel AW, Fatehi F, Kovner C. Nurses' sleep, work hours, and patient care quality, and safety. *Sleep Health*. 2020;6:314–320.
131. Kaliyaperumal D, Elango Y, Alagesan M, Santhanakrishanan I. Effects of sleep deprivation on the cognitive performance of nurses working in shift. *JCDR*. 2017;11:CC01.
132. Institute of Medicine (U.S.), Committee on the Work Environment for Nurses and Patient Safety; Page A, ed. *Keeping Patients Safe: Transforming the Work Environment of Nurses*. National Academies Press; 2004.
133. Reichard AA, Marsh SM, Moore PH. Fatal and nonfatal injuries among emergency medical technicians and paramedics. *Prehosp Emerg Care*. 2011;15:511–517.
134. Patterson PD, Weaver MD, Frank RC, et al. Association between poor sleep, fatigue, and safety outcomes in emergency medical services providers. *Prehosp Emerg Care*. 2012;16:86–97.
135. Drake CL, Wright KP. Shift work, shift-work disorder, and jet lag. In MH Kryger, T Roth, WC Dement, eds. *Principles and Practice of Sleep Medicine*, Fifth Edition. Saunders, (2011):784–798.
136. Patterson PD, Suffoletto BP, Kupas DF, Weaver MD, Hostler D. Sleep quality and fatigue among prehospital providers. *Prehosp Emerg Care*. 2010;14:187–193.
137. Harvey B. Firefighter sleep deprivation in the Raleigh (NC) Fire Department: An objective test. *Fire Eng*. 2013;166:20–20.
138. Kim KH, Kim JW, Kim SH. Influences of job stressors on psychosocial well-being, fatigue and sleep sufficiency among firefighters. *Korean J Occup Environ Med*. 2006;18:232–245.
139. Domrachev A, Savchenkov YI, Mikhailova L. Some personality characteristics of fire service specialists under conditions of prolonged intense workloads. *Human Physiol*. 2004;30:581–584.
140. Clack J. *The Management Effects of Firefighters Working a Consecutive 48-Hour Shift*. National Fire Academy; 2003.
141. Pfefferbaum B, North CS. Mental health and the COVID-19 pandemic. *N Engl J Med*. 2020;383:510–512.
142. Holmes EA, O'Connor RC, Perry VH, et al. Multidisciplinary research priorities for the COVID-19 pandemic: A call for action for mental health science. *Lancet Psychiatry*. 2020;7:547–560.
143. Karasek RA Jr. Job demands, job decision latitude, and mental strain: Implications for job redesign. *Adm Sci Q*. 1979:285–308.
144. Chew NW, Lee GK, Tan BY, et al. A multinational, multicentre study on the psychological outcomes and associated physical symptoms amongst healthcare workers during COVID-19 outbreak. *Brain Behav Immun*. 2020;88:559–565.
145. Akkermans J, Richardson J, Kraimer ML. The Covid-19 crisis as a career shock: Implications for careers and vocational behavior. *J Vocat Behav*. 2020;119:103434.
146. Drosos N, Theodoroulakis M, Antoniou AS, Rajter ICe. Career services in the post-COVID-19 era: A paradigm for career counseling unemployed individuals. *J Employ Couns*. 2021;58:36–48.
147. Brooks SK, Dunn R, Amlôt R, Greenberg N, Rubin GJ. Social and occupational factors associated with psychological distress and disorder among disaster responders: A systematic review. *BMC Psychol*. 2016;4:016–0120.
148. Rossi R, Socci V, Pacitti F, et al. Mental health outcomes among front and second line health workers associated with the COVID-19 pandemic in Italy. *MedRxiv*. 2020;2004.
149. Pappa S, Ntella V, Giannakas T, Giannakoulis VG, Papoutsi E, Katsaounou P. Prevalence of depression, anxiety, and insomnia among healthcare workers during the COVID-19 pandemic: A systematic review and meta-analysis. Brain Behav Immun. 2020;88:901–907.
150. Huang Y, Zhao N. Generalized anxiety disorder, depressive symptoms and sleep quality during COVID-19 outbreak in China: A web-based cross-sectional survey. *Psychiatry Res*. 2020;288:112954.
151. Altman MT, Knauert MP, Pisani MA. Sleep disturbance after hospitalization and critical illness: A systematic review. *Ann Am Thorac Soc*. 2017;14:1457–1468.
152. Lutchmansingh D, Knauert M, Antin-Ozerkis D. A clinic blueprint for post-coronavirus disease 2019 RECOVERY. Learning from the past, looking to the future *Chest*. 2021;159(3):949–958.

153. Bozan Ö, Atiş ŞE, Çekmen B, Şentürk M, Kalkan A. Healthcare workers' sleep quality after COVID-19 infection: A cross-sectional study. *Int J Clin Pract*. 2021;75:e14772.
154. Martínez-Caballero CM, Cárdaba-García RM, Varas-Manovel R, et al. Analyzing the impact of COVID-19 trauma on developing post-traumatic stress disorder among emergency medical workers in Spain. *Int J Environ Res Public Health*. 2021;18:9132.
155. Huang CL-C, Wu M-P, Ho C-H, Wang J-J. Risks of treated anxiety, depression, and insomnia among nurses: A nationwide longitudinal cohort study. *PLoS One*. 2018;13:e0204224.
156. Robbins R, Affouf M, Weaver MD, et al. Estimated sleep duration before and during the COVID-19 pandemic in major metropolitan areas on different continents: Observational study of smartphone app data. *J Med Internet Res*. 2021;23:e20546.
157. Epstein LJ, Cai A, Klerman EB, Czeisler CA. Resolving delayed sleep-wake phase disorder with a pandemic: two case reports. *J Clin Sleep Med*. 2022;18:315–318.
158. Lerman SE, Eskin E, Flower DJ, et al. Fatigue risk management in the workplace. *J Occup Environ Med*. 2012;54:231–258.
159. Moore-Ede M, Miller M, Trutschel U, Guttkuhn R, Aguirre A, Fassler I. *BostonInternational Conference on Fatigue Management in Transportation*; 2009.
160. Patterson PD, Higgins JS, Van Dongen HP, et al. Evidence-based guidelines for fatigue risk management in emergency medical services. *Prehosp Emerg Care*. 2018;22:89–101.
161. Di Muzio M, Diella G, Di Simone E, et al. Comparison of sleep and attention metrics among nurses working shifts on a forward-vs backward-rotating schedule. *JAMA Network Open*. 2021;4:e2129906-e.
162. Dawson D, Campbell SS. Timed exposure to bright light improves sleep and alertness during simulated night shifts. *Sleep*. 1991;14:511–516.
163. Sallinen M, Härmä M, Åkerstedt T, Rosa R, Lillqvist O. Promoting alertness with a short nap during a night shift. *J Sleep Res*. 1998;7:240–247.
164. Brice C, Smith A. The effects of caffeine on simulated driving, subjective alertness and sustained attention. *Hum Psychopharmacol Clin Exper*. 2001;16:523–531.
165. Philip P, Taillard J, Moore N, et al. The effects of coffee and napping on nighttime highway driving: a randomized trial. *Ann Intern Med*. 2006;144:785–791.
166. Schweitzer PK, Randazzo AC, Stone K, Erman M, Walsh JK. Laboratory and field studies of naps and caffeine as practical countermeasures for sleep-wake problems associated with night work. *Sleep*. 2006;29:39–50.
167. Liira J, Verbeek J, Ruotsalainen J. Pharmacological interventions for sleepiness and sleep disturbances caused by shift work. *JAMA*. 2015;313:961–962.
168. Talmage JB, Hudson TB, Hegmann KT, Thiese MS. Consensus criteria for screening commercial drivers for obstructive sleep apnea: evidence of efficacy. *J Occup Environ Med*. 2008:324–329.
169. Hartenbaum N, Collop N, Rosen IM, et al. Sleep apnea and commercial motor vehicle operators: Statement from the joint task force of the American College of Chest Physicians, the American College of Occupational and Environmental Medicine, and the National Sleep Foundation. *Chest*. 2006;130:902–905.

Chapter 31

Sleep in Underserved Populations

Andrew R. Spector

INTRODUCTION

Sleep is of critical importance to all people, but due to a combination of socially mitigated factors, certain groups of people suffer from a greater burden of insufficient or otherwise inadequate sleep. These differences, referred to as "disparities," are prevalent in the United States among sexual and gender minorities (SGM), socioeconomically disadvantaged populations (e.g., homeless, incarcerated), and racial and ethnic minorities, including Black, Hispanic/Latinx, American Indian and Alaska natives, Asian, and Native Hawaiian and Pacific Islanders.[1] Importantly, people often fall into more than 1 of these populations, which is referred to as "intersectionality," and the impact of being a member of multiple underserved groups could have additive consequences; however, for organizational purposes, in this chapter, these populations will be considered individually. Furthermore, we are defining "underserved" in an American context and thus the research presented in this chapter will pertain specifically to American subjects. This chapter will review what is known about sleep disparities related to routine and disordered sleep in adults, as well as the various causes for these disparities.

SEXUAL AND GENDER MINORITIES

Sleep Quality and Duration

Poor sleep has been mentioned in reports of health concerns among sexual and gender minorities (SGM) dating back to the 1990s,[2–4] but much of the research specifically examining sleep health and sleep disparities in this population has taken place since 2015.[5] Thanks to this new attention, we are starting to learn much more about sleep in lesbian, gay, bisexual, and transgender populations. A recent review of this literature found that most research to date has shown sleep to be a health disparity in SGM adults, with the most consistent finding being short sleep time.[5] Additionally, studies have shown that SGM adults have a higher risk of reporting poor sleep quality or sleep disturbances (e.g., not feeling rested, trouble falling asleep, nocturnal awakenings) than cisgender, heterosexual adults,[6–9] with homosexual women more likely to wake up at night than homosexual men.[6] One large study found that SGM adults who were also members of underserved racial groups had even higher rates of sleep problems, suggesting that multiple social factors were playing a large role in affecting sleep.[10]

The consequences of poor sleep in SGM adults are many. Sleep problems among SGM adults have been linked to an increase in several chronic health conditions,[11] an increase in drug and alcohol use,[12] more risky sexual behaviors,[12] and decreased quality of life.[7] It is noteworthy that studies of sleep in SGM populations often rely on single-item and self-report study designs, with few studies using validated questionnaires or polysomnography.[5] Nevertheless, there is adequate evidence to conclude that SGM status confers added risk of insufficient and poor qualify sleep.

Sleep Disorders

Little data exists on sleep dysfunction in SGM adults that rises to the level of a diagnosable sleep disorder. While many of the subjects included in the studies noted earlier would likely have met criteria for chronic insomnia, they were not classified in this manner by the authors. For other sleep disorders, such as obstructive sleep apnea (OSA), we are just starting to see studies addressing these topics. There is evidence that homosexual women are more likely to have obesity than heterosexual women, raising their risk for OSA, but a direct link between sexual orientation and OSA in women has not been studied.[13] One study comparing HIV-positive to HIV-negative homosexual men did look for OSA but found none of the 10 subjects in either arm of their study met polysomnographic criteria for this diagnosis.[4] Even less is known about OSA in transgender patients, but 1 case series of 3 patients reported that female sex hormones successfully treated long-standing OSA in a transgender woman, and male sex hormones appeared to trigger OSA in transgender men upon initiation of gender-affirming therapy.[14] These findings are consistent with what is known about the effects of sex hormones on OSA,[15,16] although much of what is known about sex hormones and OSA comes from studies in which hormone therapy is concordant with sex (e.g., estrogen for cisgender women). Data on SGM populations regarding restless legs syndrome and hypersomnias are lacking.

With the exception of exogenous hormone therapy for transgender men, it is not thought that there is a biological basis for the sleep disparities of SGM adults. Rather, adverse social environments and both implicit and explicit discrimination are felt to be more likely causes. The impact of social environments on sleep will be explored further in a subsequent section of this chapter.

SOCIOECONOMICALLY DISADVANTAGED POPULATIONS

Sleep Quality and Duration

This section will review what is known about the sleep of 2 specific socioeconomically disadvantaged populations: incarcerated and homeless. It is not difficult to imagine that sleep quality in both groups would be poor due to the environments in which they live. Conditions in jails, for instance, can be so disruptive to sleep as to rise to a constitutional violation. In 1 such case, the jail had scheduled mandatory awakenings throughout the night.[17] Other jails only schedule a 6-hour block of time for sleep.[18] In addition to the operations of the jail, the environment of being incarcerated impairs sleep quality. Light, temperature, noise, bed quality, lack of privacy, and the threat of violence all create an environment that is not conducive to sleep. The problem is widespread in the prison population. Poor sleep quality affects greater than 70% of incarcerated women, who cite ruminations, environment, physical health, nightmares/flashbacks, and lack of access to hypnotic medications as their primary reasons for poor sleep.[19] This number is markedly higher than the number reporting sleep problems upon admission (21.5% of male inmates and 45.2% of females[20]); thus the prison environment is likely responsible for the sleep trouble of many of the inmates.

Individuals experiencing homelessness face a similar array of barriers to good sleep. Those who are able to obtain a bed in a shelter can find their sleep impaired by light, noise, and threat of theft or violence, and shelter rules often require early departures that limit potential sleep duration.[21,22] While *Martin v. City of Boise* established the rights of individuals to sleep outside when no other option exists within the jurisdiction of the Ninth Circuit, many cities across the rest of the United States still criminalize sleeping outdoors. In fact, the National Law Center on Homelessness & Poverty has identified city-wide bans on sleeping in public in 34% of American cities.[23] Furthermore, those sleeping outside face potential police harassment and the deployment of measures to make sleeping even more difficult, such as dividers on benches to prevent lying down or fencing off partially sheltered areas under bridges, collectively referred to as "hostile architecture."[24] All of these factors combine to cause severe sleep deprivation in individuals experiencing homelessness, with reports indicating that the total sleep time in this population can be as low as 3.6 hours per night, of which 2.9 hours is uninterrupted.[25] Whether sheltered or unsheltered, 26% of respondents in a survey of individuals between ages 18 and 25 who were currently unhoused reported moderate to severe sleep disturbances.[26] The availability of shelter did not correlate with sleep disturbance, but feeling unsafe in the sleeping environment did, which is important to note as it indicates that simply providing a bed and a roof is not adequate to address sleep concerns in this population.

Sleep Disorders

The prevalence of sleep apnea in incarcerated individuals is unknown. Furthermore, it is unknown if the environment of prison contributes to the development of sleep apnea, though it has been established that weight gain is a consequence of incarceration,[27] so there is potential for the risk of sleep apnea to increase as well. In the 1 study to examine the risk of sleep apnea in incarcerated women, 10% of subjects screened positive on the Multivariable Apnea Prediction Score (MAPS) to indicate a need for further sleep apnea testing.[19] In general, prisons do allow inmates with known sleep apnea to have access to positive airway pressure (PAP) devices, though some facilities suspended use of this therapy during the COVID-19 pandemic due to concerns regarding viral dissemination.

Access to sleep apnea therapy is possibly more difficult for individuals experiencing homelessness. PAP devices require access to electricity, which might not be available near enough to a shelter bed or if sleeping outside. Additionally, individuals without a stable residence could have difficulty transporting a PAP device from location to location each night.

Although insomnia is the most studied sleep disorder in incarcerated populations, even this literature is sparse, particularly for U.S. prisons. Must of the research done in this area is on interventions to improve sleep, rather than the incidence or prevalence of insomnia.[28] While various therapies have been attempted (relaxation training,[29,30] stimulus-control therapy,[29] meditation,[31,32] cognitive-behavioral therapy for insomnia[33]), the optimal treatment strategy for insomnia in incarcerated populations has not been established. Given the environmental impediments to sleep noted previously, it is likely difficult to overcome endogenous insomnia in the prison setting.

It is similarly difficult to imagine meaningful therapy for insomnia taking place while individuals remain homeless, as the external factors that disrupt sleep will persist even after addressing any endogenous reasons for insomnia, such as anxiety and dysfunctional beliefs about sleep. However, homelessness need not be a long-term condition. When adults transition to permanent supportive housing, insomnia rates significantly decline without additional insomnia intervention, and this effect is sustained for at least 12 months.[34]

There are no studies on the prevalence of narcolepsy in prison populations or in individuals experiencing homelessness. The most likely interaction of narcolepsy and other hypersomnias with the carceral system is the difficulty that prisoners might face when attempting to access amphetamine-based stimulants for therapy, a phenomenon noted in the literature on attention deficit disorder.[35] Otherwise, there are no data to support a causal link between narcolepsy and subsequent incarceration or vice versa. While narcolepsy is associated with lower household income,[36] it has not been shown to be associated with increased rates of homelessness.

RACIAL AND ETHNIC MINORITIES

Terminology

Before proceeding with a discussion of sleep in racial and ethnic minorities, we must first discuss terminology. As race is a social rather than biological construct, there is no indisputably correct way to classify people into races. Therefore, for the purposes of this chapter, we will rely upon the National Institutes of Health definitions.[37] Furthermore, the use of the term "minority" is currently heavily debated, with writers suggesting that this term be abandoned.[38] Other phrases, including "non-White," "people of color," and "BIPOC" (Black, Indigenous, and other people of color) are all debated and often rejected as replacements.[39] Given the heterogeneity of the populations included in these terms, it is not surprising that there is no consensus regarding terminology. Therefore, in the absence of a universally accepted alternative, we have elected to use the term "minority" as we will be discussing populations that are currently in the minority in the United States. While we do not believe than any individual is "a minority," as this is demeaning, we use the term here in a strictly numerical sense in referring to populations.

Sleep Duration

Of all underserved populations, racial and ethnic minority (RM) groups have been the best studied. In the United States, RM groups experience both subjectively and objectively worse sleep than White people.[40] Population-based studies have shown higher risks of both inadequate or excessive sleep to varying degrees in all RM groups in the United States.[41–48] In fact, race—specifically, being Black—has been shown to be more predictive of extreme sleep than any medical condition, income, sex, age, or geographic region.[45,49] Some of this disparity between Black and White survey respondents could be due to a reporting bias. White respondents tend to overestimate how much they actually sleep by a greater degree than Black respondents do.[50] Therefore, it is important to confirm the subjective reports of inadequate sleep with objective data.

The finding of inadequate sleep duration in Black Americans was tested with actigraphy and polysomnography, confirming 30 minutes less sleep and a lower sleep efficiency in the Black group compared to the combined White and Asian group.[51] Thus both objective and subjective data support the finding of shorter sleep duration in Black Americans. Black Americans are not alone among RM groups reporting short sleep. Native Hawaiians and Other Pacific Islanders also reported particularly short sleep durations in a large survey that also confirmed short sleep in Black participants.[52]

To tease out race from socioeconomic status, studies have added additional socioeconomic variables, such as neighborhood economics, and have shown that sleep duration does not vary between Black and White residents of government-assisted rental housing or mobile homes/trailers, but disparities are evident among Black subjects in higher socioeconomic classes.[53,54] Thus Black people suffer impaired sleep due to factors that are independent of the effects of poverty.

Sleep Quality

Aside from the duration of sleep, sleep quality is also decreased among RM groups. While little is known about sleep quality or subjective sleep difficulties in American Indian/Alaska native or Native Hawaiian and Pacific Islander populations, several studies have looked at these factors in Black, Hispanic, and Asian populations in the United States. Multiple studies have concluded that sleep quality, as determined by actigraphy-derived sleep efficiency, is worse in Black participants compared to Hispanic, Asian, and non-Hispanic White participants.[44,51] Subjectively, Black and Hispanic respondents rate their sleep to be lower quality than White respondents.[55] As would be expected, lower socioeconomic status was associated with an even lower sleep quality score. Consistent with research on sleep duration that showed a smaller gap between races in the lowest socioeconomic groups, White subjects in the low socioeconomic group had the highest risk of poor sleep quality. Wealth, it can be concluded, is most beneficial for sleep among respondents who do not have the added burdens of being a member of an RM group.

Sleep Apnea

Racial and ethnic minorities, regardless of socioeconomic status, are at increased risk of sleep disorders, particularly OSA. The degree of difference between races has been studied in a variety of manners, leading to different conclusions about the exact nature of racial disparities in OSA.[56] Early research into racial disparities in OSA suggested that the largest gap is in Black Americans below age 26.[57] Later research found that the disparities existed in older subjects as well. One study of middle-aged adults showed large racial disparities, with Hispanic and Black subjects demonstrating a 3 times higher likelihood of sleep disordered breathing than White subjects, and Asian subjects showing the same condition nearly 4 times as often as White subjects.[58] Another study of elderly adults showed a 2-fold risk of OSA in Black compared to White subjects.[59] Subsequent research found that American Indians were nearly twice as likely as White Americans to have at least moderately severe OSA, while the Black versus White comparison was not significant.[60] Although overall, RM groups seem more likely to have OSA, there is debate as to whether race predicts OSA severity when comparing Black and White subjects, with mixed findings in the literature.[59,61]

One hypothesis for the cause of racial health disparities in OSA is the differential rates of obesity. For example, Black people have been shown to have higher rates of obesity, and research suggests that Black women have the highest rates of obesity in the United States.[63] Obesity could, therefore, be a mediator for the higher risk of OSA in this population. However, studies on obesity almost invariably utilize body mass index (BMI) as their metric, which was not calibrated to measure obesity in Black women when it was first derived in 19th century Belgium, so studies relying on BMI in non–White male populations need to be evaluated with caution. Likewise, there is evidence that traditionally accepted BMI cutoffs for obesity in the United States do not adequately address the risk of obesity-related complications such as OSA in Asian populations.[64] This leads to a dramatic risk of underdiagnosing OSA in Asian populations in the United States, where medical providers are cued to investigate OSA based on a conception of obesity that might apply better to White or Black patients.[44] Therefore, obesity rates are likely to play a role in racial health disparities for OSA, but the nature of this interaction requires further exploration.

Another potential cause of racial disparities in OSA is genetics. The role of genetics in OSA has been explored in both White and Black families, with evidence suggesting that OSA is heritable in both groups.[65] Genetics could play a role in OSA through obesity, ventilatory control, soft tissue factors, or craniofacial features.[56] For instance, ethnically Chinese patients with OSA showed more skeletal restriction in their airways than White patients.[66] Craniofacial differences could account for the increased rate of OSA in Asian compared to White populations at the same BMI.[44] In a search for specific loci that control OSA, research on White families identified chromosomes 2p and 19p as being linked to sleep apnea severity,[67] while in Black families, it was 8q.[68] Other studies have searched for a variety of different mutations,[56] but most do not indicate how White and Black subjects were identified as such. This is a concern because there is only a moderate correlation between self-reported race and European versus African genetic ancestry in Americans.[69] Thus, genetic studies that attempt to assign genetic causes of diseases to Black or White Americans (groups that are socially, not genetically defined) need to be interpreted with caution. Overall, despite family history being predictive of OSA,[70] no genetic variant has been consistently identified to account for known racial disparities in OSA prevalence.[56]

Once OSA has been identified, treatment often includes continuous positive airway pressure (CPAP). Differential effects of OSA on health could result from racial disparities in adherence to therapy, but research on CPAP adherence has shown variable results with regard to race.[71–73] The little data that exists on Hispanic populations demonstrated that CPAP acceptance was lower than in non-Hispanic White patients at the same healthcare system.[74] In studies where Black race has been predictive of CPAP non-adherence, controlling for neighborhood and socioeconomic status eliminated that effect.[75] The majority of studies on CPAP adherence rates has focused specifically on Black and White populations, with little known about CPAP adherence in other RM groups. It is not likely that there is an intrinsic quality among any RM group that would limit

CPAP usage; thus the value of relying on race as opposed to other social factors in explaining CPAP adherence rates is probably low.

For patients who fail CPAP therapy, surgical intervention is sometimes an option. Racial disparities have been noted in surgical OSA patients, with Hispanic and Asian populations overrepresented in the surgical versus non-surgical group.[76] It is possible that this is related to the lower prevalence of obesity in these populations, with a bias toward surgical referrals of non-obese patients. Income and insurance status also played a role in predicting who received surgery, but these factors were not reported with respect to each racial group to be able to determine if economics would account for the observed racial difference.

In summary, the bulk of the evidence indicates that OSA is more common but not necessarily more severe in RM groups in the United States. Certain populations risk underdiagnosis of OSA due to recognition of risk (e.g., normal BMI for Asian patients with OSA). Overall, socioeconomic factors are more important than race in adherence to therapy.[77]

Insomnia

Insomnia is the most prevalent sleep disorder in the United States, with 1 large study estimating its prevalence at 27.3% in a 12-month period during 2012–2013.[78] While sleep quality can be defined in a variety of ways, chronic insomnia is specifically defined as difficulty falling asleep, difficulty staying asleep, waking up too early, or relying on medications to sleep for at least 3 times per week for at least 3 months.[79] When assessing racial disparities in insomnia, it is important to consider that insomnia is a subjective condition and thus dependent on responses by research participants. As a result, there is a possibility that there is a response bias, with some populations less likely to admit to sleep problems due to fear of cultural stereotyping (e.g., Black participants do not want to be labeled as lazy[80] for sleeping during the day) or due to interpreting what constitutes a sleep problem in a culturally specific manner. It's likely that a response bias is at least partially responsible for the wide range of findings in studies of racial disparities in insomnia.

With that caveat in mind, we can review the divergent results of insomnia research by race. One study showed that women of different ethnic backgrounds had highly disparate rates of insomnia, ranging from 33% (Haitian) to 77% (Eastern European).[81] This same study found Dominican and American-born Black participants with rates similar to self-identified European-Americans (70%–73%), while native English speakers from the Caribbean were more similar to Haitians (34%). This study illustrates how difficult it can be to obtain reliable, subjective data from a multicultural population. Taken at face value, though, it confirms that culture and ethnicity are more important than race in determining the prevalence of insomnia in different groups, as would be expected.

Other studies have shown contradictory results, with 1 study finding that non-Hispanic White and Hispanic adults have higher insomnia severity scores than Black adults,[82] while another found that the rate is lower in Hispanic than non-Hispanic White adults.[83] Still another found a lower rate of insomnia in Chinese (16%) than White (22.5%), Black (25%), or Hispanic (26.5%) participants.[44] In 1 of the only studies to assess this population, American Indian/Alaskan Natives in the American military showed the highest rates of insomnia (33.7%) while Asian participants showed the lowest (15.1%).[84] Native Americans were significantly more likely than any other racial group to report insomnia in this study. None of the other groups were significantly different from each other. When all RM populations were combined, there was a clear increase in incident chronic insomnia among RM participants compared to White participants.[85]

Overall, there is ample evidence that formally diagnosed insomnia, like subjectively disturbed sleep, is more common in RM populations. However, the role of biases in the instruments used to identify insomnia and the cultural variance in defining difficulty falling and staying asleep may affect our understanding of racial disparities in insomnia.

Narcolepsy

Narcolepsy is a condition that is thought to have a genetic predisposition, namely, the presence of the HLA-DQB1*06:02 allele,[86] but twin studies have shown low concordance, and most people with the allele do not have narcolepsy, implicating environmental triggers.[87] Early studies of narcolepsy identified higher rates of the disease among Black military recruits.[88] This finding has been confirmed more recently with rates of 0.0322% in White people, 0.0428% in Black people, 0.015% in Asian people, and 0.0279% in those identified as another race.[89] In this study, the HLA-DQB1*06:02 allele was found in relative proportion to the rates of narcolepsy as would be expected.

Another study comparing narcolepsy across races showed higher rates of the HLA-DQB1*06:02 allele in Black patients with narcolepsy than in White, Asian, or Hispanic patients.[90] Black patients also reported more sleepiness and had shorter mean sleep latencies on multiple sleep latency tests, which could indicate either a more severe phenotype or a recruitment bias in the study if Black patients with less severe phenotypes are not presenting for evaluation. As expected in the setting of higher frequencies of the HLA-DQB1*06:02 allele, Black patients showed lower levels of cerebrospinal fluid hypocretin, a marker for narcolepsy and a common finding in patients with cataplexy.[91] Intriguingly, despite the associations between HLA-DQB1*06:02, low hypocretin, and cataplexy,[86,91] Black patients showed lower rates of cataplexy.[90] The authors of this study speculate that since Black patients may be at higher risk of sleep apnea, the presence of OSA and absence of cataplexy could lead to sleep medicine providers missing a comorbid diagnoses of narcolepsy type 2 (without cataplexy) in patients with OSA. Thus, the study would have a higher ratio of patients with narcolepsy type 1 (with cataplexy) and fewer with type 2, which would give the false appearance of cataplexy being less common in Black patients. The variation in symptoms seen in this study has not been confirmed in other studies, though. For instance, 1 study showed no significant variability in symptomatology or age of onset across racial groups, comparing Black, White, Asian, Hispanic, and mixed race/ethnicity patients with narcolepsy.[92]

As noted earlier, only a small percentage of narcolepsy can be accounted for by genetics. Thus, we must look to other factors that could contribute to the difference in prevalence we see in Black Americans versus all other racial and ethnic groups. Narcolepsy is thought to be more common in those born in March than in September, which raises the possibility of a fetal or perinatal exposure in the etiology of narcolepsy.[93] Whether that factor is an infectious disease, nutritional deficiency, maternal trauma, or any of a number of other possibilities is unknown. An analysis of childhood illnesses showed that adults with narcolepsy were more likely to have been diagnosed with strep throat as a child, but not pneumonia, hepatitis, mononucleosis, or encephalitis or exposure to the antibiotics commonly used to treat these conditions.[36] Likewise, there was no association between any of the investigated non-infectious diseases (aside from night terrors), number of head traumas, or vaccinations in the narcolepsy group versus controls. Thus, of all the childhood factors, the presence of strep throat could have the most impact on the subsequent development of narcolepsy, as there is no clear mechanism by which night terrors could cause narcolepsy. Further evidence for a streptococcal-mediated etiology for narcolepsy is the presence of immune markers for recent streptococcal infection at narcolepsy onset with dwindling levels later in the course of the disease.[94] Streptococcal infection could activate an autoimmune response, resulting in damage to the hypothalamus and symptoms of narcolepsy.

If streptococcal infection contributed to the development of narcolepsy, we would expect to see higher rates of infection in Black children, for whom narcolepsy rates are highest. This is not the case, though. Black and Hispanic children are substantially less likely than White children in the United States to be diagnosed with streptococcal pharyngitis.[95] However, streptococcal infections typically lead to immune-mediated complications only if untreated.[96] So if the reason for low rates of streptococcal pharyngitis in Black children is due to underdiagnosis, there could be more untreated cases and thus more risk for narcolepsy as a complication, particularly if there is a streptococcal infection interaction with the immune response mediated by the underlying HLA-DQB1*06:02 haplotype. Therefore, it is possible that some of the observed racial disparity in narcolepsy prevalence is due to untreated streptococcal infections, but this possibility is still speculative at this time. As we learn more about the etiology of narcolepsy, we will also discover why some RM groups are more affected by it.

In summary, narcolepsy rates are slightly but significantly higher in Black Americans than in other racial groups, but the phenotype is relatively similar. While there is some evidence that

Black subjects might have more severe symptoms, this is not consistent across studies. The higher prevalence of the HLA-DQB1*06:02 allele in Black patients could indicate that people with certain ancestries are more likely to develop narcolepsy for genetic reasons, but differential environmental factors, such as exposure to streptococcal infection, almost certainly play a key role. The full spectrum of environmental factors that might lead to racial disparities in narcolepsy has not yet been elucidated.

Restless Legs Syndrome (RLS)

One of the early studies examining the prevalence of RLS in different racial groups was prompted by the general observation that there were fewer Black patients presenting to an RLS clinic.[97] When examined rigorously, though, the rate of RLS was not significantly different between White and Black patients in this community sample once other variables were controlled. This suggests the absence of Black patients from RLS clinic that the researchers had observed had more to do with access to or desire for care than any inherent difference in the disease. More recently, though, studies have found that Black and other RM participants were significantly less likely than White participants to endorse RLS symptoms during direct interviews[98–100] and less than half as likely to have periodic limb movements of sleep on polysomnography.[101] The cause for the difference in findings could relate to study methodology (e.g., community or primary care office location), sample size (over 1000 participants in the community study and fewer than 200 in the office-based study), or the general health status of the population, as RLS has been linked to numerous other conditions.[102] Another possible confounder is the genetic homogeneity of the study population. For instance, in the primary care study showing a 3 times higher rate of RLS in the White subjects,[98] if the White subjects shared a common ethnic ancestry (e.g., Icelandic, Portuguese), there could be genetic factors raising the rates of RLS compared to the Black subjects in the study that might not have been observed with different White populations. A more genetically heterogeneous sample, therefore, would be more likely to show equal rates between racial groups.

Very little has been written about the prevalence of RLS in other RM populations. One primary care–based study showed a lower rate of RLS in Hispanic compared to White subjects.[100] As RLS is a subjective condition, language and culture could play a role in the reporting of RLS symptoms. Evidence of this was seen in a study that showed lower rates of RLS in Hispanics of Mexican descent in the United States with low acculturation versus those with high acculturation (defined by the Short Acculturation Scale for Hispanics).[103] This study also showed lower rates of RLS in Hispanic participants compared to non-Hispanic White participants. No studies to date have included high enough numbers of other RM populations in the United States to be able to analyze prevalence rates.

CAUSES OF DISPARITIES

Socioeconomics

For each of the underserved populations, the combination of social and environmental factors and intentional and unintentional discrimination are felt to be the leading causes of the noted disparities. Poverty is a concern for all of the underserved populations, and while socioeconomic status alone does not explain all of the variance in sleep health noted earlier, poverty does play a significant role in sleep health in myriad ways, so we will begin our discussion of causes of sleep disparities with economic factors.

One of the most direct ways in which poverty affects sleep is through longer work hours, such as from working multiple jobs, or from working overnight shifts, which could reduce the opportunity for sleep. Most effects of poverty on sleep are less direct, though no less important. A substantial body of research has linked neighborhoods—often a proxy marker for both wealth and race—and sleep problems.[104] Early work in this field found that increased neighborhood disorder, a metric derived from social and structural disorganization and disrepair,[105] was associated with poorer sleep quality.[106] This finding has been replicated, strongly implicating neighborhood factors in reducing sleep quality.[107]

A 3-part model for neighborhood effects on sleep has been proposed: "ambient hazards and physical exposures, psycho-physiological pathways, and health behavior."[107] The physical environment poses a threat to sleep through artificial light,[108,109] noise,[110] air pollution,[111,112] and thermoregulation.[113,114] One study from New York City identified disparities in light and noise pollution as disruptive influences on sleep for Hispanic compared to non-Hispanic White populations.[115] Sleep duration and quality are not the only aspects of sleep that are worse due to environmental factors. Studies have found that air pollution and warmer temperatures also worsen sleep apnea.[111,113,114] Another physical factor that can impact sleep is neighborhood walkability. Sleep apnea is slightly less severe in patients residing in locations that are more conducive to outdoor activities.[116] Predictably, there is evidence that exposure to these sleep-disrupting environmental factors is associated with being a member of an RM population and being in a lower socioeconomic tier.[117]

The physical environment is only 1 piece of the puzzle when it comes to how neighborhoods can affect sleep. Another large driver of poor sleep health involves community safety and neighborhood resources; these are the social elements of the environment.[118] When a neighborhood is safer and has more social cohesion, sleep improves in both duration and earlier timing, findings that are independent of age, race, socioeconomic status, or marital status.[119] Similar studies also showed less daytime sleepiness among people living in neighborhoods with fewer adverse social factors.[120,121] Neighborhood violence also mediates sleep, with both objectively and subjectively worse sleep in both Black and Hispanic people living in higher-violence locations.[122,123] Beyond race, the perceived safety of neighborhoods affects the sleep of men who have sex with men.[124] There is also an association between a healthy diet and reduced OSA severity,[125] so patients living in neighborhoods without ready access to healthy food ("food deserts") would likely be at higher risk of OSA.

Discrimination

A common theme in each of these socioeconomic factors is that they can all increase stress, such as fear, hypervigilance, and ruminations. Another source of stress is discrimination. In fact, even anticipating discrimination can trigger a stress response.[126] A review of discrimination and sleep revealed that all 17 studies on the subject found a relationship between discrimination and negative effects on sleep.[127] There is evidence of this effect in multiple populations, such as Hispanic,[128] Black,[129] and Chinese Americans.[130] While the role of discrimination on RM groups is well-studied, the impact of discrimination on sleep in SGM populations is not known.

The negative impact of socioeconomic status on sleep is powerful enough to affect all racial groups, including White. Therefore, the role of racial discrimination on sleep becomes more apparent at higher socioeconomic levels. While White people in professional occupations slept more than White people classified as laborers, the opposite was true for Black people,[131] perhaps a manifestation of the concept that Black people need to "work twice as hard to get half as far."[132]

One study looking at discrimination and sleep demonstrated a significant association between being treated unfairly and both subjective and objective measures of sleep quality.[133] Furthermore, Black people were significantly more likely to report being treated unfairly than White people. This finding was supported by additional research using the Everyday Discrimination Scale[130] and the Scale of Ethnic Experience, which yields a perceived discrimination score.[134] These studies revealed both changes in self-reported sleep quality as well as objective changes in sleep quality, including increased polysomnographic wake after sleep onset and reduced stage N3 sleep. Future research should elucidate how discrimination affects the sleep of other underserved populations.

Access to Care

Many populations are at risk for inadequate care of sleep disorders due to difficulty accessing care. The first sleep center to be located on a Self-Determination Native American Reservation and to be accredited by the American Academy of Sleep Medicine did not open until 2017.[135] This is significant because the distance a patient must travel to a sleep center is positively correlated with more severe sleep apnea upon initial presentation.[136]

The availability of sleep testing can be a substantial barrier to care, with wait times in the United States ranging from 2 to 10 months for in-lab polysomnography,[137] though the rise of home sleep apnea testing has likely shortened these numbers by shunting some patients to alternative pathways of care.[138] Furthermore, sleep centers are not accessible for all patients due to geographic distance. For example, at the time of publication, only 5 sleep specialists were listed in the American Academy of Sleep Medicine directory for the State of Wyoming, and they were located in only 3 cities. This could leave people hundreds of miles from the nearest sleep medicine specialist. Furthermore, as of 2016, 4 states and 105 of the largest 167 cities did not have a single behavioral sleep medicine provider.[139] Sleep medicine faces both a shortage of providers and a geographically imbalanced distribution. The rising prevalence of telehealth services could improve healthcare accessibility for many, but technological limitations such as internet speed and computer availability mean that even telehealth cannot eliminate all disparities in access to care.[140]

For patients able to reach a sleep center, they still face the barrier of cost. No systematic studies of polysomnogram costs have been performed, but they are popularly reported to range from $600 to over $7000 depending on the location and type of test.[141] Uninsured patients would most likely depend on charity care by their local health system to cover these costs. Insured patients would be subjected to copays, deductibles, and co-insurance values, which could keep the test financially out of reach. For those who are able to afford testing, treatments such as cognitive behavioral therapy, pharmacotherapy for narcolepsy, or CPAP machines and supplies for obstructive sleep apnea represent another level of cost burden. Not all insurance plans will cover therapy with a behavioral sleep medicine provider. And while insurance plans will cover CPAP machines and medications in theory, documentation burdens including prior authorization rules, step therapy, and out of pocket costs for patients can keep these treatments inaccessible even to insured patients. These location and cost barriers hit underserved patients the hardest as they are most likely to be uninsured, underinsured, or geographically distant from medical care.

Clinical Decision-Making

While many of the factors that affect underserved populations occur prior to the clinical visit, sleep medicine providers can also contribute to healthcare disparities through biased decision-making. For example, while obesity is a known risk factor for OSA,[142] this is a much greater issue for White and Black patients than it is for Asian patients. In 1 study in multiple American cities, patients of Chinese heritage with normal BMI had 1.59 times the risk for severe OSA as their White counterparts with normal BMI, yet they were less likely to have been diagnosed with OSA prior to the study.[44] Although there are several possible reasons for this discrepancy, one possibility is that the assumption that only people with obesity develop sleep apnea could have led to inadequate care for the patients of Chinese heritage.

We also see a difference in clinical practice when it comes to hypnotic prescriptions. Being White increases the odds of being prescribed a hypnotic.[143,144] It is not known if patients of other races were offered these medications at the same rate but declined them, or if they were not offered the drugs in the first place, but it does suggest that race influences prescribing in some way. This would not be a surprise, as this finding has also been reported in several contexts for opiate medications.[145–147]

Explicit biases can factor in as much as, or more than, the implicit biases noted previously. One example of this would be if providers and their office staff do not respectfully utilize patients' preferred pronouns. This can manifest even in subtle ways, such as providing intake paperwork with a forced male/female dichotomy for patients to select one. Patients who represent SGM groups cite discrimination in the healthcare setting as a barrier to care.[148–150] Thus, while many drivers of sleep health disparities involve social determinants of health, such as neighborhood safety, racism, and costs of care, sleep medicine providers still have a large role to play in reducing disparities in their offices as they care for each individual patient.

CONCLUSION

Underserved populations, including sexual and gender minorities, those experiencing homelessness and incarceration, and those from racial and ethnic minority backgrounds have an increased risk of poor sleep, manifesting as inadequate sleep durations, poor sleep quality, and more sleep disorders. The causes of these disparities can be linked to the effects of poverty and neighborhood qualities, such as safety, light, and noise, but also to discrimination, clinical decision-making biases, and insufficient access to healthcare. Each of these issues must be addressed to improve the sleep—and thereby the health—of these vulnerable populations.

REFERENCES

1. National Institute on Minority Health and Health Disparities. Overview. December 22, 2020. https://www.nimhd.nih.gov/about/overview/.
2. Blosnich JR, Farmer GW, Lee JGL, Silenzio VMB, Bowen DJ. Health inequalities among sexual minority adults: Evidence from ten U.S. states, 2010. *Am J Prevent Med*. 2014;46(4):337–349. https://doi.org/10.1016/j.amepre.2013.11.010.
3. Rahman Q, Silber K. Sexual orientation and the sleep-wake cycle: A preliminary investigation. *Arch Sex Behav*. 2000 Apr;29(2):127–134. doi:10.1023/a:1001999821083.
4. Norman SE, Chediak AD, Kiel M, Cohn MA. Sleep disturbances in HIV-infected homosexual men. *AIDS*. 1990;4(8):775–782.
5. Butler ES, McGlinchey E, Juster R-P. Sexual and gender minority sleep: A narrative review and suggestions for future research. *J Sleep Res*. 2020;29(1):e12928. https://doi.org/10.1111/jsr.12928.
6. Chen J-H, Shiu C-S. sexual orientation and sleep in the U.S.: A national profile. *Am J Prev Med*. 2017;52(4):433–442. https://doi.org/10.1016/j.amepre.2016.10.039.
7. Auer MK, Liedl A, Fuss J, et al. High impact of sleeping problems on quality of life in transgender individuals: A cross-sectional multicenter study. *PLoS One*. 2017;12(2):e0171640. doi:10.1371/journal.pone.0171640.
8. Galinsky AM, Ward BW, Joestl SS, Dahlhamer JM. Sleep duration, sleep quality, and sexual orientation: Findings from the 2013–2015 National Health Interview Survey. *Sleep Health*. 2018;4(1):56–62. https://doi.org/10.1016/j.sleh.2017.10.004.
9. Hsieh N, Ruther M. Sexual minority health and health risk factors: Intersection effects of gender, race, and sexual identity. *Am J Prev Med*. 2016;50(6):746–755. https://doi.org/10.1016/j.amepre.2015.11.016.
10. Caceres BA, Hickey KT, Heitkemper EM, Hughes TL. An intersectional approach to examine sleep duration in sexual minority adults in the United States: Findings from the Behavioral Risk Factor Surveillance System. *Sleep Health*. 2019;5(6):621–629. https://doi.org/10.1016/j.sleh.2019.06.006.
11. Dai H, Hao J. Sleep deprivation and chronic health conditions among sexual minority adults. *Behav Sleep Med*. 2019;17(3):254–268. doi:10.1080/15402002.2017.1342166.
12. Duncan DT, Goedel WC, Mayer KH, et al. Poor sleep health and its association with mental health, substance use, and condomless anal intercourse among gay, bisexual, and other men who have sex with men. *Sleep Health*. 2016;2(4):316–321. https://doi.org/10.1016/j.sleh.2016.07.003.
13. Boehmer U, Bowen DJ, Bauer GR. Overweight and obesity in sexual-minority women: Evidence from population-based data. *Am J Public Health*. 2007;97(6):1134–1140. doi:10.2105/AJPH.2006.088419.
14. Robertson BD, Lerner BS, Collen JF, Smith PR. The effects of transgender hormone therapy on sleep and breathing: A case series. *J Clin Sleep Med*. 15(10):1529–1533. doi:10.5664/jcsm.7992.
15. Payne K, Lipshultz LI, Hotaling JM, Pastuszak AW. Obstructive sleep apnea and testosterone therapy. *Sexual Med Rev*. 2020:296–303. https://doi.org/10.1016/j.sxmr.2020.04.004.
16. Bixler EO, Vgontzas AN, Lin H-M, et al. Prevalence of sleep-disordered breathing in women. *Am J Resp Crit Care Med*. 2001;163(3):608–613. doi:10.1164/ajrccm.163.3.9911064.
17. Flynn M. "Sleep is critical to human existence": Judge orders county jail to stop constantly waking up female inmates. *Washington Post*. March 28, 2019. https://www.washingtonpost.com/nation/2019/03/28/sleep-is-critical-human-existence-judge-orders-county-jail-stop-constantly-waking-up-female-prisoners/. Accessed January 8, 2022.
18. North Carolina Department of Public Safety. 24 hours in prison. https://www.doc.state.nc.us/dop/hours24.htm. Accessed January 8, 2022.
19. Harner HM, Budescu M. Sleep quality and risk for sleep apnea in incarcerated women. *Nurs Res*. 2014 May–Jun;63(3):158–169. doi:10.1097/NNR.0000000000000031.
20. Diamond PM, Magaletta PR, Harzke AJ, Baxter J. Who requests psychological services upon admission to prison? *Psychol Serv*. 2008;5(2):97–107. doi:10.1037/1541-1559.5.2.97.
21. Olsen HB. Homelessness and the impossibility of a good night's sleep. *The Atlantic*. Published August 14, 2014.
22. Groton DB, Spadola C. "I ain't getting enough rest": A qualitative exploration of sleep among women experiencing homelessness. *J Soc Distress Homeless*. 2021;32:1–8. doi:10.1080/10530789.2021.1961991.
23. Bauman T. *NO SAFE PLACE: The Criminalization of Homelessness in U.S. Cities*. 2019. Accessed January 8, 2022. https://homelesslaw.org/wp-content/uploads/2019/02/No_Safe_Place.pdf
24. McFadden C. 15 examples of 'anti-homeless' hostile architecture that you probably never noticed before. *Interesting Engineering*. Published April 8, 2023. https://interestingengineering.com/15-examples-of-anti-homeless-hostile-architecture-that-you-probably-never-noticed-before. Accessed January 8, 2022.
25. Hoops Calhoun K, Chassman S. Sleep quality and quantity among adults experiencing homelessness: An ecological systems approach. *J Hum Behav Soc Envi*. 2021;32(6):1–14. doi:10.1080/10911359.2021.1968556.

26. Redline B, Semborski S, Madden DR, Rhoades H, Henwood BF. Examining sleep disturbance among sheltered and unsheltered transition age youth experiencing homelessness. *Med Care*. 2021;59:S182–S186.
27. Shaw NS, Rutherdale M, Kenny J. Eating more and enjoying it less. *Women Health*. 1985;10(1):39–57. doi:10.1300/J013v10n01_04.
28. Dewa LH, Kyle SD, Hassan L, Shaw J, Senior J. Prevalence, associated factors and management of insomnia in prison populations: An integrative review. *Sleep Med Rev*. 2015;24:13–27. https://doi.org/10.1016/j.smrv.2014.12.002.
29. Toler HC. The treatment of insomnia with relaxation and stimulus-control instructions among incarcerated males. *Correctional Psychologist*. 1978;5(2):117–130. doi:10.1177/009385487800500202.
30. Lutz SJ. The effect of relaxation training on sleep, state anxiety, and sick call in a jail population. *J Prison Jail Health*. 1990;9(1):55–71.
31. Abrams AI, Siegel LM. The Transcendental Meditation® program and rehabilitation at Folsom State Prison: A cross-validation study. *Correctional Psychologist*. 1978;5(1):3–20. doi:10.1177/009385487800500101.
32. Sumter M, Monk-Turner E, Turner C. The benefits of meditation practice in the correctional setting. *J Correct Health Care*. 2009;15(1):47–57. doi:10.1177/1078345808326621.
33. Randall C, Nowakowski S, Ellis JG. Managing acute insomnia in prison: Evaluation of a "one-shot" cognitive behavioral therapy for insomnia (CBT-I) intervention. *Behav Sleep Med*. 2019;17(6):827–836. doi:10.1080/15402002.2018.1518227.
34. Henwood BF, Dzubur E, Redline B, et al. Longitudinal effects of permanent supportive housing on insomnia for homeless adults. *Sleep Health*. 2019;5(3):236–240. https://doi.org/10.1016/j.sleh.2019.01.001.
35. Applebaum KL. Assessment and treatment of correctional inmates with ADHD. *Am J Psychiatry*. 2008;165(12):1520–1524. doi:10.1176/appi.ajp.2008.08060849.
36. Koepsell TD, Longstreth WT, Ton TGN. Medical exposures in youth and the frequency of narcolepsy with cataplexy: A population-based case–control study in genetically predisposed people. *J Sleep Res*. 2010;19(Part I):80–86. https://doi.org/10.1111/j.1365-2869.2009.00756.x.
37. National Institutes of Health. Racial and Ethnic Categories and Definitions for NIH Diversity Programs and for Other Reporting Purposes. Updated April 8, 2015. https://grants.nih.gov/grants/guide/notice-files/not-od-15-089.html. Accessed December 23, 2020.
38. Lambert R. There is nothing minor about us: Why Forbes won't use the term minority to classify Black and Brown people. Forbes.com. Published October 8, 2020. https://www.forbes.com/sites/rashaadlambert/2020/10/08/there-is-nothing-minor-about-us-why-forbes-wont-use-the-term-minority-to-classify-black-and-brown-people/?sh=76bda9667e21. Accessed December 23, 2020.
39. Meraji SM, Escobar N, Devarajan K. Is it time to say R.I.P. to "POC"? NPR. Published September 30, 2020. https://www.npr.org/2020/09/29/918418825/is-it-time-to-say-r-i-p-to-p-o-c. Accessed December 23, 2020.
40. Johnson DA, Jackson CL, Williams NJ, Alcántara C. Are sleep patterns influenced by race/ethnicity - a marker of relative advantage or disadvantage? Evidence to date. *Nat Sci Sleep*. 2019;11:79–95. doi:10.2147/NSS.S169312.
41. Hale L, Do DP. Racial differences in self-reports of sleep duration in a population-based study. *Sleep*. 2007 Sep;30(9):1096–1103. doi:10.1093/sleep/30.9.1096.
42. Whinnery J, Jackson N, Rattanaumpawan P, Grandner MA. Short and long sleep duration associated with race/ethnicity, sociodemographics, and socioeconomic position. *Sleep*. 2014;37(3):601–611. doi:10.5665/sleep.3508.
43. Chapman DP, Croft JB, Liu Y, Perry GS, Presley-Cantrell LR, Ford ES. Excess frequent insufficient sleep in American Indians/Alaska natives. *J Environ Public Health*. 2013;2013(1):259645. doi:10.1155/2013/259645.
44. Chen X, Wang R, Zee P, et al. Racial/ethnic differences in sleep disturbances: The Multi-Ethnic Study of Atherosclerosis (MESA). *Sleep*. 2015;38(6):877–888. doi:10.5665/sleep.4732.
45. Carnethon MR, De Chavez PJ, Zee PC, et al. Disparities in sleep characteristics by race/ethnicity in a population-based sample: Chicago Area Sleep Study. *Sleep Med*. 2016;18:50–55. https://doi.org/10.1016/j.sleep.2015.07.005.
46. Krueger PM, Friedman EM. Sleep duration in the United States: A cross-sectional population-based study. *Am J Epidemiol*. 2009;169(9):1052–1063. doi:10.1093/aje/kwp023.
47. Kalmbach DA, Pillai V, Arnedt JT, Drake CL. DSM-5 insomnia and short sleep: Comorbidity landscape and racial disparities. *Sleep*. 2016;39(12):2101–2111. doi:10.5665/sleep.6306.
48. Stamatakis KA, Kaplan GA, Roberts RE. Short sleep duration across income, education, and race/ethnic groups: Population prevalence and growing disparities during 34 years of follow-up. *Ann Epidemiol*. 2007 Dec;17(12):948–955. doi:10.1016/j.annepidem.2007.07.096.
49. Nunes J, Jean-Louis G, Zizi F, et al. Sleep duration among Black and White Americans: Results of the National Health Interview Survey. *J Natl Med Assoc*. 2008;100(3):317–322. https://doi.org/10.1016/S0027-9684(15)31244-X.
50. Jackson CL, Patel SR, Jackson WB II, Lutsey PL, Redline S. Agreement between self-reported and objectively measured sleep duration among White, black, Hispanic, and Chinese adults in the United States: Multi-Ethnic Study of Atherosclerosis. *Sleep*. 2018;41(6):zsy057. doi:10.1093/sleep/zsy057.
51. Mezick EJ, Matthews KA, Hall M, et al. Influence of race and socioeconomic status on sleep: Pittsburgh SleepSCORE project. *Psychosom Med*. 2008;70(4):410–416. doi:10.1097/PSY.0b013e31816fdf21.
52. McElfish PA, Narcisse M-R, Selig JP, Felix HC, Scott AJ, Long CR. Effects of race and poverty on sleep duration: Analysis of patterns in the 2014 Native Hawaiian and Pacific Islander National Health Interview Survey and General National Health Interview Survey data. *J Racial Ethn Health Disparities*. 2020;4(5):420–428. doi:10.1007/s40615-020-00841-4.
53. Gaston SA, Jackson WB, Williams DR, Jackson CL. Sleep and cardiometabolic health by

government-assisted rental housing status among Black and White men and women in the United States. *Sleep Health*. 2018;4(5):420–428. https://doi.org/10.1016/j.sleh.2018.07.010.

54. Johnson DA, Thorpe RJ, McGrath JA, Jackson WB, Jackson CL. Black-White differences in housing type and sleep duration as well as sleep difficulties in the United States. *Int J Environ Res Public Health*. 2018 Mar 21;15(4):564. doi:10.3390/ijerph15040564.
55. Patel NP, Grandner MA, Xie D, Branas CC, Gooneratne N. "Sleep disparity" in the population: Poor sleep quality is strongly associated with poverty and ethnicity. *BMC Public Health*. 2010;10(1):475. doi:10.1186/1471-2458-10-475.
56. Dudley KA, Patel SR. Disparities and genetic risk factors in obstructive sleep apnea. *Sleep Med*. 2016;18:96–102. https://doi.org/10.1016/j.sleep.2015.01.015.
57. Redline S, Tishler PV, Hans MG, Tosteson TD, Strohl KP, Spry K. Racial differences in sleep-disordered breathing in African-Americans and Caucasians. *Am J Resp Crit Care Med*. 1997;155(1):186–192. doi:10.1164/ajrccm.155.1.9001310.
58. Kripke DF, Ancoli-Israel S, Klauber MR, Wingard DL, Mason WJ, Mullaney DJ. Prevalence of sleep-disordered breathing in ages 40–64 years: A population-based survey. *Sleep*. 1997;20(1):65–76. doi:10.1093/sleep/20.1.65.
59. Ancoli-Israel S, Klauber MR, Stepnowsky C, Estline E, Chinn A, Fell R. Sleep-disordered breathing in African-American elderly. *Am J Resp Crit Care Med*. 1995;152(6):1946–1949. doi:10.1164/ajrccm.152.6.8520760.
60. Young T, Shahar E, Nieto FJ, et al. Predictors of sleep-disordered breathing in community-dwelling adults: The Sleep Heart Health Study. *Arch Intern Med*. 2002;162(8):893–900. doi:10.1001/archinte.162.8.893.
61. Alkhazna A, Bhat A, Ladesich J, Barthel B, Bohnam AJ. Severity of obstructive sleep apnea between Black and White patients. *Hosp Pract*. 2011;39(4):82–86. doi:10.3810/hp.2011.10.926.
62. Sjoding MW, Dickson RP, Iwashyna TJ, Gay SE, Valley TS. Racial bias in pulse oximetry measurement. *N Engl J Med*. 2020;383(25):2477–2478. doi:10.1056/NEJMc2029240.
63. Baskin ML, Ard J, Franklin F, Allison DB. Prevalence of obesity in the United States. *Obesity Rev*. 2005;6(1):5–7. https://doi.org/10.1111/j.1467-789X.2005.00165.x.
64. Low S, Chin MC, Ma S, Heng D, Deurenberg-Yap M. Rationale for redefining obesity in Asians. *Ann Acad Med Singap*. 2009 Jan;38(1):66–69.
65. Buxbaum SG, Elston RC, Tishler PV, Redline S. Genetics of the apnea hypopnea index in Caucasians and African Americans: I. Segregation analysis. *Genet Epidemiol*. 2002;22(3):243–253. https://doi.org/10.1002/gepi.0170.
66. Sutherland K, Lee RWW, Cistulli PA. Obesity and craniofacial structure as risk factors for obstructive sleep apnoea: Impact of ethnicity. *Respirology*. 2012;17(2):213–222. https://doi.org/10.1111/j.1440-1843.2011.02082.x.
67. Palmer LJ, Buxbaum SG, Larkin E, et al. A whole-genome scan for obstructive sleep apnea and obesity. *Am J Hum Genet*. 2003;72(2):340–350. https://doi.org/10.1086/346064.
68. Palmer LJ, Buxbaum SG, Larkin EK, et al. Whole genome scan for obstructive sleep apnea and obesity in African-American families. *Am J Resp Crit Care Med*. 2004;169(12):1314–1321. doi:10.1164/rccm.200304-493OC.
69. Bryc K, Durand EY, Macpherson JM, Reich D, Mountain JL. The genetic ancestry of African Americans, Latinos, and European Americans across the United States. *Am J Hum Genet*. 2015;96(1):37–53. doi:10.1016/j.ajhg.2014.11.010.
70. Redline S, Tishler PV, Tosteson TD, et al. The familial aggregation of obstructive sleep apnea. *Am J Resp Crit Care Med*. 1995;151(3 Pt 1):682–687. doi:10.1164/ajrccm/151.3_Pt_1.682.
71. May AM, Gharibeh T, Wang L, et al. CPAP adherence predictors in a randomized trial of moderate-to-severe OSA enriched with women and minorities. *Chest*. 2018;154(3):567–578. https://doi.org/10.1016/j.chest.2018.04.010.
72. Scharf SM, Seiden L, DeMore J, Carter-Pokras O. Racial differences in clinical presentation of patients with sleep-disordered breathing. *Sleep Breath*. 2004 Dec;8(4):173–183. doi:10.1007/s11325-004-0173-5.
73. Hsu N, Zeidler MR, Ryden AM, Fung CH. Racial disparities in positive airway pressure therapy adherence among veterans with obstructive sleep apnea. *J Clin Sleep Med*. 16(8):1249–1254. doi:10.5664/jcsm.8476.
74. Tran D, Wallace J. Obstructive sleep apnea syndrome in a publicly funded healthcare system. *J Natl Med Assoc*. 2005;97(3):370–374.
75. Billings ME, Auckley D, Benca R, et al. Race and residential socioeconomics as predictors of CPAP adherence. *Sleep*. 2011;34(12):1653–1658. doi:10.5665/sleep.1428.
76. Ruthberg J, Summerville L, Cai Y, Boas S, Otteson T, Kumar A. Utilization of surgical treatment for sleep apnea: A study of health disparities. *Am J Otolaryngol*. 2020;41(6):102670. https://doi.org/10.1016/j.amjoto.2020.102670.
77. Wallace DM, Williams NJ, Sawyer AM, et al. Adherence to positive airway pressure treatment among minority populations in the US: A scoping review. *Sleep Med Rev*. 2018;38:56–69. doi:10.1016/j.smrv.2017.04.002.
78. Olfson M, Wall M, Liu SM, Morin CM, Blanco C. Insomnia and impaired quality of life in the United States. *J Clin Psychiatry*. 2018 Sep 11;79(5):9151. doi:10.4088/JCP.17m12020.
79. American Academy of Sleep Medicine. *International Classification of Sleep Disorders*. 3rd ed. AASM; 2014.
80. Katz D, Braly K. Racial stereotypes of one hundred college students. *J Abnorm Soc Psychol*. 1933;28(3):280–290. doi:10.1037/h0074049.
81. Jean-Louis G, Magai C, Casimir GJ, et al. Insomnia symptoms in a multiethnic sample of American women. *J Womens Health*. 2008;17(1):15–25. doi:10.1089/jwh.2006.0310.
82. Kaufmann CN, Mojtabai R, Hock RS, et al. Racial/ethnic differences in insomnia trajectories among U.S. older adults. *Am J Geriatr Psychiatry*. 2016;24(7):575–584. https://doi.org/10.1016/j.jagp.2016.02.049.
83. Grandner MA, Petrov MER, Rattanaumpawan P, Jackson N, Platt A, Patel NP. Sleep symptoms, race/ethnicity, and socioeconomic position. *J Clin Sleep Med*. 2013;9(09):897–905. doi:10.5664/jcsm.2990.

84. Taylor DJ, Pruiksma KE, Hale WJ, et al. Prevalence, correlates, and predictors of insomnia in the US Army prior to deployment. *Sleep*. 2016;39(10):1795–1806. doi:10.5665/sleep.6156.
85. Singareddy R, Vgontzas AN, Fernandez-Mendoza J, et al. Risk factors for incident chronic insomnia: A general population prospective study. *Sleep Med*. 2012;13(4):346–353. https://doi.org/10.1016/j.sleep.2011.10.033.
86. Mignot E, Hayduk R, Black J, Grumet FC, Guilleminault C. HLA DQB1*0602 is associated with cataplexy in 509 narcoleptic patients. *Sleep*. 1997;20(11):1012–1020. doi:10.1093/sleep/20.11.1012.
87. Mignot E. Genetic and familial aspects of narcolepsy. *Neurology*. 1998;50(2 Suppl 1):S16. doi:10.1212/WNL.50.2_Suppl_1.S16.
88. Solomon P. Narcolepsy in Negroes. *Dis Nerv Syst*. 1945 Jun;6(6):179–183.
89. Longstreth WT, Ton TGN, Koepsell T, Gersuk VH, Hendrickson A, Velde S. Prevalence of narcolepsy in King County, Washington, USA. *Sleep Med*. 2009;10(4):422–426. https://doi.org/10.1016/j.sleep.2008.05.009.
90. Kawai M, O'Hara R, Einen M, Lin L, Mignot E. Narcolepsy in African Americans. *Sleep*. 2015;38(11):1673–1681. doi:10.5665/sleep.5140.
91. Kanbayashi T, Inoue Y, Chiba S, et al. CSF hypocretin-1 (orexin-A) concentrations in narcolepsy with and without cataplexy and idiopathic hypersomnia. *J Sleep Res*. 2002;11(1):91–93. https://doi.org/10.1046/j.1365-2869.2002.00284.x.
92. Okun ML, Lin L, Pelin Z, Hong S, Mignot E. Clinical aspects of narcolepsy-cataplexy across ethnic groups. *Sleep*. 2002;25(1):27–35. doi:10.1093/sleep/25.1.27.
93. Dauvilliers Y, Carlander B, Molinari N, et al. Month of birth as a risk factor for narcolepsy. *Sleep*. 2003;26(6):663–665. doi:10.1093/sleep/26.6.663.
94. Aran A, Lin L, Nevsimalova S, et al. Elevated anti-streptococcal antibodies in patients with recent narcolepsy onset. *Sleep*. 2009;32(8):979–983. doi:10.1093/sleep/32.8.979.
95. Shay S, Shapiro NL, Bhattacharyya N. Pediatric otolaryngologic conditions: Racial and socioeconomic disparities in the United States. *Laryngoscope*. 2017 Mar;127(3):746–752. doi:10.1002/lary.26240.
96. Darrow DH, Buescher ES. Group A streptococcal pharyngitis. *Curr Opin Otolaryngol Head Neck Surg*. 2002;10(6):449–454.
97. Lee HB, Hening WA, Allen RP, Earley CJ, Eaton WW, Lyketsos CG. Race and restless legs syndrome symptoms in an adult community sample in east Baltimore. *Sleep Med*. 2006;7(8):642–645. https://doi.org/10.1016/j.sleep.2006.03.015.
98. Alkhazna A, Saeed A, Rashidzada W, Romaker AM. Racial differences in the prevalence of restless legs syndrome in a primary care setting. *Hosp Pract (1995)*. 2014 Aug;42(3):131–137. doi:10.3810/hp.2014.08.1127.
99. Molnar MZ, Lu JL, Kalantar-Zadeh K, Kovesdy CP. Association of incident restless legs syndrome with outcomes in a large cohort of US veterans. *J Sleep Res*. 2016;25(1):47–56. https://doi.org/10.1111/jsr.12335.
100. Alattar M, Harrington JJ, Mitchell CM, Sloane P. Sleep problems in primary care: A North Carolina Family Practice Research Network (NC-FP-RN) Study. *J Am Board Fam Med*. 2007;20(4):365. doi:10.3122/jabfm.2007.04.060153.
101. Scofield H, Roth T, Drake C. Periodic limb movements during sleep: Population prevalence, clinical correlates, and racial differences. *Sleep*. 2008;31(9):1221–1227.
102. Innes KE, Selfe TK, Agarwal P. Prevalence of restless legs syndrome in North American and Western European populations: A systematic review. *Sleep Med*. 2011;12(7):623–634. https://doi.org/10.1016/j.sleep.2010.12.018.
103. Sawanyawisuth K, Palinkas LA, Ancoli-Israel S, Dimsdale JE, Loredo JS. Ethnic differences in the prevalence and predictors of restless legs syndrome between Hispanics of Mexican descent and Non-Hispanic Whites in San Diego County: A population-based study. *J Clin Sleep Med*. 2013;09(01):47–53. doi:10.5664/jcsm.2338.
104. Hunter JC, Hayden KM. The association of sleep with neighborhood physical and social environment. *Public Health*. 2018;162:126–134. https://doi.org/10.1016/j.puhe.2018.05.003.
105. Ross CE, Mirowsky J. Disorder and decay: The concept and measurement of perceived neighborhood disorder. *Urban Aff Rev*. 1999;34(3):412–432. doi:10.1177/107808749903400304.
106. Hill TD, Burdette AM, Hale L. Neighborhood disorder, sleep quality, and psychological distress: Testing a model of structural amplification. *Health Place*. 2009;15(4):1006–1013. https://doi.org/10.1016/j.healthplace.2009.04.001
107. Hale L, Hill TD, Friedman E, et al. Perceived neighborhood quality, sleep quality, and health status: Evidence from the Survey of the Health of Wisconsin. *Soc Sci Med*. 2013;79:16–22. https://doi.org/10.1016/j.socscimed.2012.07.021.
108. Yamauchi M, Jacono FJ, Fujita Y, et al. Effects of environment light during sleep on autonomic functions of heart rate and breathing. *Sleep Breath*. 2014 Dec;18(4):829–835. doi:10.1007/s11325-014-0951-7.
109. Cho C-H, Lee H-J, Yoon H-K, et al. Exposure to dim artificial light at night increases REM sleep and awakenings in humans. *Chronobiol Int*. 2016;33(1):117–123. doi:10.3109/07420528.2015.1108980.
110. Perron S, Plante C, Ragettli MS, Kaiser, DJ, Goudreau S, Smargiassi A. Sleep disturbance from road traffic, railways, airplanes and from total environmental noise levels in Montreal. *Int J Environ Res Public Health*. 2016;13(8):809.
111. Zanobetti A, Redline S, Schwartz J, et al. Associations of PM10 with sleep and sleep-disordered breathing in adults from seven U.S. urban areas. *Am J Resp Crit Care Med*. 2010;182(6):819–825. doi:10.1164/rccm.200912-1797OC.
112. Fang SC, Schwartz J, Yang M, Yaggi HK, Bliwise DL, Araujo AB. Traffic-related air pollution and sleep in the Boston Area Community Health Survey. *J Expo Sci Environ Epidemiol*. 2015;25(5):451–456. doi:10.1038/jes.2014.47.
113. Weinreich G, Wessendorf TE, Pundt N, et al. Association of short-term ozone and temperature

with sleep disordered breathing. *Eur Respir J*. 2015;46(5):1361. doi:10.1183/13993003.02255-2014.
114. Valham F, Sahlin C, Stenlund H, Franklin KA. Ambient temperature and obstructive sleep apnea: Effects on sleep, sleep apnea, and morning alertness. *Sleep*. 2012;35(4):513–517. doi:10.5665/sleep.1736.
115. Teoh T, Olson C. Effects of ambient noise on sleep in New York City. *J Transport Health*. 2018;9:S15. https://doi.org/10.1016/j.jth.2018.05.068.
116. Billings ME, Johnson DA, Simonelli G, et al. Neighborhood walking environment and activity level are associated with OSA: The Multi-Ethnic Study of Atherosclerosis. *Chest*. 2016;150(5):1042–1049. https://doi.org/10.1016/j.chest.2016.06.012.
117. Casey JA, Morello-Frosch R, Mennitt DJ, Fristrup K, Ogburn EL, James P. Race/ethnicity, socioeconomic status, residential segregation, and spatial variation in noise exposure in the contiguous United States. *Environ Health Perspect*. 2017;125(7):077017. doi:10.1289/EHP898.
118. Billings ME, Hale L, Johnson DA. Physical and social environment relationship with sleep health and disorders. *Chest*. 2020;157(5):1304–1312. https://doi.org/10.1016/j.chest.2019.12.002.
119. Johnson DA, Simonelli G, Moore K, et al. The neighborhood social environment and objective measures of sleep in the Multi-Ethnic Study of Atherosclerosis. *Sleep*. 2017;40(1):zsw016. doi:10.1093/sleep/zsw016.
120. DeSantis AS, Diez Roux AV, Moore K, Baron KG, Mujahid MS, Nieto FJ. Associations of neighborhood characteristics with sleep timing and quality: The Multi-Ethnic Study of Atherosclerosis. *Sleep*. 2013;36(10):1543–1551. doi:10.5665/sleep.3054.
121. Johnson DA, Brown DL, Morgenstern LB, Meurer WJ, Lisabeth LD. The association of neighborhood characteristics with sleep duration and daytime sleepiness. *Sleep Health*. 2015;1(3):148–155. https://doi.org/10.1016/j.sleh.2015.06.002.
122. Johnson DA, Lisabeth L, Hickson D, et al. The social patterning of sleep in African Americans: Associations of socioeconomic position and neighborhood characteristics with sleep in the Jackson Heart Study. *Sleep*. 2016;39(9):1749–1759. doi:10.5665/sleep.6106.
123. Simonelli G, Dudley KA, Weng J, et al. Neighborhood factors as predictors of poor sleep in the Sueño Ancillary Study of the Hispanic Community Health Study/Study of Latinos. *Sleep*. 2017;40(1):zsw025. doi:10.1093/sleep/zsw025.
124. Duncan DT, Park SH, Goedel WC, et al. Perceived neighborhood safety is associated with poor sleep health among gay, bisexual, and other men who have sex with men in Paris, France. *J Urban Health*. 2017;94(3):399–407. doi:10.1007/s11524-017-0148-z.
125. Reid M, Maras JE, Shea S, et al. Association between diet quality and sleep apnea in the Multi-Ethnic Study of Atherosclerosis. *Sleep*. 2019;42(1):zsy194. doi:10.1093/sleep/zsy194.
126. Sawyer PJ, Major B, Casad BJ, Townsend SSM, Mendes WB. Discrimination and the stress response: Psychological and physiological consequences of anticipating prejudice in interethnic interactions. *Am J Public Health*. 2012;102(5):1020–1026. doi:10.2105/AJPH.2011.300620.
127. Slopen N, Lewis TT, Williams DR. Discrimination and sleep: A systematic review. *Sleep Med*. 2016;18:88–95. https://doi.org/10.1016/j.sleep.2015.01.012.
128. Alcántara C, Patel SR, Carnethon M, et al. Stress and sleep: Results from the Hispanic Community Health Study/Study of Latinos Sociocultural Ancillary Study. *SSM Population Health*. 2017;3:713–721. https://doi.org/10.1016/j.ssmph.2017.08.004.
129. Cheng P, Cuellar R, Johnson DA, et al. Racial discrimination as a mediator of racial disparities in insomnia disorder. *Sleep Health*. 2020;6(5):543–549. https://doi.org/10.1016/j.sleh.2020.07.007.
130. Lewis TT, Troxel WM, Kravitz HM, Bromberger JT, Matthews KA, Hall MH. Chronic exposure to everyday discrimination and sleep in a multiethnic sample of middle-aged women. *Health Psychol*. 2013 Jul;32(7):810–819. doi:10.1037/a0029938.
131. Jackson CL, Redline S, Kawachi I, Williams MA, Hu FB. Racial disparities in short sleep duration by occupation and industry. *Am J Epidemiol*. 2013;178(9):1442–1451. doi:10.1093/aje/kwt159.
132. DeSante CD. Working twice as hard to get half as far: Race, work ethic, and America's deserving poor. *Am J Polit Sci*. 2013;57(2):342–356.
133. Beatty DL, Hall MH, Kamarck TA, et al. Unfair treatment is associated with poor sleep in African American and Caucasian adults: Pittsburgh SleepSCORE project. *Health Psychol*. 2011;30(3):351–359. doi:10.1037/a0022976.
134. Tomfohr L, Pung MA, Edwards KM, Dimsdale JE. Racial differences in sleep architecture: The role of ethnic discrimination. *Biol Psychol*. 2012;89(1):34–38. doi:10.1016/j.biopsycho.2011.09.002.
135. American Academy of Sleep Medicine. Sleep health for Apaches. Published September 18, 2018. https://aasm.org/sleep-health-for-apaches-v3i3/. Accessed January 29, 2021.
136. Allen AJMH, Amram O, Tavakoli H, Almeida FR, Hamoda M, Ayas NT. Relationship between travel time from home to a regional sleep apnea clinic in British Columbia, Canada, and the severity of obstructive sleep. *Ann Amer Thorac Soc*. 2016;13(5):719–723. doi:10.1513/AnnalsATS.201509-613BC.
137. Flemons WW, Douglas NJ, Kuna ST, Rodenstein DO, Wheatley J. Access to diagnosis and treatment of patients with suspected sleep apnea. *Am J Resp Crit Care Med*. 2004;169(6):668–672. doi:10.1164/rccm.200308-1124PP.
138. Stewart SA, Skomro R, Reid J, et al. Improvement in obstructive sleep apnea diagnosis and management wait times: A retrospective analysis of a home management pathway for obstructive sleep apnea. *Can Respir J*. 2015;22:516580. doi:10.1155/2015/516580.
139. Thomas A, Grandner M, Nowakowski S, Nesom G, Corbitt C, Perlis ML. Where are the behavioral sleep medicine providers and where are they needed? A geographic assessment. *Behav Sleep Med*. 2016;14(6):687–698. doi:10.1080/15402002.2016.1173551.
140. Pierce RP, Stevermer JJ. Disparities in use of telehealth at the onset of the COVID-19 public health emergency. *J Telemed Telecare*. 2020;29(1):3–9. doi:10.1177/1357633X20963893

141. Babu AR, Herdegen J, Fogelfeld L, Shott S, Mazzone T. Type 2 diabetes, glycemic control, and continuous positive airway pressure in obstructive sleep apnea. *Arch Intern Med*. 2005;165:447–452. doi:10.1001/archinte.165.4.447.
142. Vgontzas AN, Tan TL, Bixler EO, Martin LF, Shubert D, Kales A. Sleep apnea and sleep disruption in obese patients. *Arch Intern Med*. 1994;154(15):1705–1711. doi:10.1001/archinte.1994.00420150073007.
143. Blazer D, Hybels C, Simonsick E, Hanlon JT. Sedative, hypnotic, and antianxiety medication use in an aging cohort over ten years: A racial comparison. *J Am Geriatr Soc*. 2000;48(9):1073–1079. https://doi.org/10.1111/j.1532-5415.2000.tb04782.x.
144. Kaufmann CN, Spira AP, Alexander GC, Rutkow L, Mojtabai R. Trends in prescribing of sedative-hypnotic medications in the USA: 1993–2010. *Pharmacoepidem Drug S*. 2016;25(6):637–645. https://doi.org/10.1002/pds.3951.
145. Tamayo-Sarver JH, Hinze SW, Cydulka RK, Baker DW. Racial and ethnic disparities in emergency department analgesic prescription. *Am J Public Health*. 2003;93(12):2067–2073. doi:10.2105/ajph.93.12.2067.
146. Janakiram C, Chalmers NI, Fontelo P, et al. Sex and race or ethnicity disparities in opioid prescriptions for dental diagnoses among patients receiving Medicaid. *J Am Dent Assoc*. 2019;150(10):e135–e144. doi:10.1016/j.adaj.2019.06.016.
147. Swift SL, Glymour MM, Elfassy T, et al. Racial discrimination in medical care settings and opioid pain reliever misuse in a U.S. cohort: 1992 to 2015. *PLoS One*. 2019;14(12):e0226490. doi:10.1371/journal.pone.0226490.
148. Safer JD, Coleman E, Feldman J, et al. Barriers to healthcare for transgender individuals. *Curr Opin Endocrinol Diabetes Obes*. 2016 Apr;23(2):168–171. doi:10.1097/med.0000000000000227.
149. Bradford J, Reisner SL, Honnold JA, Xavier J. Experiences of transgender-related discrimination and implications for health: Results From the Virginia Transgender Health Initiative Study. *Am J Public Health*. 2012;103(10):1820–1829. doi:10.2105/AJPH.2012.300796.
150. Jaffee KD, Shires DA, Stroumsa D. Discrimination and delayed health care among transgender women and men. *Med Care*. 2016;54(11):1010–1016. doi:10.1097/MLR.0000000000000583.

SECTION VII

The Field of Sleep Medicine

Chapter 32

The History of Sleep Medicine

Surina Sharma and Nancy Collop

INTRODUCTION

Sleep was considered a passive process during early times, which eventually gave way to notions of sleep as a more active process.[1] Before the discovery of sleep-related rapid eye movements (REMs), sleep was regarded universally as an inactive state of the brain, which occurred as the inevitable result of reduced sensory input, while waking up and being awake were considered a reversal of this process, occurring mainly because of bombardment of the brain by stimulation from the environment.[1] No clear distinction was seen between sleep and other inactive states, such as coma, intoxication, hypnosis, anesthesia, and hibernation. Since early times, it has been postulated that compounds like alcohol and opium induced a sleep-like state and that coffee and tea have the power to prevent sleep.[1]

In addition to reduction of stimulation, there was a "hypnotoxin theory," where fatigue products, or toxins, were accumulated during the day, finally causing sleep, during which they were eliminated gradually.[1,2] In the 1920s, University of Chicago physiologist Nathaniel Kleitman performed a series of sleep-deprivation studies and observed that individuals who stayed up all night were generally less impaired and sleepy the next morning than in the middle of their sleepless night.[1,2] Kleitman argued that this was against the theory of continual buildup of hypnotoxin in the brain or blood. He also suggested that humans get very impaired after about 60 hours of wakefulness, and longer periods of sleep deprivation produce negligible change in their level of impairment.[1,2]

ELECTRICAL ACTIVITY OF THE BRAIN

In 1875, the Scottish physiologist Richard Caton demonstrated electrical rhythms in the brains of animals.[3] In 1929, Hans Berger recorded electrical activity of the human brain, and further differentiated these rhythms when subjects were awake or asleep.[3,4] In 1937, Alfred Loomis, working from his private laboratory in New York, first documented the characteristic electroencephalogram (EEG) patterns of what is now called NREM (non-rapid eye movement) sleep: vertex waves, sleep spindles, K complexes, and delta slowing.[5] He divided sleep into 5 stages of increasing depth, from A through E, which formed the basis for the current classification of NREM sleep.[5] In 1953, a new sleep stage, stage REM (rapid eye movement sleep) was described with a correlation of dreaming by Kleitman, with the assistance of his graduate student, Eugene Aserinsky, at the University of Chicago.[6] In 1957, William Dement and Kleitman described human sleep cycles of NREM sleep followed by REM sleep, with cycles repeating throughout the night.[5–7] They proposed a new classification of sleep, using 4 stages of NREM and REM sleep. These classifications are still used today with very few alterations. This electrophysiological analysis of human sleep has been the basis of the immense literature on sleep available to us today.

THE ASCENDING RETICULAR SYSTEM

Insulated implantable electrodes were developed after World War II, after which sleep research on animals began.[1] In 1949, "Brain stem reticular formation and activation of EEG," one of the most influential studies dealing with sleep and wakefulness, was published by Moruzzi and Magoun. Transitions from sleep to wakefulness, or from states of relaxation and drowsiness to alertness and attention, are all characterized by an apparent breaking up of the synchronization of discharge of elements of the cerebral cortex.[8,9] In the seminal paper by Moruzzi and Magon, the authors studied cats that had received chloralosane anesthesia and concluded that transitions from sleep to wakefulness were characterized by a disruption of the synchronization of discharge of elements of the cerebral cortex, and alteration were marked in the EEG by the replacement of high-voltage slow waves with low-voltage fast activity.[9]

High-frequency electrical stimulation with electrodes implanted in the brainstem reticular formation produced EEG activation and arousal.[9] These findings indicated that EEG activation, wakefulness, and consciousness were at one end of spectrum, and EEG synchronization, sleep, and lack of consciousness were at the other end.[1,9]

Another conclusion from the Moruzzi paper was the possibility of maintained activity within the ascending brainstem accounting for wakefulness, while reduction of its activity, either naturally, with drugs like barbiturates, or by experimental injury and disease, may respectively precipitate normal sleep, contribute to anesthesia, or produce pathological somnolence.[9]

Starzl and coworkers demonstrated that sensory collaterals into reticular formation suggested that sensory stimulation could cause prolonged activation of the brain and sustained wakefulness.[1] By this they were able to account for the fact that wakefulness outlasts and can be maintained in the absence of sensory stimulation.

The theory of reticular activating system was an anatomically based passive theory of sleep or active theory of wakefulness. In conclusion, experiments on cats identified a cephalically directed brainstem system, the stimulation of which desynchronizes and activates the EEG, replacing high slow waves with low-voltage fast activity.[9]

This system is in the central core of the brainstem, comprising a series of reticular relays ascending to the basal diencephalon. Its effects are exerted upon the cortex and are mediated, in part at least, by the diffuse thalamic projection system.[9]

HISTORY OF SPECIFIC SLEEP DISORDERS

Includes the history and origin of common sleep disorders that we encounter in clinical practice.

Movement Disorders

RESTLESS LEGS/ANXIETAS TIBIARUM

Restless legs syndrome (RLS) was initially coined Anxietas Tibiarum in the medical literature in 1861 by Whitmaack[12] and was thought to be a manifestation of hysteria. However, the term *restless legs syndrome* was extensively described with a full clinical picture by

Karl-Axel Ekbom.[10] In 1943, he first encountered patients with peculiar paresthesia-like sensation in their legs, with relief on movement, and in 1944, he reported on 8 cases in a series.[11] In 1945, "Restless legs: A clinical study of a hitherto overlooked disease in the legs characterized by peculiar paresthesia ['Anxietas tibiarum'], pain and weakness and occurring in two main forms, asthenia crurum parasethetica and asthenia crurum dolorosa," his doctoral thesis, was published.[12]

In the 19th and 20th centuries, other neurologists, including Wittmaack, along with Romberg, Gilles de la Tourette, Bing, and Oppenheim, published about restless legs in textbooks.[13]

For many years following Ekbom's description, RLS was thought to be a rare disorder. Current data suggests that it may be one of the most common sleep-related disorders with prevalence as high as 10%.

Duncan (1854) and Levick (1862) independently described cases of RLS in pregnancy, an association which is currently well established.[14] Opioids and iron were used as treatment in these patients, a therapy that is still used to the present day.[14] Though these patients had similar symptoms, they incorrectly classified this disorder as a mild form of chorea.[14]

Macdonald Critchley in 1955 noted that in the 17th century, famous English physician and anatomist Sir Thomas Willis described symptoms like RLS. He described restlessness of arms and legs of sufferers which prevented them from falling asleep. The symptoms were thought to originate from the spinal cord.[15] Because of this early description, many sources use the term *Willis-Ekbom disease* to describe RLS.

JACTATION CAPITIS NOCTURNA: RHYTHMIC MOVEMENTS

Rhythmic movement during sleep of an 18-month-old child was first described by Mary Putaman-Jacobi in 1880. This case report discussed "nocturnal rotatory head movement" and was read before the New York Medical Society.[16] "The mother described that after the child had been asleep for a couple of hours, he would turn over on his right side, drawing the right arm above his head, and applying the left hand over the left ear. Once in this position, he would begin to oscillate his head on the pillow from right to left, in a perfectly rhythmical manner. The oscillation would be maintained for about half an hour, and then the child slept quietly again."[16p390-401] Later, "head banging" in children was reported by Zappert at the Society of Internal Medicine and Pediatrics in Vienna.[17] These episodes were also described by Cruchet as "tics"; he differentiated between those which occur selectively at sleep onset and those which occur during sleep.[18]

The largest case series at that time included 15 cases published by Steir, of which 75%–80% of the cases were of head banging.[19] From early observation, it was not very clear when these symptoms resolved, in adolescence or adulthood.

Insomnia

Although insomnia is one of the most common sleep disorders, the diagnostic concept of insomnia fluctuates between insomnia as a symptom or a disorder. Boissier de Sauvages, in his book *Nosologia methodica morborum*, cited from the medical literature about 11 different diseases, all causing insomnia.[20] Boissier noted that reduced forces (*vires imminuuntur*), restlessness (*inquietudo*), and anxiety all may result in increased sensitivity to nighttime awakening, a concept similar to what is described as hyperarousal today.[20] In the 19th century, Durham[21] and Hammond [22] concluded from experiments in animals and from observations in infants and patients that sleep is caused by diminished circulation of blood in the brain. Based on this assumption, potassium bromide was used as a pharmacological sleep aid, a substance which was assumed to exert an anemic action on the brain and to reduce its reactivity to stimuli.[23] In the second half of the 19th century, new substances with sedating properties, such as chloral hydrate, were synthesized.[24] During these times, opinions were divided on appropriate treatment of sleeplessness and if medications should be given or not. In 1861, strong argument about non-pharmacological therapy was made by James Russell. His reasoning was not to rely on medicines and to focus on self-discipline and managing the mind.[25]

A new era of pharmacological treatment of insomnia began with the synthetization of the first compound of a new class of hypnotics, the barbiturates, at the beginning of the

20th century.[26] Barbiturates became the leading class of hypnotics until the mid-20th century. In the 1960s, barbiturate hypnotics were replaced by the newly developed benzodiazepines, starting with chlordiazepoxide in 1960 and diazepam in 1963.[27]

Benzodiazepines interact mainly with the neurotransmitter gamma-aminobutyric acid (GABA) at the GABA-A receptor site.[27] Hypnotic drugs which bind to subsets of the GABA receptor were developed later, frequently summarized as "z-drugs" (zopiclone, zolpidem, and zaleplon). More recently, a newer class of drugs acting on the neurotransmitter orexin/hypocretin, have been developed which are involved in the regulation of wakefulness.[28]

Although the pharmacological treatments were effective, challenges like loss of efficacy, unresponsiveness to treatment, rebound insomnia, and daytime sleepiness or hangover effect were commonly noted. Two main alternatives to drug therapy were developed in the middle of the past century, including issues relating to sleep hygiene and use of principles of behavioral and cognitive therapy, developed in psychology.[29] Methods used included sleep restriction, cognitive therapies, stimulus control, and rules for sleep hygiene.[30,31] Studies have suggested a similar efficiency of pharmacological and behavioral/cognitive therapies; however, the latter showed outlasting effects of the non-pharmacological treatments in comparison to drug therapy.

Hypersomnia

In 1829, a book was published by Bruno Shindler describing various case reports of patients with sleepiness, documenting variable patterns of sleepiness: sleepiness in short intervals, periodic sleep episodes, continuous sleepiness; as well as its duration (days, months, even years).[32] Some of these cases were combined with a characteristic inability to awaken the person from pathological sleep. However, given the limited knowledge of neurological, psychiatric, or infectious causes of sleepiness, this condition remained obscure. In the late 19th and early 20th centuries, the medical community became aware of 3 disorders which had pathological sleepiness as their predominant symptom.

AFRICAN SLEEPING SICKNESS

Sleeping sickness, or trypanosomiasis, was an epidemic illness which affected the African population. It was first described by colonial authorities. An English physician and abolitionist, Thomas Masterman Winterbottom, who had practiced for 4 years in Sierra Leone, found sleeping sickness among the inhabitants of Benin.[32] Some years later, when he practiced again in England, he gave an impressive account of the fatal course of the illness.[32] He published a case report in 1803 documenting the characteristic sign of swollen lymph glands along the back of the neck in the early stage of the disease, and noting other symptoms, including increased appetite, squinting, convulsions, and excessive sleepiness, ultimately followed by death within 3–4 months. He also mentioned that the symptom of swollen lymph glands was noted long ago by Arabian slave traders, who then refrained from buying slaves with this sign.

NARCOLEPSY

The first description of this disorder was by Jean Baptiste Edourad Gelineau in 1880.[8] Gélineau (1880) called the disease *narcolepsy*, derived from the Greek, which meant "somnolent seized."[33] He was the first to publish a clear description of the constellation of components that constitute the syndrome. Late in the 19th century, 2 case reports were published on patients who fell asleep repeatedly in inadequate situations with sudden loss of muscle tone, typically evoked by surprise or laughter.[34–36] Subsequently, in 1916, Richard Hennberg coined the term *cataplexy* for the emotionally induced muscle weakness that we now know is seen in most patients with type 1 narcolepsy[8]

In 1960, Vogel recognized that REM sleep happened at sleep onset in narcoleptics rather than the normal 1–2 hours later.[37] Japanese narcoleptics were observed to carry HLA haplotype DR2, a finding later confirmed in American Caucasians.[38] A lower frequency of HLA DR2 in African Americans led to the discovery that the antigen responsible was DQ1 rather than DR2.[39] The responsible subtype was identified as HLA DQB1*0602,[40] present in 85%–90% of narcoleptics who have cataplexy.[41]

Molecular genetic studies in animal models of the disease led to the detection of orexin/hypocretin, a transmitter of hypothalamic origin which is unusually low or absent in the majority of patients with narcolepsy-cataplexy.[42] In 1998, 2 peptides were identified in the hypothalamus: hypocretin 1 (Hrct-1) and Hrct-2, their names revealing the hypothalamic origin and homology to secretin.[43] Simultaneously, another group of investigators identified the same peptides and called them orexin-A and orexin-B, based on their appetite-stimulating function.[44] These molecules arise from a precursor called preprohypocretin (synthesized by a small number of cells in the posterior and lateral hypothalamus). They project to the brain and spinal cord, specifically the monoaminergic and cholinergic fields of the brainstem tegmentum, comprising the ascending reticular activating system.[45,46] Two receptors were identified, with Hrct-1 receptors with high affinity for Hrct-1 and Hrct-2 receptors with high affinity for Hrct-2.

In 1999, research in a canine model at Stanford led by Dr. Mignot led to the discovery that narcolepsy was caused by deletion in the Hrct-2 receptor gene[47]and was found to be an autosomal recessive trait. Another group of investigators studying orexin knockout mice showed that mice developed either REM sleep or cataplexy while awake.[48] Subsequent autopsy studies of the brains of human narcoleptics showed that Hcrt was absent in the hypothalamus, cortex, and pons, and Hcrt neurons were reduced by 90% compared to controls.[49.50] It was also found that CSF Hrct was low in patients with cataplexy (87%) and in some patients without cataplexy (14%), with normal levels in control subjects (0%) or in patients with neurological disorders (2%).[51]

ENCEPHALITIS LETHARGICA

The third event contributing to much of the understanding of daytime sleepiness and sleep pathology was the epidemic occurrence of a new infectious disease, encephalitis lethargica (also known as sleeping sickness) in 1916–1927 in Europe, described by Constantin von Economo.[52,53] Sleep was a major symptom of the disease, either in the form of hypersomnia, agrypnia, or sleep inversion. Based on the study of the brainstem lesions in encephalitis lethargica, Economo came to the conclusion that it is the brain stem centers that control wakefulness and sleep[53] Lesions of the anterior area (basal forebrain) produced wakefulness, those of the posterior area produced sleep. The inverse was true for stimulation of these areas. Further knowledge on the interplay between cortical and subcortical structures for the regulation of sleep and wakefulness was the late 1940s when Moruzzi and Magoun recognized the key role of the brainstem reticular formation (ascending reticular activating system, ARAS) for the regulation of wakefulness and sleep. Of note, no recurrence of the epidemic has since been reported, though isolated cases still continue to occur.

RECURRENT HYPERSOMNIA

Two early Russian case reports by Anfimoff (1898) and Kabanich (1923)[54,55] described persons with recurrent sleep attacks and protracted sleep and were reproduced in some detail by Kaplinsky and Schulmann.[56] In the early 20th century, Willi Kleine[57] and Max Levin[58] both reported on cases of periodic sleepiness, mostly in young males, with episodes of hyperphagia, sexual disinhibition, and other signs of abnormal behavior, which were noted in the subject between episodes. The term *Kleine-Levin syndrome* was first used by Critchley and Hoffman for this rare syndrome of recurrent hypersomnia, suggesting the involvement of hypothalamus for the clinical picture.[59] It has been documented by Dauvillers et al. that human leukocyte antigen DQB1*0201 allele is associated with Kleine-Levin syndrome. Diffuse brain hypoperfusion, mainly in thalamic and frontotemporal areas, has been found on single-photon emission computed tomography (SPECT). Functional neuroimaging during the symptomatic period of Kleine-Levin showed transient hypoactivity in the thalamic region and lesser degree of hypoactivity noted in hypothalamus, frontal and temporal regions, with resolution of thalamic hypoperfusion during asymptomatic periods. [60]

In 1990, the diagnostic criteria for Kleine-Levin syndrome were modified by the International Classification of Sleep Disorders (ICSD) where it was defined by recurring episodic daytime sleepiness, and may or may not be associated with hyperphagia and abnormal behavior.[60]

Parasomnias

Although the term *parasomnia* is relatively new, the sleep disturbances belonging to this category have been known since ancient times. The term *parasomnia* was first used in 1905 by the Swiss psychologist Edouard Claparède,[61] who differentiated 3 forms of pathological sleep: insomnia, hypersomnia, and parasomnia. A few years later, Albert Salmon described nightmares, sleep walking, and sleep talking as parasomnias.[62]

SLEEPWALKING

The 19th century was the peak time for publications on sleep walking due to a widespread interest in animal magnetism or "magnetic sleep," described as a sleep-like state, frequently associated with a somnambulistic episode, which was induced by magnetizers or hypnotists.[63] Early in the 20th century, Sadger, a Viennese psychiatrist and disciple of Freud, published a monograph *Sleep Walking and Moon Walking*,[64] describing an analysis of sleep walking in his patients and as seen in novels. He described sleepwalking as a "motor outbreak of the unconscious and serves like the dream, the fulfillment of secret, forbidden wishes, mostly of a sexual erotic nature."[64]

Later, EEG studies showed that the sleep walking episodes began during slow wave sleep, and the EEG during somnambulistic incidents was low voltage with mixed frequencies.[65] If the alpha waves occurred, they were not blocked by eye opening. During these incidents, sleepwalkers appeared to be aware of their environment but indifferent to it, with eyes open, a blank stare, and rigid movements. The EEG studies also confirmed that these incidents occurred early during sleep.

INCUBUS: NIGHTMARE DISORDERS

A detailed description of incubus in medieval theology and medicine can be found in a book by Van der Lugt.[66] Paulus Aegineta, a 7th century surgeon of the island of Aegina, gave his version of a detailed description of the disorder as "persons suffering the attack experience incapable of motion, a torpid sensation in their sleep, a sense of suffocation, and oppression, as if from one pressing them down, with inability to cry out, or they utter inarticulate sounds."[67] He further notes that some often imagine that they even hear the person who is pressing them down and offers lustful violence to them, but he flies away when they attempt to grasp him with their fingers.

The concept of nightmare disorder has changed substantially with time. Previously, nightmare disorder was thought to be caused by an outside force or person, an explanation which in present time does not exist, and such explanations were identified as superstition. From the medical point of view, the "evil" was assumed to be caused by indigestion[68] or stagnation of the blood.[69] Later, Ernest Jones understood the nightmare as the expression of the deepest mental conflict.[70] After the identification of REM and NREM as 2 different states of sleep, the symptoms complex of an incapability to move, associated with anxiety, was split into 2 different disorders. The diagnostic system of the Association of Sleep Disorders Centers (the precursor to the International Classification of Sleep Disorders [ICSD]) separated incubus under the diagnostic category "Sleep Terror," distinct from the category "Dream Anxiety Attacks" (nightmares).[71]

In the revised classification system of the ICSD (ICSD 3, 2005) [60], the term *incubus* was canceled. Components of the historical symptom complex are now divided in 3 different categories: Recurrent Isolated Sleep Paralysis, Sleep Terrors, and Nightmare Disorder.[72]

PAVOR NOCTURNUS: SLEEP TERRORS

Since the 17th century, Pavor Nocturnus, or sleep terrors, have been described in textbooks.[73] In 1845, Dr. Hesse was one of the first to write a monograph on sleep terrors in children, giving a clear description of these attacks and separating them from sleep walking and nightmares.[74] As he described, these attacks occurred abruptly, lasting for 15–20 minutes, and came to an end slowly; many children were not able to describe what was horrifying to them. The victims of these attacks are in panic and do not recognize their environment.[74]

Rey (1897) assumed "adenoid vegetations" as the main cause for nightly attacks.[75] Comparable observations were made earlier by Warrington Haward, who observed disappearance of what he called "nightmare" after the removal of the tonsils in 4 children.[76] Braun (1896) regarded the disease as a form of neurasthenia, defined as an increased irritability of the nervous system.[77]

Much later, in the EEG era of sleep medicine, it was established that somnambulism and night terrors arise out of deep NREM sleep, and both represented disorders of arousal.[78]

REM Sleep Behavior Disorder (RBD)

This disorder was first reported by Schenck, Mahowald, and colleagues in 1986.[79] Prior to this, Jouvet and Morrison described an RBD equivalent in animals, where they experimentally lesioned cat's brains (pontine tegmentum lesions) and described "oneiric behaviors."[79]Hishikawa's group in the 1970s described a peculiar sleep state in alcoholics and other subjects of drug withdrawal with rapid eye movements and increased chin muscle activity (described as "stage 1-REM with tonic EMG."[79] In 1981, this "stage-1 REM" was also described in patients with Shy Drager syndrome.[79]

After 1990, more extensive studies on RBD revealed that about half of RBD cases were associated with neurological disorders, especially neurodegenerative diseases pathologically known as synucleiopathies (Parkinson disease [PD], Lewy body dementia, and multiple system atrophy).[79]

More recently, it was reported that RBD is also often noted in narcolepsy, although the pathophysiological mechanism of this state was still unknown.[79]

OBSTRUCTIVE SLEEP APNEA (OSA)

Reports on respiratory pauses (apneas) were rare before the 19th century. One of the first medical dissertations on this topic was published by Alberti and Lust in 1745; these authors described risk factors such as corpulence, short neck, and other risk factors affecting the airways during sleep.[80] Observation of sleep-disordered breathing was written about by Charles Dickens in 1836, where he described Joe, "an obese boy noted to be lazy" and a loud snorer in his published case series entitled *Posthumous Papers of the Pickwick Club*.[81]

Original descriptions of sleep apnea were made in independent medical publications in 1965 by Gastaut, Tassinari, and Duron in France and by Jung and Kuhlo in Germany.[1]

A case report published in 1960 by Heidelberg University Hospital described a patient who had come for investigation of recurring morning headache and was observed to have respiratory pauses during sleep with recovery breathing, followed with a loud snore. Drachman and Gummit described evaluation of EEG and blood gas analysis in an obese woman who demonstrated repetitive stoppage of air exchange despite persistence of thoracoabdominal movements.[1]

Guilleminault was the first to describe obstructive sleep apnea (OSA) as a clinical syndrome. Alberto Tassinari, Elio Lugaresi, in addition to Giorgio Coccagna and Guilleminault, provided a complete description of sleep apnea syndrome, including the occurrence of sleep apnea in nonobese patients, an account of the cardiovascular correlates, and the importance of snoring and hypersomnolence as diagnostic indicators.

Historic literature on therapeutic interventions of OSA were rare in early times; however, it was advised to avoid sleeping in supine sleep position as it promoted snoring and mouth breathing.

A few cases of resection of parts of the soft palate successfully eliminated obstruction of respiration in sleep,[82,83,84] In 1978, Remmers et al. documented the relationship between intraluminal airway pressure and elevtromyography (EMG) activity of the genioglossus muscle in the pathophysiology of upper airway collapse in the pharyngeal segment of the airway, and tracheostomy was recognized as an effective treatment.[85] Before the 1980s, tracheostomy remained the only effective, though undesirable, treatment of OSA. This highly effective approach was replaced in 1981 by 2 new procedures, 1 surgical (uvulopalatopharyngoplasty [UPPP]) and other mechanical (use of continuous nasal airway pressure).

In 1981, Fujita et al. introduced UPPP, involving trimming and reorientation of the posterior and anterior tonsillar pillars and excision of the uvula and posterior palate.[86] This was aimed to enlarge the airspace in the oropharynx, thus preventing the airway from collapsing at night.

A breakthrough in therapy came in 1981 when Sullivan et al. were the first to treat sleep apnea mechanically by continuous positive airway pressure, a method which soon became the treatment of choice.[87] In the 1990s, the use of oral appliances was first published in the journal *Sleep* as a potential treatment for

OSA, but became more popular as a potential treatment option in the early 2000s.[88]

More recently, upper airway stimulation as a treatment alternative for those who fail prior therapy has been gaining popularity. First publication of transcutaneous submental stimulation was in 1988 in Japan and was shown to improve daytime sleepiness and snoring; however, there was only minimal improvement in AHI (apnea hypopnea index).[89] A few other studies involving submaxillary stimulation have been published but with variable results. Hypoglossal nerve stimulation (HNS) emerged as an alternative to muscle stimulation. In 1993, studies demonstrated that HNS was capable of keeping the airway open during sleep but could not eliminate apnea once established.[90] The initial trial of efficacy was reported in 2001. In the United States the pivotal trial for HNS, also known as Inspire therapy, was completed in 2013 and gained Food and Drug Administration approval in April 2014.

Circadian Rhythm Sleep Disorders

The assessment of rest-activity cycle was made by Syzmanski, a Viennese biologist who innovated an actimetric device to measure activity across the 24-hour period in all animal and human babies.[91,92] This helped to differentiate between monophasic and polyphasic sleep among different species, and between day-active animals which use light, and night-active animals that use odor for orientation. Miniature actimetric portable devices became popular in the 1980s, which were used in circadian rhythm research and sleep medicine.

In 1972, anatomic destruction of the suprachiasmatic nucleus (SCN) in rats, located in the hypothalamus, was shown to eliminate circadian rhythms in adrenal corticosterone. It was noted to affect the drinking and locomotor activity in rats.[93,94] Moore and Lenn identified the retinohypothalamic tract that serves the important function of connecting the SCN with the photic environment.[95] Another finding suggesting the central role of SCN in the circadian rhythmicity was that individual neurons dissociated from the SCN could maintain rhythmic circadian firing patterns when cultured in vitro.[96]

The circadian rhythm research expanded rapidly in 1978, when the SCN was recognized as the central locus of circadian timing.[92] The interaction between sleep and circadian rhythms was studied intensively in the following years, with results of the experimental studies then integrated into a theoretical frame by the most influential 2-process model of sleep regulation.

The first gene coding for clock protein, the "*per* gene," was found in 1975 in Drosophila.[97] mRNA transcript of the *per* gene was found to oscillate in a circadian fashion because of transcriptional regulation.[98] Another gene, *tim*, [99] the timeless gene, was found later, and mRNA of the *tim* gene oscillated in synchrony with the *per* gene. *CLOCK* and *BMAL1*[100,101]genes were identified later.

In 1999, Jones[102] found a profound phase advance of the sleep-wake cycle, melatonin, and body temperature rhythm in association with a very short circadian period. The inheritance of this trait was found to be an autosomal dominant pattern. Toh et al.[103] established that the familial advanced sleep phase syndrome resulted in mis-sense mutation of the clock component of hPER2 protein which alters the circadian periodicity. Observations from these studies suggested that people with delayed sleep phase likely had a similar genetic basis, except that the subjects had a delayed circadian period instead of advanced sleep phase.

Light was found to be the dominant synchronizing force affecting the circadian rhythm.[104] In 1963, Wurtman et al. reported that melatonin synthesis in the pineal gland was under the inhibitory control of light.[105] The retinohypothalmic tract connecting the retina to the SCN was first documented in 1971.[106] Moore et al. subsequently went on to identify the neural pathway by which output from the SCN reaches the pineal gland.[107]

DEVELOPMENT OF ACADEMIC SLEEP MEDICINE AND SLEEP MEDICINE ORGANIZATIONS

American Academy of Sleep Medicine (AASM)

The AASM was originally called the Association of Sleep Disorders Centers (ASDC) and was founded in 1975. The original leadership group included Drs. Dement, Edward Bixler, Ismet Karacan, Milton Kramer, David Kupfer, Howard Roffwarg, Thomas Roth, and Elliot Weitzman.

The first sleep disorders center was established as a narcolepsy clinic at Stanford University in 1964. By 1975, in addition to Stanford, Montefiore Medical Center in New York, Ohio State University, Baylor College in Houston, University of Cincinnati Medical Center, and the University of Pittsburgh Medical School were doing overnight sleep studies.

The ASDC Accreditation Committee, previously known as the Certification Committee, accredited the first sleep center at Montefiore Hospital in New York on April 27, 1977.

The ASDC appointed a Nosology Committee in February 1976 to begin the task of creating a diagnostic system for sleep and arousal disorders that would include all conditions encountered clinically. A complete revision, begun in 1985 under the direction of Dr. Michael Thorpy, ended in publication of *The International Classification of Sleep Disorders: Diagnostic and Coding Manual* (ICSD) in 1990.

In 1999, the name of the organization was changed to the American Academy of Sleep Medicine (AASM).

The Sleep Research Society (SRS) was founded in 1961, when a group of researchers met in 1961 to discuss ideas and data. In 1962, group selected its first secretary-treasurer, Dr. Joseph Kamiya.

In 1972, Dr. Michael Chase began the annual publication of *Sleep Research* that included abstracts and articles published during the year. In 1998, the journal *Sleep* took over publication of the abstracts from the annual meeting, which by then had evolved into the current combined meeting including the SRS and the AASM.

On January 13, 1986, the ASDC and the SRS, along with the Association of Polysomnographic Technologists (APT), formed a federation—the Association of Professional Sleep Societies (APSS). A few years later, the APT withdrew from the APSS partnership, leading to yet another name change to Associated Professional Sleep Societies from the Association of Professional Sleep Societies in 1989.

In 1988, an international organization was founded, the World Sleep Federation (WSF). At the time of collaboration, it comprised AASM, Asian Sleep Research Society, Australasian Sleep Association, Canadian Sleep Society, European Sleep Research Society, Latin American Sleep Societies, and Sleep Research Society. The World Association of Sleep Medicine (WASM) was another international organization. In 2016, both WSF and WASM collaborated to form the World Sleep Society.

The American Academy of Dental Sleep Medicine (AADSM) was originally founded as the Sleep Disorders Dental Society in 1991. The initial team included 8 dentists with interest in treating sleep-disordered breathing. In 1998, the AADSM established a certification program in dental sleep medicine and administered its first examination in 1999; it has offered an examination each year thereafter.

Sleep Medicine Fellowship Training

A Sleep Medicine fellowship training committee was formed by the AASM in 1988. The committee was responsible for developing formal guidelines for the comprehensive training of physicians in sleep medicine. Trainees had various backgrounds, including internal medicine, psychiatry, neurology, pulmonary, and pediatrics.

Board eligibility is typically a requirement for individuals completing fellowship training. The original certifying organization for sleep medicine providers was the American Board of Sleep Medicine (ABSM). It required its candidates to have the equivalent of 1 year of formal fellowship training in sleep medicine or, through a clinical waiver, with limited formal training.

To encourage the accreditation process, the ABSM decided to phase out the clinical waiver option by 2003, and to require a full year of sleep medicine training in an AASM-accredited fellowship by the year 2005.

As the ABSM and AASM fellowship accreditation was ongoing, in 2002, AASM applied within the Accreditation Council on Graduate Medical Education (ACGME) for the establishment of sleep medicine training programs within the ACGME. In the spring of 2003, the ACGME appointed a Sleep Medicine Working Group (SMWG). The SMWG developed training requirements for ACGME-approved 1-year Sleep Medicine fellowships. These initial training requirements were approved in June 2004.

For many years prior to 2004, the sleep medicine organizations requested ABMS (American Board of Medical Specialties) for a certification examination but had been consistently rebuffed. However, finally the ACGME, under the leadership of the late Dr. Marvin Dunn, accredited sleep medicine training and subsequently, the ABMS agreed to offer a sleep medicine certification examination.

PhD trainees in sleep medicine have made noteworthy contributions, especially in the field of behavioral sleep medicine (BSM). The focus of BSM is on the evaluation and treatment of insomnia, especially cognitive behavioral therapy, the evaluation and treatment of circadian rhythm disorders and parasomnias, as well as improving the compliance of patients with various treatment measures such as positive airway pressure for sleep-disordered breathing. The first review course in Behavioral Sleep Medicine was offered by the AASM in April 2004.

The first examination in ABSM was given in 2003 by a committee led by Dr. Edward Stepanski, resulting in 31 candidates being certified. This examination was focused on psychologists and physicians interested in this field.

HIGHLIGHTS OF THE IMPORTANT MILESTONES IN SLEEP MEDICINE

1880: Gelineau, a French neurologist, recognizes narcolepsy and cataplexy as a condition associated with sudden sleep attacks, distinct from epilepsy.

1937: Loomis and colleagues document the characteristics on an EEG of what is now known as NREM (non-rapid eye movement) sleep. Loomis outlines 5 stages of the increasing depth of sleep, classified as A through E.

1953: A new sleep stage called REM (rapid eye movement) sleep is discovered by Dement and Kleitman. This stage of sleep is believed to be associated with dreaming.

1957: Dement and Kleiman propose a new classification of sleep, which proposes 4 stages of NREM sleep as well as REM sleep.

1964: A Narcolepsy Center is established at Stanford University.

1966: Researchers in Europe describe the clinical entity of sleep apnea syndrome. At that time, the only treatment available is tracheostomy.

1968: A manual is developed for the scoring of sleep.

1970: Stanford University develops the first comprehensive sleep center, and the ability to perform nocturnal polysomnography (sleep study) is developed.

1975: At this time there are now 5 sleep centers. The need for an organization that would be oriented around the sleep center and that would also provide medical and research direction is recognized. The Association of Sleep Disorders Centers (ASDC) is founded. This organization today is known as the American Academy of Sleep Medicine (AASM).

1976: The ASDC forms a nosology committee to develop a diagnostic system that will

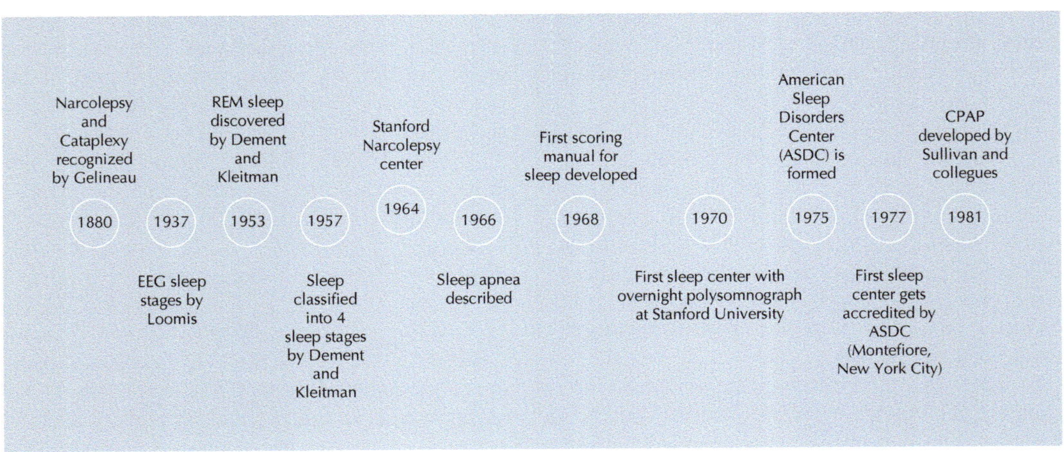

consider all the sleep and arousal disorders that are seen clinically.

1977: The ASDC accredits the first sleep center at Montefiore Hospital in New York City.

1978: The first issue of the journal *Sleep* is published.

1980: The first report on the successful use of an oral appliance is published.

1981: Sullivan and colleagues introduce a new treatment for sleep apnea: continuous positive airway pressure (CPAP). CPAP became the mainstay of treatment in the early days, and has continued to be the gold standard for the management of sleep apnea.

1986: The first scientific meeting dedicated to sleep and sleep disorders is held in Columbus, Ohio.

1987: Ancoli-Israel and colleagues use home testing devices.

1987: The ASDC changes its name to the American Sleep Disorders Association (ASDA) and will eventually be known as the AASM.

1989: AASM begins to accredit fellowship programs in sleep medicine for physicians with an interest in this field.

1990: The first copy of *International Classification of Sleep Disorders* is published (ICSD-1).

1992: The first practice parameters document is published by the AASM.

1994: The American Medical Association (AMA) recognizes sleep medicine as a subspecialty

REFERENCES

1. Pelayo R, Dement WC. *History of Sleep Physiology and Medicine: Principles and Practices of Sleep Medicine*. 6th ed. Elsevier; 2015:3–14.
2. Inoué S, Honda K, Komoda Y. Sleep as neuronal detoxification and restitution. *Behav Brain Res*. 1995 Jul–Aug;69(1-2):91–96. doi:10.1016/0166-4328(95)00014-k. PMID: 7546322.
3. Rechtschaffen A, Bergmann BM, Everson CA, et al. Sleep deprivation in the rat: X. Integration and discussion of the findings. *Sleep*. 1989;12:68–87.
4. Everson CA. Sustained sleep deprivation impairs host defense. *Am J Physiol*. 1993;265(5 Pt 2):R1148–R1154.
5. Bonnet MH. Sleep deprivation. In: Kryger MH, Roth T, Dement W, eds. *Principles and Practice of Sleep Medicine*. 3rd ed. WB Saunders; 2000:53–71.
6. Kripke DF, Simons RN, Garfinkel L, et al. Short and long sleep and sleeping pills. Is increased mortality associated? *Arch Gen Psychiatry*. 1979;36:103–116.
7. Kripke DF, Garfinkel L, Wingard DL, et al. Mortality associated with sleep duration and insomnia. *Arch Gen Psychiatry*. 2002;59:131–136.
8. Shepard JW Jr, Buysse DJ, Chesson AL Jr, et al. History of the development of sleep medicine in the United States. *J Clin Sleep Med*. 2005;1(1):61–82.
9. Moruzzi G, Magoun HW. Brainstem reticular formation and activation of the EEG. *Electroencephalogr Clin Neurophysiol*. 1949;1:455–473.
10. Ekbom KA. Restless legs syndrome. *Neurology*. 1960;10:868–873.
11. Ekbom KA. Asthenia crurum paraesthetica (Irritable legs). *Acta Med Scand*. 1944;118:197–209.
12. Ekbom KA. Restless legs. *Acta Med Scand*. 1945;158:1–123.
13. Romberg MH. *Lehrbuch der Nervenkrankheiten des Menschen. Ersten Bandes erste Abtheilung*. Alexander Duncker, 1840.
14. Levick JJ. Remarks on chorea with notices of some allied disorders. *Am J Med Sci*. 1862;85:40–54.
15 Willis T. *The London Practice of Physick*. Thomas Basset and William Crook; 1685.
16. Putman-Jacobi M. Case of nocturnal rotary spasm. J Nerv Ment Dis. 1880;7: pages 390–401.
17. Zappert J. Über rhythmische Kopfbewegungen im Schlafe. *Mitteilungen Ges Inn Med Kinderheilk Wien*. 1904;3:231–233.
18. Stier E. Über das gewohnheitsmäßige nächtliche Kopfschütteln der Kinder. *Z ges Neurol Psychiat*. 1924;90:213–234.
19. Cruchet R. *Contribution à l'étude des rythmies d'habitude du sommeil*. Gaz hebdom sci méd Bordeaux; 1906; Fev 18.
20. Boissier de Sauvages F. Nosologia methodica morborum. Classes, genera et species. Amsterdam, 1763. Boissier de Sauvages F. *Nosologie methodique, dans laquelle les maladies sont rangées par classes, suivant le systême de Sydenham, & l'ordre des Botanistes*. Traduite du Latin. Hérissant et le Fils; 1771.
21. Durham AE. The physiology of sleep. *Guy Hosp Rep*. 1860;6:149–173.
22 Hammond WA. On Wakefulness: With an Introductory Chapter of the Physiology of Sleep. JB Lippincott and Co.; 1866.
23. Lewitzky. Ueber die Wirkung des Bromkalium auf das Nervensystem. *Virchows Arch Path Anat Physiol*. 1869;45:183–197.
24. Liebreich O. *Das Chloralhydrat ein neues Hypnoticum und Anaestheticum und dessen Anwendung in der Medicin*. GF Otto Müller's Verlag; 1869.
25. Russell J. On sleepiness. *Br Med J*. 1861;1:545–548, 2:488–490, 2:527–529.
26. Fischer E, von Mering J. Über eine neue Klasse von Schlafmitteln. *Therap Gegenw*. 1903;44:97–101.
27. López-Muñoz F, Ucha-Udabe R, Alamo C. The history of barbiturates a century after their clinical introduction. *Neuropsychiatr Dis Treat*. 2005;1:329–343.
28. Mignot E. History of narcolepsy at Stanford. *Immunol Res*. 2014;58:315–339.
29. Spielman AJ, Caruso LS, Glovinsky PB. A behavioral perspective on insomnia treatment. *Psychiat Clin North Am*. 1987;10:541–543.
30. Miller CB, Espie CA, Epstein DR, et al. The evidence base of sleep restriction therapy for treating insomnia disorder. *Sleep Med Rev*. 2014;18:415–424.
31. Riemann D, Perlis ML. The treatments of chronic insomnia: A review of benzodiazepine receptor agonists and psychological and behavioral therapies. *Sleep Med Rev*. 2009:13:205–214.

32. Winterbottom TM. *An account of the native Africans in the neighbourhood of Sierra Leone, to which is added an account of the present state of medicine among them*. C Whittingham; 1803.
33. Gélineau JBE. De la narcolepsie. *Gaz des Hôp Civ et Milit Empire Ottoman*. 1880;53:626–628, 635–637.
34. Westphal C. Zwei Krankheitsfälle, vorgetragen in der Berliner Medicinisch Psychologischen Gesellschaft. I. Anfälle larvierter Epilepsie, dem Ausbruche paralytischer Geistesstörung Jahre lang vorausgehend. II. Eigenthümliche mit Einschlafen verbundene Anfälle. *Arch Psychiat Nervenkr*. 1877;7:622–635.
35. Schenck CH, Bassetti CL, Arnulf I, Mignot E. English translation of the first clinical reports on narcolepsy by Westphal and Gélineau in the late 19th century, with commentary. *J Clin Sleep Med*. 2007; 3:301–311.
36. Lennox WG. Thomas Willis on narcolepsy. *Arch Neurol*. 1939; 41:348–351.
37. Rechtschaffen A, Wolpert E, Dement W, et al. Nocturnal sleep in narcoleptics. *Electroencephal Clin Neurophysiol*. 1963; 15:599–609.
38. Juji T, Sataki M, Honda Y, Doy Y. HLA-antigens in Japanese patients with narcolepsy. *Tissue Antigens*. 1984; 24:316–319.
39. Matsuki K, Grumet FC, Lin X, et al. DQ (rather than DR) gene marks susceptibility to narcolepsy. *Lancet*. 1992;339(8800):1052.
40. Mignot E, Lin X, Arrigoni J, et al. DQB1*0602 and DQA1*0102 (DQ1) are better markers than DR2 for narcolepsy in Caucasian and Black Americans. *Sleep*. 1994;17(Suppl 8): S60–S67.
41. Mignot E, Hayduk R, Black J, et al. HLA DQB1*0602 is associated with cataplexy in 509 narcoleptic patients. *Sleep*. 1997; 20:1012–1020.
42. Mignot E. History of narcolepsy at Stanford. *Immunol Res*. 2014; 58:315–339.
43. de Lecea L, Kilduff TS, Peyron C, et al. The hypocretins: Hypothalamus-specific peptides with neuroexcitatory activity. *Proc Natl Acad Sci U S A*. 1998; 95:322–327.
44. Sakurai T, Amemiya A, Ishii M, et al. Orexins and orexin receptors: A family of hypothalamic neuropeptides and G protein-coupled receptors that regulate feeding behavior. *Cell*. 1998; 92:573–585.
45. Marcus JN, Aschkenasi CJ, Lee CE, et al. Differential expression of orexin receptors 1 and 2 in the rat brain. *J Comp Neurol*. 2001;18(435):6–25.
46. Kilduff TS, Peyron C. The hypocretin/orexin ligand-receptor system: Implications for sleep and sleep disorders. *Trends Neurosci*. 2000; 23:359–365.
47. Lin L, Faraco J, Li R, et al. The sleep disorder canine narcolepsy is caused by a mutation in the hypocretin (orexin) receptor 2 gene. *Cell*. 1999; 98:365–376.
48. Chemelli RM, Willie JT, Sinton CM, et al. Narcolepsy in orexin knockout mice: Molecular genetics of sleep regulation. *Cell*. 1999; 98:437–451.
49. Peyron C, Faraco J, Rogers W, et al. A mutation in a case of early onset narcolepsy and a generalized absence of hypocretin peptides in human narcoleptic brains. *Nat Med*. 2000; 6:991–997.
50. Thannickal TC, Moore RY, Nienhuis R, et al. Reduced number of hypocretin neurons in human narcolepsy. *Neuron*. 2000; 27:469–474.
51. Nishino S, Ripley B, Overeem S, Lammers GJ, Mignot E. Hypocretin (orexin) deficiency in human narcolepsy. *Lancet*. 2000;355(9197):39–40.
52. Von Economo C. *Die encephalitis lethargica*. Deuticke, 1917.
53. Von Economo C. Der Schlaf als Lokalisationsproblem. In: Sarason D (Hrsg). *Der Schlaf. Mitteilungen und Stellungnahme zum derzeitigen Stande des Schlafproblems*. JF Lehmanns; 1929:38–54.
54. Macnish R. *The Philosophy of Sleep*. M'phun; 1830.
55. Gimson WG. Case of prolonged and profound sleep, occurring at intervals during twenty years. *Br Med J*. 1863;1:616.
56. Kaplinsky MS, Schulmann ED. Über die periodische Schlafsucht. *Acta Med Scand*. 1935;85:107–128.
57. Kleine W. Periodische Schlafsucht. *Monatsschr Psychiat Neurol*. 1925;57:285–320.
58. Levin M. Periodic somnolence and morbid hunger: A new syndrome. *Brain*. 1936;59:494–504.
59. Critchley M, Hoffman H. The syndrome of periodic somnolence and morbid hunger (Kleine-Levin syndrome). *Br Med J*. 1942;1:137–139.
60. American Academy of Sleep Disorders, International Classification of Sleep disorders, 1990, First edition.
61. Claparède E. Esquisse d'une théorie biologique du sommeil. *Arch Psychol*. 1905;4:246–349.
62. Salmon A. *La fonction du sommeil*. Vigot Frères; 1910.
63. Schulz H, Salzarulo P. The evolution of sleep medicine in the 19th and the early 20th century. In: Chokroverty S, Billiard M, eds. *Sleep Medicine: A Comprehensive Guide to Its Development, Clinical Milestones and Advances in Treatment*. Springer; 2015:75–89.
64. Sadger J. *Über Nachtwandeln und Mondsucht. Eine medizinisch-literarische Studie*. Franz Deuticke; 1914. (Engl. transl., *Sleep Walking and Moon Walking*, http://www.gutenberg.org/ebooks/30556).
65. Jacobson A, Kales A, Lehmann D, Zweizig JR. Somnambulism: All-night electroencephalographic studies. *Science*. 1965;148:975–977.
66. Van der Lugt. The incubus in scholastic debate: Medicine, theology, and popular belief. In: Biller P, Ziegler J, eds. *Religion and Medicine in the Middle Ages*. York Studies in Medieval Theology III. Boydell Press; 2001:175–200.
67. Adams F, ed. *The medical work of Paulus Aegineta, the Greek physician, transl. into English with a copious commentary containing a comprehensive view of the knowledge possessed by the Greeks, Romans, and Arabians, on all subjects connected with medicine and surgery*. Vol. I. Welsh, Treuttel, Würtz, & Co.; 1884.
68. Chirac P. *Dissertatio academica, in qua disquiritur an incubo ferrum rubiginosum, afferm*. Pech; 1692.
69. Bond J. *An Essay on the Incubus or Nightmare*. D. Wilson and T. Durham; 1753.
70. Jones E. *On the Nightmare*. Institute of Psychoanalysis, 1931.
71. Association of Sleep Disorders Centers. Diagnostic classification of sleep and arousal disorders: Sleep Disorders Classification Committee, Roffwarg HP (Chairman). *Sleep*. 1979;2:1–137.
72. American Academy of Sleep Medicine. *International Classification of Sleep Disorders*. 3rd ed. American Academy of Sleep Medicine, 2014.
73. Timaeus von Guldenklee B. *Casus medicinales praxi trigenta sex annorum observati. Accessere et modicamentorum singularium quae in casibus proponuntur descriptiones*. Christian Kirchner; 1667. http://opacp

lus. bsb-muenchen.de/metaopac/search?db=100&id=BV001700507.
74. Hesse CG. *Über das nächtliche Aufschrecken der Kinder im Schlafe und die psychisch-gerichtliche Bedeutung des Aufschreckens in den späteren Lebensaltern*. HA Pierer; 1845.
75. Rey JG. Beiträge zur pathogenese und ätiologie des pavor nocturnus. *Jahrb Kinderheilk*. 1897;45:247–264.
76. Warrington Haward J. On enlargement of the tonsils as a cause of nightmare. *Br Med J*. 1873;649.
77. Braun L. Über das nächtliche Aufschrecken der Kinder. *Jahrb Kinderheilk*. 1896;43:407–456.
78. Broughton R. Sleep disorders: Disorders of arousal? *Science*. 1968;159:1070–1078.
79. Tachibana N. [Historical overview of REM sleep behavior disorder in relation to its pathophysiology]. *Brain Nerve*. 2009 May;61(5):558–568. Japanese. PMID: 19514516.
80. Alberti M, Lust, Fridericus W. *Diss. inaug. med. de rhoncho dormientium. Vom Schnarchen der Schlafenden*. JC Hendelii; 1745.
81. Dickens, Charles. *The Posthumous Papers of the Pickwick Club*. Porter.
82. Boswoth FH. *Disease of the Nose and Throat*. William Wood & Co.; 1896.
83. Henoch E. Vorlesungen über Kinderkrankheiten. 11. Aufl.; 1903.
84. Cline CL. The effects of intra-nasal obstruction on the general health. *Med Surg Rep*. 1892; 67:259–260.
85. Remmers JE, deGroot WJ, Sauerland EK, et al. Pathogenesis of upper airway occlusion during sleep. *J Appl Physiol*. 1978;44:931–938.
86. Fujita S, Conway W, Zorick F, Roth T. Surgical correction of anatomic azbnormalities in obstructive sleep apnea syndrome: Uvulopalatopharyngoplasty. *Otolaryngol Head Neck Surg*. 1981 Nov–Dec;89(6):923–934. doi:10.1177/019459988108900609. PMID: 6801592.
87. Sullivan GE, Issa FG, Berthon-Jones M, Eves L. Reversal of obstructive sleep apnoea by continuous positive airway pressure applied through the nares. *Lancet*. 1981;1:862–865.
88. Practice parameters for the treatment of snoring and obstructive sleep apnea with oral appliances. American Sleep Disorders Association Sleep. 1995;18(6):511–513.
89. Miki H, Hida W, Inoue H, et al. A new treatment for obstructive sleep apnea syndrome by electrical stimulation of submental region. *Tohoku J Exp Med*. 1988;154:91–92.
90. Decker MJ, Haaga J, Arnold JL, et al. Functional electrical stimulation and respiration during sleep. *J Appl Physiol*. (1985) 1993;75:1053–1061.
91. Szymanski JS. Aktivität und Ruhe bei Tieren und Menschen. *Z allg Physiol*. 1918;18:105–162.
92. Kawamura H, Ibuka N. The search for circadian rhythm pacemakers in the light of lesion experiments. *Chronobiol*. 1978;5:69–88.
93. Moore RY, Eichler VB. Loss of a circadian adrenal corticosterone rhythm following suprachiasmatic lesions in the rat. *Brain Res*. 1972;42:201–206.
94. Stephan FK, Zucker I. Circadian rhythms in drinking behavior and locomotor activity of rats are eliminated by hypothalamic lesions. *Proc Natl Acad Sci U S A*. 1972;69:1583–1586.
95. Moore RY, Lenn NJ. A retinohypothalamic projection in the rat. *J Comp Neurol*. 1972;146:1–14.
96. Welsh DK, Logothetis DE, Meister M, et al. Individual neurons dissociated from rat suprachiasmatic nucleus express independently phased circadian firing rhythms. *Neuron*. 1995;14:697–706.
97. Konopka RJ, Benzer S. Clock mutants of Drosophila melanogaster. *Proc Natl Acad Sci U S A*. 1971;68:2112–2116.
98. Hardin PE, Hall JC, Rosbash M. Feedback of the Drosophila period gene product on circadian cycling of its messenger RNA levels. *Nature*. 1990;343(6258):536.
99. Sehgal A, Rothenfluh-Hilfiker A, Hunter-Ensor M, et al. Rhythmic expression of timeless: A basis for promoting circadian cycles in period gene autoregulation. *Science*. 1995;270(5237):808–810.
100. Darlington TK, Wager-Smith K, Ceriani MF, et al. Closing the circadian loop: CLOCK-induced transcription of its own inhibitors per and tim. *Science*. 1998;280(5369):1599–1603.
101. Gekakis N, Staknis D, Nguyen HB, et al. Role of the CLOCK protein in the mammalian circadian mechanism. *Science*. 1998;280(5369):1564–1569.
102. Jones CR, Campbell SS, Zone SE, et al. Familial advanced sleep-phase syndrome: A short-period circadian rhythm variant in humans. *Nat Med*. 1999;5:1062–1065.
103. Toh KL, Jones CR, He Y, et al. An hPer2 phosphorylation site mutation in familial advanced sleep phase syndrome. *Science*. 2001;291(5506):1040–1043.
104. Czeisler CA, Khalso SBS. The human circadian timing system and sleep-wake regulation. In: Kryger MH, Roth T, Dement W, eds. *Principles and Practice of Sleep medicine*. 3rd ed. WB Saunders; 2000:353–375.
105. Wurtman RJ, Axelrod J, Phillips LS. Melatonin synthesis in the pineal gland: Control by light. *Science*. 1963;142:1071–1073.
106. Moore RY, Lenn NJ. A retinohypothalamic projection in the rat. *J Comp Neurol*. 1972;146:1–14.
107. Moore RY, Heller A, Wurtman RJ, et al. Visual pathway mediating pineal response to environmental light. *Science*. 1967;155(759):220–223.

Chapter 33

Patient-Centered Sleep Care

Using Technology to Amplify Our Clinical Reach

Barry G. Fields and Ilene M. Rosen

INTRODUCTION

Although there is increased recognition of importance of sleep health, there is a scarcity of appropriately trained providers to ensure it.[1] Providing patient-centered care in sleep medicine requires reconsideration of the current model of care, which presently involves nearly automatic referral of patients with a sleep complaint to a sleep specialist, or to a sleep center for testing, with subsequent referral to a sleep specialist for management. The future of sleep medicine lies in *precision* sleep medicine whereby a patient can be identified, diagnosed, and treated in ways that best suit the patient's needs, sleep disorder pathophysiology, and lifestyle. This will require an innovative approach that truly focuses on the individual patient and how they might engage with the healthcare system for their sleep care. With the increased availability and proliferation of smartphone applications, patients are increasingly self-identifying themselves as needing additional sleep evaluation and management. Unfortunately, not everyone has access to a sleep medicine specialist or a sleep center, which is increasing the expectation that non-specialty trained providers will evaluate and manage straightforward sleep disorders. Advances in telemedicine and machine learning in recent years might be leveraged to improve the experience of care.

SCREENING FROM THE PALM OF A PATIENT'S HAND

The field of sleep medicine has long sought to optimize sleep disorder screening by employing such questionnaires such as the Berlin Questionnaire,[2] STOP-Bang Questionnaire,[3] International Restless Legs Syndrome (RLS) Questionnaire,[4] and Epworth Sleepiness Scale.[5] But in order for patients to fill out these questionnaires, they typically must already be in the healthcare setting in which they are offered. That is, a *healthcare provider* has decided that they should fill them out. Future care pathways will need to start with the patient, who will dictate where, when, and why they feel it is necessary to evaluate their sleep. Often, this nudge will come from the palm of their hands. Smartphone-based, sleep-related applications (apps) are a specific type of consumer sleep technology (CST). The American Academy of Sleep Medicine (AASM) defines CST as "non-prescription devices directly marketed to consumers that may make an assertion to perform sleep monitoring, tracking, or sleep-related interventions."[6] Apps are "typically a small, specialized program downloaded onto mobile devices."[6] Our discussion will focus on apps due to their burgeoning presence within all strata of society, though their advantages and limitations can be applied to any other type of CST (e.g., wearable health tracker, non-mobile device monitors, etc.).

Given the heavy societal burden of obstructive sleep apnea (OSA),[7] a smartphone app that can detect it and related disorders accurately could be particularly helpful.[7] Technology has already advanced in the wireless sleep-recording realm that may allow patients to test themselves for sleep disorders while simply placing their smartphone next to their bed during sleep. One study examined an app incorporating specialized radiofrequency sensors and artificial intelligence (AI) algorithms. It demonstrated a sensitivity of 88.3% and specificity of 80.0% to detect an apnea hypopnea index (AHI) of ≥15 events/hour of detected sleep time when compared to simultaneous polysomnograph (PSG) recording.[8] Another study showed similarly promising results regarding app-based snore detection. Manually measured snore time and intensity based on conventional audio recording during polysomnography (gold standard) was compared to the app's determination of the same variables. The authors found a high correlation—a 95% mean accuracy rate—between the app and the manual method. The findings suggest that this app, and similar ones, may be particularly useful for single sleepers who wish to screen themselves for the presence of snoring or sleep-related breathing disorder in the absence of a bed partner to inform them of it.[9]

Patients will also likely continue and expand utilization of apps to measure overall sleep quality, quantity, and pattern. Hundreds of these apps now exist through Google Play and Apple's App Store with these functions, and more will likely be developed. This potential treasure trove of patient-generated health data brings with it serious questions and concerns. If clinicians are to incorporate app data into their assessments and treatment plans, they must (1) trust its veracity, (2) possess the skills needed to interpret the data, and (3) ensure that the data collection in and of itself has not harmed patients physically (e.g., screen viewing degrading sleep hygiene, minimization of false negatives, and disease burden underestimation) and/or psychologically (e.g., undue anxiety concerning overestimated abnormalities).[10] Indeed, a recent examination of simultaneous sleep stage designation among several popular apps revealed significant inaccuracies in comparison to a gold-standard sleep diary.[11] Therefore, the role of the clinician will also be to determine when *not* to base treatment plans on app data and when to pursue more conventional home and in-laboratory sleep testing. Clinicians will need to stay up to date on sleep app technology and their validations studies as more patients bring these data into daily clinical conversations.

ENLARGING THE POOL OF SLEEP PROVIDERS: BOARD CERTIFIED AND NON-BOARD CERTIFIED

As many more individuals identify themselves as potential sleep medicine patients through the use of apps, the current pool of board-certified sleep medicine physicians (BCSMPs) is not large enough to meet their needs; it is estimated that 23.5 million Americans suffer from undiagnosed OSA and 24.2 million Americans have chronic insomnia.[12] Due to the relative scarcity of BCSMPs, and despite the expansion of sleep team members,[13] future sleep medicine care pathways will likely incorporate other healthcare professionals such as primary care providers (PCPs). PCP-based management of OSA has received particular attention in the literature; many more PCPs than BCSMPs exist, and they may be ideally situated to diagnose and manage the common disorder. A number of studies have shown PCP-based OSA management to be at least as effective as BCSMP-based care in terms of treatment adherence and efficacy.[14–17] Furthermore, at least 2 studies have suggested significant cost savings utilizing a PCP- based approach as opposed to a sleep center–based approach.[14,17]

Nevertheless, PCP involvement in OSA management is fraught with inherent limitations and complexities often left unaddressed in research studies. High patient volume and wide scope of practice already constrain PCPs' ability to take on this additional role. Furthermore, real concern exists, even among PCPs, regarding their fund of knowledge. In a recent mixed methods study, researchers interviewed patients, PCPs, and BCSMPs about PCP-based management of OSA.[18] While PCPs were generally confident diagnosing OSA (especially with BCSMP guidance), they were generally less confident about OSA treatment and their role in providing it. Patient interviews revealed that they perceived their PCP's uncertainty, which can impact the PCP-patient alliance.[18] Such perceived knowledge gaps among both patients and their PCPs are not surprising given the many options for sleep-testing tools, treatments, and even styles of each treatment (e.g., various styles of PAP facial interfaces). Perhaps it is most realistic to consider PCPs' future role in sleep medicine as similar to their role for other chronic diseases[19]; they could screen for OSA (with patient-driven app data as a common conversation-starter), order diagnostic testing (if there is a high pretest probability of OSA), and, if appropriate, initiate and manage treatment (assuming symptom improvement and stabilization). In this model, BCSMPs could be consulted again if treatment loses efficacy or new symptoms emerge,[20] similar to how a provider might refer a patient with difficult to control diabetes or asthma to a diabetologist or pulmonologist, respectively.[19]

Similar clinical paradigms have been considered for insomnia, a common sleep disorder that could be an even more ideal candidate for PCP-driven management than OSA.[21–23] Most patients with insomnia first present their symptoms to a PCP.[24] Furthermore, evidence-based cognitive behavioral therapy for insomnia (CBTi) can be delivered in a standardized, manual-based format. This feature lends CBTi well to non-sleep-medicine professionals delivering the therapy to patients. Research has shown promising results when primary care nurses and nurse practitioners provide CBTi to patients.[21,22,25] Self-directed digital CBTi within the primary care setting has also been shown to be effective in a Veterans Affairs (VA) population.[26] Nevertheless, many non-sleep providers rarely provide such therapies outside of research environments due to a lack of knowledge,[27–29] training,[28,30] and time.[27,31] Similar constraints limit PCP involvement in more neurologically oriented sleep disorders such as narcolepsy; there is no literature to support their management in a primary care setting.

In summary, there is growing literature that PCPs could play a significant future role in sleep disorder management. However, there are 2 major limiting factors: time and knowledge. Finding more time in PCPs' schedules is a complex feat beyond the scope of this chapter. However, providing them with more sleep medicine knowledge appears to be a more attainable goal. The object of this endeavor should not be to supplant the specialized training of BCSMPs, but rather to allow integration of common sleep disorder management into the purview of the PCP. Working toward this aim, the Veterans Administration (VA) system developed Specialty Care Access Network-Extension for Community Healthcare Outcomes (Scan-ECHO), subsequently relabeled VA-ECHO. The program, developed in 2003, was originally designed to improve rural patient access to specialty care. Project ECHO educates PCPs so they may become more informed partners in specialty care (not only in sleep medicine), subsequently improving improves veterans' access to that care.

Using telehealth, VA-ECHO specialists present short didactic sessions to PCPs. Later in the program, PCPs may engage in case discussions with the specialists. Other healthcare team members, such as nurses, pharmacists, and technicians, are often involved.[32] VA-ECHO has been deployed in many specialties, such as hepatology,[33] geriatrics,[34] and pain management.[35] One program has even adapted VA-ECHO into a more focused "Sleep VA-ECHO." The VA Puget Sound Health Care System (VAPSHCS) found rural providers receptive to its curriculum over the 3-month course. Participants reported enhanced comfort managing common sleep complaints (e.g., sleep-disordered breathing, insomnia, PTSD-related sleep problems) and providing appropriate patient education.[36]

Programs such as VA-ECHO require that PCPs have the time and institutional support to complete them; the VAPSHCS authors found that lack of protected time was the most common reason for rural PCPs not to take part in the training.[36] Since the future of sleep medicine likely includes PCP involvement, it behooves BCSMPs and related sleep team members to assist their colleagues in building strong business cases showing that patient healthcare expenditures could be optimized if more non-subspecialist providers could integrate sleep medicine care into that which they already provide.

A VIRTUAL SLEEP MEDICINE ENVIRONMENT

Access to future sleep medicine paradigms relies not only on the number of sleep providers, but also on how patients access them; patients in any urban, suburban, or rural area may find it difficult to receive care in person due to disability, work schedule, or other socioeconomic factors. While there is increasing attention paid to improving sleep training among non-sleep-specialty practitioners and growing the number of BCSMPs,[37] the AASM asserted, "none of these solutions has more immediate potential to overcome these challenges than telemedicine, which can dramatically increase sleep medicine accessibility and clinical efficacy."[37,38] That immediate potential remained largely untapped until the COVID-19 pandemic brought it into many more clinical settings.[39]

Telemedicine is a relatively broad term, defined by the Federation of State Medical Boards as " the practice of medicine using electronic communication, information technology or other means of interaction between a licensee in one location and a patient in another location, with or without an intervening healthcare provider." [40] It is distinguished from the broader term "telehealth" because "telemedicine" specifically refers to patient-provider interactions. Because this chapter focuses on the future of sleep patient care, we will use the "telemedicine" terminology. Furthermore, it is important to differentiate between *synchronous* and *asynchronous* telemedicine. Asynchronous telemedicine includes patient-provider messaging through secure patient portals and store-and-forward technologies such as those now available through most PAP device manufactures' websites. In contrast, synchronous telemedicine involves real-time communication between patients and providers. Synchronous telemedicine includes the audio-visual interactions used for clinical video telehealth (CVT).

These terminology distinctions are important to understand. Before the COVID-19 pandemic, only certain types of telemedicine (usually CVT, often in specific locations) could be reimbursed by state, federal, or private insurer funding. Those decisions severely limited its deployment. However, the COVID-19-associated public health emergency, declared in March 2020, loosened restrictions significantly. For instance, the Centers for Medicare and Medicaid Services (CMS) will now reimburse sleep medicine CVT visits that originate from a patient's home; reimbursement had previously been limited to CVT visits originating from clinical settings in prespecified rural areas. Furthermore, CMS currently recognizes asynchronous telemedicine—so-called "e-visits" and "virtual check-ins"—as reimbursable patient-provider interactions.[41] There is no guarantee that these changes will persist indefinitely, but the future of sleep telemedicine—and indeed sleep medicine as a whole—relies heavily upon their longevity. Both the Senate and the House of Representatives are considering a "Telehealth Modernization Act" that would allow many of them to become permanent.[42]

As questions regarding the financial feasibility of telemedicine are further addressed, so too are concerns about clinical efficacy. There is a growing body of research that clinical outcomes do not differ whether clinical care is delivered in person or via telemedicine. Research has shown that OSA patients' PAP adherence, functional outcomes, and satisfaction do not differ when assessed through in-person versus CVT-based care.[43,44] Recent insomnia literature also reveals encouraging results with cognitive behavioral therapy for insomnia (CBT-I) provided through CVT producing similar clinical improvements as CBT-I provided in person.[45] Although CVT-based treatment outcome studies in other sleep disorders remain lacking, an Italian study is currently exploring the role of CVT for the diagnosis and treatment of narcolepsy in adolescents and adults.[46] A nonrandomized feasibility study previously showed no difference.[47]

Due these growing demonstrations of financial and clinical feasibility, it is extremely likely that sleep telemedicine will retain its role as a patient accessibility tool within our field. One can imagine patients discussing their sleep concerns with a non-sleep-specialty practitioner through telemedicine. The non-sleep-specialty practitioner may use artificial intelligence (AI; see "Artificial Intelligence/Machine Learning" section) within the electronic medical record (EMR) to guide further evaluation choices and whether a BCSMP needs to be consulted. The patient could then access BCSMP care through telemedicine once again from initial evaluation through follow-up. Although questions about physical exam utility and accuracy persist,[48] many sleep medicine patients may receive equivalent care to in-person evaluation without ever traveling to a sleep center.

ARTIFICIAL INTELLIGENCE/MACHINE LEARNING: FROM SCREENING TO TESTING TO TREATMENT

Given the pressures on both sleep-trained and non-sleep-trained clinicians, access to patient-centered sleep medicine care will require innovative models of care inclusive of more robust clinical tools to guide clinicians and streamline the patient experience. AI will fill this vital role by utilizing large data sets to enable computers to perform tasks traditionally completed by humans.[49] Machine learning (ML), a term often used interchangeably with AI, possesses algorithms that learn from previous experience to enhance future performance on tasks such as disease identification and classification. Indeed, AI/ML will likely touch future patients at each point along their sleep medicine journey.

Screening and Evaluation

Patients provide large amounts of data, even at initial presentation, to non-sleep-specialty practitioners and BCSMPs alike: demographics, physical examination, specific complaints, and—increasingly commonly—smartphone app and wearable device data. AI may leverage EMR data to identify individuals at risk for a sleep disorder who may benefit from a more thorough evaluation.[50] For instance, OSA symptom phenotypes can be clustered into disturbed sleep, slightly sleepy, moderately sleepy, and excessively sleepy subtypes.[51,52] The excessively sleepy subtype was associated with increased risk of congestive heart failure (CHF), cardiovascular disease (CVD), and coronary artery disease (CAD).[53] An ML system integrated into the EMR could alert a non-sleep-specialty practitioner that a patient's objective (e.g., age, gender, and BMI) and subjective (e.g., sleepiness) phenotype places that individual at greater risk of CHF, CVD, and CAD if found to have OSA. The non-sleep-specialty practitioner could then prioritize these individuals for OSA testing or BCSMP referral, even in the absence of receiving any specialized education to complete the workup; a similar model has been demonstrated in a neurology practice taking care of an epilepsy population.[54] This situation illustrates one example where AI utilizes a growing evidence base to *personalize* care in a more *precise* fashion for the patient who is seeking it.

Testing

AI's involvement in sleep medicine will continue to expand as a patient moves from the screening/evaluation to the testing part of their journey. An AASM Position Statement addressing AI suggests that multi-channel PSG data lends itself well to these ML analyses.[49] AI-guided PSG analyses could reduce human data interpretation error, mitigate unconscious biases, and reduce technical staff time to manually score PSG recordings. Recently, the AASM introduced a pilot program to auto-scoring software programs' sleep staging accuracy. The programs' scoring will be compared to that of a panel of experts, and only programs with similar or greater accuracy than the experts will obtain AASM certification.[55]

AI's future application to sleep medicine may extend beyond sleep-disordered breathing to other disorders such as narcolepsy. A gold standard for its diagnosis, Multiple Sleep Latency Testing (MSLT), itself has limited specificity, especially for type 2 narcolepsy patients.[56] This finding is due (at least in part) to inconsistencies among individuals who score the individual 30-second epochs.[57] The suboptimal interrater reliability that results has significant implications for patient care and livelihood; a "false-negative" MSLT-based diagnosis can limit patients' access to life-altering medication and workplace accommodations. To address these limitations, researchers have leveraged ML to stage as little as 5 seconds of sleep, a level of precision much greater than the conventional 30-second epoch scoring. They demonstrated 96% sensitivity and 91% specificity for narcolepsy type 1, a specificity that rises to 99% when adding HLA-DQB1*06:02 typing to their model.[58]

Treatment

In addition to screening and testing, AI will also inform treatment. Returning to the previous theme of phenotypic OSA subtyping, emerging data suggest that OSA is a common endpoint of many sleep-induced pathophysiological processes. Finnsson et al. describe 4 respiratory endotypes—loop gain, upper airway collapsibility, arousal threshold, and upper airway dilator muscle response—that can identify unique traits of each patient's OSA pathophysiology. They can be estimated through ventilation analyses during periods of airway obstruction using parameters already present on PSG.[59] Recent work by Sands et al.[60] shows how careful analysis of nasal pressure transducer data can expose these specific endotypes of phenotypic pathology leading to a patient's OSA development. The researchers surmise that these phenotypic insights—including muscle compensation to pharyngeal collapsibility—can lead to more targeted, personalized therapies that reflect these underlying pathologies.[59,60] ML incorporating these elements could guide clinicians to more effective, personalized treatment options a given patient may tolerate best.[61] For example, AI may help identify patients who could benefit most from positive airway pressure (PAP) therapy in terms of CVD risk reduction. Although some studies have cast doubt on the CVD benefits of PAP, many of the sleepiest patients were excluded from these analyses.[62,63]An ML paradigm that incorporates symptoms (sleepier vs. less sleepy) could guide BSCMPs and non-BCSCPs alike as to who would benefit most from this therapy. By using AI technology in this manner, clinicians would also be better positioned to prioritize patients for regular cloud-based PAP adherence monitoring,

AI/ML in Sleep Medicine: A Broad Future View

While AI-guided diagnosis should not supplant BCSMP review and judgment, it holds promise to impact sleep management positively for both BCSMPs and non-sleep-specialty practitioners. AI may be thought of as an additional member of the healthcare team that allows them to focus on the most complex patient management issues within a larger population. As discussed earlier, one can foresee AI assisting both BCSMPs and non-sleep-specialty practitioners at multiple points in the screening, evaluation, and testing process. Indeed, it could facilitate non-sleep-specialty practitioners' ordering home sleep apnea testing (HSAT) or PSG in patients at risk for OSA. BCSMPs could then utilize AI while interpreting those studies and deciding on a more personalized treatment plan. Chronic disease management and treatment monitoring could be shared among BCSMPs and non-BSCSMPs as is feasible and appropriate, with AI continuing to assist clinicians with ongoing follow-up (e.g., anticipating needed changes in PAP settings or to other modes of treatment).

ENHANCED SLEEP TESTING PRECISION

Since sleep medicine relies so heavily on testing, it is important to consider advances in this area beyond those already discussed in the previous section. Polysomnography (PSG) and the Multiple Sleep Latency Test (MSLT) remain gold standards for the diagnosis of sleep-disordered breathing and central disorders of hypersomnolence, respectively. Both tools utilize electroencephalogram (EEG), electromyogram (EMG), electrocardiogram (ECG), and electrooculogram (EOG) derivations to define sleep stages, while PSG also employs an oro-nasal thermistor, nasal pressure transducer, pulse oximetry, and respiratory inductance plethysmography (RIP). Many of these parameters have existed for decades, but their accuracy, precision, and utility in sleep disorder diagnosis have come into question. These shortcomings, particularly in regard to precision, will continue to be studied and improved upon as sleep medicine moves through the 21st century.

Advancements in PSG analysis will serve an important role in advancing "Precision Sleep Medicine," heralding improved personalization of both diagnosis and treatment.[64] Enhanced, automated EEG analysis may allow us more insight into sleep quality differences, particularly for individuals with sleep fragmentation due to narcolepsy or insomnia. Sleep stages are currently defined by the majority of a stage present in a 30-second epoch. This strategy, accepted for decades, ignores the subtler intra-epoch stage variation that could have serious implications on perceived sleep quality. Patients with significant sleep fragmentation are particularly vulnerable to the imprecision of this "one size fits all" scoring model. Enhancements in spectral analysis will make it increasingly possible to characterize EEG power density. In one recent meta-analysis, the authors found that patients with insomnia disorder (ID) demonstrated increased alpha and sigma power during rapid eye movement (REM) sleep. In addition, ID was associated with decreased delta power and increased theta, alpha, and sigma power during non-rapid eye movement (NREM) sleep. These findings are important because they may assist future BCSMPs in differentiating ID subtypes and devising more tailored treatment plans for patients.[65]

Sleep testing advancements in narcolepsy diagnosis are being sought due to the time consumption and relatively complexity of gold-standard MSLT. Progress in PSG-based narcolepsy diagnosis (without relying on MSLT) is nascent but promising. Younes et al. has developed a method of continually measuring sleep depth: the odd-ratio product (ORP).[66] Using spectral EEG analysis, the ORP evaluates the relative power of different frequencies (alpha, beta, delta, theta) in 3-second continuous epochs. The frequencies are ranked from least to most intense, and a 4-digit Bin # is generated for each epoch. The lower the ORP, the deeper the sleep. Conversely, higher levels of ORP during NREM sleep (lighter sleep) on overnight PSG have been correlated with excessive daytime sleepiness, determined the following day on MSLT.[67] It is hypothesized that further work with ORP could lead to useful diagnostic paradigms for narcolepsy that no longer rely on MSLT.

Additional attempts to characterize narcolepsy without the use of MSLT come through machine learning. As noted previously, ML utilizes various computational approaches with large, complex data to complete tasks without needing specific instructions. ML has previously demonstrated utility in auto-scoring sleep stages.[68] Of particular importance to hypersomnia research is how those abilities can be leveraged to diagnose narcolepsy through PSG alone. Studies have previously demonstrated that the degree of sleep/wake stage mixing/dissociation can differentiate narcolepsy patients from non-narcolepsy patients.[69] In a study of type 1 narcolepsy patients, an ML algorithm was utilized to measure this sleep/wake stage mixing/dissociation on raw PSG signals using 5-second scoring epochs.[58] They achieved a specificity of 96% and a sensitivity of 91% to diagnose type 1 narcolepsy. With the addition of HLA-DQB1*06:02 to their algorithm, specificity reached 99%.

Taken together, these advancements in EEG spectral analysis, ORP, and ML elicit many implications for the future of sleep medicine testing. The 30-second hand-scored epoch, central to our understanding and analysis of sleep staging for decades, may be replaced by much shorter (1–3 second) epochs scored through ML that allow more precise sleep staging than ever before. Indeed, the very nature of current staging may be replaced by characterizations of sleep that more accurately reflect normal and abnormal structure and function. The result will advance precision sleep medicine while leveraging the power of technology already available to optimize sleep disorder diagnosis and personalize treatment plans.[64]

BIG DATA

Much of the effort to advance patient-centered, precision sleep medicine model is not actually predicated on individual or even small group studies and analysis. On the contrary, developing this healthcare model depends on big data to optimize patient evaluation and treatment pathways. As noted earlier, 21st-century sleep medicine will rely more heavily on AI/ML, which in turn rely on thousands or even millions of observations to enhance independent analyses.

Data Warehouses

Large data sets, also known as data warehouses, will continue to play a major role in this big data acquisition, storage, and development. These data warehouses can include EMRs, health insurance claims, and registries. Many data warehouses have already been explored to inform sleep care. Cistulli et al.[70] examined PAP adherence patterns among 2.62 million users of a cloud-based database containing information remotely transmitted from the patients' PAP devices. Although their focus was PAP adherence (75% of patients met the Centers for Medicare and Medicaid Services [CMS] definition for such), one can imagine the copious data points present in the database, from mask leak rates and residual respiratory events to contours of breathing patterns and minute ventilation rates. This data can be used similarly to PSG data, creating phenotypes delineating physiologic responses to PAP and predicting which patients will respond best to the therapy.[70] Data warehouses are also changing how we learn about sleep-related side effects of medication. Revol et al.[71–73] have utilized VigiBase, the WHO Global database of Individual Case Safety Reports (ICSR), to identify medications previously unknown to cause or exacerbate central sleep apnea (CSA). The database of more than 17 million ICSR from 131 countries allowed the authors to uncover the CSA-triggering effects of baclofen,[71] ticagrelor,[72] and gabapentinoids[73]; these adverse effects might not have been recognized without this big data source. Ongoing analyses of similar data sets will enhance future "pharmacovigilance" as it pertains to sleep disorders.[74]

Industry Partnerships

Over the past several years, collaboration between sleep professionals and technology companies has grown. This trend will likely continue into the future as sleep medicine relies more on industry to harness and apply the "big data," as noted previously. For example, AASM leadership has met with companies such as Fitbit, Verily, and Google to hasten this process.[75] In 2021, the AASM announced a unique partnership with Google.[76] The company's second-generation Nest Hub now incorporates a Sleep Sensing feature that generates a low-energy radar to detect an individual's movements during the sleep period.[77] That information, in addition to snore and light sensor data, allows Nest Hub to provide users with personalized feedback about their sleep patterns and potential disruptors.[77] It then offers evidence-based recommendations and tips based on sleep science. Although the product is not meant to diagnose or treat any disorder, it does engage patients about their sleep patterns and potential problems. This information can then be interwoven into conversations with various healthcare providers and, ultimately, increases the likelihood that otherwise latent sleep disorders will be addressed.

CONCLUSION

A primary goal of 21st-century sleep medicine should be to improve access to patient-centered, personalized care while maintaining optimal clinical outcomes. To attain this goal, we must implement innovative care models that employ the latest technical advances. A major limiting factor is the size of the current subspecialty workforce; it is too small to the meet demand for sleep medicine care. Although the concept of expanding BCSMP reach via the sleep team has long been applied to advanced practice providers such as physician assistants and nurse practitioners, perhaps now is the time to think more broadly. In the 21st century, AI/ML has the potential to be the amplifier that utilizes EMR data to suggest personalized next steps in management. Likewise, the modern-day sleep team includes the spectral analysis during PSG that allows more precise delineation of pathophysiologic phenotypes. And it includes the smartphone app that places access to these care advancements in the palm of a patient's hand. The future of sleep medicine relies on how we leverage and integrate these tools among large populations, within our own practices and with non-sleep-specialty practitioners, who may be the first point of contact for patients who might benefit from addressing a sleep complaint. Extending our clinical reach through technology has the potential to transform how individuals view sleep as a pillar of health and how patients are identified and diagnosed, and how they receive personalized treatment for sleep disorders.

REFERENCES

1. Plante DT, Epstein LJ, Fields BG, Shelgikar AV, Rosen IM. Competency-based sleep medicine fellowships: Addressing workforce needs and enhancing educational quality. *J Clin Sleep Med*. 2020;16(1):137–141. doi:10.5664/jcsm.8138.
2. Netzer NC, Stoohs RA, Netzer CM, Clark K, Strohl KP. Using the Berlin Questionnaire to identify patients at risk for the sleep apnea syndrome. *Ann Intern Med*. 1999;131(7):485–491. doi:10.7326/0003-4819-131-7-199910050-00002.
3. Chung F, Yegneswaran B, Liao P, et al. STOP Questionnaire. *Anesthesiology*. 2008;108(5):812–821. doi:10.1097/ALN.0b013e31816d83e4.
4. Walters AS, LeBrocq C, Dhar A, Hening W, Rosen R, Allen RP, Trenkwalder C; International Restless Legs Syndrome Study Group. Validation of the International Restless Legs Syndrome Study Group rating scale for restless legs syndrome. *Sleep Med*. 2003;4(2):121–132. doi:10.1016/s1389-9457(02)00258-7.
5. Johns MW. A new method for measuring daytime sleepiness: The Epworth sleepiness scale. *Sleep*. 1991;14(6):540–545. doi:10.1093/sleep/14.6.540.
6. Khosla S, Deak MC, Gault D, et al. Consumer sleep technology: An American Academy of Sleep Medicine position statement. *J Clin Sleep Med*. 2018;14(5):877–880. doi:10.5664/jcsm.7128.
7. Peppard PE, Young T, Barnet JH, Palta M, Hagen EW, Hla KM. Increased prevalence of sleep-disordered breathing in adults. *Am J Epidemiol*. 2013;177(9):1006–1014. doi:10.1093/aje/kws342.
8. Tiron R. Screening for obstructive sleep apnea with novel hybrid acoustic smartphone app technology. *J Thorac Dis*. 2020;12(8):4476–4495. doi:10.21037/jtd-20-804.
9. Chiang J-K, Lin Y-C, Lin C-W, Ting C-S, Chiang Y-Y, Kao Y-H. Validation of snoring detection using a smartphone app. *Sleep Breath*. 2022;26(1):81–87. doi:10.1007/s11325-021-02359-3.
10. Khosla S, Deak MC, Gault D, et al. Consumer sleep technology: An American Academy of Sleep Medicine position statement. *J Clin Sleep Med*. 2018;14(5):877–880. doi:10.5664/jcsm.7128.
11. Khosla S, Deak MC, Gault D, et al. Consumer sleep technologies: How to balance the promises of new technology with evidence-based medicine and clinical guidelines. *J Clin Sleep Med*. 2019;15(1):163–165. doi:10.5664/jcsm.7598.
12. Sullivan F. *Hidden Health Crisis Costing America Billions: Underdiagnosing and Undertreating Obstructive Sleep Apnea Draining Health Care System*. 2016. https://aasm.org/resources/pdf/sleep-apnea-economic-crisis.pdf. American Academy of Sleep Medicine. Accessed April 28, 2025.
13. Rosen IM. Change is the only constant in life (and in sleep medicine). *J Clin Sleep Med*. 2018;14(6):1025–1030.
14. Sanchez Quiroga MÁ, Corral Penafiel J, Carmona Bernal C, et al. Primary care physicians can comprehensively manage sleep apnea patients using a semi-automatic algorithm. ERS International Congress 2018 abstracts: European Respiratory Society; 2018:PA2259.
15. Sanchez-de-la-Torre M, Nadal N, Cortijo A, et al. Role of primary care in the follow-up of patients with obstructive sleep apnoea undergoing CPAP treatment: A randomised controlled trial. *Thorax*. 2015;70(4):346–352. doi:10.1136/thoraxjnl-2014-206287.
16. Chai-Coetzer CL, Antic NA, Rowland LS, et al. Primary care vs specialist sleep center management of obstructive sleep apnea and daytime sleepiness and quality of life: A randomized trial. *JAMA*. 2013;309(10):997-1004. doi:10.1001/jama.2013.1823.
17. Tarraubella N, Sánchez-de-la-Torre M, Nadal N, et al. Management of obstructive sleep apnoea in a primary care vs sleep unit setting: A randomised controlled trial. *Thorax*. 2018;73(12):1152–1160. doi:10.1136/thoraxjnl-2017-211237.
18. Pendharkar SR, Blades K, Kelly JE, et al. Perspectives on primary care management of obstructive sleep apnea: A qualitative study of patients and health care providers. *J Clin Sleep Med*. 2021;17(1):89–98. doi:10.5664/jcsm.8814.
19. Fields BG, Rosen IM. The future of sleep medicine: A patient-centered model of care. In: Badr MS, Martin JL, eds. *Essentials of Sleep Medicine: A Practical Approach to Patients with Sleep Complaints*. Springer International; 2022:69–87.
20. Kuna ST. Diagnosis and management of patients with obstructive sleep apnea in primary care: Ready or not? *Am J Resp Crit Care Med*. 2018;198(5):557–558. doi:10.1164/rccm.201803-0555ED.
21. Espie CA, MacMahon KMA, Kelly H-L, et al. Randomized clinical effectiveness trial of nurse-administered small-group cognitive behavior therapy for persistent insomnia in general practice. *Sleep*. 2007;30(5):574–584. doi:10.1093/sleep/30.5.574.
22. Bothelius K, Kyhle K, Espie CA, Broman J-E. Manual-guided cognitive-behavioural therapy for insomnia delivered by ordinary primary care personnel in general medical practice: A randomized controlled effectiveness trial. *J Sleep Res*. 2013;22(6):688–696. doi:10.1111/jsr.12067.
23. Chai-Coetzer CL, Antic NA, McEvoy RD. Identifying and managing sleep disorders in primary care. *Lancet Resp Med*. 2015;3(5):337–339. doi:10.1016/S2213-2600(15)00141-1.
24. Morin C, Leblanc M, Daley M, Gregoire J, Merette C. Epidemiology of insomnia: Prevalence, self-help treatments, consultations, and determinants of help-seeking behaviors. *Sleep Med*. 2006;7(2):123–130. doi:10.1016/j.sleep.2005.08.008.

25. Sandlund C, Hetta J, Nilsson GH, Ekstedt M, Westman J. Improving insomnia in primary care patients: A randomized controlled trial of nurse-led group treatment. *Int J Nurs Studies*. 2017;72:30–41. doi:10.1016/j.ijnurstu.2017.03.007.
26. Hermes EDA, Rosenheck RA, Burrone L, Dante G, Lukens C, Martino S. *Implement Res Pract*. 2021;2:1–15. doi 10.1177/26334895211053659.
27. Koffel E, Bramoweth AD, Ulmer CS. Increasing access to and utilization of cognitive behavioral therapy for insomnia (CBT-I): A narrative review. *J Gen Intern Med*. 2018;33(6):955–962. doi:10.1007/s11606-018-4390-1.
28. Ulmer CS, Bosworth HB, Beckham JC, et al. Veterans Affairs primary care provider perceptions of insomnia treatment. *J Clin Sleep Med*. 2017;13(08):991–999. doi:10.5664/jcsm.6702.
29. Maire M, Linder S, Dvořák C, et al. Prevalence and management of chronic insomnia in Swiss primary care: Cross-sectional data from the "Sentinella" practice-based research network. *J Sleep Res*. 2020;29(5):e13121. doi:10.1111/jsr.13121.
30. Davy Z, Middlemass J, Siriwardena AN. Patients' and clinicians' experiences and perceptions of the primary care management of insomnia: Qualitative study. *Health Expect*. 2015;18(5):1371–1383. doi:10.1111/hex.12119.
31. Cheung JM, Atternäs K, Melchior M, Marshall NS, Fois RA, Saini B. Primary health care practitioner perspectives on the management of insomnia: A pilot study. *Aust J Prim Health*. 2014;20(1):103–112. doi:10.1071/PY12021.
32. Stevenson L, Ball S, Haverhals LM, Aron DC, Lowery J. Evaluation of a national telemedicine initiative in the Veterans Health Administration: Factors associated with successful implementation. *J Telemed Telecare*. 2018;24(3):168–178. doi:10.1177/1357633X16677676.
33. Su GL, Glass L, Tapper EB, Van T, Waljee AK, Sales AE. Virtual consultations through the Veterans Administration SCAN-ECHO Project improves survival for veterans with liver disease. *Hepatology*. 2018;68(6):2317–2324. doi:10.1002/hep.30074.
34. Guzman-Clark J, Harrell K, Leff A, et al. Implementation of an ECHO-based program to provide geriatric specialty care consultation and education to remote primary care teams. *Fed Pract*. 2016;33(4):40–45.
35. Ball S, Wilson B, Ober S, Mchaourab A. SCAN-ECHO for pain management: Implementing a regional telementoring training for primary care providers. *Pain Med*. 2018;19(2):262–268. doi:10.1093/pm/pnx122.
36. Parsons EC, Mattox EA, Beste LA, et al. Development of a sleep telementorship program for rural Department of Veterans Affairs primary care providers: Sleep Veterans Affairs Extension for community healthcare outcomes. *Ann Am Thorac Soc*. 2017;14(2):267–274. doi:10.1513/AnnalsATS.201605-361BC.
37. Watson NF. a unified plan to strengthen the sleep medicine pipeline and maximize our workforce. *J Clin Sleep Med*. 2016;12(06):781–784. doi:10.5664/jcsm.5864.
38. Watson NF, Rosen IM, Chervin RD. The past is prologue: The future of sleep medicine. *J Clin Sleep Med*. 2017;13(01):127–135. doi:10.5664/jcsm.6406.
39. Johnson KG, Sullivan SS, Nti A, Rastegar V, Gurubhagavatula I. The impact of the COVID-19 pandemic on sleep medicine practices. *J Clin Sleep Med*. 2021;17(1):79–87. doi:10.5664/jcsm.8830.
40. Federation of State Medical Boards. House of Delegates Annual Business Meeting. 2018. Published 2022. https://www.fsmb.org/siteassets/advocacy/policies/fsmb-workgroup-on-telemedicineapril-2022-final.pdf. Accessed 4/28/25.
41. Centers for Medicare and Medicaid Services. Medicare telemedicine health care provider fact sheet. 2020. https://www.cms.gov/newsroom/fact-sheets/medicare-telemedicine-health-care-provider-fact-sheet. Accessed April 28, 2025.
42. Khosla S, Beam E, Berneking M, et al. The COVID-19 pandemic and sleep medicine: A look back and a look ahead. *J Clin Sleep Med*. 2022;18(8):2045–2050. doi:10.5664/jcsm.10102.
43. Fields BG, Behari PP, McCloskey S, et al. Remote ambulatory management of veterans with obstructive sleep apnea. *Sleep*. 2016;39(3):501–509. doi:10.5665/sleep.5514.
44. Parikh R, TouVelle MN, Wang H, Zallek SN. Sleep telemedicine: Patient satisfaction and treatment adherence. *Telemed e-Health*. 2011;17(8):609–614. doi:10.1089/tmj.2011.0025.
45. Arnedt JT, Conroy DA, Mooney A, Furgal A, Sen A, Eisenberg D. Telemedicine versus face-to-face delivery of cognitive behavioral therapy for insomnia: A randomized controlled noninferiority trial. *Sleep*. 2021;44(1):zsaa136. doi:10.1093/sleep/zsaa136.
46. Ingravallo F, Vignatelli L, Pagotto U, et al. Protocols of a diagnostic study and a randomized controlled non-inferiority trial comparing televisits vs standard in-person outpatient visits for narcolepsy diagnosis and care: TElemedicine for NARcolepsy (TENAR). *BMC Neurology*. 2020;20(1):176. doi:10.1186/s12883-020-01762-9.
47. Pizza F, Vignatelli L, Oriolo C, et al. Multidisciplinary care of patients with narcolepsy during coronavirus disease 2019 pandemic in Italy via televisit: The TElemedicine for NARcolepsy feasibility study. *Sleep*. 2022;45(12):zsac228. doi:10.1093/sleep/zsac228.
48. Yurcheshen ME, Pigeon W, Marcus CZ, et al. Interrater reliability between in-person and telemedicine evaluations in obstructive sleep apnea. *J Clin Sleep Med*. 2021;17(7):1435–1440. doi:10.5664/jcsm.9220.
49. Goldstein CA, Berry RB, Kent DT, et al. Artificial intelligence in sleep medicine: An American Academy of Sleep Medicine position statement. *J Clin Sleep Med*. 2020;16(4):605–607. doi:10.5664/jcsm.8288.
50. Cade BA-O, Hassan SM, Dashti HS, et al. Sleep apnea phenotyping and relationship to disease in a large clinical biobank. *JAMA Open*. 2022;11(5):ooab117. doi: 10.1093/jamiaopen/ooab117.
51. Keenan BT, Kim J, Singh B, et al. Recognizable clinical subtypes of obstructive sleep apnea across international sleep centers: A cluster analysis. *Sleep*. 2018;41(3):zsx214. doi: 10.1093/sleep/zsx214. doi:10.1093/sleep/zsx214.

52. Kim J, Keenan BT, Lim DC, Lee SK, Pack AI, Shin C. Symptom-based subgroups of Koreans with obstructive sleep apnea. *J Clin Sleep Med*. 2018;14(03):437–443. doi:10.5664/jcsm.6994.
53. Mazzotti DR, Keenan BT, Lim DC, Gottlieb DJ, Kim J, Pack AI. Symptom subtypes of obstructive sleep apnea predict incidence of cardiovascular outcomes. *Am J Resp Crit Care Med*. 2019;200(4):493–506. doi:10.1164/rccm.201808-1509OC.
54. Mulvey MA, Veerapandiyan A, Marks DA, Ming X. Electronic health record cue identifies epilepsy patients at risk for obstructive sleep apnea. *Neurol Clin Pract*. 2018;8(6):468–471.
55. American Academy of Sleep Medicine. AI/Autoscoring Pilot Certification is coming soon. 2021. https://aasm.org/american-academy-of-sleep-medicine-google-help-people-improve-their-sleep/. Accessed April 28, 2025.
56. Ruoff C, Pizza F, Trotti LM, et al. The MSLT is repeatable in narcolepsy type 1 but not narcolepsy type 2: A retrospective patient study. *J Clin Sleep Med*. 2018;14(1):65–74. doi:10.5664/jcsm.6882.
57. Johns MW. Sensitivity and specificity of the multiple sleep latency test (MSLT), the maintenance of wakefulness test and the Epworth Sleepiness Scale: Failure of the MSLT as a gold standard. *J Sleep Res*. 2000;9(1):5–11. doi:10.1046/j.1365-2869.2000.00177.x.
58. Stephansen JB, Olesen AN, Olsen M, et al. Neural network analysis of sleep stages enables efficient diagnosis of narcolepsy. *Nature Comm*. 2018;9(1):5229. doi:10.1038/s41467-018-07229-3.
59. Finnsson E, Ólafsdóttir GH, Loftsdóttir DL, et al. A scalable method of determining physiological endotypes of sleep apnea from a polysomnographic sleep study. *Sleep*. 2021;44(1):zsaa168. doi:10.1093/sleep/zsaa168.
60. Sands SA, Edwards BA, Terrill PI, et al. Phenotyping pharyngeal pathophysiology using polysomnography in patients with obstructive sleep apnea. *Am J Resp Crit Care Med*. 2018;197(9):1187–1197. doi:10.1164/rccm.201707-1435OC.
61. Eckert DJ. Phenotypic approaches to obstructive sleep apnoea: New pathways for targeted therapy. *Sleep Med Rev*. 2018;37:45–59. doi:10.1016/j.smrv.2016.12.003.
62. McEvoy RD, Antic NA, Heeley E, et al. CPAP for prevention of cardiovascular events in obstructive sleep apnea. *N Engl J Med*. 2016;375(10):919–931. doi:10.1056/NEJMoa1606599.
63. Peker Y, Glantz H, Eulenburg C, Wegscheider K, Herlitz J, Thunström E. Effect of positive airway pressure on cardiovascular outcomes in coronary artery disease patients with nonsleepy obstructive sleep apnea: The RICCADSA randomized controlled trial. *Am J Resp Crit Care Med*. 2016;194(5):613–620. doi:10.1164/rccm.201601-0088OC.
64. Lim DC, Mazzotti DR, Sutherland K, et al. Reinventing polysomnography in the age of precision medicine. *Sleep Med Rev*. 2020;52:101313. doi:10.1016/j.smrv.2020.101313.
65. Zhao W, Van Someren EJW, Li C, et al. EEG spectral analysis in insomnia disorder: A systematic review and meta-analysis. *Sleep Med Rev*. 2021;59:101457. doi:10.1016/j.smrv.2021.101457.
66. Younes M, Ostrowski M, Soiferman M, et al. Odds ratio product of sleep EEG as a continuous measure of sleep state. *Sleep*. 2015;38(4):641–654. doi:10.5665/sleep.4588.
67. Younes M, Giannouli E, Meza S. Enhancements to the multiple sleep latency test. *Nat Sci Sleep*. 2016:145. doi:10.2147/NSS.S103596.
68. Zhang L, Fabbri D, Upender R, Kent D. Automated sleep stage scoring of the Sleep Heart Health Study using deep neural networks. *Sleep*. 2019;42(11):zsz159. doi:10.1093/sleep/zsz159.
69. Olsen AV, Stephansen J, Leary E, et al. Diagnostic value of sleep stage dissociation as visualized on a 2-dimensional sleep state space in human narcolepsy. *J Neurosci Methods*. 2017;282:9–19. doi:10.1016/j.jneumeth.2017.02.004.
70. Cistulli PA, Armitstead J, Pepin J-L, et al. Short-term CPAP adherence in obstructive sleep apnea: A big data analysis using real world data. *Sleep Med*. 2019;59:114–116. doi:10.1016/j.sleep.2019.01.004.
71. Revol B, Jullian-Desayes I, Bailly S, et al. Baclofen and sleep apnoea syndrome: Analysis of VigiBase, the WHO pharmacovigilance database. *Eur Respir J*. 2018;51(1). doi:10.1183/13993003.01855-2017.
72. Revol B, Jullian-Desayes I, Tamisier R, et al. Ticagrelor and central sleep apnea. *J Am Coll Cardiol*. 2018;71(20):2378–2379. doi:10.1016/j.jacc.2018.03.447.
73. Revol B, Jullian-Desayes I, Cracowski JL, et al. Gabapentinoids and sleep apnea syndrome: A safety signal from the WHO pharmacovigilance database. *Sleep*. 2019;42(2):zsy242. doi:10.1093/sleep/zsy242.
74. Pépin JL, Bailly S, Tamisier R. Big data in sleep apnoea: Opportunities and challenges. *Respirology*. 2020;25(5):486–494. doi:10.1111/resp.13669.
75. Kirsch DB, Khosla S. Public awareness, medical integration, and innovation in sleep medicine. *J Clin Sleep Med*. 2019;15(05):799–801. doi:10.5664/jcsm.7786.
76. AASM. American Academy of Sleep Medicine partners with Google to help people understand and improve their sleep. March 15, 2021. https://aasm.org/american-academy-of-sleep-medicine-google-help-people-improve-their-sleep/.
77. Nest. https://blog.google/products/google-nest/new-nest-hub-soli/. March 16, 2021.

Index

For the benefit of digital users, indexed terms that span two pages (e.g., 52–53) may, on occasion, appear on only one of those pages.

Tables, figures, and boxes are indicated by an italic *t*, *f*, and *b* following the page number.